D1249136

Catalog of Prenatally Diagnosed Conditions

Catalog of Prenatally Diagnosed Conditions

Third Edition

David D. Weaver, M.D.

Professor and Director of Clinical Genetic Services
Department of Medical and Molecular Genetics
Indiana University School of Medicine
Indianapolis, Indiana

with the assistance of

Ira K. Brandt, M.D.

Emeritus Professor and Former Director of the Section of Metabolism,
Departments of Pediatrics and of Medical and Molecular Genetics
Indiana University School of Medicine
Indianapolis, Indiana

WITHDRAWN

Rock Valley College
Educational Resources
Center

The Johns Hopkins University Press
Baltimore and London

© 1989, 1992, 1999 The Johns Hopkins University Press
All rights reserved. Published 1999
Printed in the United States of America on acid-free paper

9 8 7 6 5 4 3 2 1

The Johns Hopkins University Press
2715 North Charles Street
Baltimore, Maryland 21218-4363
www.press.jhu.edu

A catalog record for this book is available from the British Library.

Library of Congress Cataloging-in-Publication Data

Weaver, David D., 1939–
   Catalog of prenatally diagnosed conditions / David D. Weaver ; with the assistance of
Ira K. Brandt.—3rd ed.
      p.   cm.
   Includes bibliographical references and index.
   ISBN 0-8018-6044-X (alk. paper)
   1. Fetus—Diseases.   2. Fetus—Abnormalities.   3. Prenatal diagnosis.   I. Brandt,
Ira K.   II. Title.
   [DNLM: 1. Prenatal Diagnosis.   2. Abnormalities—diagnosis.   3. Fetal Diseases—
diagnosis.   WQ 209 W363c 1999]
   RG626.W35   1999
   618.3'2075—dc21
   DNLM/DLC
   for Library of Congress   98-17788
                                                                              CIP

Ry
RG
626
W35
1999

$106.25

900423

To the five most important women in my life: Bess Eugene Weaver, my mother; Florence Lucy Marshall and Margaret Catherine Sinclair, my aunts; Margaret Elizabeth Brickey, my sister; and Pamela Kae Weaver, my wonderful wife.

Contents

Acknowledgments

The support and effort of the following individuals in making this third edition possible are gratefully acknowledged:

— Ira K. Brandt, M.D., Professor Emeritus of Pediatrics and Medical Genetics, Indiana University School of Medicine, for his assistance, particularly in updating Chapter 6, Inborn Errors of Metabolism. In doing so, he added 35 additional disorders, 212 new references, and revised most of the other entries;

— Merrill Benson, M.D., Professor and Chairperson, Department of Medical and Molecular Genetics, Indiana University School of Medicine for his financial and administrative support;

— Jennifer Peet, M.S., Genetic Counselor, St. Christopher Hospital for Children, Philadelphia, for her editorial assistance;

— Dorothy Quinlan, Gerry Adams, Karen Lisby, and Belynda Gilbert for their excellent secretarial and editorial contributions;

— Wendy A. Harris, Medical Editor, the Johns Hopkins University Press, for her sound advice and guidance during the preparation and production of all three editions of this catalog;

— And finally, to my wife, Pamela K. Weaver, for tolerance in preparing this revision, for her efforts in editing the introduction, and for her moral support and guidance during this project.

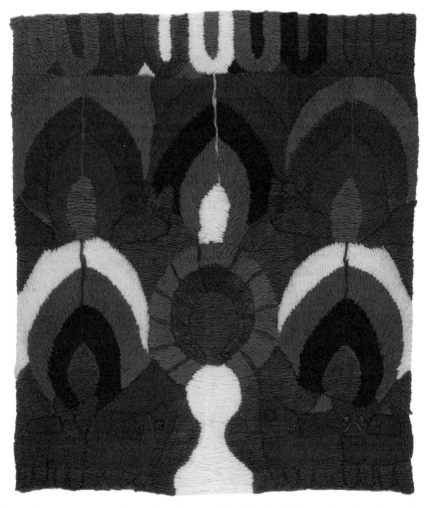

The above figure is a crewel-stitched piece made by a Guatemalan Mayan Indian and donated to me by Dr. Luis F. Escobar. The picture tells the story of a pregnant Mayan princess (small center figure), who is united to her fetus by a cord (center to top). The fetus and its intrauterine life are represented by the nine U-shaped structures at the top of the work. Surrounding the princess are trees, represented by the four arch-shaped structures at the sides. The top two arches symbolize physical life, while the bottom two symbolize spiritual life. Among the trees are wild, ferocious animals (bottom) that have the potential to harm the pregnancy and the fetus. These animals are prevented from doing so by God (lower center in white) and other animals (to the right and left of the mother), all of whom represent worldly goodness.

In Guatemala, the custom is that the maternal grandmother constructs the stitchery during the pregnancy of her granddaughter. The stitchery is hung in the granddaughter's home, where it protects her pregnancy from complications while protecting the fetus from birth defects.

Introduction

In a limited fashion, human beings probably have been making prenatal diagnoses since the age of reasoning. For instance, we suspect that mothers and their physicians or midwives have always been able to diagnose fetal demise by the lack of fetal movement or the inability to detect the fetal heartbeat. Although not especially accurate, estimating fetal size by external palpation of the fetus has been a time-honored practice. Furthermore, the diagnosis of hydramnios (polyhydramnios), oligohydramnios, and intrauterine growth retardation by determining inappropriate uterine size were done long before the development and use of ultrasound. Widespread use of prenatal diagnosis did not occur until the 1970s, however, when rapid advances in technology during the 1960s allowed for accurately diagnosed fetal disorders. These advances occurred primarily in the fields of biochemistry, cytogenetics, clinical genetics, and the physical sciences. Additional advances in these fields have continued and other technologies such as chorionic villus sampling and molecular genetic technology have emerged as primary players. All areas of prenatal technology now provide a varied and fascinating array of approaches to the diagnosis of embryonic and fetal conditions.

Amniocentesis apparently was accomplished first by Schatz in 1883, and was performed for the treatment of hydramnios. The oldest reference to the prenatal diagnosis of a condition included in this catalog is craniorachischisis (PD 120000), published in 1917 by James T. Case. Dr. Case detected absence of cranial bones by radiographic means in a pregnancy complicated by hydramnios. Although his diagnosis prenatally was anencephaly, at autopsy, the fetus had both anencephaly and rachischisis (craniorachischisis). His observation appears to be the first radiographic report of an abnormal fetal condition.

During the 1930s and 1940s, and into the 1950s, there were limited publications reporting prenatal abnormalities. The paucity of publications during this period probably was due not only to a lack of interest in and an inability to make prenatal diagnoses, but also to the nearly total lack of *in utero* treatment of fetal conditions. The interest in prenatal diagnosis changed rapidly in the 1950s, however, with the development of a method to diagnose and to treat prenatally erythroblastosis fetalis (PD 204000). The reader may recall that prior to the development of RhoGAM^R in the late 1960s, Rh incompatibility between the mother and the fetus was a relatively common and occasionally lethal fetal disorder. Fetal death occurred because of maternal Rh–antibody induced, severe fetal hemolysis, which in turn led to severe anemia, congestive heart failure, and finally fetal death. In the early 1950s, Bevis demonstrated that the severity of the fetal anemia could be assessed accurately by analyzing the liquor amnii (the amniotic fluid) for the concentrations of nonhematin iron and urobilinogen (Bevis, 1950, 1952). He demonstrated convincingly that the greater the concentration of these substances in the amniotic fluid, the greater was the severity of the erythroblastosis fetalis (Bevis, 1956; Liley, 1961; Freda, 1965). Because testing for these substances required amniotic fluid, the assessment of erythroblastosis fetalis entailed third-trimester amniocentesis and resulted in a surge of interest in the procedure. Further interest in the prenatal diagnosis of erythroblastosis fetalis was stimulated by reports by Liley (1963) and subsequently others (Queenan and Adams, 1965; Queenan and Douglas, 1965; Queenan and Wyatt, 1965) of the successful treatment of this condition by intrauterine transfusion of erythrocytes into the fetal abdomen. One of the authors (DDW) vividly recalls a personal involvement with this prenatal treatment. As a third-year medical student at the University of Oregon School of Medicine in Portland, Oregon, I had the opportunity to assist with the transfusion of several severely affected fetuses. The procedures were essentially failures, but the excitement generated by attempting to save the lives of fetuses was intoxicating and intense.

Although the *in utero* treatment of erythroblastosis fetalis in the 1960s was of limited success and fraught with major complications, the procedure created major interest in prenatal testing and treatment, and most importantly provided an impetus for doing second-trimester amniocentesis. Interest in second-trimester amniocentesis (sometimes called *paracentesis* in the 1950s and 1960s) was stimulated further by the development of a method to determine fetal sex. The determination was accomplished by detection in females, or lack of detection in males, of sex chromatin (Barr) bodies in amniotic fluid cells (Serr et al., 1955; Fuchs and Riis, 1956; Makowski et al., 1956; Shettles, 1956; Serr and Margolis, 1964). In 1960, Riis and Fuchs first made clinical application of the procedure. These investigators determined the sex of fetuses at risk for the X-linked recessive disorder, hemophilia. They offered to terminate any pregnancy with a male fetus. Several years later, further excitement about amniocentesis and prenatal diagnosis occurred with the demonstration that chromosomal analysis was possible on cultured amniotic fluid cells (Steele and Breg, 1966; Thiede et al., 1966). This inventive discovery was followed quickly by the publication of an article about the prenatal detection of chromosomal abnormalities (balanced D/D translocation carrier and chromosomal breakage secondary to fetal rubella infection) (Jacobson and Barter, 1967). The following year, the first reports of the *in utero* diagnosis of Down syndrome were published (Nadler, 1968; Valenti et al., 1968).

Fetal biochemical disorders were also reported during this period. The first actual biochemical disorder diagnosed prenatally was congenital adrenal hyperplasia. Jeffcoate and associates (1965) established the diagnosis by finding elevated levels of 17-ketosteroid and pregnanetriol in the amniotic fluid of an affected fetus. In 1968, Nadler reported the prenatal diagnosis of galactosemia by identifying the absence of galactose-1-phosphate uridyl transferase activity in cultured amniotic fluid cells. Nadler's article appears to be the first to detect a prenatal condition by direct enzyme assay.

With the advent of the more frequent use of amniocentesis, the successful development of amniotic fluid cell culture and karyotyping techniques, and the diagnosis of a number of fetal disorders in the late 1960s and early 1970s, the prenatal diagnosis "floodgates" were opened. Prenatal diagnosis in the 1970s become commonplace, and there were hundreds of publications describing dozens of ways to diagnose fetal/embryonic conditions. These methodologies now permit the prenatal detection of a large array of different fetal conditions. In addition to the rapid development of technology in the 1970s, there also was a rapid increase in the number of prenatal diagnostic centers throughout the world (Levine et al., 1975). Furthermore, as a result of the liberalization of abortion statutes, changes in cultural attitudes toward family size, quality of life issues, and freedom of choice, as well as extensive media coverage and publicity given to prenatal diagnosis, demand for these services soared in this period (Kaback, 1973). Today, prenatal diagnostic services are well accepted, and in most developed nations they have become the standard of care and are available to most women desiring these services.

A number of other techniques for doing prenatal diagnosis were also introduced in the 1970s. For instance, the ability to screen for neural tube defects (NTDs) was first demonstrated by Brock and Sutcliffe (1972). They accomplished this by determining amniotic fluid concentrations of alpha-fetoprotein (AFP), a normal fetal protein. These researchers were able to demonstrate that elevated levels of the AFP were associated with anencephaly and spina bifida cystica in the fetus. Subsequently we have learned that elevation in the amniotic fluid AFP level occurs with many disorders, not only those associated with disruption of the integrity of the skin as with NTDs, omphalocele (PD 144000), and aplasia cutis congenita (PD 194920), but also with other conditions, such as congenital nephrosis, Finnish type (PD 176000), or duodenal atresia (PD 133000), that do not involve the skin. Elevated amniotic fluid AFP levels now have been documented in 60 different conditions (see *Alpha-fetoprotein, elevated in amniotic fluid* in the Index).

As an extension of the amniotic fluid AFP work, Brock and associates (1973) also demonstrated the feasibility of screening for fetal conditions by detecting elevated levels of AFP in maternal serum. In this article, they reported the detection of an anencephalic fetus whose mother's serum AFP level was greater than six times the mean for her gestational age. Subsequent studies have shown that maternal serum AFP levels are also elevated in most of the same fetal conditions that are associated with elevated amniotic fluid AFP levels (see *Alpha-fetoprotein, elevated in maternal serum* in the Index). A further major advance in the use of maternal serum AFP occurred with the observation that lower-than-average levels of maternal serum AFP were associated with Down syndrome (PD 101000). This insight was first published by Merkatz and associates in 1984, and confirmed subsequently by others (Wald and Cuckle, 1981; Cuckle et al., 1984; Fuhrmann et al., 1984; Seller, 1984; Tabor et al., 1984; Voigtlander and Vogel, 1985). Low levels of maternal serum AFP have also been found in association with other trisomies and chromosomal abnormalities, fetal demise, and a host of other conditions and syndromes (see *Alpha-fetoprotein, reduced levels in maternal serum* in the Index). Although amniotic fluid and maternal serum AFP testing have become widely used as a screening procedure for the detection of fetal abnormalities in the United States and else-where, the detection of an abnormally high or low AFP value in itself is never diagnostic of a specific fetal disorder. The presence of abnormal levels of AFP, however, is an indication for further prenatal testing.

With the success of the AFP screening program, other chemical substances were sought that would indicate fetal abnormalities and that could be used to screen pregnancies. One of the first discovered was acetylcholinesterase (AChE), an en-zyme that normally hydrolyzes acetylcholine to choline and is particularly abundant in nervous tissue, especially at nerve endings. Smith et al. (1979) and Chubb et al.

(1979) originally reported the use of this enzyme for the detection of NTDs. They demonstrated a quantitative increase in AChE in the amniotic fluid of fetuses with anencephaly and spina bifida cystica. Later, other reports showed that AChE could be distinguished reliably from pseudocholinesterase (cholinesterase), a normal constituent of amniotic fluid, by gel electrophoresis (Smith et al., 1979; Wald and Cuckle, 1981). The distinction can be accomplished because AChE migrates more rapidly than pseudocholinesterase on gel electrophoresis (Seller and Cole, 1980).

Gel electrophoresis normally is used when the amniotic fluid AFP concentration is found to be elevated. If an AChE isozyme band also is present, then the chance that the fetus has an NTD is greatly increased. Other conditions, however, may be associated with the presence of amniotic fluid AChE isozyme on gel electrophoresis. As listed in the Index (see *Acetylcholinesterase isozyme, rapidly migrating amniotic fluid*), there are 29 other disorders that have been reported with this finding. Detection of fetal disorders by demonstrating fetal AChE in the maternal serum has not yet been accomplished.

Other biochemical substances that have been used successfully to screen for disorders in the fetus include gamma-glutamyltranspeptidase (Brock et al., 1984a; Aitkin et al., 1985), aminopeptidase M (Brock et al., 1984a), phenylalanine-resistant alkaline phosphatase (Brock et al., 1984a; Aitkin et al., 1985), human chorionic gonadotropin (hCG) (Bogart et al., 1987; Arab et al., 1988; Muller and Boue, 1990), and unconjugated estriol (Canick et al., 1987). hCG and unconjugated estriol have been used for maternal serum screening of Down syndrome (Sheldon and Simpson, 1991a), and when these two hormonal assays are combined with maternal serum AFP screening, often referred to as the "triple test" or "triple screening" for Down syndrome, the detection rate for Down syndrome is increased appreciably—75% in one study (Bradley et al., 1994). However, because of the false-positive rates and the cost of triple testing, controversy over the use of this testing procedure has been voiced (Bogart, 1991; Keatinge and Williams, 1991; Macri et al., 1991; Sheldon and Simpson, 1991b; Wishart, 1991a,b).

The 1970s also saw an explosion in the number of different inborn errors of metabolism for which prenatal testing was available. Although much of the analysis involves testing for enzyme deficiencies, metabolic precursors or breakdown products were also used in various ways. For instance, the increased or prolonged retention of ^{35}S-cystine in cultured amniotic fluid cells or homogenized chorionic villi from fetuses with cystinosis (PD 213000) has been used to establish this diagnosis (Schneider et al., 1974; States et al., 1975; Smith et al., 1987). For more extensive discussions of the prenatal diagnosis of metabolic disorders, the reader is directed to two reviews by Desnick and associates (1985, 1992) and one by Winchester (1990), as well as various chapters in Milunsky's *Genetic Disorders and the Fetus: Diagnosis, Prevention and Treatment* (1992).

Another modality that has become a cornerstone in prenatal diagnosis is ultrasound, the use of high frequency sound waves to generate a visual picture. Ultrasound was first used in obstetrics, gynecology, and prenatal diagnosis in the mid-1950s (Donald et al., 1958; Donald, 1962, 1969; Sunden, 1964; Holmes, 1983). The visualization of the placenta, the fetal head, hydramnios, and twins were reported first by Donald and associates in 1958. Since its introduction as a prenatal diagnostic technique, the use of ultrasound has expanded rapidly. The primary reasons for its rise in popularity are based on the noninvasive nature of the procedure; the refinement of ultrasound technology, particularly with regard to improved resolution; and the ease with which the equipment can be used. Because of these advances, ultrasound and related techniques such as echocardiology and Doppler are now among the most widely used technologies providing prenatal assessment and prenatal diagnoses. These technologies have essentially replaced the use of prenatal radiography.

The feasibility of diagnosing fetal heart conditions was originally reported in the early and mid-1970s, when reports of ultrasound imaging of the fetal heart began to appear (Garrett and Robinson, 1970; Winsberg, 1972; Suzuki et al., 1974; Egeblad et al., 1975). A host of articles in the late 1970s and the beginning of the 1980s were published at that time describing the detection of fetal heart abnormalities. The abnormalities reported were mainly fetal arrhythmias (Hackeloer, 1979; Klein et al., 1979; Madison et al., 1979; Newburger and Keane, 1979; Crowley, 1980; Harrison, 1980; Kleinman et al., 1980, 1982, 1983) and congenital anomalies of the fetal heart (Henrion and Aubry, 1979; Allan et al., 1981a,b). Detection of heart conditions prenatally is important in that doing so affords the opportunities for termination of pregnancies with affected fetuses, and in continued pregnancies, better management of the pregnancies. Furthermore, if treatment of fetal congenital heart abnormalities is not available prenatally, treatment may be available postnatally (Kleinman et al., 1983).

As a direct result of our abilities to diagnose cardiac problems prenatally, a number of prenatal treatment modalities have been conceived and implemented for these problems. Although most of the treatments have involved problems with arrhythmias of one type or another (Kleinman et al., 1983; Bertrand et al., 1986; Carpenter et al., 1986; Killeen and Bower, 1987), congestive heart failure resulting from severe fetal anemia also has been treated successfully (Peters and Nicolaides, 1990; Sahakian et al., 1991).

Along with the development of ultrasound and echocardiography to assess the fetal heart, Doppler ultrasound techniques also have been adopted to analyze fetal blood flow (Wolfson et al., 1977; Stuart et al., 1980; Gill et al., 1981). Initially, these techniques were applied to the umbilical arteries and the blood velocity waveforms generated by blood flow through these arteries. The types of waveforms found in the vessels have been shown to correlate with the health of the fetus. Abnormal waveforms have been seen in fetuses who have had intrauterine growth retardation, who have been stressed, or who subsequently experienced fetal demise (Friedman, 1985; Reuwer et al., 1987; Rizzo et al., 1987a). Doppler ultrasound also has been applied to the evaluation of certain congenital heart defects such as aortic valvar stenosis (Hata et al., 1990) and vascular defects like pulmonary atresia (Allan et al., 1986) and premature constriction of the fetal ductus arteriosus (Huhta et al., 1987b). Because of its unique ability to assess blood flow, Doppler ultrasound appears to have a promising future in prenatal diagnosis.

Fetoscopy, the direct visualization of the fetus using an optical instrument, was first accomplished by Westin in 1954 via a transcervical approach. Abdominal fetoscopy was subsequently introduced (Mandelbaum et al., 1967; Valenti, 1972, 1973; Scrimgeour, 1973). Early application of fetoscopy included fetal skin biopsy, reported originally by Valenti in 1972; fetal blood sampling by the same investigator in 1973 and later by others (Hobbins and Mahoney, 1974; Patrick et al., 1974; Benzie and Doran, 1975; Hobbins and Mahoney, 1975); and direct visualization of the fetus. The first diagnoses established by fetoscopy were β-thalassemia (PD 211000) and sickle cell anemia (PD 209000). These diagnoses were made by analyzing fetal blood obtained by fetoscopy in at-risk fetuses (Alter et al., 1976). The first dysmorphic condition, Ellis-van Creveld syndrome (PD 158000) diagnosed with the aid of fetoscopy was reported by Mahoney and Hobbins (1977), who diagnosed the condition by visualizing polydactyly in a fetus at risk. Fetal skin biopsy obtained by fetoscopy first was used to determine dermatologic diagnoses in 1980 (Golbus et al., 1980; Rodeck et al., 1980). With the use of fetoscopy, direct intravascular fetal transfusion was accomplished first in 1981, in the treatment of severe erythroblastosis fetalis (Rodeck et al., 1981). In this case, fetoscopy was used to localize and to guide the insertion of a needle into an umbilical vein.

Although fetoscopy has been used to visualize the fetus directly, to obtain fetal blood, to give transfusions, and to perform fetal skin biopsies, only the last procedure remains a viable function of fetoscopy today. Because of improvement in sonography, the difficulty encountered in visualizing the entire fetus, and the attendant risk, fetoscopy now is used infrequently for direct visualization of the fetus. Fetal blood sampling and fetal transfusion previously done by fetoscopy essentially have been replaced by cordocentesis using an ultrasound-guided needle. As a result of this advance, fetal skin biopsy remains the only viable function of fetoscopy today, and this function is rapidly being replaced by molecular genetic techniques for diagnosis of severe skin disorders.

In 1975, Kan and coworkers were the first to report the direct diagnosis of β-thalassemia using fetal blood. They obtained fetal blood samples by *in utero* aspiration of blood from the placenta, followed by partial separation of the fetal and maternal bloods by differential agglutination. As noted previously, Alter and associates (1976) reported the diagnosis of sickle cell anemia and β-thalassemia from fetal blood obtained by fetoscopy. In 1979, Rodeck and Campbell, using fetoscopy, reported that fetal blood sampling could be more reliably obtained by puncturing the umbilical vessels at the point where the umbilical cord inserts into the placenta. Here the vessels are relatively large and fixed. A major advance in fetal blood sampling was reported in 1983 by Daffos and collaborators (1983a,b), who obtained pure fetal blood by aspirating the umbilical vein with a needle inserted through the maternal abdomen and uterine wall, capitalizing on ultrasound to guide the needle into the vein. Advantages of this method are that it is safer, more rapid, and easier to perform than obtaining blood by fetoscopy (Weiner, 1987). Subsequently, Hobbins and associates (1985) named this procedure *percutaneous umbilical blood sampling* (PUBS), a term that has enjoyed considerable popularity. Worldwide, however, *cordocentesis* now appears to have a wider usage, and thus, we use this term throughout the catalog. Because of its relative ease of use and safety, cordocentesis now is used extensively throughout the world not only for fetal blood sampling, but also for fetal transfusion. Diagnoses that have been established by use of cordocentesis include chromosomal abnormalities, fetal infections, coagulation defects, hemoglobin and red cell disorders, metabolic problems, and immunologic conditions (Nicolaides et al., 1986a; Weiner, 1988).

Whereas the 1970s saw the fruition of amniocentesis, ultrasound, and biochemical and molecular testing, the 1980s will be remembered for the development of chorionic villus sampling (CVS). Specifically, CVS ushered in the era of first-trimester testing. Although CVS became widely used in the 1980s, the technique actually was first introduced in 1968 using biopsy forceps to sample placental tissue under hysteroscopic guidance (Hahnemann and Mohr, 1968; Hahnemann, 1974). However, it was not until the adaptation of sonographically directed biopsy used in conjunction with either flexible biopsy forceps (Kazy et al., 1980, 1982) or a suction catheter (Old et al., 1982) that the procedure achieved an acceptable level of safety, ease of use, and reliability. With these advances the procedure gained widespread popularity. CVS has two major advantages over standard amniocentesis—that is, amniocentesis done at 14 weeks or later of gestational age. The first is that chorionic villus cells grow more rapidly in culture than do amniotic fluid cells. Therefore, the results of the analysis may be obtained more rapidly. Second is that CVS can be done in the first trimester, allowing for earlier termination of the pregnancy when termination is safer and may be less emotionally trying to parents.

Up until 1984, CVS reportedly had been done only by a transcervical approach. In that year, Smidt-Jensen and Hahnemann (1984) introduced a transabdominal technique. One of the advantages to this approach is that CVS can be done throughout the pregnancy, beginning late in the first trimester. In many centers today, transabdominal CVS has gained such acceptance that its use over transcervical testing is determined by the position of the placenta and/or by the preference of the woman undergoing testing.

Beginning in the 1970s, molecular genetic technology has changed not only the practice of genetics, but also that of medicine as a whole. Similarly, the technology has changed significantly the practice of prenatal diagnosis by either allowing the diagnosis of certain conditions, such as cystic fibrosis (PD 256000), to be more accurately and simply made; or for the diagnosis to be established in the first place, as is the case with phenylketonuria (PKU) (PD 218750). Before the development of modern molecular genetic methodology, PKU had not been diagnosed either from amniotic fluid cells or chorionic villi. The reason the diagnosis had not been established previously was because the enzyme in this condition, phenylalanine hydroxylase, is expressed normally only in liver. By 1985, the gene coding for this enzyme had been linked to various restriction-fragment–length polymorphisms (RFLPs), and the prenatal diagnosis of the disorder had been made using both amniotic fluid cells and chorionic villi (Lidsky et al., 1985). Similarly, before 1986, cystic fibrosis was diagnosed indirectly by the demonstration of a deficiency of phenylalanine-inhibitable alkaline phosphatase activity in amniotic fluid cells (Brock, 1983). With first the localization and then the discovery of the gene on chromosome 7, the diagnosis could be established by RFLP linkage (Spence et al., 1986; Feldman et al., 1989), and then subsequently by direct testing for various mutations within the gene (Novelli et al., 1990).

From a historical standpoint, the first reported prenatal diagnosis ever established by molecular genetic techniques was reported by Kan and associates in 1976, who cited the diagnosis of alpha-thalassemia by means of DNA linkage assessment. The prenatal diagnosis of sickle cell anemia by molecular genetic methodology first was made 2 years later (Kan and Dozy, 1978).

Unquestionably, the importance of molecular genetics and our ability to establish prenatal diagnoses for Mendelian conditions by this technology will continue to expand in the future. As a result, many more inherited disorders will be amenable to diagnosis. In addition, it is also likely that a number of the genes involved in many common conditions such as depression, alcoholism, schizophrenia, hypertension, and inherited cancers will be discovered, and prenatal testing of these conditions will become available.

In the 1980s, several other techniques for obtaining prenatal diagnoses were also introduced. Among these were "early" amniocentesis, computerized axial tomography (CT scan), magnetic resonance imaging (MRI), preconception genetic analysis, preimplantation embryo biopsy, and isolation of fetal cells in maternal blood. The technique of early amniocentesis simply means doing the procedure prior to 14 weeks of gestation. With advances in ultrasound and tissue culture techniques, earlier amniocentesis has become routine in some centers (Johnson and Godmilow, 1988) and can be done as early as 11 weeks of gestation (Eiben et al., 1997). The relative safety of this procedure is still being debated, however (Brumfield et al., 1996; Wilson et al., 1996; Eiben et al., 1997). CT scans have been used to make or assist in the diagnosis of several conditions, including conjoined twins (PD 255000), Dandy-Walker syndrome (PD 121000), fetal demise (PD 260000), hydrocephalus (PD 125000), and teratoma of the brain (PD 281000). In the future, CT scanning probably will see limited use because of the fetal radiation exposure involved. Because magnetic waves are not known to be deleterious to the fetus, and because there has been improvement in the technology, MRI scanning, however, probably will see increased use, and likely will replace CT scans for the purposes of prenatal diagnosis. In the past, MRI scanning has been involved in the diagnosis of cerebellar lobe hypoplasia (PD 119380), conjoined twins (PD 255000), craniopharyngioma (PD 272460), abdominally located ectopic pregnancy (PD 257500), and other disorders. To date, MRI scanning for prenatal diagnosis has been used primarily as an adjunct to ultrasound for either confirmation of findings or when the quality of ultrasound has been reduced, as may happen with oligohydramnios (Mattison and Angtuaco, 1988). For extensive reviews of MRI applied to prenatal diagnosis, the reader should consult publications by Weinreb et al. (1985), Daffos et al. (1988b), and Mattison and Angtuaco (1988).

Preconception genetic analysis is the method of analyzing the polar body to predict the makeup of the egg. This approach has had limited use in prenatal diagnosis but has been used to test for the delta F508 cystic fibrosis gene mutation (Strom et al., 1990). Preimplantation embryo biopsy is the technique of removing one or more blastomeres from the blastocyst in order to do cytogenetic or genetic analyses. Embryonic sex (PD 265000) (Penketh et al., 1989) and cystic fibrosis (PD 256000) (Strom et al., 1990) have been determined by this technique. Finally, the presence of fetal cells in the maternal blood has raised the possibility of doing prenatal diagnosis via maternal blood sampling (Gray et al., 1988; Bianchi et al., 1989). Considerable effort has been put forth to develop this procedure and as of this writing, a limited number of diagnoses have been accomplished by this approach. The procedure, however, is still considered experimental, and is not available for general use (Nakagome et al., 1991). For more details, the reader may wish to consult Ganshirt et al. (1995), Simpson and Elias (1995), Steele et al. (1996), and Lamvu and Kuller (1997).

ETHICAL ISSUES IN PRENATAL DIAGNOSIS

Each religious, racial, or cultural group most likely has its own beliefs concerning prenatal testing, prenatal treatment, and termination of pregnancies for fetal defects. Because of the diversity of beliefs globally, it is only reasonable to raise some of the ethical dilemmas that occur in the United States. These dilemmas are also discussed by Wertz and Fletcher (1989), who have presented a cross-cultural survey of medical geneticists and how they deal with ethical issues.

For both medical and legal reasons in the United States, many physicians, clinical geneticists, and genetic counselors believe that women have the right to know about and receive prenatal testing. For the most part, women in the United States have access to prenatal testing regardless of their reasons for wanting to be tested. However, paying for these services may create problems for many individuals because both private and federal funding of such services vary throughout the country. In most states, women currently have the legal right to terminate a defective fetus regardless of the seriousness of the fetal problem, and can do so until the fetus reaches the age of viability. Depending on the locality, the age limit varies from 20 to 26 weeks of menstrual age. Fetuses who are found to have lethal or grave conditions that can be diagnosed with reasonable certainty, such as anencephaly, often can be terminated even after the "age of viability" by early labor induction (Chervenak et al., 1984f). Equally important to note is that women in the United States also have the right not to terminate a pregnancy despite the diagnosis of fetal problems. Furthermore, most health-care workers would agree that neither our society nor our government has the right to force women to terminate a prenancy. This is so even though the fetal problems are perceived to be serious and later will place a significant burden on society; for example, a child who will develop severe retardation and whose care ultimately will be assumed by society. Women also have the right not to undergo prenatal testing regardless of their risk of having a defective fetus. For example, a 36-year-old woman who has experienced previous miscarriages finally succeeds in carrying a pregnancy to 11 weeks of gestation. Because of the inherent risks involved in testing, she may be less likely to undergo chromosomal testing, even though she has an increased risk of having a fetus with a trisomy. Also of note is the general belief among most physicians, counselors, and others that the risks involved in prenatal testing need to be presented in a relatively nonbiased fashion, and that we respect and support the mother's (couple's) decision to either have or not have testing done. Now that maternal serum alpha-fetoprotein screening or triple screening is common practice, however, this last tenet is less likely to be followed, and women who have abnormal maternal serum screening results will have greater pressures brought to bear on them to have further testing.

A number of ethical issues arise as a direct result of prenatal testing. For instance, justification for termination of a pregnancy is probably the greatest single ethical issue in prenatal diagnosis in the United States. Although many physicians and other health-care providers have little difficulty accepting the termination of a fetus with a lethal disorder, such as anencephaly, only a few would accept the termination when, for example, the fetus is not the sex of the parent(s)'s choice (Wertz and Fletcher, 1989). The greatest dilemma for couples and physicians seems to occur either when the fetal disorder is not lethal, or when the diagnosis of a lethal condition cannot be made with certainty. The latter situation arises with a number of skeletal dysplasias. For instance, if the fetus has short limbs and a small chest, a neonatal lethal bone dysplasia is likely. Unless there is a family history of such a condition, the situation is problematic because the prenatal diagnosis of most bone dysplasias still cannot be made with certainty (Escobar et al., 1990). However, because the genes involved in many of the bone dysplasias have or are likely to be discovered in the near future, this scenario is changing rapidly.

Another ethical issue that is continually debated concerns what routine fetal testing should be done, and which tests, if any, should be mandatory. For instance, should a woman ever be forced to participate in any prenatal testing? Should, for example, ultrasound examination and maternal serum alpha-fetoprotein or triple screening be mandated for all pregnancies? By doing so, would we be creating more anxiety in parents than that which is offset by the benefits of the testing? Do we have the right to impose prenatal testing? Johnson and Elkins (1988) have proposed guidelines for mandatory prenatal testing. These guidelines state that testing be considered for disorders that are serious or life-threatening, that testing be accurate, that effective *in utero* treatments be available, and finally, that testing be of minimal risk to the mother. Although it may sound strange to be suggesting mandatory prenatal testing, if fetal damage from whatever cause can be prevented by *in utero* or immediate postnatal treatment, then mandatory testing may become a reality. The same arguments that have been used to justify mandatory newborn screening can be used for justifying mandatory prenatal testing.

Additional ethical problems involve who should pay for prenatal testing and whether third parties who pay for testing should have access to the information obtained. Because greater numbers of individuals in this country have no health insurance coverage, the former problem is becoming more acute. Another issue that needs consideration is, when is it justified to test for a particular condition? For instance, should prenatal testing be offered for Huntington disease (PD 265700), because the average age of onset is 37 years, and rarely does the condition develop before the person is in their twenties. A further question that occasionally arises is how much information should be conveyed to parents when an abnormality is found in their fetus or arises in the testing for fetal problems? Should all details about testing and an abnormal detected condition be given to them, or only those details that the counselor believes are important to the immediate situation? Should artifacts that arise as the result of cell culture done for chromosomal analysis of the fetus be discussed? Should follow-up evaluation of an abnormal fetus prenatally, following termination, or after delivery be required? What should be done if the rights of the fetus conflict with rights of the mother? For example, suppose there is an effective prenatal treatment for a particular fetal condition, but the mother refuses treatment. Whose rights should be given precedence, especially as treatment would require violation of the mother's body and might involve substantial risk to her and/or her fetus?

With regard to these ethical issues, there are no absolute principles for resolving them. Each situation must be evaluated individually and a decision reached by the parties involved on the basis of the particular circumstances, and with respect for the human and legal rights of all parties involved. However, there are a number of excellent publications that set forth guidelines to those who are attempting to resolve ethical conflicts. Suggested reading includes material on pregnancy termina-tions (Fineman and Gordis, 1982; Motulsky and Murray, 1983; Beeson and Golbus, 1985), fetal versus maternal rights (Chervenak and McCullough, 1985), prenatal screening (Powledge and Fletcher, 1979; Fletcher et al., 1985; Fost, 1989), fetal therapy (Ruddick and Wilcox, 1982; Fletcher, 1985), and general ethical issues regarding prenatal diagnosis (Powledge and Fletcher, 1979; Fletcher, 1986; Johnson and Elkins, 1988; Wertz and Fletcher, 1989; Clarke et al., 1994). Ethical issues associated with prenatal diagnosis of hemoglobinopathies (Fletcher, 1979) and Huntington disease (Smurl and Weaver, 1987) are also recommended for these specific conditions.

ON THE DEVELOPMENT OF THIS BOOK

By the mid-1970s, the literature about prenatal diagnosis was becoming extensive. At this time, one of the authors (DDW) occasionally would be asked if a particular condition had been or could be diagnosed prenatally. Because there were no avail-able comprehensive listings of diagnosed conditions, and because the question frequently required an immediate answer, the author had to spend considerable time and effort searching the literature. It became evident that an abstract of the available literature and a comprehensive listing of disorders that had been diagnosed prenatally would be of value not only to us, but perhaps also to others.

In 1979, Sharon Stephenson, then a graduate student in the Department of Medical Genetics, Indiana University School of Medicine, and one of the authors (DDW) began a systematic review and abstraction of the literature. These efforts culminated in the publication of a review article on this topic in the early 1980s (Stephenson and Weaver, 1981). The article summarized the then current information on prenatal diagnosis. Subsequently, Stephenson left graduate school for medical school, and I continued the review process. These ongoing efforts culminated in the publication of the first edition of this catalog (1989). Doing the second edition was made possible in part by a sabbatical leave by one of us (DDW) at the University of New South Wales, Sydney, Australia. This leave was sponsored and made possible by Dr. Max Nicholls, who was on the faculty of this institute. Dr. Nicholls also was instrumental in editing that edition in part. The third edition has been done by a collective effort of the authors, with one of us (IKB) handling the review of metabolic disorders.

STATISTICAL ASPECTS OF THE BOOK

In an article published in 1981 (Stephenson and Weaver, 1981), we presented information on 182 prenatally diagnosed conditions and included 301 citations. Contained within the first edition of this catalog were 445 conditions and 1221 references (Table 1). In the second edition, there were 601 disorders and 1848 references. In this revision, there are 940 conditions and 2730 references. Needless to say, these data indicate a substantial growth in our overall knowledge of prenatal diagnosis since the publication of that first article.

The number of conditions in each section and subsection of all three editions is presented in Table 2. This information indicates a continued growth in the number of disorders diagnosed across all categories. Physical birth defects and dysmorphic syndromes still represent the greatest number of disorders in any one category, with 399 conditions listed (42% of the total). The percentage of disorders in this category is down slightly from 44%, the total in the second edition.

STATEMENT OF PURPOSE

Physicians, counselors, and other health-care providers are sometimes faced with the situation of needing to know if a birth defect or genetic condition can be diagnosed prenatally. Unless this information is known and available to them, these individuals cannot provide appropriate advice to women, couples, or families wishing to make informed reproductive decisions. The major goal of this book,

Table 1. Increases in the Number of Conditions and References Included in the Various Editions of This Catalog

	1981 Article*	First Edition (1989)	Second Edition (1992)	Third Edition (1998)
Number of conditions	182	445 (244%)[#]	601 (35%)[#]	940 (56%)[#]
Number of references	301	1221 (406%)[#]	1848 (51%)[#]	2730 (48%)[#]

* Stephenson and Weaver, 1981.
[#] Increase over the previous publication.

Table 2. Number of Conditions Listed by Sections and Subsections

	Subsection Total	Section Total
Chromosomal anomalies		153 (84)
Congenital malformations, deformations, disruptions, and related disorders		399 (265)
Cardiovascular system	57 (39)	
Central nervous system	36 (32)	
Gastrointestinal and related systems	34 (27)	
Skeletal system	94 (58)	
Urogenital system	30 (23)	
Other malformations, deformations, disruptions, and related disorders	148 (86)	
Dermatologic disorders		14 (12)
Fetal infections		38 (11)
Hematological disorders and hemoglobinopathies		37 (25)
Hematologic disorders	25 (15)	
Hemoglobinopathies	12 (10)	
Inborn errors of metabolism		131 (96)
Disorders of amino acid metabolism	31 (20)	
Disorders of carbohydrate metabolism	15 (8)	
Disorders of lipid metabolism	32 (26)	
Disorders of mucopolysaccharide metabolism	8 (7)	
Other metabolic disorders	45 (35)	
Tumors and cysts		98 (50)
Other prenatal conditions		61 (58)
Multiple congenital anomalies of unknown etiology— single case reports		9 (0)
	Grand Total	940 (601)

Note: Numbers in parentheses represent the number of conditions reported in the second edition.

then, is to provide a single source for obtaining much of the information needed for evaluation, counseling, and decision making. More specifically, the catalog is intended to provide abstracted information about conditions that have been diagnosed prenatally. References are included for each condition to afford the reader access to more extensive discussion of the condition, if needed. Other uses of this catalog include determining if a condition has been diagnosed prenatally, the specific techniques used to detect prenatal findings, the specific prenatal findings associated with each diagnosed condition, the gestational age when the diagnosis was established or the finding observed prenatally, and the differential diagnosis of abnormalities detected prenatally. Some information on prenatal treatment is also included. The catalog also may be helpful as a reference source for a variety of research projects.

For a condition to be included in this catalog, the disorder had to meet three criteria. First, the information about the condition has to be published. Second, the diagnosis or finding(s) has to have been made or detected during the pregnancy, in the embryo, or, in one case, prior to conception (see cystic fibrosis [PD 256000]). Finally, the condition has to be an abnormality of the embryo, fetus, umbilical cord, or placenta. Because maternal disorders do not meet all of the above criteria, they are not included in the catalog *per se.* However, fetal conditions that result from maternal disorders are listed. An example is diabetic macrosomia (PD 243500), which results from maternal diabetes. For the most part, chromosomal abnormalities also are not included unless noncytogenetic findings have been reported. For instance, in Turner syndrome (PD 105000), cystic hygromas and other physical problems frequently have been observed, and therefore, these findings are included under this disorder.

THE ORGANIZATION AND USE OF THE BOOK

Information in this book is divided into text, references, and index sections. The following discussion is intended to explain the organization of each of these sections.

The text is partitioned into chapters, with each chapter representing a separate disease category; for example, dermatologic disorders. Certain chapters, namely Chapter 2, Congenital Malformations, Deformations, Disruptions, and Related Disorders; Chapter 5, Hematologic Disorders and Hemoglobinopathies; and Chapter 6, Inborn Errors of Metabolism, are further subdivided into subsections. The rationale for this organization is first, to group related disorders together in order to be able to compare similar conditions, and second, to allow the reader to determine which disorders in a particular disease category have been diagnosed prenatally. For example, only six of the seven classic mucopolysaccharidoses and three of the four subtypes of Sanfilippo disease have been diagnosed prenatally. If the text of the book were not organized into chapters and subsections, this type of assessment could not be made as readily. As it is organized, the text also can assist in finding conditions. Because each disorder is listed alphabetically within each chapter or subsection, the reader can easily locate the disorder of interest by turning to the chapter or subsection under which the disorder is listed, and then finding it in its alphabetical position.

Each condition listed in the text has been assigned a reference number. The numbering system used here was modeled after the one used by Victor A. McKusick in his *Mendelian Inheritance in Man: Catalogs of Autosomal Dominant, Autosomal Recessive, and X-linked Phenotypes,* seventh edition (McKusick, 1986). The advantage of this system is that it allows conditions to be kept in numerical order while still affording the insertion of new disorders in their appropriate alphabetical order. Having conditions in numerical order makes it easier to locate rapidly the condition within the text. To distinguish reference numbers used here from those used by McKusick in his catalogs, the letters PD, which stand for prenatal diagnosis, have been added in front of each reference number in this catalog. Unfortunately, McKusick numbers cannot be used for all of the conditions included in this catalog because not all prenatal conditions listed here are monogenic and listed in his book. For example, twin transfusion syndrome (PD 115500), a condition normally only affecting monozygotic twins, is not listed by McKusick, but has been diagnosed prenatally.

In the first edition of this catalog, the PD number was a five-digit number. Because a deficiency of sequential numbers developed in several of the chapters during the preparation of the second edition, it became necessary to go to a six-

Table 3. Changes in PD Numbers and Names since the Second Edition

Former PD Numbers and Name	New PD Numbers and Name
PD 100510 Deletion chromosome Xp	PD 100504 Deletion chromosome X(p22.31pter)
PD 100512 Deletion chromosome 1q	PD 100513 Deletion chromosome 1(q42q44)
PD 100515 Deletion chromosome 4p	PD 105275 Wolf–Hirschhorn syndrome
PD 100800 Deletion chromosome 13q	PD 100840 Deletion chromosome 13(q12.1q12.3)
PD 101280 Extra embryonic/fetal chromosomal discordance	Deleted
PD 101290 Interstitial deletion chromosome 1	PD 100510 Deletion chromosome 1(q25q32)
PD 101485 Isochromosome 12p mosaicism	PD 101680 Tetrasomy 12p
PD 105270 45,X male	PD 105355 45,X male
PD 105320 XXXXY syndrome	PD 100160 Chromosome XXXXY syndrome
PD 106500 Arrhythmia, cardiac	Deleted
PD 128000 Microcephaly, unspecified type	PD 128300 Microcephaly, unspecified type
PD 130880 Werdnig–Hoffmann disease	PD 271100 Spinal muscular atrophy, type I
PD 166000 Osteopetrosis	PD 166000 Osteopetrosis, autosomal recessive, infantile form
PD 169000 Sacral agenesis	PD 169040 Sacral dysgenesis
PD 179120 Premature rupture of fetal membranes	PD 264100 Fetal membranes, premature rupture
PD 188000 Body wall defects with reduction limb anomalies	PD 191900 Limb–body wall complex
PD 191250 Goldenhar syndrome	PD 192775 Oculoauriculovertebral spectrum
PD 192880 Pena–Shokeir phenotype	PD 191232 Fetal akinesia/hypokinesia sequence
PD 198250 Lowry hyperkeratosis syndrome	PD 198250 Restrictive dermopathy, lethal
PD 207850 Neonatal alloimmune thrombocytopenia	PD 207850 Thrombocytopenia, neonatal alloimmune
PD 209500 Sickle-β-thalassemia	PD 208950 Sickle-β-thalassemia
PD 247700 Marfan syndrome	PD 267470 Marfan syndrome
PD 250000 Testicular feminization	PD 249800 Testicular feminization
PD 265120 Fetomaternal transfusion	PD 109750 Fetomaternal transfusion

(*continues*)

Table 3. (*continued*)

Former PD Numbers and Name	New PD Numbers and Name
PD 265620 Hematoma, retroplacental	PD 265480 Hematoma, retroplacental
PD 267500 Martin–Bell syndrome	PD 265270 Fragile-X syndrome
PD 271520 Schwartz–Jampel syndrome	PD 271075 Schwartz–Jampel syndrome
PD 271550 Transplacental hemorrhage, massive bidirectional	PD 109800 Fetomaternal transfusion, massive, chronic, and bidirectional
PD 272000 Werdnig–Hoffman disease	PD 271100 Spinal muscular atrophy, type I

digit number in the second edition. There has been no change in the numbering system in this edition. Changes in PD numbers and names made during the preparation of this edition are presented in Table 3.

Following the PD number of each entry in the text is the preferred name of the condition, and by which name the disorder is listed elsewhere in the catalog. In parentheses following the preferred name may be one or more alternative names, acronyms, or abbreviations for the condition. Finally, we have included in the heading of each entry the McKusick number for the disorder, if available. This latter item is denoted by "McKusick No.," followed by the six-digit indexing number found in McKusick's book (McKusick, 1997). If no number is available, then "None" is inserted in place of the number. If we are uncertain to which McKusick number an entry should be assigned, then an "Unknown" is recorded, followed by one or more McKusick numbers that could apply to the entry. For instance, atrial septal defect, PD 107500, has been detected prenatally, but it could not be determined which atrial septal defect of the three disorders (108800, 108900, 600309) listed by McKusick applied to this condition in this catalog.

Following the heading of each entry in the text is presented one or more methods used to diagnose the disorder or to detect the abnormalities associated with the conditions. The methods cited are listed in alphabetical order. Following each method are the abnormal findings that have been detected by that particular technique. The reference(s) reporting the finding(s) is placed underneath the findings. These references are arranged according to their year of publication, with the older article appearing first.

In this catalog only those features that have been detected prenatally and reported in the literature are included in the section following the techniques and in the Index.

Superscripts are often used in the text. Their definitions are presented in the "Definition of Superscript Letters" following this section. If the superscript letter "g" has been placed behind a technique used for prenatal detection or following a finding, then the condition was diagnosed or the findings were observed in the first trimester. If the superscript letter "d" appears behind a technique or following a finding, the condition was diagnosed or the finding has been only observed in the third trimester. If neither "g" nor "d" is present, then the diagnosis or observation was made during the second trimester.

For a number of the disorders in the catalog, additional information is included about the condition. This information is under specific headings. The first heading will have one of the following titles: "Syndrome Note," "Disease Note," "Dysplasia

Note," "Sequence Note," "Situation Note," or "General Comments." The next heading is normally "Prenatal Diagnosis." Under this last section the preferred method(s) of diagnosing the condition prenatally is stated. The "Prenatal Diagnosis" section may be followed by a "Differential Diagnosis" entry, listing other conditions that should be considered in making the diagnosis of the particular disorder. The list of disorders in this section is not exhaustive, however, and other conditions may need to be considered in the differential. Following the "Differential Diagnosis" section, a prenatal treatment section, if prenatal treatment has been accomplished successfully, may be included. When a prenatal treatment segment is cited, the information normally is divided into "Prenatal Treatment" and "Treatment Modality" sections. The former presents general information about prenatal treatment and states the most efficacious means of treatment. The latter entry lists those methods in which treatment has had some degree of success. Appropriate references also are included in each treatment section. At various places in the text are inserted statements denoted by "Comment(s)." These statements contain information about or explain the text material immediately preceding the statements. The "Comment(s)" sections normally are indented one tab in from the text to which they refer.

References to all the articles referred to in the introductory material and text are placed in alphabetic order by author in the reference section. This section immediately follows the chapter section. When there are two or more articles with the first authors having the same last name, the references are listed according to the following scheme: Articles written by only one author are listed first according to the year of publication, with the oldest one being presented first. Articles by two authors follow and are listed alphabetically according to the second author's last name, with the oldest one (by year) listed first if the same two authors have two or more published articles. Finally included are those articles written by three or more authors arranged by year of publication and alphabetically by the second, third, and so on, author's name. In any of the three categories, if the same authors have two or more articles published in the same year, then following the year of publication is added "a," "b," "c," and so on, to distinguish between these articles. Note also should be made that in ordering the authors alphabetically, the initials of the authors are ignored. This reference system is necessitated by the manner in which the references are cited in the text.

The final section of the book is the Index, in which all prenatally diagnosed conditions included in the text are listed in alphabetic order. The PD number following each entry is the reference number for locating the condition in the text. The alternative names of each condition have also been placed in the Index, with the preferred term for the disorder and its corresponding PD number in parentheses following the name. In addition, the prenatal findings for each condition included in the text and the conditions that have been associated with these findings have been incorporated into the Index. For example, hydramnios, a relatively common finding in abnormal pregnancies, has been associated with 220 separate prenatal disorders. These disorders are cited in the Index following the entry of hydramnios. This latter information is useful because by looking up a finding such as hydramnios in the Index, one can arrive at a differential diagnosis for that finding.

STYLISTIC CONSIDERATIONS

Greek letters are used when appropriate. Greek letters used include: α = alpha, β = beta, γ = gamma, τ = tau, Δ or δ = delta, Ψ = psi, and σ = sigma.

In most instances, the naming of a disorder essentially is arbitrary, and the use of a particular name for a condition is, to some extent, at the discretion of the author. The selection of a disorder's primary name listed in this book has been based on our preference of the names that are in common use. In general, the preferred term—that is, the one in common use among geneticists—has been selected. When an individual's name is used for the condition, only the person's last name is used. For example, de Lange syndrome (PD 191200), rather than Cornelia de Lange syndrome, is used. The exception to this rule is Treacher Collins syndrome (PD 194500), which is such a widely used eponym that it is justifiable to use Dr. Collins' first name. Furthermore, the possessive forms of individuals' names are not used. Thus, Down syndrome (PD 101000), rather than Down's syndrome, is preferred here. A dash has been placed between conditions that are named after two or more individuals; for example, Ellis–van Creveld syndrome (PD 158000). Hyphens are also placed between conditions named after abnormal anatomical structures when the name of the defect is completely spelled out, as in agnathia-microstomia-synotia syndrome (PD 183000). However, hyphens have been eliminated when anatomic parts are used to name a syndrome. For example orofaciodigital syndrome, type II, an alternative name for Mohr syndrome (PD 192620), is used in preference to oro-facio-digital syndrome, type II. Ultrasound, rather than sonography or sonar, has been used for the most part.

CONCLUDING REMARKS

The rapidity with which prenatal diagnostic information is appearing and the diversity of the journals in which articles on this topic are being published makes it difficult to keep this catalog up to date. As a result, a number of articles and conditions have yet to be included. The reader is advised not to use this book as the sole source of information about the diagnosis of prenatal conditions. Furthermore, we would be grateful to receive reprints of published articles on prenatal diagnosis or any comments about this book or the information found or not found within it.

Finally, it is anticipated that our knowledge of prenatal diagnosis will continue to grow at a rapid pace, particularly in light of the speed of identification of new genes; that new techniques for making additional prenatal diagnoses will be developed; and that our facilities to see patients will continue to expand. Thus, we as a medical community will be providing more diagnostic services to a larger number of women who carry fetuses with a wider array of problems. In turn, we will have a greater opportunity for *in utero* fetal treatment and/or to deliver affected fetuses at facilities qualified to handle these problems. Perhaps more important, we shall also be reassuring more couples that their fetuses appear to be normal!

Definitions of
Superscript Letters

Throughout the various chapters of this catalog, superscript letters have been incorporated to convey specific information about the conditions or findings. To improve the accessibility to the definition of these letters, this section has been printed on a separate page highlighted by a blackened margin.

The definitions of superscript letters include the following:

[a] All conditions diagnosed or abnormal findings detected in the second trimester, unless otherwise indicated.

[b] Diagnosis confirmed or made by conventional cytogenetic methods.

[c] Specific diagnosis not made by the indicated procedure or finding(s).

[d] Specific diagnosis made or abnormality found, so far, only in the third trimester.

[e] Defect not revealed on a routine second trimester ultrasonic scan.

[f] Timing of amniocentesis for the determination of bilirubin level dictated by the severity of previously affected fetuses; i.e., the procedure normally is done at 20–24 weeks in severe cases and later in milder ones.

[g] Diagnosis made or abnormality found in the first trimester.

[h] Gestational age at the time of diagnosis or detection of findings not stated.

[i] The testing was done or the diagnosis assumed correct because the condition occurred or is present in a sibling or parent, a parent is known to be a gene carrier, or the embryo or fetus has been exposed to a specific and recognized teratogen.

[j] Treatment done, so far, only in the third trimester.

Abbreviations Used in this Catalog

Listed below are most of the abbreviations that are used in this catalog.

Abbreviation	Definition
ACDHPA	Acyl-CoA-dihydroxyacetone phosphate acyltransferase
ACTH	Adrenocorticotropic hormone
AFP	Alpha-fetoprotein
ASA	Argininosuccinic acid
ASD	Atrial septal defect
ASH	Asymmetric septal hypertrophy
AV	Atrioventricular
beta hCG	beta human chorionic gonadotropin
CAH	Congenital adrenal hyperplasia
CHD	Congenital heart defect
CMT	Charcot–Marie–Tooth (disease)
CMV	Cytomegalovirus
CNS	Central nervous system
CT	Computerized tomography
CVS	Chorionic villus sampling
DMD	Duchenne muscular dystrophy
DNA	Deoxyribonucleic acid
DSS	Dosage-sensitive sex
EBL	Epidermolysis bullosa letalis
ECG	Electrocardiogram
ECMO	Extracorporeal membrane oxygenation
EFE	Endocardial fibroelastosis
ELISA	Enzyme-linked immunosorbent assay
ETF	Electron transferring flavoprotein
E3	Estriol
FBN1	Fibrillin 1 (gene)
FISH	Fluorescence *in situ* hybridization
FSH	Follicle stimulating hormone
HbF	Fetal hemoglobin
hCG	Human chorionic gonadotropin

HEM	Highly echogenic meconium
HIV	Human immunodeficiency virus
HPL	Human placental lactogen
IGF-I	Insulin-like growth factor I
IGFBP-3	Insulin-like growth factor binding protein 3
IHSS	Idiopathic hypertrophic subaortic stenosis
IUGR	Intrauterine growth retardation
IVG	Isovalerylglycine
LDL	Low-density lipoprotein
L/S ratio	Lecithin/sphingomyelin ratio
L1CAM	L1 cell adhesion molecule
MASA	Mental retardation-aphasia-shuffling gait-adducted thumbs (syndrome)
MCAD	Median-chain acyl-coenzyme A dehydrogenase
MOM	Multiple of the median
MRI	Magnetic resonance imaging
MT	Mitochondria
mtDNA	Mitochondrial DNA
NBT	Nitroblue tetrazolium
OFC	Occipitofrontal circumference
OFD	Orofaciodigital (syndrome)
PCR	Polymerase chain reaction
PD	Prenatal diagnosis
PEE	Phosphate-eliminating enzyme
PNP	Purine nucleoside phosphorylase
PUBS	Percutaneous umbilical blood sampling
RFLP	Restriction-fragment–length polymorphism
RNA	Ribonucleic acid
SD	Standard deviation
SLE	Systemic lupus erythematosus
SMA	Spinal muscular atrophy
SUA	Single umbilical artery
SVT	Supraventricular tachycardia
TEM	Transmission electron microscope
TGV	Transposition of the great vessels
TSH	Thyroid stimulating hormone
UPD	Uniparental disomy
VNTR	Variable number tandem repeats
VSD	Ventricular septal defect
WT1	Wilms tumor 1 (gene)
21-HO	21-hydroxylase
17-HOP	17-hydroxyprogesterone

Catalog of
Prenatally Diagnosed
Conditions

Chapter 1

Chromosomal Anomalies[a]

General References: Wladimiroff et al., 1988a; Eydoux et al., 1989

General Comments: Chromosomal abnormalities in the fetus and/or placenta are relatively common. Chromosomal studies can be done on almost any living tissue of the fetus, including amniotic fluid cells (amniocytes), chorionic villi, and fetal white cells, and on cells from fetal urine, ascitic fluid, and cystic hygroma fluid. The usual indications for doing a fetal chromosomal study include parental chromosomal abnormalities, previous sibling with a trisomy, a low level of maternal serum alpha-fetoprotein (AFP) or estriol, elevated human chorionic gonadotropin (hCG), fetal structural abnormalities of unknown etiology, and most commonly, advanced maternal age.

In a study reported by Wladimiroff and co-workers (1988a), 35 of 170 fetuses (20.5%) with structural abnormalities were detected to have chromosomal aberrations. The chromosomal abnormalities found were autosomal trisomies (54%), Turner syndrome (45,X) (23%), triploidy (11.5%), other sex chromosomal anomalies {46,X,i(q), 47,XXY, and 47,XYY} (8.5%), and an unbalanced familial translocation (6;9). Seven other chromosomal abnormalities were found in the postnatal period from fetuses on whom a chromosomal analysis was not performed.

Specific antenatal indications for doing chromosomal analyses as suggested by Wladimiroff and associates (1988a) include: (1) a specific structural defect known to be associated with chromosomal abnormalities, such as hydrocephalus, cardiac defects, duodenal atresia, omphalocele, and cystic hygroma; (2) multiple structural anomalies; (3) intrauterine growth retardation (IUGR); (4) hydramnios; (5) nonimmune hydrops fetalis; and (6) rare defects such as teratomas, abdominal cysts, and facial clefts.

Eydoux and associates (1989) reported on another larger series of chromosomally abnormal fetuses. They did karyotypes on 936 fetuses with abnormalities detected in utero and another 6,515 done for maternal age, and found chromosomal aberrations in 4.4% of cases with amniotic fluid disorders (i.e., hydramnios, oligohydramnios, and so forth), 6.7% in fetal growth retardation, 15.8% in fetal or placental abnormalities, and 3.2% in advanced maternal age. When multiple abnormalities were detected in the fetuses, 80% of them were trisomy 13, trisomy 18, trisomy 21, or monosomy X; whereas 4.9% were triploidies; and 3.3% were balanced and 9.8% were unbalanced, non-Robertsonian structural abnormalities.

Chromosomal discordance between chorionic villi and the fetus occurs in

1–2% of pregnancies evaluated by first trimester chorionic villus sampling (CVS) (Kalousek, 1990). Various combinations of aneuploidy and placental/fetal mosaicism have been reported. These combinations in general include placental mosaicism with normal fetal chromosomal constitution, with mosaic fetal aneuploidy, or with nonmosaic fetal aneuploidy; nonmosaic placental aneuploidy with either normal fetal chromosomal makeup or mosaic fetal aneuploidy; and normal placental chromosomal constitution with either mosaic fetal chromosomal composition or nonmosaic fetal aneuploidy. Monosomic, trisomic, and polyploidic mosaicisms have been reported with these kinds of mosaicisms (Callen et al., 1988).

The most commonly found fetoplacental chromosomal discordance is placental mosaicism with normal fetal chromosomal constitution, now called *confined placental mosaicism*. The concept and term was first proposed by Kalousek and Dill in 1983. Confined placental mosaicism appears to arise most frequently by "trisomy rescue" (Delozier-Blancher et al., 1995), a situation where the conceptus is initially trisomic but one of the trisomic chromosomes is lost during later cell divisions in those cell(s) that form the embryo proper. Although the embryonic karyotype is now numerically correct, the embryo may still face an adverse outcome because of uniparental disomy (UPD) of the previously trisomic chromosomes. Uniparental disomy is the presence of two homologous chromosomes inherited from the same parent; normally one of each of the homologous chromosomes comes from each parent (biparental disomy). Theoretically, UPD will occur in a third of fetuses undergoing trisomy rescue because loss of the trisomic chromosome is probably random. Uniparental disomy may lead to an abnormal phenotype when genes on the involved chromosomes are subject to imprinting. For example, Prader–Willi syndrome is the result of maternal uniparental disomy in 20% of cases, and this situation probably arises as a result of the above mechanism.

The following convention has been adopted in listing chromosomal mosaicisms in this catalog: (1) confined placental mosaicism with no apparent fetal chromosomal aberration and, if known, biparental disomy is cited as trisomy (monosomy) (chromosome involved), confined placental mosaicism with diploid fetus; (2) confined placental mosaicism with maternal uniparental disomy is cited as trisomy (chromosome involved), confined placental mosaicism with maternal uniparental disomy; (3) confined placental mosaicism with paternal uniparental disomies cited as trisomy (chromosome involved) confined placental mosaicism with paternal uniparental disomy; (4) placental and fetal mosaic aneuploidy is cited as trisomy (monosomy) (chromosome involved), both placental and fetal mosaicism; (5) placental mosaicism with pure fetal trisomy (monosomy) is cited as trisomy (monosomy) (chromosome involved), placental mosaicism with nonmosaic fetal trisomy (monosomy); (6) placental nonmosaic aneuploidy with normal fetal chromosomal makeup is cited as trisomy (monosomy) (chromosome involved), placental nonmosaic trisomy (monosomy) with normal fetal chromosomes; (7) placental nonmosaic aneuploidy with mosaic fetal aneuploidy is cited as trisomy (monosomy) (chromosome involved), placental nonmosaic trisomy (monosomy) with fetal mosaic trisomy (monosomy); (8) normal placental chromosomal constitution with fetal mosaic chromosomal composition is cited as trisomy (monosomy) (chromosome involved), fetal mosaicism with normal placental chromosomes; and (9) normal placental chromosomal constitution with fetal nonmosaic chromosomal aneuploidies cited as trisomy (monosomy) (chromosome involved), fetal nonmosaic trisomy (monosomy) with normal placental chromosomes. Pure (nonmosaic) trisomy (monosomy) in both the placenta (if this information is known) and the fetus is referenced as trisomy (monosomy) (chromosome involved).

As with most conventions, there may be exceptions to the standard rules. One exception is confined trisomy 16 mosaicism of the amnion and umbilical cord (see Trisomy 16, amnion and umbilical cord mosaicism only [PD 103500]).

PD 010000 CAT-EYE SYNDROME {Chromosome 22 partial tetrasomy; inv dup 22(q11); Schmid-Fraccaro syndrome}[b] (McKusick No. 115470)

Syndrome Note: Clinically the cat-eye syndrome is characterized by coloboma of the iris, downslanting palpebral fissures, dysmorphic ears, preauricular tags and/or pits, congenital heart defects, and anal atresia. Cytogenetically, the condition is caused by a supernumerary marker chromosome that is an inverted and duplicated 22q11.

Amniocentesis: 46,XX/47,XX,+mar found in amniotic fluid cells.[c] Marker was bisatellited, dicentric, NOR positive and Distamycin-DAPI negative.
Driscoll et al., 1993b
by fluorescence in situ hybridization (FISH) marker positive for 22q11
Driscoll et al., 1993b

PD 100000 CHROMOSOMAL ANOMALIES, GENERAL[b] (McKusick No. None)

Karyotypic analysis of cultured amniotic fluid cells, or chorionic villi, the latter either from cultured or from direct preparation
Simpson and Martin, 1976; Schmid, 1977; Hsu et al., 1978; Simoni et al., 1983, 1984, 1986

PD 100100 CHROMOSOME XXX SYNDROME[b] (Triple X syndrome; Trisomy X; 47,XXX) (McKusick No. None)

Alpha-fetoprotein[c]: elevated in maternal serum
Burton, 1987; Warner et al., 1988
elevated in maternal serum but not in amniotic fluid
Warner et al., 1988
Amniocentesis[c]: decreased level of aminopeptidase M activity in amniotic fluid
Brock et al., 1984a
Maternal blood sampling[c]: elevated level of beta human chorionic gonadotropin (beta hCG)
Barkai et al., 1991
reduced levels of unconjugated estriol (E3)
Barkai et al., 1991
Preimplantation embryo biopsy[g]: FISH demonstrated 3 X chromosomes
Weier et al., 1993
Ultrasound: ascites,[c,d] elevation of the diaphragm,[c,d] sonolucent mass; in the fetal pelvis,[c,d] minimal fetal movements,[c,d] fetal demise[c,d]
Spear and Porto, 1988
Comments: At autopsy the fetus reported on by Spear and Porto (1988) had extensive ascites, a dilated bladder with an abnormal urethra that opened on the perineum between the vagina and anus, an imperforate

hymen with distended vagina, and a bicornuate uterus. There was ovarian dysgenesis and evidence of meconium peritonitis.
> no visualization of fetal kidney or bladder,[c] oligohydramnios[c]
>> Hogge et al., 1989a
>> Comments: In addition to the bilateral renal agenesis noted prenatally in the fetus reported by Hogge and colleagues (1989a), at autopsy there were hypoplastic ovaries, absence of the uterus and fallopian tubes, and a small bladder.
> increase echogenicity of fetal bowel
>> Strasberg et al., 1995

PD 100150 CHROMOSOME XXX/DOWN SYNDROME[b] (48,XXX,+21)
(McKusick No. None)

> Ultrasound[c]: nuchal thickening, large ventricular septal defect, 2-vessel umbilical cord
>> Park et al., 1995

PD 100160 CHROMOSOME XXXXY SYNDROME (XXXXY SYNDROME; 49,XXXXY; 49,XXXXY SYNDROME)[b] (McKusick No. None)

Syndrome Note: With poly-X plus Y chromosomal disorders, there are more severe growth deficiency, mental deficiency, and hypoplastic genitalia, and increased number of malformations including congenital heart defects, and clubfoot deformities with increasing number of X chromsomes.
> Hovav et al., 1993
> Doppler ultrasound[c]: decreased umbilical artery blood flow
>> Reuwer et al., 1987
> Ultrasound[c]: thickened skin over the scalp, hydrops fetalis, pleural effusion, thickened placenta, bilateral clubfoot deformity, hydramnios
>> Hovav et al., 1993

PD 100200 CHROMOSOME XYY SYNDROME[b] (McKusick No. None)

> Alpha-fetoprotein[c]: elevated in maternal serum
>> Ryynanen et al., 1983
>> low level in maternal serum
>>> Rajendra et al., 1986
> Maternal blood sampling[i]: after immunomagnetic removal of maternal lymphocytes and flow cytometry sorting utilizing antitrophoblast monoclonal antibodies, YY chromosomal constitution determined by FISH using biotin-labeled alpha-satellite centromeric probes for the Y chromosome.
>> Cacheux et al., 1992
> Ultrasound[c]: third-degree atrioventricular heart block, complex congenital heart disease, right heart dilatation
>> Wladimiroff et al., 1988a

PD 100350 COMPLEX CHROMOSOME REARRANGEMENT NO. 1
{46,XX,t(1;8)(8;9)(1pter → 1q43::8q13 → 8qter;1qter → 1q43::8p12 → 8q13::9p21 → 9pter;8pter → 8p12::9p21 → 9qter),t(4;7)(4pter → 4q21.3::7q22 → 7q31.2::4q25 → 4qter;7pter → 7q22::4q21.3 → 4q25::7q31.2 → 7qter),del(12)(pter → q13.3::q21.1 → qter)} (McKusick No. None)

Syndrome Note: The diagnosis of the above chromosomal problem was accomplished by FISH using whole chromosomal painting and repetitive sequence probes.
> Spikes et al., 1995

Ultrasound[c,d]: IUGR, oligohydramnios
    Spikes et al., 1995
    Comments: The child reported by Spikes and associates (1995) had multiple congenital anomalies, none of which were major. The child subsequently experienced growth deficiency and developed microcephaly. At the age of 5-1/2 years, she was moderately to severely intellectually retarded.

PD 100500 CRI DU CHAT SYNDROME (del 5p; Monosomy 5p)[b] (McKusick No. None)

Chorionic villus sampling[g,i]: partial deletion of chromosome 5p detected by appropriate DNA probes in an at-risk embryo
    Wasmuth et al., 1988
    Comments: Various members in three generations of this family carried a balanced translocation that could be detected only by DNA analysis. The family originally was studied both cytologically and by DNA analysis because the proband, two of her half-siblings, and a paternal cousin each had features of the cri du chat syndrome. The mother of the embryo cited above, who carried the balanced translocation, also had had a meiotic recombination event between the small translocation segment of 5p and the homologous region on the normal chromosome 5.

Maternal blood drawing[c,h]: low level of serum estriol
    Berlin et al., 1995
Ultrasound[c]: abnormally abrupt fetal movements
    Boue et al., 1982

PD 100502 DELETION CHROMOSOME X/Xq26.1qter {45,X/ 45,X,dic(X;15)(XpterXq26.1::15p11;15q}[b] (McKusick No. None)

Alpha-fetoprotein[c,h]: elevated in maternal serum
    Scheuerle et al., 1995
Maternal report[c,h]: decreased fetal movements
    Scheuerle et al., 1995
    Comments: The child reported with the above translocation had normal birth weight and postnatal growth. She, however, experienced developmental delay and was dysmorphic. Her abnormal features included dolichocephaly, frontal hair whorl, frontal bossing, midfacial hypoplasia, telecanthus, epicanthal folds, upslanting palpebral fissures, and Wolfflin–Kruckmann spots in both irides.

PD 100504 DELETION CHROMOSOME X(p22.31pter) {46,del(X)(p22.31),Y}[b] (McKusick No. None)

Condition Note: Bick and associates (1989, 1992) have reported on a male fetus with chondrodysplasia punctata, X-linked recessive form; X-linked ichthyosis; and Kallmann syndrome produced by the terminal deletion of the p arm of the X chromosome. The mother was a carrier of this chromosomal aberration, and previously an affected male sibling had been born to her.

Prenatal Diagnosis: A karyotype of appropriate fetal tissue is the only definitive method of diagnosing the condition in a de novo situation. Elevated levels of amniotic fluid dehydroepiandrosterone sulfate and/or deficiency of steroid sulfatase in culture amniotic fluid cells is probably sufficient for the diagnosis in an at-risk fetus.

Differential Diagnosis: Chondrodysplasia punctata, rhizomelic type (PD 150050); Conradi–Hunermann syndrome; Placental steroid sulfatase deficiency (PD 24900); Kallmann syndrome that is not associated with a deletion of chromosome X.

Amniocentesis[i]: elevated level of dehydroepiandrosterone sulfate in amniotic fluid

Bick et al., 1989; Bick et al., 1992

low level of steroid sulfatase in cultured amniotic fluid cells

Bick et al., 1989; Bick et al, 1992

Ultrasound[i]: nasal hypoplasia

Bick et al., 1989; Bick et al, 1992

PD 100506 DELETION CHROMOSOME 1p/15p {45,XY,-1,-15, +der(1)t(1;15)(p36.3;q11.1)}[b] (McKusick No. None)

Ultrasound[c]: isolated situs inversus, decreased biparietal diameter to femur length ratio

Coss et al., 1995

PD 100509 DELETION CHROMOSOME 1(p36.3pter) {Deletion Chromosomes 1 (p36.31pter), (p36.32pter) and (p36.33pter)} (McKusick No. None)

Syndrome Note: The clinical features associated with deletion of chromosome 1 (p36.3pter) include microcephaly, prominent forehead, deep-set eyes, depressed nasal bridge, flat midface, relative prognathism, abnormal ears, small hands and feet, self-abusive behavior, and mental retardation (Reish et al., 1995).

In the patients reported by Reish and co-workers (1995), the deletion on chromosome 1 was detected by high resolution G-banding chromosomal analysis and confirmed by FISH assessment.

Ultrasound[c,h]: IUGR

Reish et al., 1995

PD 101510 DELETION CHROMOSOME 1(q25q32) {Interstitial deletion chromosome 1(q25q32); 46,XY,del(1)(q25q32)} (McKusick No. None)

Ultrasound[c,d]: ascites, oligohydramnios, IUGR

Scarbrough et al., 1988

Comments: The fetus reported above by Scarbrough and co-workers (1988) was thought to have partial obstruction of the urethra with resulting ascites. The ascites resolved by the 38th week of gestation, leaving a soft abdomen with wrinkled abdominal skin at birth. The authors (Scarbrough et al., 1988) believe that this child had the urethral obstruction malformation sequence or prune belly syndrome.

PD 100512 DELETION CHROMOSME 1(q41qter) {46,XX,del(1)(q41qter)}[b] (McKusick No. None)

Ultrasound[c]: posterior fossa cyst that compressed the cerebellum, increased nuchal skin thickness, abdominal wall defect

Rotmensch et al., 1991

Comments: After termination, the fetus reported by Rotmensch and co-workers (1991) had multiple congenital anomalies including an arachnoid cyst in the posterior fossa and an omphalocele.

PD 100513 DELETION CHROMOSOME l(q42q44) {46,XX,del(1)(q42q44)}
(McKusick No. None)

Ultrasound[c]: increased nuchal fold thickness
Van Dyke et al., 1989

PD 100516 DELETION CHROMOSME 4(q21.1q25) {Interstitial deletion
4q21.1q25; 46,XY,del(4)(q21.1q25)}[b] (McKusick No. None)

Ultrasound[c,d]: hydramnios
Kulharya et al., 1995

PD 100518 DELETION CHROMOSOME 4(q21.2q25), inversion 4(p15.3q21.2)
{46,XY,der(4)inv ins(3;4)(p21.32;q25q21.2),inv(4)(p15.3q21.2)}[b] (McKusick No.
None)

Maternal report[c,d]: decreased fetal movements
Hegmann et al., 1996
Method not stated[c,d]: slowing of fetal growth, oligohydramnios
Hegmann et al., 1996
Comments: The father of the child reported by Hegmann and associates
(1996) carried an insertional translocation between chromosomes 3 and
4 in which a segment from 4q was inserted into 3p, and a pericentric
inversion of chromosome 4. His chromosomal makeup was 46,XY, inv
ins(3;4)(p21.32;q25q21.2),inv(4)(p15.3q21.2).

PD 100520 DELETION CHROMOSOME 6q {46,XY,del(6)(q23)}[b] (McKusick
No. None)

Condition Note: Deletion of the long arm of chromosome 6 is a relatively
uncommon chromosomal problem. The deletion may be either a terminal or an
interstitial deletion of 6q, or it may involve a ring chromosome of 6. Clinical
features include microcephaly, abnormal facial features, cleft palate, short stature, clinodactyly, camptodactyly, congenital heart defect, and mental retardation.
Shen-Schwarz et al., 1989
Prenatal Diagnosis: A partial or complete deletion of the long arm of chromosome 6 in the fetus is diagnostic. It may be a chance finding during prenatal
screening, detected in a fetus with other abnormalities who is screened for
chromosomal problems, or discovered because one parent has a balanced translocation involving 6q.
Differential Diagnosis: Deletions involving other chromosomes.
Ultrasound[c]: IUGR; large, fluid-filled, mobile mass extending from the occiput
along the back to the first thoracic vertebra; mild hydrocephalus with the
lateral ventricular hemispheric width ratio of 85.7%; bilateral hydrothorax;
hypoplastic left lung; nonvisualization of the right lung; diaphragmatic hernia,
malposition of the liver
Shen-Schwarz et al., 1989
Comments: The fetus reported by Shen-Schwarz and associates (1989) was
found to have a de novo terminal deletion of chromosome 6. Following
termination of the pregnancy at 21 weeks of gestation, the fetus was found
to have an asymmetrical sloping forehead, flat nasal bridge, anteverted
nares, long philtrum, micrognathia, cleft palate, cystic hygroma, bilateral
diaphragmatic hernias, hypoplastic lungs, persistent atrioventricular canal,
agenesis of the corpus callosum, and absence of the olfactory bulbs.

PD 100600 DELETION CHROMOSOME 7q22 {Interstitial deletion 7q22; 46,X, del(7)(q22.1q22.3)}[b] (McKusick No. None)

Alpha-fetoprotein[c]: elevated in maternal serum
Stevenson et al., 1989
Ultrasound[c]: anencephalus
Stevenson et al., 1989

PD 100650 DELETION CHROMOSOME 7q32 {46,XY,del(7q)(q32); 7q del; 7q del(q32); 46,XY,7q del}[b] (McKusick No. None)

Ultrasound[c]: ventriculomegaly
Drugan et al., 1989a; Drugan et al., 1989b; Evans et al., 1989
encephalocele
Drugan et al., 1989b; Evans et al., 1989

PD 100700 DELETION CHROMOSOME 7q35 {del(7)(q34q36); Interstitial deletion (7)(pterq34::q36qter)}[b] (McKusick No. None)

Ultrasound[c,d]: severe, symmetric IUGR
Fryns et al., 1988
Comments: In addition to the interstitial deletion of chromosome 7q35, the fetus also had a de novo reciprocal translocation {t(3;7)(q27;q35)} (Fryns et al., 1988)

PD 100710 DELETION CHROMSOME 8(p11.1pter) MOSAICISM {46,XX/ 46,XX, del(8p) (p11.1pter)}[b] (McKusick No. None)

Alpha-fetoprotein[c,h]: elevated in maternal serum
Laudon and Buchanan, 1993
Maternal blood sampling[c,h]: low levels of maternal serum free beta hCG
Laudon and Buchanan, 1993
Comments: At autopsy, the fetus reported by Laudon and Buchanan (1993) was dysmorphic and found to have downslanting palpebral fissures, deformed right ear, high arched palate, micrognathia, and an increased number of Hassall's corpuscles in the thymus.

PD 100715 DELETION CHROMOSOME 8q[b] (McKusick No. None)

Ultrasound[c]: cystic hygroma
Neu et al., 1993

PD 100720 DELETION CHROMOSME 8(q24.11q24.13) {Langer–Giedion syndrome; Persistent cloaca; Trichorhinophalangeal syndrome, type II; Urethral obstruction malformation sequence; 46,XX,del (8)(q24.11q24.13)} (McKusick Nos. 100100, 150230)

Condition Note: Langer–Giedion syndrome or trichorhinophalangeal syndrome, type II is characterized by sparse hair, bulbous "pear-shaped" nose, cone-shaped epiphyses of the phalanges of the hands, multiple exostoses, and mental retardation. Normally, the condition has a sporadic occurrence in a family, and is associated with a microdeletion in the long arm of chromosome 8 {8q24.11q24.13}. Persistent cloaca and associated urethral obstruction malformation sequence is not normally part of Langer–Giedion syndrome, nor of deletion of 8q, and may be just a nonrandom association in the case reported by Ramos and co-workers (1992).
Ramos et al., 1992; McKusick, 1996

Ultrasound[c,d]: megaureters, megacystis, oligohydramnios
Ramos et al., 1992

Comments: In the fetus reported by Ramos and associates (1992), there was spontaneous decompression of the bladder between 29 weeks of gestation and birth at 39 weeks. The female child had persistent cloaca with a single perineal opening, and very lax and redundant skin of the abdomen. At the age of 9 years, she was diagnosed with Langer–Giedion syndrome and found to have the 8q deletion (46,XX,del 8q24.11q24.13)

PD 100730 DELETION CHROMOSOME 9(p24pter)/duplication 5(q31qter)[b] {46,XY,-9,+der(9),t(5;9)(q32;p24)} (McKusick No. None)

Ultrasound[c,d]: complex cardiac malformations, oligohydramnios
Schimmenti et al., 1995

PD 100740 DELETION CHROMOSOME 10p {46,XY,del(10)(p13)}[b] (McKusick No. None)

Ultrasound[c]: hydramnios[h]
Eydoux et al., 1989

PD 100750 DELETION CHROMOSOME 10q {46,XX,del(10)(q25.1)}[b] (McKusick No. None)

Alpha-fetoprotein[c]: low level in maternal serum
Dickerman et al., 1987
Ultrasound[c]: microcephaly
Dickerman et al., 1987

PD 100820 DELETION CHROMOSOME 13, RING 13 {Ring Chromosome 13; 46,XX, r(13)}[b] (McKusick No. None)

Ultrasound[c]: anencephaly
Palmer et al., 1987
ventriculomegaly of the brain[h]
Eydoux et al., 1989
ocular hypertelorism[h]
Eydoux et al., 1989
clubfoot deformity
Eydoux et al., 1989

PD 100824 DELETION CHROMOSME 13, RING 13, + MARKER {45,XX,-13/46,XX,-13,r(13)/46,XX,-13,+mar}[b] (McKusick No. None)

Ultrasound[c,d]: "strawberry-shaped" skull, cystic hygroma, polydactyly
Luthardt et al., 1993

Comments: In the fetus cited by Luthardt and co-authors (1993), the ring 13 and marker chromosome were found in amniotic fluid cells, chorionic villi, and fetal blood cells. The ring 13 was confirmed by alpha satellite probe and whole chromosomal painting probes; the origin of the marker chromosome was not determined.

PD 100830 DELETION CHROMSOME 13q[b] (McKusick No. None)

Ultrasound[c]: cystic hygroma
Neu et al, 1993

PD 100840 DELETION CHROMOSOME 13(q12.1q12.3) {46,XY/ 46,XY,del(13)(q12.1q12.3); 46,XX,del(13)(q12)}[b] (McKusick No. None)

Ultrasound[c,d]: hydrocephalus
> Palmer et al., 1987
> anencephalus
> Evans et al., 1989

PD 100845 DELETION CHROMSOME 13(q13)[b] (McKusick No. None)

Ultrasound[c,h]: anencephaly
> Drugan et al., 1989b
Amniocentesis[c,h]: acetylcholinesterase present in amniotic fluid
> Drugan et al., 1989b

PD 100870 DELETION CHROMOSOME 13(q21.2q22)
{46,XY,del(13)(q21.2q22)}[b] (McKusick No. None)

Monitoring fetal heart tones[c,d]: 30-second episode of fetal heart deceleration and subsequent prolonged bradycardia
> Khong et al., 1994
Examination of amniotic fluid after artificial rupture of membranes[c,d]: heavily blood-stained liquor
> Khong et al., 1994
Ultrasound[c,d]: double bubble sign
> Khong et al., 1994

> *Comments*: After the fetus reported by Khong and associates (1994) was delivered in a very depressed state, the neonate was found to have thinning and ulceration of one of the umbilical arteries. The ulcer had bled into the umbilical cord and amniotic fluid. In addition, the neonate had multiple atresias of the small intestine, Hirschsprung disease of the colon, and anemia. At 9 months, after a complicated clinical course and multiple bouts of aspirations, the infant died. Chromosomal analysis revealed an interstitial deletion of the long arm of chromosome 13 {46,XY,del(13)-(q21.2q22)}.

PD 100900 DELETION CHROMOSOME 13(q22q32) {Interstitial deletion chromosome 13q; 46,XY,del(13)(q22q32)}[b] (McKusick No. None)

Ultrasound[d,i]: markedly enlarged fetal head, large intracranial cystic structure occupying most of the cranial vault, no midline brain structures
> Simpson et al., 1988

> *Comments*: The fetus reported by Simpson and co-workers (1988) had a previous sibling with the same chromosomal aberration. However, both parents had normal chromosomal constitutions and the recurrence of this chromosomal problem probably represents germ-line mosaicism in one parent.

PD 100915 DELETION CHROMOSOME 13(q23.3qter)[b] (McKusick No. None)

Ultrasound[c]: oligohydramnios
> Urioste et al., 1995

> *Comments*: The fetus reported by Urioste and associates (1995) developed oligohydramnios because of fetal membrane leakage. After birth the child was thought to have Opitz–Frias syndrome (PD 192800). In addition there

was deficiency of coagulation factors VII and X, the genes for which are located in the chromosomal region 13q34.

PD 100920 DELETION CHROMOSOME 13(q32.1q32.3)[b] (McKusick No. None)

Ultrasound[c]: holoprosencephaly
Brown et al., 1995

PD 100930 DELETION CHROMOSOME 14q {46,XY,del(14)(q32)}[b] (McKusick No. None)

Ultrasound[c]: IUGR,[h] oligohydramnios[h]
Eydoux et al., 1989

PD 100940 DELETION CHROMOSOME 15(q11q13) (Prader–Willi/Angelman syndrome region deletion)[b] (McKusick No. 600161, 600162, see also 105830, 176270)

Abnormality Note: Without phenotypic information or parental origin of the deleted chromosome 15, it is not possible to determine if a fetus has Prader–Willi or Angelman syndrome. Therefore in this situation, the designation of deletion chromosome 15q11-15q13 or Prader–Willi/Angelman syndrome region deletion is used.

Amniocentesis: G-band analysis showed deletion in the 15q11-q13 region
Toth-Fejel et al., 1995
FISH probes demonstrated deletion in the 15(q11q13) of a number 15 chromosome
Toth-Fejel et al., 1995

PD 100950 DELETION CHROMOSOME 17p {46,XX,del(17)(p13.1)}[b] (McKusick No. None)

Condition Note: In this condition the terminal portion of 17p is deleted and differs from the Miller–Dieker syndrome (PD 101510) in that in the latter condition there is an interstitial deletion in the number 17 chromosome at the 13.3 band only.
Prenatal Diagnosis: Chromosomal analysis of amniotic fluid cells, chorionic villi, or fetal white cells is the only method of detecting this condition with certainty.
Differential Diagnosis: Other conditions associated with a chromosomal deletion.

Echocardiogram[c,d]: small left ventricle, hypoplastic mitral valve
Greenberg et al., 1988a
Ultrasound[c,d]: small left ventricle of the heart, hypoplastic mitral valve, IUGR, hydramnios
Greenberg et al., 1988a
Comments: The fetus reported by Greenberg and associates (1988a) died at 34 weeks of gestation and labor was induced. At autopsy there was malrotation of the colon, small and nodular thymus, hypoplastic left ventricle with mitral valve atresia, a large atrial septal defect, a small ventricular septal defect, an enlarged right ventricle with a double-outlet right ventricle, and pulmonary valve stenosis with an overriding, anteriorly placed aorta. The authors felt that the fetus probably had DiGeorge syndrome although there was no interruption of the aortic arch and no detection studies of chromosome 22 were done.

PD 100960 DELETION CHROMOSOME, RING 18 (Ring 18)[b] (McKusick No. None)

Ultrasound[c,d]: alobar holoprosencephaly as indicated by no evidence of cerebral hemispheres or a brainstem, fused thalami, massive hydrocephalus, recessed nasal region, ocular hypotelorism, dilated loops of bowel, and bilateral hydronephrosis
Diehn et al., 1995

PD 100965 DELETION CHROMOSOME, RING 18(p11.23q22.1) {Double ring 18; Mosaic ring 18/monosomy 18; 46,XY, r(18)(p11.23q22.1)}[b] (McKusick No. None)

Ultrasound[c]: hypoplastic right heart, pulmonary artery tresia, cleft lip and palate, single umbilical artery
Clark et al., 1995
Comments: After the above fetal abnormalities were detected at 24 weeks of gestation (Clark et al., 1995), an amniocentesis was done with the resulting karyotype being 46,XY,r(18)/45,XY,-18 with 25% of the colonies having monosomy 18. Cordocentesis revealed 46,XY,r(18) in all fetal white cells. The fetus was delivered at 34 weeks and had other multiple congenital anomalies. A repeat blood karyotype showed 46,XY,r(18) 9p11.23q32.1) in 95/100 cells, double ring in 4 cells, and deleted ring in 1.

PD 100970 DELETION CHROMOSOME 18p {46,XY,del(18p)}[b] (McKusick No. None)

Ultrasound[c]: ventriculomegaly of the brain[h]
Eydoux et al., 1989

PD 100972 DELETION CHROMOSOME 18(p11.1)/MOSAIC TRISOMY 18q {Mosaic 46,XX,del(18)(p11.1)/46,XX,-18,+i(18q)de novo}[b] (McKusick No. None)

Ultrasound[c]: hydramnios
Qumsiyeh et al., 1995
Comments: After termination of the fetus reported by Qumsiyeh and associates (1995), the fetus was found to be dysmorphic and had brachycephaly, low posterior hairline, prominent occiput, ocular hypertelorism, depressed nasal bridge, broad nose, full lips with down-turned corners, micrognathia, slightly low-set ears, small penis, brachydactyly, broad hands, and club feet.

PD 100975 DELETION CHROMSOME 18(q22) {46,XX,del(18)(q22)}[b] (McKusick No. None)

Ultrasound[c]: no abnormalities found
Peters-Brown et al., 1995
Comments: The fetus reported by Peters-Brown and co-workers (1995) was delivered at 33 weeks of gestation and had no physical anomalies other than a cleft palate. At 10 months, she had midface hypoplasia and mild developmental delay.

PD 100978 DELETION CHROMSOME 21q[b] (McKusick No. None)

Ultrasound[c]: holoprosencephaly, congenital heart defect, type unspecified
Berry et al., 1990

PD 100980 DELETION CHROMOSOME 21(q22qter)[b] (McKusick No. None)

Ultrasound[c,h]: dilated pulmonary artery, small left ventricle
Theodoropoulos et al., 1995

PD 100990 DICENTRIC (15q11;15q11) marker {47,XX,dic(15q11;15q11)}[b]
(McKusick No. None)

Ultrasound[c]: no abnormalities found
Gray et al., 1995a

PD 100995 DIGEORGE SYNDROME (Deletion chromosome 22q11;
Hypoplasia of the thymus and parathymus)[b] (McKusick No. 188400)

Syndrome Note: DiGeorge syndrome is comprised of conotruncal heart defects, hypoplastic or absent thymus and parathyroids leading to deficiency of T cells and hypocalcemia, and abnormal facial features. A microdeletion involving chromosome 22g11 is present in most patients. There is approximately 8% familial transmission of the 22q11 deletion. The same or similar deletion is found in most individuals with the velocardiofacial (Shprintzen) syndrome (PD 194665).
McKusick, 1995; Van Hemel et al., 1995
Prenatal Diagnosis: The only definitive method of diagnosis that has been reported is that of detecting the deletion at 22q11.
Differential Diagnosis: CATCH 22; Conotruncal heart malformations; Velocardiofacial syndrome (PD 194665).
Amniocentesis[h]: presence of a deletion at 22q11 by FISH
Van Hemel et al., 1995
Comments: In the fetus reported by Van Hemel and associates (1995), a sister and the father also were found to have the 22q11 deletion; the sister had the full syndrome, whereas the father was physically normal but had mild learning disabilities and a tendency for depression and alcohol abuse.

PD 101000 DOWN SYNDROME (Trisomy 21 syndrome; 46,XX,+t(21;21);
47,XX or XY,+21)[b] (McKusick No. None)

Prenatal Diagnosis: The only definitive methods for diagnosing Down syndrome is via a chromosomal analysis of tissue obtained by amniocentesis, chorionic villus sampling or cordocentesis; or by determining the number of chromosome 21s present in these tissues or from fetal cells obtained from maternal cell sorting or from the endocervical canal by the use of chromosome (DNA) probes. The latter technique normally utilizes FISH.

The risk that the fetus has Down syndrome increases with certain maternal serum or fetal physical findings: for instance, decreased levels of maternal serums AFP for gestation increases the risk of Down syndrome with an inverse relation between the AFP level and the risk; similarly, a decrease in unconjugated estriol uE3, while an elevation of hCG is associated with an increase in risk. All three tests used concurrently can detect 75% of Down syndrome fetuses (Bradley et al., 1994). Likewise, the detection of certain fetal abnormalities also increases the likelihood of Down syndrome in the fetus (Benacerraf et al., 1994; Vintzileos and Egan, 1995). These abnormalities include nuchal thickening, shortened femur and humerus, hyperechogenic bowel, choroid plexus cysts, and major structural defects. Using these findings, Benacrerraf and associates (1994) were able to detect 73% of fetuses with Down syndrome.

Acetylcholinesterase[c]: fast migrating isozyme in amniotic fluid demonstrated by gel electrophoresis
> Crandall et al., 1989

Alpha-fetoprotein[c]: low levels in maternal serum
> Cuckle et al., 1984; Fuhrmann et al., 1984; Merkatz et al., 1984; Seller, 1984; Tabor et al., 1984; Voigtlander and Vogel, 1985; Baumgarten et al., 1985; Kaffe and Hsu, 1985; Nelson and Peterson, 1985; Schoenfeld et al., 1985; Rajendra et al., 1986; Ashwood et al., 1987; Bogart et al., 1987; Arab et al., 1988; Ben-Yishay et al., 1988; Crandall et al., 1988; Dickerman et al., 1988; Fisher et al., 1988; Redwine et al., 1988; Schneider et al., 1988; Barsel-Bowers et al., 1989; Del Junco et al., 1989; Johnson et al., 1989a; Shah et al., 1989; Carlson and Platt, 1993; Bradley et al., 1994; Benn et al., 1995

low levels in amniotic fluid
> Trigg et al., 1984; Baumgarten et al., 1985; Cuckle et al., 1985; Hullin et al., 1985; Nelson and Peterson, 1985; Cuckle and Wald, 1986; Martens and Rivas, 1986; Ashwood et al., 1987; Crandall et al., 1987; Dickerman et al., 1988; Jones and Evans, 1988; Kaffe et al., 1988; Crandall et al., 1988

Comments: In one study (Kaffe et al., 1988), the median AFP value in amniotic fluid of fetuses with Down syndrome was 0.72 multiple of the median (MOM).

elevated in maternal serum
> Fisher et al., 1988

elevated in amniotic fluid
> Weinberg et al., 1975; Fisher et al., 1981; Crandall and Matsumoto, 1984b; Kaffe et al., 1988; Crandall et al., 1989

Amniocentesis: identification of three fluorescent bodies in amniotic fluid cells following hybridization with No. 21 chromosome probes (FISH)
> Julien et al., 1986; Ward et al., 1995

Comments: According to one study (Carelli et al., 1995), the detection rate for trisomy 21 using FISH procedure is now 90.8%.

deficiency of amniotic fluid disaccharidases prior to 21 weeks of gestation in fetuses with duodenal atresia[c]
> Morin et al., 1980; Morin et al., 1987

elevation of amniotic fluid disaccharidases prior to 21 weeks' gestation[c]
> Morin et al., 1980

decreased levels of activity of amniotic fluid disaccharidases, maltase, sucrase, trehalase, and lactase[c]
> Kleijer et al., 1985b

decreased levels of gamma-glutamyltranspeptidase activity in amniotic fluid[c]
> Brock et al., 1984a; Aitkin et al., 1985; Macek et al., 1987; Morin et al., 1987; Jones and Evans, 1988

increased levels of gamma-glutamyltranspeptidase activity in amniotic fluid[c]
> Muller et al., 1988

Comments: There was duodenal atresia in the case of Muller and associates (1988). The atresia was located below the sphincter of Oddi.

aspiration of cystic hygroma fluid and culture of cystic hygroma fluid cells[c]

> Al Saadi, 1989

decreased levels of aminopeptidase M activity in amniotic fluid[c]

> Brock et al., 1984a

increased percentage of phenylalanine-resistant alkaline phosphatase activity in amniotic fluid[c]

> Brock et al., 1984a; Aitken et al., 1985; Carey and Pollard, 1986; Morin et al., 1987

decreased percentage of homoarginine-resistant alkaline phosphatase activity in amniotic fluid[c]

> Brock et al., 1984a; Aitken et al., 1985; Carey and Pollard, 1986; Morin et al., 1987

reduced levels of alkaline phosphatase in amniotic fluid[c]

> Jalanko et al., 1983

increased levels of beta hCG in amniotic fluid[c]

> Bharathur et al., 1988

decreased or absence of 36,000-Dalton glycoprotein[c]

> Pena et al., 1989

Chorionic villus sampling[c,g]: trisomy 21 karyotype in chorionic villi

> Brambati and Simoni, 1983; Besley et al., 1988; Bovicelli et al., 1988

Cordocentesis: 47,XY,+21 karyotype on fetal white cells

> Tilley et al., 1993

transient myeloproliferative disorder as indicated by a white cell count in fetal blood of 108,000/mm^3 with 96% circulative blast forms

> Tilley et al., 1993

Echocardiography[c]: atrial and ventricular septal defects

> Nicolaides et al., 1986a

ostium primum and secundum atrial septal defects with the atrioventricular valves lying straight across the septum

> Allan et al., 1981b

Endocervical canal sampling[g]: trisomy 21 fetal cells found by FISH using chromosome 21 probes

> Adinolfi et al., 1995

Fetal blood drawing using fetoscopy followed by fetal blood karyotype[b]

> Nicolaides et al., 1986a

Fetal blood obtained by cardiac puncture during feticide[b]

> Pijpers et al., 1989a

Maternal blood sampling[c]: increased levels of hCG in maternal serum[c]

> Bogart et al., 1987; Arab et al., 1988; Bharathur et al., 1988; Muller and Boue, 1990; Bradley et al., 1994; Benn et al., 1995

increased levels of the subunit of human chorionic gonadotropin (alpha-hCG) in maternal serum[c]

> Bogart et al., 1987

increased levels of beta hCG in maternal serum[c]

> Del Junco et al., 1989; Knight et al., 1989

increased levels of progesterone, Schwangerschafts protein-1, and human placental lactogen[c]

Knight et al., 1989

reduced levels of maternal serum unconjugated estriol[c]

Canick et al., 1987; Bradley et al., 1994; Benn et al., 1995

utilization of triple screening (maternal serum levels of AFP, hCG, and unconjugated estriol) to increase the woman's risk for carrying a fetus with Down syndrome

Bradley et al., 1994

Comments: By using the combination of all three of the above biochemical markers, and a threshold for further testing of equal to or greater than 1:384, Bradley and associates (1994) were able to detect 75% of fetuses with Down syndrome.

decreased levels of insulin-like growth factor-I (IGF-I)

Chu and Boots, 1995

decreased levels of insulin-like growth factor binding protein-3 (IG-FBP-3)[c]

Chu and Boots, 1995

Maternal blood sampling with subsequent fetal cell sorting[h]: trisomy 21 cells detected by FISH using chromosome 21 probes

Wachtel et al., 1995

Comments: The fetuses reported by Wachtel and colleagues (1995) had been diagnosed with trisomy 21 by other methods prior to maternal blood sampling

Maternal urine sample[c]: elevated level of free beta hCG

Spencer et al., 1995

Ultrasound[c]: hydrocephalus

Chervenak et al., 1983b; Nicolaides et al., 1986a; Benacerraf et al., 1987; Redwine et al., 1988; Zerres et al., 1992; Benacerraf et al., 1994

microcephaly[d]

Hentemann et al., 1989

brachycephalus

Zerres et al., 1992

ventriculomegaly (brain)

Benacerraf et al., 1994

choroid plexus cyst

Ostlere et al., 1989; Zerres et al., 1992; Benacerraf et al., 1994; Kupferminc et al., 1994; Walkinshaw et al., 1994a

cerebellar cleft

Benacerraf et al., 1994

orbital hypotelorism[h]

Eydoux et al., 1989

cystic hygroma[g]

Benacerraf et al., 1987; Palmer et al., 1987; Cullen et al., 1988; Abramowicz et al., 1989; Eydoux et al., 1989; Hentemann et al., 1989; Vats et al., 1989

redundant nuchal skin or abnormal amount of soft tissue behind the fetal neck and occiput

Benacerraf et al., 1985; Benacerraf et al., 1987; Wolstenholme et al., 1989; Benacerraf et al., 1994

Comments: The above findings are distinct from cystic hygroma and, when present, increase the risk for Down syndrome. A nuchal skin-fold thickness of 6 mm or more was considered to be a significant finding. Chromosomal analyses of these fetuses should be considered.

occipital edema
    Wolstenholme et al., 1989
hydrops fetalis with or without cystic hygroma
    Curry et al., 1983; Pearce et al., 1984; Nicolaides et al., 1986a; Benacerraf et al., 1987; Palumbos et al., 1987; Cosper et al., 1988; Abramowicz et al., 1989; Nicolaides and Azar, 1990
pleural effusion
    Pearce et al., 1984; Nicolaides et al., 1986a; Blott et al., 1988a; Rodeck et al., 1988; Nicolaides and Azar, 1990
ventriculomegaly (heart) (atrium 710 mm in diameter)
    Carlson and Platt, 1993
atrioventricular canal defect
    Benacerraf et al., 1987
atrial septal defect
    Allan et al., 1981a; Nicolaides et al., 1986a
ventricular septal defects
    Allan et al., 1981a; Nicolaides et al., 1986a; Carlson et al., 1988; Benacerraf et al., 1994
tetralogy of Fallot[d]
    Wladimiroff et al., 1988a
incomplete interventricular septum, single leaflet of each atrioventricular valve, absent interatrial septum
    Balcar et al., 1984
    Comment: Endocardial cushion defect was confirmed at autopsy of the fetus.
congenital heart defect, undefined type
    Wolstenholme et al., 1989
sinus bradycardia[d]
    Wladimiroff et al., 1988a; Eydoux et al., 1989
diaphragmatic hernia
    Benacerraf et al., 1994
esophageal atresia
    Carlson et al., 1988; Eydoux et al., 1989
duodenal atresia
    Wladimiroff et al., 1988a; Eydoux et al., 1989; Benacerraf et al., 1994
duodenal atresia with double bubble sign, dilated stomach, hydramnios
    Zimmerman, 1978; Jassani et al., 1982; Balcar et al., 1984; Nicolaides et al., 1986a; Carlson et al., 1988; Hentemann et al., 1989
increased echogenicity of fetal bowel
    Benacerraf et al., 1994; Pallante et al., 1995; Strasberg et al., 1995
meconium peritonitis
    Benacerraf et al., 1987
omphalocele
    Nyberg et al., 1989

ascites
>Lenz et al., 1985; Nicolaides and Azar, 1990; Tilley et al., 1993

dilatation of the renal pelvis (pyelectasis)
>Benacerraf et al., 1994

decreased humeral length
>Benacerraf et al., 1994

widely spaced thumb and index finger
>Carlson et al., 1988

decreased femoral length
>Platt et al., 1988; Tilley et al., 1993; Benacerraf et al., 1994

ratio of actual femoral length to expected femoral length of 0.91 or less (expected femur length = 9.645 + 0.9338 × biparietal diameter [mm])
>Benacerraf et al., 1987

significantly greater mean biparietal diameter/femoral length ratio (1.76, 95% confidence interval, 1.66 to 1.85 in Down syndrome group; 1.65, 95% confidence interval, 1.63 to 1.69 in control group)
>Miller et al., 1989

>*Comments*: Miller and associates (1989) feel that the above finding was not efficacious enough to warrant screening for Down syndrome and do not recommend its use for screening purposes.

clubfoot deformity
>Benacerraf et al., 1987

dilated renal pelvis, hydrops fetalis secondary to urethral valves obstructing the urethra
>Lenz et al., 1985

hydramnios
>Blott et al., 1988a; Rodeck et al., 1988; Eydoux et al., 1989; Hentemann et al., 1989; Nicolaides and Azar, 1990; Zerres et al., 1992; Tilley et al., 1993

oligohydramnios
>Lenz et al., 1985; Nyberg et al., 1989

intrauterine growth retardation
>Williamson et al., 1988; Eydoux et al., 1989; Hentemann et al., 1989

reduced crown-to-rump length[g]
>Tchobroutsky et al., 1985

abnormal fetal movements in some fetuses
>Boue et al., 1982

fetal demise
>Benn et al., 1995

PD 101250 DUPLICATION, PARTIAL, CHROMOSOME 1q MOSAICISM
{46,XX,dir dup (1)(q12qter)/46,XX}[b] (McKusick No. None)

Ultrasound[c,d]: hydrocephaly, renal agenesis, oligohydramnios
>Stevenson et al., 1986

>*Comments*: At birth, the child reported by Stevenson and associates (1986) was also found to have sirenomelia.

PD 101251 DUPLICATION Xp21pter {Gonadal dysgenesis, XY female type; Swyer syndrome; 46,dup(X)(p21pter)Y} (McKusick No. None)

Syndrome Note: Swyer syndrome is present in patients with an XY or similar chromosomal constitution with gonadal dysgenesis and normal female genitalia.

At puberty these individuals do not develop secondary sexual characteristics, do not menstruate, and have "streak" gonads. Except for these latter features, they do not have any somatic stigmata of Turner syndrome. Individuals with this syndrome probably are lacking the testis-determining factor or other genes involved in testicular development.

McKusick, 1995

In the family reported by Bernstein and coworkers (1980), there were three females in three generations who had a 46,XXp+ karyotype and were normal. One female child and a female fetus in the third generation had 46,Xp+Y karyotypes. Both latter individuals had multiple congenital anomalies. The 46,Xp+Y sister also was profoundly retarded and died at age 5. An autopsy disclosed normal female internal genitalia and ovarian gonadal dysgenesis. The X chromosomal abnormality was thought to be 46,dup(X)(p21pter)Y.

Bernstein et al., 1980

Amniocentesis[i]: karyotype of amniotic fluid cells revealed 46,Xp+Y.

Bernstein et al., 1980

Comments: In the two affected individuals reported by Bernstein and associates (1980), serologic testing indicated absence of H-Y antigen in skin fibroblasts of the fetus, and blood leukocytes and skin fibroblasts in the sister.

PD 101252 DUPLICATION 1q MOSAICISM {46,XY/ 46,XY,dup(1)(pterqter::q32q12::q12qter)}[b] (McKusick No. None)

Ultrasound[c]: anencephaly, facial cleft

Robbins-Furman et al., 1995

Comments: In the fetus reported by Robbins-Furman and associates (1995), the complex duplication cited above was found in 4 of 31 amniotic fluid cells.

PD 101253 DUPLICATION 5(q15q22) {46,XX,dup(5)(q15q22)}[b] (McKusick No. None)

Ultrasound[c]: cystic hygroma

Li et al., 1995

Comments: Amniocentesis at 16 weeks of gestation was done on alleged monozygotic twins after one was found to have a cystic hygroma. Both twins had dup(5)(q15q22). At birth the twin with the cystic hygroma died in the neonatal period from a complex congenital heart disease; the other twin had a cleft palate and a duplicated ureter. The father, who was phenotypically normal, possessed the same chromosomal duplication.

Li et al., 1995

PD 101255 DUPLICATION 6q {46,XX,dup(6)(q16qter)}[b] (McKusick No. None)

Ultrasound[c]: IUGR[h]

Eydoux et al., 1989

PD 101260 DUPLICATION 18p {46,XX,dup(18)(p11.1pter)}[b] (McKusick No. None)

Alpha-fetoprotein[c]: elevated levels in maternal serum but not in amniotic fluid

Wolff et al., 1989

Comments: A chromosomal analysis on amniotic fluid cells of the above fetus was undertaken because of elevation of maternal serum AFP. The fetus was found to have a duplication of the p arm of chromosome 18. The mother carried the same duplication. The chromosomal abnormality was not an 18ph+ variant. Both the resulting child and the mother were physically normal and the mother was intellectually normal.

PD 101280 HAPLOID EMBRYO (McKusick No. None)

Preimplantation embryo biopsy[g]: Fluoresence in situ hybridization demonstrated only one number 8 and 18 chromosomes, and only one sex chromosome, an X chromosome
Weier et al., 1993

PD 101295 INVERSION, DUPLICATION CHROMOSOME 1 {46,XX,inv dup(1)(p11q31)}[b] (McKusick No. None)

Ultrasound[c,h]: IUGR, oligohydramnios
Eydoux et al., 1989

PD 101300 INVERSION CHROMOSOME 1 {46,XX,inv(1)(p13q21)mat}[b] (McKusick No. None)

Alpha-fetoprotein[c]: reduced level in maternal serum
Redwine et al., 1988

PD 101400 INVERSION CHROMOSOME 7 {46,XX,inv(7)(p13q22)mat}[b] (McKusick No. None)

Alpha-fetoprotein[c]: reduced level in maternal serum
Redwine et al., 1988

PD 101450 INVERSION CHROMOSOME 15, DUPLICATION CHROMOSOME 15, TRISOMY 18 {48,XY+inv dup(15),+18}[b] (McKusick No. None)

Condition Note: The most consistent clinical findings of inverted duplication of chromosome 15 include mental retardation, speech problems, hypotonia, behavioral disturbances, seizures, strabismus, and abnormal dermatoglyphics. Some individuals with the inverted duplication of chromosome 15 are phenotypically normal.
Phelan et al., 1989

Prenatal Diagnosis: Chromosomal analysis is probably the only method available for the diagnosis of the inverted duplication of chromosome 15. Trisomy 18 may be suspected by ultrasonic findings but can only be definitively diagnosed by cytogenetic means.

Differential Diagnosis: Cytogenetically, the marker chromosome present in this condition needs to be differentiated from bisatellited marker chromosomes. This can be done by in situ hybridization in many cases. Trisomy 13 syndrome (PD 103000), Trisomy 18 syndrome (PD 104000), and other chromosomal anomalies also need to be considered.

Ultrasound[c,d]: shortened forearms, nonvisualization of the stomach, hydramnios
Phelan et al., 1989

Comments: Most of the features in the above reported case were probably

due to the trisomy 18 rather than the inversion and duplication of chromosome 15.

PD 101475 ISOCHROMOSOME 5p MOSAICISM {46,XX/47,XX,+i(5p)}[b]
(McKusick No. None)

Ultrasound[c]: structural abnormalities of the kidney,[h] hydramnios[h]
Eydoux et al., 1989

PD 101490 ISOCHROMOSOME 18q {46,XX,i(18q)}[b] (McKusick No. None)

Condition Note: Isochromosome 18q results in trisomy for the q arm and mono-
somy for the p arm of chromosome 18.
Ferre et al., 1993
Ultrasound[c]: microcephaly[d]
Spinner et al., 1991
intracranial cystic mass[d]
Spinner et al., 1991
holoprosencephaly
Berry et al., 1990
cerebral anomalies suggestive of alobar holoprosencephaly
Ferre et al., 1993
Comments: At autopsy in the case reported by Ferre and co-authors
(1993), there were cyclopia, arhinia, and alobar holoprosencephaly.
orbital hypotelorism[d]
Spinner et al., 1991
single orbit
Ferre et al., 1993
proboscis[d]
Spinner et al., 1991
Comments: The fetus reported by Spinner and associates (1991) postnatally and at autopsy was found to have holoprosencephaly, microphthalmia, a short and webbed neck, radial and thumb hypoplasia, a single ventricle of the brain, and a 7-cm in diameter brain cyst
in the posterior cerebral hemispheres.
omphalocele[h]
Eydoux et al., 1989
prominent heel
Berry et al., 1990
intrauterine growth retardation[d]
Eydoux et al., 1989; Spinner et al., 1991; Ferre et al., 1993
hydramnios[h]
Eydoux et al., 1989

PD 101495 ISOCHROMOSOME 20q MOSAICISM {46,XX/46,XX,i(20q);
46,XY/46,XY,i(20q)}[b] (McKusick No. None)

Alpha-fetoprotein[c]: elevated levels in maternal serum
Richkind et al., 1991
reduced levels in maternal serum
Richkind et al., 1991

PD 101497 ISOCHROMOSME 22q, PLACENTAL MOSAICISM WITH FETAL NONMOSAICISM {i(22q); 46,XY/46,XY,-22,+t(22:22)(p11;q11)}[b] (McKusick No. None)

Ultrasound[c]: cystic hygroma
Spinner et al., 1992

PD 101500 KLINEFELTER SYNDROME (Chromosome XXY syndrome; XXY syndrome; 46,XY/47,XXY; 47,XXY)[b] (McKusick No. None)

Alpha-fetoprotein[c]: elevated in maternal serum
Ryynanen et al., 1983; Wheeler et al., 1987; Hajianpour et al., 1989; Fejgin et al., 1990; Cervetti et al., 1995
Amniocentesis: decreased levels of gamma-glutamyltranspeptidase activity in amniotic fluid[c]
Brock et al., 1984a
decreased levels of aminopeptidase M activity in amniotic fluid[c]
Brock et al., 1984a
identification of two Y chromosomes using biotinylated chromosome-specific DNA probe in uncultured amniotic fluid cells
Guyot et al., 1988
Chorionic villus sampling[g]: 47,XXY karyotype of chorionic villi
Nicolaides et al., 1986b; Bovicelli et al., 1988
Comments: Sampling by the transabdominal approach has been done as early as 9 weeks of gestation (Bovicelli et al., 1988) and as late as 37 weeks (Nicolaides et al., 1986b).
Maternal blood sampling with fetal cell enrichment by cell sorting and FISH for X and Y chromosomes: mosaic 46,XY/47,XYY plus maternal 46,XX cells
Bischoff et al., 1995a
Ultrasound[c]: cystic hygroma
Neu et al., 1993
multicystic and dysplastic kidney located in the pelvis[d]
Kanaan et al., 1995
Comments: The fetus reported by Kanaan and associates (1995) in addition to the kidney abnormalities and XXY chromosomal constitution detected prenatally, had an ectodermal dysplastic lesion of the scalp and congenital aganglionic megacolon postnatally.

PD 101510 MILLER–DIEKER SYNDROME {Deletion chromosome 17p13; 46,XX,der(17)t(17;?)(p13?)mat; 46,XX,-17,+der(17),t(7;17)(p22.3;p13.2)}[b] (McKusick No. 247200)

Amniocentesis[i]: fetus possessed the same balanced translocation {46,XX,-17,+der)(17),t(7;17)(p22.3;p13.2)pat} as did an affected sibling.
Stratton et al., 1984
Ultrasound[i]: smooth gyral pattern, head circumference lagging behind normal growth for gestational age,[d] hydramnios[d]
Krauss et al., 1988
Comments: The mother of the fetus reported by Krauss and co-authors (1988) carried an apparent balanced translocation involving chromosome 7 and another unknown chromosome (46,XX,t(17;?)(p13?). The fetus in this pregnancy apparently had a deletion of 17p13 {46,XX,der(17)-

t(17;?)(p13;?)}. After birth at 36 weeks of gestation, the child had features consistent with the Miller–Dieker syndrome.

Prenatally, the presence of a smooth gyral pattern and a diminishing head size was thought by Krauss and associates (1988) to represent lissencephaly.

omphalocele[c]
>Toi et al., 1995

PD 101530 MONOSOMY 1q {del(1q); Deletion chromosome 1q; 46,XX,1q-}[b] (McKusick No. None)

Alpha-fetoprotein[c]: elevated in maternal serum
>Burton, 1987
>elevated in maternal serum but not in amniotic fluid
>Warner et al., 1988

PD 101550 MONOSOMY 4p/PARTIAL TRISOMY 20p
{46,XX,der(4),t(4;20)(p16;p12),inv(18)(pll;q11)pat}[b] (McKusick No. None)

Alpha-fetoprotein[c]: elevated in amniotic fluid
>Vamos et al., 1985
Ultrasound[c]: oligohydramnios secondary to severe renal hypoplasia, IUGR
>Vamos et al., 1985

PD 101560 MONOSOMY 18 (45,XY,-18) (McKusick No. None)

Preimplantation embryo biopsy[q]: FISH demonstrated only one number 18 chromosome
>Weier et al., 1993

PD 101564 MONOSOMY 18/X (McKusick No. None)

Preimplantation embryo biopsy[q]: FISH demonstrated only one number 18 chromosome, only one sex chromosome (an X chromosome), but two number 8 chromosomes
>Weier et al., 1993

PD 101570 MONOSOMY 22 MOSAICISM (45,XY,-22/46,XY)[b] (McKusick No. None)

Doppler flow studies[c,d]: absent diastolic flow in the internal carotid and middle cerebral arteries[c,d]
>Lewinsky et al., 1990
Ultrasound[c]: abdominal wall defect with loops of intestine protruding through the defect and no membrane covering the protruding bowel (gastroschisis),[d] hydramnios[d]
>Lewinsky et al., 1990

PD 101585 PENTASOMY X (Penta X syndrome; 49,XXXXX)[b] (McKusick No. None)

Amniocentesis[d]: FISH for X and Y chromosomes indicated five X chromosomes and no Y chromosomes
>Myles et al., 1995

Ultrasound[c,d]: massive hydrocephalus, a Dandy–Walker malformation suggested by the third and fourth ventricles being dilated and splaying of the cerebellum, hydramnios
>Myles et al., 1995

PD 101595 SATELLITED 4q (Extra ribosomal DNA)[b] (McKusick No. None)

Condition Note: Occasionally a nonacrocentric human chromosome contains satellited material from a translocation involving the p arm of an acrocentric chromosome. Providing that the derived chromosome has not lost a significant amount of chromosomal material, the individual will be phenotypically normal. This occurs because the satellited segment (p arm of acrocentric chromosomes) codes for ribosomal RNA, and humans apparently tolerate some excess or deficiency of ribosomal RNA.
>Miller et al., 1995

Amniocentesis: identification of ribosomal RNA by ribosomal DNA probes tagged with biotin
>Miller et al., 1995

Comments: In the family reported by Miller and cohorts (1995), a fetus was diagnosed at 16 weeks' gestation as having a satellited 4q. Further genetic analysis of all phenotypically normal family members revealed that the father of the baby, the fetus's paternal aunt, and the fetus's paternal grandmother also carried the derived 4q.

PD 101597 SMITH–MAGENIS SYNDROME {Interstitial deletion 17(p11.2p11.2)}[b] (McKusick No. 182290)

Syndrome Note: The Smith–Magenis syndrome is produced by an interstitial deletion of 17p11.2p11.2. Molecular genetic studies indicate that this syndrome probably is a contiguous gene deletion syndrome. The characteristics of the disorder include brachycephaly, midfacial hypoplasia, cleft palate, prognathism, congenital heart defect, and growth deficiency. Neurologic problems seen are mental retardation, hyperactivity, self-destructive behavior, and onychotillomania.
>Fan and Farrell, 1994; McKusick, 1996

Alpha-fetoprotein[c]: low level in maternal serum
>Fan and Farrell, 1994

PD 101600 TETRAPLOIDY (92,XXXX; 92,XXYY/46,XY mosaicism)[b] (McKusick No. None)

Amniocentesis: FISH using chromosome 13, 18, 21, X, and Y probes revealed that 70% or greater of amniotic fluid cells had four signals for each the 13, 18, 21, and X chromosomes.
>Goyert et al., 1993

Cordocentesis (percutaneous umbilical blood sampling, or PUBS): fetal white cells revealed cell to have tetraploidy (92,XXXX).
>Sagot et al., 1993

Fetal blood drawing using fetoscopy followed by fetal blood karyotype
>Nicolaides et al., 1986a

Ultrasound[c]: hydrops fetalis
>Nicolaides et al., 1986a

hydrocephalus, agenesis of the corpus callosum, cerebellar hypoplasia
Sagot et al., 1993
no gastric pattern
Sagot et al., 1993
tiny urinary bladder
Sagot et al., 1993
asymmetrical IUGR
Sagot et al., 1993
oligohydramnios
Sagot et al., 1993

PD 101650 TETRAPLOIDY MOSAICISM OF THE PLACENTA (92,XXXX/ 46,XX mosaicism of the placenta)[b] (McKusick No. None)

Alpha-fetoprotein[c]: elevated in maternal serum
Nyland et al., 1987
Comments: In this case a woman was found to have elevated maternal serum AFP, normal amniotic fluid AFP, no acetylcholinesterase in the amniotic fluid, and low-level tetraploidy mosaicism of amniotic fluid cells (7% and 9% on two occasions). Karyotype on fetal blood showed 100 cells with 46,XY chromosome constitution. The conclusion of Nyland and associates (1987) was that this situation represented placental mosaicism.

PD 101660 TETRAPLOID TURNER SYNDROME (90,XX)[b] (McKusick No. None)

Condition Note: Complete tetraploidy is a lethal disorder produced by the presence of four haploid sets of chromosomes. Occasionally a fetus with tetraploidy does survive to term and subsequently dies. These individuals usually have tetraploidy/diploidy mosaicism.
  In the condition listed here, the fetus had many features of Turner syndrome. Two of the expected sex chromosomes were also missing, giving the fetus the same ratio of autosomes to sex chromosomes (44:1) as seen in the usual case of Turner syndrome (PD 105000).
Fryns et al., 1987
Prenatal Diagnosis: This very rare condition probably cannot be separated from Turner syndrome (PD 105000) based on the prenatal physical findings alone. Diagnosis is established only by chromosomal analysis.
Differential Diagnosis: Tetraploidy (PD 101600), Turner syndrome (PD 105000), Turner syndrome, isochromosome Xp (PD 105250), Turner syndrome, isochromosome Xq (PD 105260), see also other conditions associated with cystic hygroma (see Cystic hygroma and Hydrops fetalis in the Index).
Alpha-fetoprotein[c]: elevated in the amniotic fluid
Fryns et al., 1987
Ultrasound[c]: hydrops fetalis, cystic hygroma
Fryns et al., 1987

PD 101662 TETRASOMY 1q {Isochromosome 1q; 47,XX,+i(1q)}[b] (McKusick No. None)

Ultrasound[c]: intrauterine fetal demise; prominent nuchal translucency
Robbins-Furman et al., 1995
Comments: All amniotic fluid cells examined had a 47,XX+i(1q) chromo-

Rock Valley College - ERC

somal constitution; there was no mosaicism found (Robbins-Furman et al., 1995).

PD 101664 TETRASOMY 1q MOSAICISM {Isochromosome 1q; 46,XY/ 47,XY,+i(1q)}[b] (McKusick No. None)

Ultrasound[c]: anencephaly
    Robbins-Furman et al., 1995
Comments: Amniotic fluid cells in the case reported by Robbins-Furman and co-authors (1995) showed 46,XY/47,XY,+i(1q) (24 and 6 cells, respectively).

PD 101670 TETRASOMY 9p SYNDROME {47,XY,+dup(9p)}[b] (McKusick No. None)

Syndrome Note: Tetrasomy 9p is usually produced by the presence of an extra chromosome that contains duplication of the 9p arms {47,XY or XX,+dup(9p)}. The resulting phenotype includes IUGR with low birth weight; psychomotor retardation; failure to thrive; brachycephaly, microcephaly, or hydrocephaly; widely separated sutures; enlarged fontanels; ocular hypertelorism; skeletal anomalies; severely malformed extremities; ambiguous genitalia; and congenital heart defects.
    Jalal et al., 1991
Prenatal Diagnosis: At present, the diagnosis can be made only from a chromosomal analysis. In most situations, a fetus with multiple anomalies of unknown etiology should have a chromosomal analysis done prior to birth.
Differential Diagnosis: This disorder needs to be differentiated from other tetrasomies such as tetrasomy i(12p) (PD 101680).
    Ultrasound[c,d]: mild hydrocephaly, cleft palate, clubfoot deformity
        Jalal et al., 1991
        dilated posterior horns of the lateral ventricles, cystic malformation in the posterior fossa
        McDowall et al., 1989

PD 101680 TETRASOMY 12p {Isochromosome 12p; Isochromosome 12p mosaicism; Pallister–Killian syndrome; Pallister mosaic syndrome; Teschler–Nicola/Killian syndrome; 46,XY/47,XY,+i(12p)}[b] (McKusick No. None

General Comments: The diagnosis of tetrasomy i(12p) in the fetus reported by Shivashankar and colleagues (1988) was confirmed not only by standard cytogenetic means prenatally but also by autoradiograph postnatally, utilizing ^{3}H-labeled probe for the KRAS2 gene. No mosaicism was found in this case. In the case reported by Cangany and associates (1995), the chromosome abnormally was detected by G-banded metaphases and confirmed by FISH.
    Ultrasound[c]: increased orbital diameters
        Shivashanker et al., 1988
        diaphragmatic hernia
        Eydoux et al., 1989; Bresson et al., 1991
        femoral and humeral lengths diminished relative to gestational and other fetal measurements, increased orbital diameters
        Shivashankar et al., 1988
        short limbs,[d] sacral appendage,[d] Dandy–Walker malformation[d]
        Cangany et al., 1995

hydrops fetalis
    Sharland et al., 1991
hydramnios
    Shivashankar et al., 1988; Eydoux et al., 1989; Bresson et al., 1991; Cangany et al., 1995

PD 101687 TRANSLOCATION CHROMSOME X;X
{45,X,t(X;X)(qter→cen::p11.3→qter)[b] (McKusick No. None)

Amniocentesis: Geimsa (G) and reverse (R) staining of culture amniotic fluid cells showed one normal X and one rearranged X chromosome with asymmetric banding around the pericentromeric region.
    Tachdjian et al., 1995
    fluorescence in situ hybridization utilizing X chromosome alpha satellite DNA probe indicated three hybridization signals in metaphase and interphase nuclei of cultured amniotic fluid cells.
    Tachdjian et al., 1995
    localization of X;X break points by analysis of hybridization signals with laser scanning image cytometry
    Tachdjian et al., 1995
    Comments: The case reported by Tachdjian and co-authors (1995) had no unusual pre- or postnatal physical findings other than gonadal dysgenesis noted at 1 year. The parents had normal chromosomes.

PD 101690 TRANSLOCATION CHROMOSOME X;22 {46,XX,-22,+der(22),t(X;22)(p11;p11)mat; 46,XX,-22+der,t(X;22)(22qter to Xpter)mat}[b] (McKusick No. None)

Alpha-fetoprotein[c]: low level in maternal serum
    Ben-Yishay et al., 1988

PD 101700 TRANSLOCATION CHROMOSOME Y;14 {t(Y;14)}[b] (McKusick No. None)

Alpha-fetoprotein[c]: elevated level in maternal serum
    McMorrow et al., 1987

PD 101710 TRANSLOCATION CHROMOSOME 1;8
{46,XY,t(1;8)(p34.1;q24.1)pat}[b] (McKusick No. None)

Alpha-fetoprotein[c]: reduced levels in maternal serum
    Redwine et al., 1988
    Comments: The translocation was balanced in the fetus reported by Redwine and associates (1988).

PD 101714 TRANSLOCATION 1;11 {46,XX/46,XX,t(1;11) (p34;q15) confined placental mosaicism}[b] (McKusick No. None)

Ultrasound[c]: oligohydramnios, fetal demise
    Adam et al., 1993
    Comments: In the fetus reported by Adam and associates (1993), the translocation was de novo.

PD 101720 TRANSLOCATION CHROMOSOME 2;10 {46,XY,-10,+der(10),t(2;10)(p24;q26)mat}[b] (McKusick No. None)

Ultrasound[c,i]: anencephaly
    Singer et al., 1986

PD 101740 TRANSLOCATION CHROMOSOME 4;14
{46,XY,der(14),t(4;14)(p15.2;p11.2)pat}[b] (McKusick No. None)

Ultrasound[c]: bladder outlet obstruction with distention
Palmer et al., 1987

PD 101780 TRANSLOCATION CHROMOSOME 5;7
{46,XX,der(7),t(5;7)(p13;q34)}[b] (McKusick No. None)

Ultrasound[c]: cystic hygroma
Palmer et al., 1987

PD 101800 TRANSLOCATION CHROMOSOME 10;16
{46,XX,der(10)t(10;16)(q26;p13.1); 46,XY,der(10)t(10;16)(q26;p13.1)}[b] (McKusick No. None)

Condition Note: Bofinger and associates (1991) reported on a family in which nine family members in three generations carried a balanced reciprocal translocation {46,XX or XY, rcp(10;6)(q26;p13.1)}. Four of these carriers produced six affected children {46,XX or XY,der(10)t(10:16)(q26;p13.1)}. Associated findings in these children included hydrops fetalis, ascites, congenital heart defects, psychomotor retardation, failure to thrive, hypotonia, narrow palpebral fissures, abnormal ears, cleft palate, thumb abnormalities, hypogenitalism, inguinal hernia, and sparse hair.

Ultrasound[c]: tachycardia,[d] irregular heartbeat,[d] dilated and overriding aorta,[d] ventricular septal defect (VSD)[d]
Bofinger et al., 1991
ascites
Bofinger et al., 1991
hydrops fetalis[d]
Bofinger et al., 1991
hydramnios[d]
Bofinger et al., 1991

PD 101850 TRANSLOCATION CHROMOSOME 11;22
{47,XY+der(22),t(11;22)(q23;q11)}[b] (McKusick No. None)

Fetal blood drawing utilizing fetoscopy, followed by fetal blood karyotype
Nicolaides et al., 1986a
Ultrasound[c]: hydrops fetalis
Nicolaides et al., 1986a
severe symmetrical IUGR
Dickerman et al., 1987
hydramnios
Clark et al., 1989

PD 101900 TRANSLOCATION CHROMOSOME 13;14 {45,XY,t(13q14q) de novo}[b]

Alpha-fetoprotein[c]: reduced in maternal serum
Redwine et al., 1988
Comments: The translocation reported by Redwine and associates (1988) appeared to have been balanced.

PD 102000 TRIPLOIDY (46,XX/69,XXY mosaicism; 69,XXX; 69,XXY; 69,XYY)[b] (McKusick No. None)

Condition Note: Human triploidy is essentially a nonviable chromosomal disorder that occurs in about 1% of recognized human pregnancies resulting from the incorporation of three sets of haploid chromosomes in the conceptus. Only a few of these pregnancies survive beyond the first trimester and still fewer to term. The vast majority of term infants with nonmosaic triploidy die during the first few days or weeks of life. However, when fetuses with triploidy mosaicism reach term, the likelihood of survival is better, but the vast majority of these individuals are severely or profoundly retarded. The typical dysmorphic features found in pure triploidy include unusual facies with ocular hypertelorism, flat nasal bridge, cleft lip and palate, and micrognathia; syndactyly of the third and fourth fingers; atrial and ventricular septal defects; genital abnormalities; and hydrocephalus and partial hydatidiform molar degeneration of the placenta with cystically dilated villi.

Parental origin of the extra haploid set in triploidy fetuses was reported by Miny and associates (1995). In their investigation, these workers found 10 of 17 cases with maternal origin of the extra set of chromosomes. They also observed 5 of 7 cases of paternal origin of the triploidy had partial moler degeneration of the placenta, whereas only 1 in 10 was the finding in the maternal triploidy. The biparietal-to-thoracic diameters in paternal triploidy cases were always 1:1 or below, whereas in the maternal ones, the ratios were greater than 1:1.

Meisner et al., 1987

Prenatal Diagnosis: The definitive diagnosis can be established only by chromosomal studies of fetal tissue. However, the condition should be considered whenever there is intrauterine growth deficiency with a relatively large placenta whether in the presence of hydatidiform molar degeneration or not.

Differential Diagnosis: Other conditions causing IUGR should be considered (see Intrauterine growth retardation in the Index).

Acetylcholinesterase[c]: present in amniotic fluid
   Freeman et al., 1988
      fast migrating isozyme on gel electrophoresis
         Crandall et al., 1989; Freeman et al., 1989
            Comments: In the cases of Crandall and associates (1989) and Freeman and colleagues (1989), the above finding was found in association with open spina bifida.

Alpha-fetoprotein[c]: elevated in amniotic fluid
   Porreco et al., 1980; de Elejalde and Elejalde, 1985b; Crandall et al., 1989
      elevated in maternal serum
         Berkeley et al., 1983; Israel et al., 1986; Burton, 1987; Freeman et al., 1988; Warner et al., 1988; Freeman et al., 1989; Rogers and Phelan, 1989; Benn et al., 1995; Evans et al., 1995a; Miny et al., 1995; Smith et al., 1995
      elevated levels in maternal serum but normal levels in amniotic fluid
         Warner et al., 1988; Freeman et al., 1989; Kazazian et al., 1989
      reduced in maternal serum
         Hentemann et al., 1989

Amniocentesis[c]: elevated pregnancy-specific beta$_1$-glycoprotein (SP1) in amniotic fluid
   Heikinheimo et al., 1984

decreased level of gamma-glutamyltransferase activity in amniotic fluid
> Macek et al., 1987

Amniograph[c]: shortened trunk, disparity between fetal head size and trunk size, with relatively large fetal head
> Bocian et al., 1978; Crane et al., 1985

Chorionic villus sampling[c,g]: hydropic villi
> Rupp et al., 1989

Computerized scan of the fetal head[c]: rostrally displaced boomerang-shaped cerebral cortex characteristic of holoprosencephaly
> Filly et al., 1984

Cordocentesis (PUBS): fetal blood karyotype showed 69 chromosome count
> Bieber et al., 1987

Doppler ultrasound[c]: decreased umbilical arterial blood flow
> Reuwer et al., 1987

Endocervical canal sampling[g]: triploid cells found by FISH using various autosomal probes
> Adinolf et al., 1995

Fetal blood drawing utilizing fetoscopy followed by fetal blood karyotype
> Nicolaides et al., 1986a

Maternal blood sampling[c]: elevated hCG
> Freeman et al., 1989; Benn et al., 1995; Miny et al., 1995; Smith et al., 1995

low levels of hCG
> Smith et al., 1995

low levels of unconjugated estriol
> Smith et al., 1995

elevated levels of unconjugated estriol
> Miny et al., 1995

Maternal history[c,g]: vaginal bleeding
> Kazazian et al., 1989; Rupp et al., 1989

Preimplantation embryo biopsy[g]: FISH demonstrated three number 18 chromosomes, two X chromosomes, and one Y chromosome
> Weier et al., 1993

Radiograph[c]: disproportionately short trunk, thin ribs
> Bocian et al., 1978

Ultrasound[c]: disproportionate measurement between fetal head and trunk, with relatively large head, intrauterine growth deficiency, large placenta, sonolucence of the fetal head
> Bocian et al., 1978; Porreco et al., 1980; Broekhuizen et al., 1983b; Pierce et al., 1984; de Elejalde and Elejalde, 1985b; Marchese et al., 1985b; Nicolaides et al., 1986a; Reuwer et al., 1987; Spirt et al., 1987

decreased ratio of head circumference to abdominal circumference
> Freeman et al., 1989

hydranencephaly
> Broekhuizen et al., 1983b

absence of septum pellucidum
> Edwards et al., 1986

holoprosencephaly detected by monoventricular fluid-filled cavity in the head that communicated with a dorsal sac, fused thalamus
> Filly et al., 1984

holoprosencephaly
    Smith et al., 1995
central echolucencies of the brain that proved to be hydrocephalus
secondary to aqueductal stenosis
    Bendon et al., 1988
ventriculomegaly (brain)
    Miny et al., 1995
hydrocephaly[c]
    Quinlan et al., 1983; de Elejalde and Elejalde, 1985b; Edwards
    et al., 1986; Nicolaides et al., 1986a; Palmer et al., 1987; Eydoux
    et al., 1989
microcephaly
    Freeman et al., 1989
macrocephaly
    Miny et al., 1995
long, wide forehead, relatively small face
    de Elejalde and Elejalde, 1984
cleft lip and palate
    Miny et al., 1995; Smith et al., 1995
nuchal edema
    Miny et al., 1995
cystic hygroma[c,g]
    Neu et al., 1993
cardiomegaly
    Benn et al., 1995
atrial septal defect[h]
    Eydoux et al., 1989
omphalocele
    Freeman et al., 1988; Eydoux et al., 1989; Miny et al., 1995
duodenal atresia
    Quinlan et al., 1983
increased echogenicity of fetal bowel
    Pallante et al., 1995
polycystic kidneys, hydronephrosis
    Broekhuizen et al., 1983b; de Elejalde and Elejalde, 1985b; Nico-
    laides et al., 1986a
meningomyelocele
    Broekhuizen et al., 1983b; Edwards et al., 1986; Crandall et al.,
    1989; Eydoux et al., 1989; Freeman et al., 1989; Miny et al., 1995
meningomyelocele seen as a sac over the skin, lack of spinous process
in the lumbar region of the spine
    de Elejalde and Elejalde, 1985b
hypoplastic male genitalia
    Nicolaides et al., 1986a
syndactyly
    Smith et al., 1995
shortened femur
    Rupp et al., 1989
clubfeet
    Rupp et al., 1989

asymmetrical fetal growth
>Smith et al., 1995

enlarged uterus with large multicystic placenta
>Berkeley et al., 1983

partial molar degeneration of the placenta
>Miny et al., 1995

large or thickened placenta with or without sonolucent lesions
>Colwill et al., 1987; Spirt et al., 1987; Bendon et al., 1988; Freeman et al., 1988; Eydoux et al., 1989; Freeman et al., 1989; Kazazian et al., 1989; Benn et al., 1995; Miny et al., 1995

normal placental morphology
>Smith et al., 1995

oligohydramnios
>Berkeley et al., 1983; Pierce et al., 1984; Crane et al., 1985; Nicolaides et al., 1986a; Gembruch and Hansmann, 1988; Wladimiroff et al., 1988a; Eydoux et al., 1989; Kazazian et al., 1989; Hentemann et al., 1989; Rogers and Phelan, 1989; Miny et al., 1995

hydramnios
>Broekhuizen et al., 1983b; Crane et al., 1985; Edwards et al., 1986; Palmer et al., 1987; Eydoux et al., 1989; Freeman et al., 1989

preeclampsia
>Broekhuizen et al., 1983b

intrauterine growth deficiency
>Freeman et al., 1988; Wladimiroff et al., 1988a; Eydoux et al., 1989; Freeman et al., 1989; Hentemann et al., 1989; Kazazian et al., 1989; Rogers and Phelan, 1989; Rupp et al., 1989; Benn et al., 1995; Miny et al., 1995

PD 102050 TRIPLOIDY, XX ANEUPLOIDY (68,XX)[b] (McKusick No. None)

Ultrasound[c]: reduced abdominal circumference, shortened femur length
>Kaffe et al., 1989

PD 102100 TRIPLOIDY, XXYY ANEUPLOIDY (70,XXYY)[b] (McKusick No. None)

Condition Note: This disorder is a sex chromosomal variant of the usual triploidy. The chromosomal condition would have required two abnormal events such as dispermy, with one sperm being diploid for the Y chromosome.
>Meisner et al., 1987

Prenatal Diagnosis: Chromosomal analysis of fetal tissue is the only means of diagnosing this condition at this time.

Alpha-fetoprotein[c]: elevated levels in the maternal serum
>Meisner et al., 1987

elevated levels in amniotic fluid
>Meisner et al., 1987

Amniography[c]: no fetal swallowing or respiratory movements
>Meisner et al., 1987

Ultrasound[c]: no fetal swallowing or respiratory movements
>Meisner et al., 1987

PD 102150 TRISOMY Xq {46,XX/47,XX,+i(Xq); Isochromosome Xq mosaicism}[b] (McKusick No. None)

Ultrasound[c,d]: hydramnios
Palmer et al., 1987

PD 102200 TRISOMY 1(q42qter)[b] (McKusick No. None)

Ultrasound[c]: fetal movements increased and jerky with hyperextension and hyperflexion of the trunk, IUGR
Boue et al., 1982
Comments: The mothers of the two fetuses with the above trisomy were sisters and each carried a balanced translocation {46,XX,t(1:17)(q42;p13)}.

PD 102250 TRISOMY 1q/19p {47,XX,+der(1),t(1;19)(p11;q11)(q11;q11)}[b] (McKusick No. None)

Acetylcholinesterase[c]: rapidly migrating isozyme present in amniotic fluid
Schwartz et al., 1989a
Alpha-fetoprotein[c]: elevated level in amniotic fluid
Schwartz et al., 1989a
Ultrasound[c]: large facial cleft, facial teratoma, brain teratoma, enlarged head (macrocephaly)
Schwartz et al., 1989a
Comments: In the above case that was reported by Schwartz and co-workers (1989), the chromosomal abnormality was detected by amniocentesis done for increased maternal age. In situ culture of amniotic fluid cells revealed three clones with a balanced translocation involving chromosomes 1 and 19 {46,XX,t(1;19)(p11;q11)} and 27 clones that were trisomic for 1q and 19p. The mother was found to carry a balanced translocation. The cells with the balanced translocation in the amniotic cell culture probably represent maternal cell contamination.

Ultrasound examination at 17 weeks was thought to indicate a dysmorphic fetus with teratomas of the face and brain. Repeat examination at 24 weeks indicated rapid growth of the intracranial tumor with marked enlargement of the fetal head. The pregnancy was terminated and an autopsy confirmed the presence of an oropharyngeal teratoma with intracranial extension. Histologically the tumor was an immature teratoma.

PD102260 TRISOMY 2, CONFINED PLACENTAL MOSAICISM WITH DIPLOID FETUS[b] (McKusick No. None)

Chorionic villus sampling[h]: trisomy 2 confined placental mosaicism
Barrett et al., 1995
Ultrasound[c]: IUGR[h]
Barrett et al., 1995
Comments: Golabi and co-workers (1995) have found placental mosaicism for trisomy 2 in 11 of 10,500 fetuses tested by CVS. Of these pregnancies, five had follow-up amniocenteses, each of which had normal fetal chromosomes. All 11 original fetuses with trisomy were found to be physically normal at birth.

lumbosacral spina bifida, ventriculomegaly
Pappas et al., 1995
Comments: Amniocentesis at 17 weeks' gestation as reported on

by Pappas and colleagues (1995) revealed 46,XY/47,XY,+2. Culture of various tissues after termination showed mosaic trisomy 2 only in the placenta and amnion.

PD 102270 TRISOMY 2, CONFINED PLACENTAL MOSAICISM WITH FETAL MATERNAL UNIPARENTAL DISOMY[b] (McKusick No. None)

Maternal blood sampling: human chorionic gonadotrophin elevated in maternal serum[c]

Harrison et al., 1995

Ultrasound[c,d]: IUGR, oligohydramnios

Harrison et al., 1995

Comments: Postnatally, the case reported by Harrison and co-authors (1995) had a normal cord blood cell chromosomal makeup, while trisomy 2 mosaicism was present in all placental tissue tested. At a later date, uniparental disomy for chromosome 2 was determined by molecular markers. The latter test was undertaken because of growth delay in the child and the placental mosaicism.

PD 102275 TRISOMY 2, FETAL MOSAICISM, PLACENTAL CHROMOSOMAL CONSTITUTION UNKNOWN[b] (McKusick No. None)

Alpha-fetoprotein[c]: elevated in maternal serum

Golabi et al., 1995

Amniocentesis: trisomy 2 mosaicism in 15 of 56 amniotic fluid cells

Golabi et al., 1995

Comments: The fetus reported by Golabi and co-workers (1995) was found to have multiple congenital anomalies after delivery at 30 weeks of gestation. Although blood, skin fibroblasts, and ascitic fluid cells had normal chromosome constitutions, hepatic fibroblasts obtained by liver biopsy showed 4 of 100 cells with trisomy 2.

Ultrasound[c]: double outlet right ventricle[d]

Golabi et al., 1995

atrial septal defect[d]

Golabi et al., 1995

ventricular septal defect[d]

Golabi et al., 1995

hydronephrosis[d]

Golabi et al., 1995

intrauterine growth retardation

Golabi et al., 1995

oligohydramnios

Golabi et al., 1995

PD 102278 TRISOMY 2, NONMOSAIC PLACENTAL TRISOMY WITH BIPARENTAL DISOMIC FETAL CHROMSOMES[b] (McKusick No. None)

Ultrasound[c]: IUGR

Main et al., 1993

Comments: Chromosomal analysis of the case reported by Main and co-authors (1993) revealed normal amniotic fluid cell and fetal blood cell chromosomal constitutions, but nonmosaic trisomy 2 in chorionic villi. Placental DNA testing indicated maternal meiosis nondisjunction. Study of the neonate's peripheral blood demonstrated biparental disomy. The infant had normal mental and motor development during the first year, but during this time experienced significant growth delay.

PD 102280 TRISOMY 2, NONMOSAIC PLACENTAL TRISOMY WITH NORMAL FETAL CHROMSOSOMES[b] (McKusick No. None)

Amniocentesis: trisomy 2 in one of two colonies (7/30 and 0/30) from cultured amniotic fluid
>Webb et al., 1995

Comments: The study reported by Webb and associates (1995) was prompted by finding trisomy 2 in all chorionic villus cells analyzed. Cordocentesis demonstrated a normal chromosome constitution (46,XX) in 100 cells examined. Blood taken at delivery and skin fibroblasts showed a normal chromosome constitution. The infant at birth was small for gestational age, had no dysmorphic features, and had some undefined renal functional abnormality. She also required surgery to close a patent ductus arteriosus.

Ultrasound[c]: abnormal umbilical Doppler wave forms
>Webb et al., 1995
>intrauterine growth retardation
>Webb et al., 1995
>reduced fetal movements
>Webb et al., 1995
>oligohydramnios
>Webb et al., 1995

PD 102285 TRISOMY 2(p13q12)MOSAIC (46,XX/47,XX,+mar)[b] (McKusick No. None)

Amniocentesis[d]: regular chromosomal analysis showed 46,XX/47,XX,+mar
>Grevengood et al., 1993
>fluorescence in situ hybridization probes revealed marker to be 2(p13q12)
>Grevengood et al., 1993

Comments: At birth the fetus/neonate reported by Grevengood and associates (1993) had an unusual face, single umbilical artery, and a diaphragmatic hernia.

Ultrasound[c,d]: diaphragmatic hernia
>Grevengood et al., 1993

PD 102290 TRISOMY 3/KLINEFELTER-TRISOMY 18 MOSAICISM (47,XX,+3/48,XXY,+18 mosaicism)[b] (McKusick No. None)

Ultrasound[d]: bilateral cleft lip, IUGR, hydramnios
>Tuerlings and Nijhuis, 1995

Comments: At birth the neonate reported by Tuerlings and Nijhuis (1995) had features of trisomy 18 that included malformed and low-set ears, bilateral cleft lip and palate, atrioventricular canal, cryptorchidism, micropenis, clenched hands with overlapping fingers, and rocker-bottom feet. Blood karyotype showed 48,XXY,+18, whereas fibroblast analysis demonstrated 47,XY,+3/48,XXY,+18 (13:19). Karyotype from amniotic fluid cells obtained at 38 weeks' gestation showed the same mosaic pattern.

PD 102300 TRISOMY 3q (46,XY,-9,+der 3,+t(3;9)(q24;p24)[b] (McKusick No. None)

Ultrasound[c,d]: Shortening of all long bones, ambiguous genitalia as determined by the detection of two round structures (labia majora or bifid scrotum with undescended testes), and midline perineal structure representing either a small penis or enlarged clitoris
Cooper et al., 1985
Comments: The ambiguous genitalia but not the chromosomal abnormality were diagnosed prenatally in the patient reported by Cooper and co-workers (1985). Anomalies found after birth included hypospadias, undescended testes, abnormal sacrococcygeal vertebrae, imperforate anus with perineal fistula, and cleft palate. The father carried a t(3;9) balanced translocation.

PD 102400 TRISOMY 4p[b] (McKusick No. None)

Ultrasound[c]: fetal movements jerky with hyperextension of trunk
Boue et al., 1982
Comments: The chromosomal problem in this fetus arose from a pericentric inversion of chromosome 4(p14;q35) that was carried by the mother.

PD 102450 TRISOMY 5, FETAL MOSAICISM, PLACENTAL CHROMOSOMAL CONSTITUTION UNKNOWN[b] (McKusick No. None)

Alpha-fetoprotein[c]: low level in maternal serum
Grace et al., 1995
Ultrasound[c]: encephalocele, microcephaly, hydrocephaly, three-chambered heart, atrioventricular canal
Grace et al., 1995
Comments: Amniotic fluid cell evaluation of the fetus reported by Grace and associates (1995) revealed 11 cells with 46,XY and 9 with 47,XY,+5; the latter were from three separate clones. Postmortem exam of the fetus also demonstrated left postaxial hexadactyly and a Meckel diverticulum.

PD 102500 TRISOMY 5p[b] (McKusick No. None)

Chorionic villus sampling[g,i]: partial trisomy of chromosome 5p detected by DNA probe analysis in at-risk embryo
Wasmuth et al., 1988; Overhauser et al., 1989
Comments: Various members in three generations of the family reported both by Wasmuth and associates (1988) and Overhauser and colleagues (1989) carried a balanced translocation that could be detected only by DNA analysis. The family was originally studied by cytogenetic and DNA analyses because the proband, two of her half-siblings, and a paternal cousin each had features of the cri du chat syndrome. The above cited embryo was trisomic for distal 5p. The pregnancy was spontaneously lost shortly after the CVS procedure.
Method not stated[g]: no fetal heart beat detected, fetal demise
Overhauser et al., 1989

PD 102550 TRISOMY 5(pterq11) {46,XX,dic der(15)t(5;15)(q11;p11)}[b] (McKusick No. None)

Ultrasound[c,d]: macrocephaly, hydramnios
Zhao et al., 1995

PD 102600 TRISOMY 5p/MONOSOMY 10p {46,XX,der(10)t(5;10)(p13;p15)}[b]
(McKusick No. None)

Ultrasound[c]: fetal movements extremely active and brisk with sudden jerks of the whole body and hyperextension of the head, hydramnios
Boue et al., 1982

PD 102690 TRISOMY 7, CONFINED PLACENTAL MOSAICISM WITH DIPLOID FETUS[b] (McKusick No. None)

Chorionic villus sampling[h]: trisomy 7 confined placental mosaicism of both cytotrophoblast and chorionic stroma
Barrett et al., 1995
Ultrasound[c,h]: IUGR
Barrett et al., 1995

PD 102692 TRISOMY 7, CONFINED PLACENTAL MOSAICISM WITH FETAL HETERODISOMY 7[b] (McKusick No. None)

Amniocentesis[c]: normal female karyotype
Langlois et al., 1995
Chorionic villus sampling[g]: complete nonmosaic trisomy 7
Langlois et al., 1995
Comments: In the child reported by Langlois and co-workers (1995), heterodisomy 7 was established by DNA analysis extracted from blood of both parents and the child, and from chorion and amnion. At age 2 years, her developmental milestones as assessed by the Denver Developmental Screening Test were age appropriate. Her height and weight, however, were less than −2SD.
Ultrasound[c,d]: IUGR, oligohydramnios
Langlois et al., 1995

PD 102700 TRISOMY 7, PLACENTAL MOSAICISM, FETAL CHROMOSOMAL CONSTITUTION UNKNOWN[b] (McKusick No. None)

Ultrasound: fetal demise
Reddy et al., 1989
Comments: In regard to the fetus reported by Reddy and asociaties (1989), mosaicism for trisomy 7 was found in multiple independent villus cultures. At 16 weeks, fetal demise was detected by ultrasonic examination. Repeat placental culture after delivery unexpectedly revealed pure trisomy 7. Unfortunately, there was culture failure of the fetal tissue.

PD 102775 TRISOMY 9 (47,XY,+9)[b] (McKusick No. None)

Condition Note: Most complete trisomy 9 fetuses are spontaneously aborted early in the pregnancy. This early loss is evident in the fact that miscarriages involving trisomy 9 contributed to 2.7% of all miscarriages secondary to a trisomic karyotype. Other forms of trisomy 9 include partial trisomy 9; trisomy 9 mosaicism (PD 102800); and trisomy 9 mosaicism, placenta only (PD 102825). These latter, less severe forms may be compatible with survive until term. Low birth weight, multiple congenital anomalies, and developmental delays in those that survive have been reported in these disorders.
Chitayat et al., 1995a

Ultrasound[c]: large cystic hygroma
Chitayat et al., 1995a

PD 102800 TRISOMY 9 MOSAICISM (46,XX/47,XX,+9; 47,XX,+9 mosaicism)[b] (McKusick No. None)

Amniocentesis: trisomy 9 mosaicism in cultured cells
Schwartz et al., 1989b
trisomy 9 in all amniotic fluid cells
Sherer et al., 1992
Comments: In the case reported by Sherer and colleagues (1992), there were no trisomic 9 cells in the blood of the neonate after birth. Fibroblast karyotype of skin, however, showed a mosaic pattern. In addition, the fetus carried a balanced translocation {t(1;20)(q42;p11.2)} received from his father.
Cordocentesis (PUBS): trisomy 9 mosaicism in fetal white cells
Schwartz et al., 1989b
Ultrasound[c]: right ventricular enlargement
Schwartz et al., 1989b
Comments: In the case presented by Schwartz and co-workers (1989), the pregnancy was terminated at about 22 weeks of gestation. At autopsy the fetus was found to have multiple congenital anomalies including bulbous nose, micrognathia, bilateral bilobed lungs, abnormal drainage of the left superior vena cava, and a single umbilical artery.
hydronephrosis
Sherer et al., 1992
short femur
Sherer et al., 1992
intrauterine growth retardation[d]
Hentemann et al., 1989; Sherer et al., 1992

PD 102825 TRISOMY 9 PLACENTAL MOSAICISM, CONFINED[b] (McKusick No. None)

Chorionic villus sampling[h]: all cells of the placenta examined had trisomy 9; normal chromosome compliment was present in the fetus
Barrett et al., 1995
Ultrasound[c,h]: IUGR
Barrett et al., 1995

PD 102850 TRISOMY 10[b] (McKusick No. None)

Ultrasound[c]: fetal nuchal edema of approximately 7 mm thickness
Farrall et al., 1993
Comments: In the fetus reported by Farrall and associates (1993), trisomy 10 was found in all amniotic fluid cells and fetal skin fibroblasts examined. The chromosomal makeup of the placenta apparently was not assessed.

PD 102975 TRISOMY 13, PARTIAL {46,XY,-12,+der(12),t(12;13)(p13;q14.1)}[b] (McKusick No. None)

Ultrasound[c]: unilateral choroid plexus cyst, clubfoot
Isada et al., 1994
Comments: In the fetus reported by Isade and co-workers (1994), there

was a de novo unbalanced translocation that resulted in a partial trisomy 13 in which the region specific for the pericentromeric probe was missing in the translocation segment.

PD 103000 TRISOMY 13 SYNDROME {Patau syndrome; 47,XX or XY,+13; 46,XX or XY,-13,+t(13q13q)}[b] (McKusick No. None)

Prenatal Diagnosis: The only definitive methods for diagnosing trisomy 13 is via chromosomal analysis of tissue obtained by amniocentesis, CVS or cordocentesis, or by determining the number of chromosome 13s present in these tissues by the use of chromosomal (DNA) probes. The latter technique normally utilizes FISH.

The risk that the fetus has trisomy 13 increases with lower levels of maternal serum AFP and elevated levels of hCG. The detection of certain fetal abnormalities also increases the likelihood for trisomy 13 (Benacerraf et al., 1994). Benacerraf and associates (1994) have developed a scoring system based on these abnormalities that increases the risk for the fetus to have trisomy 13.

Acetylcholinesterase[c]: rapidly migrating amniotic fluid isozyme
>   Wald and Cuckle, 1981

Alpha-fetoprotein[c]: elevated in amniotic fluid
>   Bobrow et al., 1978; Wald and Cuckle, 1981; Kaffe et al., 1988; Warner et al., 1988
>   *Comments*: In one of the cases reported by Kaffe and co-workers (1988), the amniotic fluid AFP was probably elevated because of fetal demise.
>   low levels in maternal serum
>>   Merkatz et al., 1984; Fisher et al., 1988; Subramaniam et al., 1988
>   elevated in maternal serum
>>   Fisher et al., 1988; Warner et al., 1988; Evans et al., 1995a

Amniocentesis: demonstration of three chromosome 13s by DNA probes (FISH)
>   Ward et al., 1995
>   decreased levels of gamma-glutamyltransferase activity in amniotic fluid
>>   Macek et al., 1987
>   decreased levels of activity of amniotic fluid disaccharidases, maltase, sucrase, trehalase, and lactase[c]
>>   Kleijer et al., 1985b
>   elevated amniotic fluid alkaline phosphatase activity in association with an omphalocele[c]
>>   Jalanko et al., 1983

Chorionic villus sampling[g]: trisomy 13 present in chorionic villi
>   Bovicelli et al., 1988

Cordocentesis (PUBS): fetal blood karyotype
>   Nicolaides et al., 1986a; Bieber et al., 1987; Yapar et al., 1995

Echocardiography[c,d]: pericardial effusion, pleural effusion, hypoplastic left ventricle, dilated right ventricle
>   DeVore et al., 1982b

Embryoscopy[c,g]: polydactyly
>   Cullen et al., 1988

Maternal blood sampling[c,g]: decreased levels of hCG in maternal serum
>   Johnson et al., 1989a
>   elevated levels of hCG and alpha-subunit of human chorionic gonadotropin (alpha-hCG) in maternal serum[c]
>>   Bogart et al., 1987

Ultrasound[c]: decreased ratio of fetal head to trunk diameter
> Sarti et al., 1980

microcephaly
> Benacerraf et al., 1986b; Palmer et al., 1987; Eydoux et al., 1989;
> Hentemann et al., 1989

macrocephaly
> Pilu et al., 1987

holoprosencephaly with cyclopia, centrally fused orbit
> Benacerraf et al., 1984; Benacerraf et al., 1986b

holoprosencephaly
> Saltzman et al., 1986; Pilu et al., 1987; Carlson et al., 1988; Nyberg
> et al., 1989; Zelante and Dallapiccola, 1989

absence of the cavum septi pellucidi
> Yapar et al., 1995

ventriculomegaly (brain)
> Drugan et al., 1986; Evans et al., 1989; Yapar et al., 1995

single ventricle (holoventricle)
> Pilu et al., 1987

meningomyelocele[d]
> Hentemann et al., 1989

hydrocephalus/ventriculomegaly
> Benacerraf et al., 1984; Saltzman et al., 1986; Drugan et al., 1989a;
> Murphy et al., 1989

partial fusion of the thalami
> Yapar et al., 1995

cerebellar hypoplasia
> Nyberg et al., 1989

ocular hypotelorism
> Benacerraf et al., 1986b

orbital hypotelorism[h]
> Eydoux et al., 1989; Berry et al., 1990

cyclops
> Berry et al., 1990

proboscis
> Benacerraf et al., 1986b

deformed nose
> Benacerraf et al., 1986b

absence of the nose
> Berry et al., 1990

large midline upper lip cleft
> Benacerraf et al., 1984

solid mass with cystic areas arising from the oropharyngeal region and
thought to be an epignathus (oral teratoma)
> Yapar et al., 1995

no visualization of the stomach because of esophageal atresia
> Eydoux et al., 1989

cleft lip and palate
> Savoldelli et al., 1982; Seeds and Cefalo, 1983; Benacerraf et al.,
> 1984; Benacerraf et al., 1986b; Saltzman et al., 1986

cystic hygroma[g]
>   Greenberg et al., 1983; Barsel-Bowers and Abuelo, 1986; Cullen et al., 1988; Neu et al., 1993

ventricular septal defect
>   Carlson et al., 1988; Drugan et al., 1989b; Evans et al., 1989; Nyberg et al., 1989; Wladimiroff et al., 1989

hypoplastic left ventricle[d]
>   Wladimiroff et al., 1989

double outlet right ventricle[d]
>   Wladimiroff et al., 1989

tetralogy of Fallot
>   Wladimiroff et al., 1989

truncus arteriosus
>   Nyberg et al., 1989

gastroschisis[h]
>   Eydoux et al., 1989

punctate calcification in the abdomen
>   Nyberg et al., 1989

omphalocele containing liver and bowel
>   Nyberg et al., 1989

omphalocele containing only bowel
>   Nyberg et al., 1989; Berry et al., 1990

>   *Comments:* When an omphalocele is detected prenatally, there is a higher chance that the fetus will have a chromosomal problem if the liver is located intraabdominally (Nyberg et al., 1989).

duodenal atresia[h]
>   Eydoux et al., 1989

omphalocele[h]
>   Eydoux et al., 1989

increased echogenicity of fetal bowel
>   Benacerraf et al., 1994; Strasberg et al., 1995

urethral obstruction with distended fetal bladder and abdomen (urethral obstruction malformation sequence or prune belly syndrome)
>   Savoldelli et al., 1982; McKeown and Donnai, 1986

hydronephrosis
>   Palmer et al., 1987; Murphy et al., 1989; Berry et al., 1990

renal dysplasia
>   Nyberg et al., 1989; Yapar et al., 1995

polycystic kidney disease[h]
>   Hentemann et al., 1989

partial absence of the upper extremities (meromelia)
>   Yapar et al., 1995

clenched hand
>   Carlson et al., 1988

absence of three fingers and partial fusion of the others
>   Yapar et al., 1995

polydactyly
>   Berry et al., 1990; Benacerraf et al., 1994

clubfoot deformity
>   Berry et al., 1990; Yapar et al., 1995

hydrops fetalis
>Greenberg et al., 1983; Barsel-Bowers and Abuelo, 1986; Cosper et el., 1988

single umbilical artery[d]
>Zelante and Dallapiccola, 1989

umbilical cord pseudocyst
>Zelante and Dallapiccola, 1989

>*Comments*: An umbilical cord pseudocyst is focal edema of the cord that gives the appearance of an anechoic, fluid-filled, multicystic mass on ultrasonic imaging. Although the pseudocyst may increase in size with time, no blood flow through the cyst is normally seen on Doppler examination (Jauniaux et al., 1988).

fetal demise
>Palmer et al., 1987; Cash et al., 1988

oligohydramnios
>Hentemann et al., 1989; Yapar et al., 1995

hydramnios
>Nyberg et al., 1989

intrauterine growth retardation
>Eydoux et al., 1989; Hentemann et al., 1989; Zelante and Dallapiccola, 1989

PD 103100 TRISOMY 13q+, PLACENTAL MOSAICISM (46,XX/46,XX,13q+ placental mosaicism; 46,XX,13q+ placental mosaicism)[b] (McKusick No. None)

Chorionic villus sampling[g]: sparse budding and decreased branching of the chorionic villi
>Reddy et al., 1989
>placental mosaicism (20% 46,XX,13q+; 80% 46,XX)

PD 103125 TRISOMY 13,17,20, MOSAIC (Mosaic triple trisomy 13,17,20; 46,XY/49,XY,+13,+17,+20)[b] (McKusick No. None)

General Comments: The mosaic triple trisomy reported by Clark and co-workers (1995) appeared to be confined to amniotic fluid cells because cells form fetal blood; placenta and foreskin all had a normal chromosome makeup.

Alpha-fetoprotein[c]: low level in maternal serum
>Clark et al., 1995

Maternal blood sampling[c]: low level of unconjugated estriol in maternal serum
>Clark et al., 1995
>low level of hCG in maternal serum
>Clark et al., 1995

PD 103175 TRISOMY 14q {46,XX,-14,+t(14;14)(p1;q21)}[b] (McKusick No. None)

Ultrasound[c]: omphalocele, oligohydramnios
>Duckett et al., 1990

>*Comments*: The fetus reported on by Duckett and co-authors (1990) was found after termination of the pregnancy to be small for gestational age (gestational age, 21 weeks; size equivalent to 18 weeks of gestation), and had dysplastic ears, no left external meatus, micrognathia, cleft palate, talipes calcaneovalgus, and an omphalocele. An autopsy revealed a ventricular septal defect, small multicystic kidneys, and pulmonary hypoplasia.

PD 103225 TRISOMY 15, FETAL MOSAICISM WITH MATERNAL UNIPARENTAL HETERODISOMY, PLACENTAL CONSTITUTION UNKNOWN (47,XX,+15/46,XX)[b] (McKusick No. None)

Amniocentesis[d]: trisomy 15 (four of nine colonies) mosaicism
    Milunsky et al., 1996
Comments: In the fetus reported by Milunsky and associates (1996), the postnatal peripheral lymphocyte chromosomal constitution was 46,XX in all 100 cells examined; in skin fibroblasts the makeup was 80% 47,XX+15. Molecular assessment revealed maternal uniparental heterodisomy for chromosome 15 in the 46,XX cell line.
Maternal blood sampling[c]: low level of serum unconjugated estriol
    Milunsky et al., 1996
Ultrasound[c,d]: IUGR
    Milunsky et al., 1996

PD 103250 TRISOMY 15q11/17q25[b] {47,XY,-15,+der(15),t(15;17)(q11;q25)}[b] (McKusick No. None)

Ultrasound[c,d]: hydrops fetalis
    Schwanitz et al., 1988
Comments: In this fetus reported on by Schwanitz and associates (1988), the father had a balanced translocation between chromosome 15 and 17 {46,XY,t(15;17)(q11;q25)}. The fetus had two derived chromosome 15s plus the translocation making him trisomic for 15q11, as well as for 17q25, an unusual chromosomal constitution.
    At birth, the child was dysmorphic and had hypoplastic midface, low set and dysplastic ears, micrognathia, short neck, and hydrops fetalis. Development was poor, and when he was 18 months old, a developmental quotient was between 20 and 37. At this time he also had microcephaly, a broad mouth with a thin upper lip, short limbs with primary shortening of the humeri and femora, and hypotonia.

PD 103475 TRISOMY 16[b] (McKusick No. None)

Alpha-fetoprotein[c]: elevated in maternal serum
    Benn et al., 1995
Maternal blood sampling[c]: elevated hCG in maternal serum
    Benn et al., 1995
Ultrasound[c]: polycystic kidneys, oligohydramnios, fetal demise
    Benn et al., 1995

PD 103500 TRISOMY 16, AMNION AND UMBILICAL CORD MOSAICISM ONLY[b] (McKusick No. None)

Ultrasound[c]: oligohydramnios
    Watson et al., 1988
Comments: The fetus reported on by Watson and associates (1988) had trisomy 16 in amniotic fluid cells in 7 of 22 colonies; the other colonies had normal chromosomal constitutions. Fetal blood cells obtained by umbilical blood sampling were 46,XX. The pregnancy was continued until the 35th week, when the mother was delivered of a 950-g female infant with renal anomalies, imperforate anus, and pulmonary hypoplasia. Normal chromosomal constitutions were found in cord blood, placenta, and skin fibro-

blasts. The umbilical cord and fetal membranes, however, were mosaic for trisomy 16 (70% trisomic cells). Because the umbilical cord is formed from the amnion, presumably the trisomy 16 originated in amniotic cells or progenitor cells.

PD 103525 TRISOMY 16, CONFINED PLACENTAL MOSAICISM WITH DIPLOID FETUS[b] (McKusick No. None)

Condition Note: Confined placental mosaicism for trisomy 16 is a situation in which there is mosaic trisomy 16 of the placenta only, with the chromosomal makeup in the fetus being normal. In this listing the presence or absence of uniparental disomy in the fetus is unknown.

> Verp et al., 1989a; Williams et al., 1989

Prenatal Diagnosis: The diagnosis is established by finding mosaic trisomy 16 in chorionic villi with normal chromosomal constitution in fetal tissue.

Differential Diagnosis: See various listings under Trisomy 16 in the Index.

Alpha-fetoprotein[c]: elevated in maternal serum
> Benn et al., 1995

Chorionic villus sampling[g]: chromosomal constitution of 47,XX,+16 in both direct chorionic villus preparations and cultured villi
> Verp et al., 1989a

Comments: In the pregnancy reported by Verp and co-authors (1989a), all chromosomal analyses from chorionic villi showed 47,XX,+16. Amniocentesis showed normal chromosomal constitution. Serial ultrasound evaluations starting at 14 weeks were normal, as was an amniotic fluid AFP level. Cord blood at delivery at 37 weeks of gestation was also chromosomally normal. The phenotype and growth indices of the neonate were normal.

mosaic trisomy in both the cytotrophoblast and chorionic stroma[h]
> Barrett et al., 1995

Maternal blood sampling[c]: elevated level of hCG
> Benn et al., 1995

Maternal history[c,d]: no fetal movement associated with fetal death at 36 weeks' gestation
> Hashish et al., 1989

Ultrasound[c]: clinodactyly
> Benn et al., 1995

slowing of fetal growth during the last half of pregnancy, multiple placental sonolucencies
> Williams et al., 1989

intrauterine growth retardation[h]
> Barrett et al., 1995

PD 103550 TRISOMY 16, FETAL MOSAICISM, PLACENTAL CHROMOSOMAL CONSTITUTION UNKNOWN[b] (McKusick No. None)

Alpha-fetoprotein[c]: elevated in maternal serum but normal in amniotic fluid
> Davies et al., 1995

Comments: The two fetuses reported by Davies and associates (1995) had trisomy 16 mosaicism of amniotic fluid cells and skin fibroblasts.

Echocardiogram[c,d]: congenital heart defect
> Ray et al., 1993

Ultrasound[c]: horseshoe kidney, two vessel umbilical cord
>Davies et al., 1995

>intrauterine growth retardation
>>Hsu et al., 1993b; Ray et al., 1993

>*Comments*: Both fetuses reported by Ray and associates (1993) had multiple congenital anomalies at birth.

>enlarged palcenta
>>Hsu et al., 1993b

>*Comments*: In the fetus reported by Hsu and co-workers (1993), no evidence was found for uniparental disomy in the fetus.

PD 103552 TRISOMY 16, FETAL MOSAICISM, PLACENTAL DISOMY (46,XY/47,XY+16)[b] (McKusick No. None)

Alpha-fetoprotein[c]: elevated in maternal serum
>Rosenblum-Vos et al., 1993

PD 103553 TRISOMY 16, FETAL MOSAICISM, PLACNETAL NONMOSAIC TRISOMY WITH BIPARENTAL DISOMY[b] (McKusick No. None)

Ultrasound[c,h]: IUGR, enlarged placenta
>Hsu et al., 1993b

Comments: In the fetus reported by Hsu and associates (1993b), amniotic fluid cells showed 10% trisomy 16; the placenta revealed all trisomy 16 cells. Molecular studies failed to show uniparental disomy for chromosome 16 in the fetus.

PD 103554 TRISOMY 16, FETAL MOSAICISM WITH BIPARENTAL DISOMY, PLACENTAL CHROMSOMAL CONSTITUTION UNKNOWN[b] (McKusick No. None)

Ultrasound[c]: IUGR
>Hsu et al., 1993b

>enlarged placenta
>>Hsu et al., 1993b

>*Comment*: In the fetus reported by Hsu and colleagues (1993), there were no trisomy cells found postnatally, and no evidence for uniparental disomy in the fetus.

PD 103555 TRISOMY 16, FETAL MOSAICISM WITH MATERNAL UNIPARENTAL DISOMY, PLACENTAL CHROMOSOMAL CONSTITUTION UNKNOWN[b] (McKusick No. None)

Alpha-fetoprotein[c]: elevated in maternal serum but normal in amniotic fluid
>Davies et al., 1995

Amniocentesis: 6 of 16 amniotic fluid cell colonies had trisomy 16
>Davies et al., 1995

Comments: An autopsy on the fetus reported by Davies and co-workers (1995) revealed a two vessel umbilical cord, partial malrotation of the gut, a double outlet right ventricle, an ectopic right kidney, and agenesis of the right external ear. Skin fibroblasts analysis indicated maternal uniparental disomy for trisomy 16.

Cordocentesis (PUBS): trisomy 16 in 2 of 200 cells
Davies et al., 1995
Maternal blood drawing[c]: elevated serum level of hCG
Davies et al., 1995

PD 103570 TRISOMY 16, PLACENTAL NONMOSAICISM, FETAL NONMOSAIC MATERNAL ISODISOMY[b] (McKusick No. None)

Ultrasound[c,d]: IUGR
Sutcliffe et al., 1993
Comments: In the fetus/child reported by Sutcliffe and associates (1993), maternal isodisomy in disomy cells from chorionic villi and cord blood was determined by various DNA probes detecting variable number tandem repeats (VNTR) polymorphisms.

PD 103600 TRISOMY 16/TRISOMY 8,16 CONFINED PLACENTAL MOSAICISM WITH FETAL BIPARENTAL DISOMY (47,XX,+16/ 48,XX,+8,+16)[b] (McKusick No. None)

Ultrasound[c]: IUGR, oligohydramnios, fetal demise
Adam et al., 1993
Comments: In the fetus reported by Adam and co-workers (1993), there was no evidence of uniparental disomy in the fetus as determined by molecular analysis.

PD 103750 TRISOMY 17(p11pter)[b] (McKusick No. None)

Condition Note: The pattern of congenital anomalies associated with trisomy 17(p11pter) includes IUGR, microcephaly, downslanting palpebral fissures, small mouth, micrognathia, dysplastic ears, short and webbed neck, congenital heart defect, hypoplasia of the genitalia, clinodactyly of the fingers, and hernias.
Lurie et al., 1995a
Ultrasound[c]: oligohydramnios
Lurie et al., 1995a

PD 104000 TRISOMY 18 SYNDROME {(Edwards syndrome; 46,XX/ 47,XX,+18; 46,XY,-18,+i(18q); 47,XX or XY,+18)}[b] (McKusick No. None)

Syndrome Note: Trisomy 18 syndrome is often associated with multiple congenital anomalies and a high prenatal or infantile mortality rate. Infants that survive beyond the first year of life are uniformly severely retarded. Most cases of trisomy 18 are produced by nondisjunction in the production of the egg or sperm. Recurrence risk for parents who have previously had an offspring with trisomy 18 is low for a sibling with trisomy 18 syndrome, but approximately 1% for trisomy 21 and other trisomies.

Prenatal Diagnosis: The only definitive methods for diagnosing trisomy 18 is via chromosomal analysis of tissue obtained by amniocentesis, CVS or cordocentesis, or by determining the number of chromosome 18s present in these tissues or from fetal cells obtained from maternal cell sorting and the endocervical canal by the use of chromosomal (DNA) probes. The latter technique normally utilizes FISH.

The risk that the fetus has trisomy 18 increases according to the level of maternal serum AFP, unconjugated estriol, and hCG levels (Palomaki et al., 1995). The detection of certain fetal abnormalities also increases the likelihood for trisomy 18 (Benacerraf et al., 1994). Benacerraf and associates (1994) have developed a scoring system based on these abnormalities that predicts the risk for trisomy 18 in the fetus.

Acetylcholinesterase[c]: rapidly migrating amniotic fluid isozyme
> Wald and Cuckle, 1981; Nevin et al.,1983b; Macri et al., 1986

elevated level in amniotic fluid
> Schmidt and Kubli, 1982

Alpha-fetoprotein[c]: elevated in amniotic fluid
> Chemke et al., 1979; Fisher et al., 1981; Wald and Cuckle, 1981; Schmidt and Kubli, 1982; Nevin et al., 1983b; Crandall and Matsumoto, 1984b; Nielsen et al., 1985; Macri et al., 1986; Lindenbaum et al., 1987

elevated in maternal serum
> Lindenbaum et al., 1987; Palmer et al., 1987; Fisher et al., 1988; Cervetti et al., 1995

decreased percentage of AFP that reacts with concanavalin A
> Nielsen et al., 1985

low levels in maternal serum
> Merkatz et al., 1984; Baumgarten et al., 1985; Nelson and Peterson, 1985; Bogart et al., 1987; Lindenbaum et al., 1987; Fisher et al., 1988; Jauniaux et al., 1988; Redwine et al., 1988; Schneider et al., 1988; Subramaniam et al., 1988; Barsel-Bowers et al., 1989; Shah et al., 1989; Canick et al., 1990; Bradley et al., 1994; Palomaki et al., 1995

Comments: The AFP levels in trisomy 18 pregnancies that are not complicated by omphaloceles and/or neural tube defects are frequently lower than the mean maternal serum values, but are usually normal in the amniotic fluid. However, both are frequently elevated when omphaloceles and/or neural tube defects are present in the trisomy 18 fetus (Lindenbaum et al., 1987; Kaffe et al., 1988). The incidence of omphalocele and neural tube defects in trisomy 18 is 6% for both (Moore et al., 1988), and these defects probably account for much of the variation in AFP levels recorded for this condition.

Amniocentesis: demonstration of three chromosome 18s in uncultured amniotic fluid cells by DNA probes (FISH)
> Ward et al., 1995

Comments: According to one study (Carelli et al., 1995), the detection rate for trisomy 18 using FISH procedure is now 95.7%.

reduced levels of alkaline phosphatase in amniotic fluid[c]
> Jalanko et al., 1983

increased percentage of phenylalanine-resistant alkaline phosphatase in amniotic fluid[c]
> Brock et al., 1984a; Aitken et al., 1985; Morin et al., 1987

decreased percentage of homoarginine-resistant alkaline phosphatase in amniotic fluid[c]
> Brock et al., 1984a; Morin et al., 1987

decreased levels of gamma-glutamyltranspeptidase activity in amniotic fluid
> Carbarns et al., 1983; Brock et al., 1984a; Aitken et al., 1985; Morin et al., 1987

decreased levels of aminopeptidase M activity in amniotic fluid
> Brock et al., 1984a

decreased levels of activity of amniotic fluid disaccharidases, maltase, sucrase, trehalase, and lactase[c]
> Kleijer et al., 1985b

decreased levels of beta hCG in amniotic fluids[c]
> Bharathur et al., 1988

Cordocentesis (PUBS): fetal blood karyotype
> Nicolaides et al., 1986a; Bieber et al., 1987

low hematocrit (anemia)[c]
> Murotsuki et al., 1992

Doppler blood flow studies[c]: normal arcuate artery wave forms but no diastolic blood flow in the umbilical arteries
> Ostlere et al., 1989

Echocardiogram[c]: double outlet right ventricle with subaortic ventricular septal defect, conal interventricular septal defect
> Kleinman and Santulli, 1983

Endocervical canal sampling[g]: trisomy 18 cells found by FISH using chromosome 18 probes.
> Adinolfi et al., 1995

External fetal monitoring[c,d]: heart variability including decreased short-term variability and late decelerations
> Jauniaux et al., 1988

Fetography[d]: prominent occiput, low set malformed ears, micrognathia, abnormal bending of wrists, flexion deformities of fingers, rocker-bottom feet
> Suzumori and Yagami, 1975

Maternal blood sampling[c]: decreased levels of hCG in maternal serum[c,g]
> Bogart et al., 1987; Arab et al., 1988; Canick et al., 1989; Johnson et al., 1989a; Suchy and Yeager, 1989; Canick et al., 1990; Bradley et al., 1994; Palomaki et al., 1995

decreased levels of unconjugated estriol in maternal serum
> Canick et al., 1989; Canick et al., 1990; Bradley et al., 1994; Palomaki et al., 1995

Maternal blood sampling with subsequent fetal cell sorting[h]: trisomy 18 cells detected by FISH using chromosome 18 probes
> Wachtel et al., 1995

Comments: The fetus reported by Wachtel and co-authors (1995) had been diagnosed with trisomy 18 by other methods prior to maternal blood sampling.

Maternal history[c,d]: decreased fetal movements
> Jauniaux et al., 1988

Preimplantation embryo biopsy[g]: FISH demonstrated three number 18 chromosomes
> Weier et al., 1993

Radiograph[c]: abnormally shaped head, compressed fetal chest
> Chemke et al., 1979

Ultrasound, abdominal[c]: unusual shaped fetal trunk, small fetal head (microcephaly) and chest, hydramnios
> Chemke et al., 1979; Fisher et al., 1981; Bowie and Clair, 1982;

Comstock and Boal, 1985; de Elejalde and Elejalde, 1985a; Bundy et al., 1986a

the fetal head could not be visualized

Nisani et al., 1981; Macri et al., 1986

Comments: After termination, the fetus was found to have anencephalus with cervical rachischisis in the case of Nisani and colleagues (1981), and only anencephalus in the case reported by Macri and associates (1986).

hydrocephalus

Benacerraf et al., 1986b; Bundy et al., 1986a; Carlson et al., 1988; Drugan et al., 1989a; Mulder et al., 1989; Palumbos and Stierman 1989; Nyberg et al., 1993; Kupferminc et al., 1994

choroid plexus cysts with or without mild dilatation of the posterior horns of the lateral ventricles

Bundy et al., 1986a; Nicolaides et al., 1986a; Farhood et al., 1987a; Farhood et al., 1987b; Furness, 1987; Camurri and Ventura, 1989; Khouzam and Hooker, 1989; Ostlere et al., 1989; Zerres et al., 1992; Bar-Hava et al., 1993; Nyberg et al., 1993; Benacerraf et al., 1994; Snijders et al., 1994; Walkinshaw et al., 1994a; Gross et al., 1995

Comments: Care needs to be taken in interpreting the significance of finding an isolated choroid plexus cyst prenatally and the relationship to trisomy 18 (Farhood et al., 1987b). In one prospective study of choroid plexus cysts, only 1 of 10 fetuses with this problem had trisomy 18 (Camurri and Ventura, 1989). Zerres and co-workers (1992) found that 4 of 832 fetuses with prenatally diagnosed growth retardation and/or physical anomalies had trisomy 18.

In another study (Snijders et al., 1994), the incidence of choroid plexus in the general fetal population was 1%; at midtrimester the incidence of choroid cysts in fetuses with trisomy 18 was 50%. The frequency of trisomy 18 in fetuses with choroid plexus cysts increased with the number of other anomalies detected. If there were two or more additional abnormalities, then the incidence of trisomy 18 was 20.5%. These authors concluded that if a choroid cyst were *isolated* then the risk for trisomy 18 was only marginally elevated, and the decision to do an amniocentesis should be based mainly on maternal age. Gross and co-workers (1995) echoed the sentiment of Snijders and associates (1994). On the other hand, Walkinshaw and associates (1994a) found that 1 in 82 fetuses with isolated choroid plexus cysts had trisomy 18. These authors recommended doing chromosomal studies on all fetuses with isolated choroid plexus cysts. Their conclusion was supported by Kupferminc and colleagues (1994). Choroid cysts can also occur in Down syndrome (PD 101000).

enlarged cerebral lateral ventricles (ventriculomegaly)

Sutro et al., 1984; Seligsohn et al., 1985; Drugan et al., 1989b; Evans et al., 1989; Snijders et al., 1994

enlarged cisterna magna characterized by a large cystic space in the posterior cranial vault which extended from the cerebellar hemispheres to the posterior calvarium

Comstock and Boal, 1985

prominent cisterna magna
   Nyberg et al., 1993
microcephaly
   Pilu et al., 1986; Eydoux et al., 1989; Snijders et al., 1994
holoprosencephaly
   Nyberg et al., 1989; Beru et al., 1990
strawberry-shaped head
   Nyberg et al., 1993; Snijders et al., 1994
cyclopia
   Nyberg et al., 1989
occipital meningocele[d]
   Muller and de Jong, 1986
encephalocele
   Nyberg et al., 1993; Benacerraf et al., 1994
prominent occiput[d]
   Muller and de Jong, 1986
brachycephaly
   Zerres et al., 1992; Snijders et al., 1994
agenesis of the corpus callosum
   Snijders et al., 1994
Arnold–Chiari malformation
   Drugan et al., 1989b; Evans et al., 1989
posterior fossa cyst
   Snijders et al., 1994
meningomyelocele
   Drugan et al., 1989b; Evans et al., 1989; Nyberg et al., 1994;
   Snijders et al., 1994
meningomyelocele presenting as a soft tissue mass protruding posteriorly from the spine
   Spirt et al., 1987
severe microphthalmia
   de Elejalde and Elejalde, 1984; de Elejalde and Elejalde, 1985a
orbital hypotelorism[d]
   Eydoux et al., 1989; Nyberg et al., 1995
exomphalos
   Snijders et al., 1994
micrognathia[d]
   de Elejalde and Elejalde, 1984; Bundy et al., 1986a; Muller and
   de Jong, 1986; Pilu et al., 1986; Snijders et al., 1994
cleft lip and/or palate[d]
   Bundy et al., 1986a; Bundy et al., 1986b; Carlson et al., 1988
increased swallowing activity, fetal regurgitation in association with esophageal atresia[d]
   Bowie and Clair, 1982
cystic hygroma
   Marchese et al., 1985b; Abramowicz et al., 1989; Eydoux et al.,
   1989; Bar-Hava et al., 1993; Neu et al., 1993; Snijders et al., 1994
lymphangiectasia
   Pearce et al., 1984; Redford et al., 1984; Marchese et al., 1985b;
   Bundy et al., 1986a; Nyberg et al., 1993

nuchal thickening
    Nyberg et al., 1993
nuchal cysts[g]
    Black et al., 1988
    Comments: The above finding was noted both by abdominal and transvaginal ultrasound during the 11th and 12th weeks of gestation. Transvaginal ultrasound screening of candidates for CVS is suggested by Black and co-authors (1988) to detect possible fetal abnormalities in suspected trisomy 18 fetuses.
diaphragmatic hernia which may be seen as a fluid-filled structure in the left chest (eventration of the diaphragm or posterolateral diaphragmatic hernia)
    Comstock and Boal, 1985; Benacerraf et al., 1986b; Comstock, 1986; Carlson et al., 1988; Eydoux et al., 1989; Berry et al., 1990; Nyberg et al., 1993
bilateral pleural effusions
    Pearce et al., 1984; Jauniaux et al., 1988
pericardial effusion[d]
    Bundy et al., 1986a; Nyberg et al., 1993
congenital heart defect
    Benacerraf et al., 1986b; Zerres et al., 1992; Snijders et al., 1994
overriding aorta[d]
    Wladimiroff et al., 1989
ventricular septal defect
    Nicolaides et al., 1986a; Saltzman et al., 1986; Carlson et al., 1988; Wladimiroff et al., 1988a; Wladimiroff et al., 1989; Nyberg et al., 1993; Kupferminc et al., 1994
atrial septal defect[d]
    Wladimiroff et al., 1989
atrioventricular canal
    Wladimiroff et al., 1989
double outlet right ventricle
    Wladimiroff et al., 1989
hypoplastic left heart with single outflow tract
    Kupferminc et al., 1994
tetralogy of Fallot
    Nicolaidas et al., 1986a; Wladimiroff et al., 1989
fused papillary muscles
    Boehmer et al., 1995
irregular tachyarrhythmia[d]
    Comstock and Boal, 1985
cardiac arrhythmias[d]
    Muller and de Jong, 1986
second degree atrioventricular canal heart block
    Wladimiroff et al., 1988a
coarctation of aorta suggested by difficulty in visualizing the aortic arch
    Colley et al., 1987
esophageal atresia[d]
    Hentemann et al., 1989
diaphragmatic hernia
    Benacerraf et al., 1994; Snijders et al., 1994

no visualization of the stomach because of esophageal atresia
> Tortora et al., 1984; Eydoux et al., 1989

nonvisualized or small stomach with decreased transient filling time
> Bundy et al., 1986b

small abdominal diameter
> Boue et al., 1982

omphalocele
> Jassani et al., 1982; Schmidt and Kubli, 1982; Marchese et al., 1985b; Muller and de Jong, 1986; Colley et al., 1987; Palmer et al., 1987; Jauniaux et al., 1988; Redwine et al., 1988; Eydoux et al., 1989; Hentemann et al., 1989; Nyberg et al., 1989; Wolstenholme et al., 1989; Zerres et al., 1992; Nyberg et al., 1993; Benacerraf et al., 1994; Boehmer et al., 1995
>
> *Comments*: When an omphalocele is detected prenatally, there is a higher chance that the fetus will have a chromosomal problem when the liver is located intraabdominally (Nyberg et al., 1989).

omphalocele with liver and bowel present in the omphalocele
> Nyberg et al., 1989

gastroschisis
> Marchese et al., 1985a; Nielsen et al., 1985

increased echogenicity of the fetal bowel
> Strasberg et al., 1995

large intraabdominal cystic structure that turned out to be a distended bladder as a result of urethral atresia
> Heller et al., 1981; Nevin et al., 1983b; Nicolaides et al., 1986a

ascites
> Bundy et al., 1986a; Palmer et al., 1987; Jauniaux et al., 1988; Nyberg et al., 1989

megacystis[d]
> Hentemann et al., 1989

allantoic cysts
> Nyberg et al., 1989; Nyberg et al., 1993

hydronephrosis
> Ostlere et al., 1989; Nyberg et al., 1993; Snijders et al., 1994

multicystic kidneys
> Nyberg et al., 1993; Snijder et al., 1994

caliectasis (pyelectasis)[d]
> Khouzam and Hooker, 1989; Boehmer et al., 1995

hydroureter[d]
> Khouzam and Hooker, 1989

bladder not visualized
> Nyberg et al., 1993

kyphoscoliosis
> Snijders et al., 1994

shortened forearms with or without absence of one of the long bones
> Benacerraf et al., 1986b; Bundy et al., 1986a

phocomelia of the arm
> Nyberg et al., 1993

radial aplasia/agenesis
> Nyberg et al., 1989; Berry et al., 1990

ankyloses of the wrists and ankles, camptodactyly with raised index fingers

Muller and de Jong, 1986

absence of the middle phalanx of the left fifth digit

Boehmer et al., 1995

hand fixed in position relative to forearm

Benacerraf et al., 1986b

severe deformity of hand, fisted or clenched hand

Benacerraf et al., 1986b; Carlson et al., 1988

clenched hand

Nyberg et al., 1993; Snijders et al., 1994

contractures and overlapping of fingers

Boue et al., 1982; Bar-Hava et al., 1993

short femur

Snijders et al., 1994

clubfoot deformities

Tortora et al., 1984; Chervenak et al., 1985a; Benacerraf et al., 1986b; Bundy et al., 1986a; Muller and de Jong, 1986; Nicolaides et al., 1986a; Zerres et al., 1992; Bar-Hava et al., 1993; Nyberg et al., 1993; Snijders et al., 1994

prominent heel (rocker-bottom foot)

Benacerraf et al., 1986b; Muller and de Jong, 1986; Snijders et al., 1994

brisk and rapid movements of arms, depressed lower extremity movements

Boue et al., 1982

intrauterine death as indicated by no detectable fetal movement and no heartbeat

Colley et al., 1987

hydrops fetalis

Curry et al., 1983; Pearce et al., 1984; Jauniaux et al., 1988; Abramowicz et al., 1989; Hentemann et al., 1989; Snijders et al., 1994

umbilical cord pseudocyst

Jauniaux et al., 1988

Comments: An umbilical cord pseudocyst is focal edema of the cord that gives the appearance of an anechoic fluid-filled multicystic mass on ultrasonic imaging. Although the pseudocyst may increase in size with time, no blood flow through the cyst is normally seen on Doppler examination (Jauniaux et al., 1988).

single umbilical artery

Tortora et al., 1984; Spirt et al., 1987; Berry et al., 1990; Nyberg et al., 1993

enlarged umbilical vein

Tortora et al., 1984; Spirt et al., 1987

intrauterine growth retardation

Boue et al., 1982; Johnson et al., 1982a; Kleinman and Santulli, 1993; Tortora et al., 1984; Benacerraf et al., 1986b; Bundy et al., 1986a; Bundy et al., 1986b; Saltzman et al., 1986; Colley et al., 1987; Williamson et al., 1988; Wladimiroff et al., 1988a; Eydoux

et al., 1989; Hentemann et al., 1989; Ostlere et al., 1989; Zerres
et al., 1992; Nyberg et al., 1993; Snijders et al., 1994
intrauterine growth retardation as indicated by decreased crown-to-
rump length[g]
    Lynch et al., 1987
hydramnios
    Tortora et al., 1984; Blundy et al., 1986b; Muller and de Jong,
    1986; Saltzman et al., 1986; Colley et al., 1987; Palmer et al., 1987;
    Spirt et al., 1987; Carlson et al., 1988; Williamson et al., 1988;
    Eydoux et al., 1989; Hentemann et al., 1989; Mulder et al., 1989;
    Nyberg et al., 1989; Ostlere et al., 1989; Zerres et al., 1992; Nyberg
    et al., 1993
oligohydramnios[d]
    Pearce et al., 1984; Bundy et al., 1986a; Nyberg et al., 1993
oligohydramnios secondary to ruptured membranes
    Mulder et al., 1989
placenta, thickened and congested
    Jauniaux et al., 1988
Ultrasound, endovaginal[g]: cystic occipital encephalocele, unilateral ventricular dilation, no detectable cerebellum, cystic hygroma, hydrops fetalis
    Grange et al., 1994
Comments: The fetus reported by Grange and co-workers (1994) was found
to have trisomy 18, and after termination the fetus physically had craniorachischisis.

PD 104250 TRISOMY 20 MOSAICISM (46,XX or XY/47,XX or XY, +20)[b]
(McKusick No. None)

Condition Note: Trisomy 20 mosaicism is one of the more common mosaicisms
found in amniotic fluid cells (Tolmie et al., 1987c). Rarely, however, is trisomy
20 found in cytogenetic surveys of spontaneous abortions or in newborns (Tolmie
et al., 1987c). Furthermore, Hsu and associates (1987) have found that 56 of 66
(85%) reported cases of trisomy 20 mosaicism were phenotypically normal. The
abnormalities found in the other 15% of abnormal individuals have had no
consistent pattern. It would appear, then, that finding trisomy 20 mosaicism
confined to amniotic fluid cells has little consequence in most fetuses. If trisomy
20 mosaicism is found in fetal tissue, for example, fetal blood, the prognosis is
probably not so good.

    Hsu and associated (1991) reviewed the findings in 101 fetuses diagnosed
with trisomy 20 mosaicism, and concluded that when this trisomic situation is
found that level II ultrasound scan of the fetus with special attention to the
cardiovascular and renal systems should be done. If abnormalities are found in
the fetus, this information is then helpful in counseling the parents and in the
parent's decision making.

    Alpha-fetoprotein[c]: elevated in maternal serum
        Tolmie et al., 1987c
    reduced level in maternal serum
        Shah et al., 1989
Ultrasound[c]: short femur and nuchal thickening
        Micale et al., 1995
    Comments: In the fetus reported by Micale and colleagues (1995), 96 of

98 clones (98%) of amniotic fluid cells had trisomy 20. After termination, fetal blood contained 6 of 50 cells (12%) with trisomy 20. Seven other tissues sources also contained trisomic cells.

PD 104450 TRISOMY 22, PLACENTAL (47,XX,+22, placenta)[b] (McKusick No. None)

Condition Note: Placental trisomy 22 is a condition in which there is complete trisomy 22 in the placenta but a normal chromosomal complement in the embryo/fetus. This situation probably arises when there is trisomy 22 at the time of conception, and the extra chromosome is lost early in the development of the definitive embryo. (For further details see discussion in the General Comments at the beginning of this chapter.) Alternatively, the trisomy may have occurred as the result of a nondisjunctional error arising early in the development of the trophoblastic tissue.

Prenatal Diagnosis: The diagnosis is suspected whenever there is trisomy 22 mosaicism in amniotic fluid cells and a normal chromosomal makeup in fetal white cells, or when there is complete trisomy 22 in the chorionic villi and normal chromosomal makeup in fetal tissue.

Differential Diagnosis: Other trisomic 22 situations should be considered such as Trisomy 22 syndrome (PD 104500) and Trisomy 22 mosaicism.

Ultrasound[c,d]: IUGR

Stioui et al., 1989

Comments: In the situation reported by Stioui and co-workers (1989), there was trisomy 22 mosaicism in the amniotic fluid cells at 16 weeks of gestation. At 19 weeks of gestation, the fetus had normal growth. A fetal white cell karyotype at that time was also normal. Intrauterine growth retardation was present at 26 weeks of gestation. At birth, the child was completely normal. Chorionic villus chromosomal analysis revealed trisomy 22 in all cells.

PD 104500 TRISOMY 22 SYNDROME (47,XX or XY,+22)[b] (McKusick No. None)

Syndrome Note: Trisomy 22 is associated with IUGR, microcephaly, broad and flat nasal bridge, epicanthal folds, ocular hypertelorism, microtic, cleft palate, pterygia of the neck, congenital heart defects including anomalous great vessels, renal and anorectal abnormalities, hypoplastic distal digits, and thumb defects.

Bacino et al., 1995

Ultrasound[c]: microcephaly

Bacino et al., 1995

cystic hygroma

Palumbos et al., 1987

cardiac anomalies

Bacino et al., 1995

ambiguous genitalia

Bacino et al., 1995

intrauterine growth retardation

Phillips et al., 1995; Ladonne et al., 1996

Comments: Ladonne and co-authors (1996) reported a fetus who had multiple congenital anomalies at birth at 32 weeks' gestation. The neonate died within minutes of birth. The pattern of abnormalities in the child was similar to that of Fryns syndrome (PD 191240). The pregnancy of this fetus was complicated by maternal diabetes, hypertension, extreme obesity, and eclampsia. Both peripheral blood and skin cells of the child indicated complete trisomy 22 (47,XY,+22).

PD 104550 TRISOMY 22(q12qter) {46,XY,-17,+der(17qter17p13::22q12qter)}[b] (McKusick No. None)

Ultrasound[c,d]: cystic hygroma, ventricular septal defect, IUGR
    Tolkendorf et al., 1991
    Comments: The mother of the fetus published by Tolkendorf and associates (1991) carried a balance translocation {46,XX,t(17;22)(p13;q12)} that apparently lead to fetal chromosomal abnormality.

PD 105000 TURNER SYNDROME (45,X; 45,X/46,XX mosaicism; 45,X/46,XY mosaicism; 45,X/46,XY/47,XYY MOSAICISM)[b] (McKusick No. None)

Prenatal Diagnosis: Detection of hydrops fetalis and/or cystic hygroma should alert one to the possibility of Turner syndrome. Under most circumstances, a chromosomal analysis of the amniotic fluid cells should be undertaken. If on the other hand a 45,X chromosomal constitution is found following analysis of embryonic or fetal tissue, the fetus should be evaluated ultrasonographically to determine if hydrops fetalis and/or cardiac defects are present. There is a direct relationship between the amount of edema and the likelihood of losing the pregnancy; the greater the edema, the higher the risk. Ultrasound assessment of the external genitalia also should be done in these situations; if male genitalia are detected, the fetus may have 45,X/46,XY mosaicism or 45,X;Y autosomal translocation (Abuelo and Barsel-Bowers, 1988). Most 45,X/46,XY fetuses turn out to have a normal male phenotype at birth (Chang et al., 1990).
Differential Diagnosis: 45,X male (PD 105335); see also Hydrops fetalis in the Index

45,X and 45,X/46,XX MOSAICISM

Acetylcholinesterase[c]: elevated in amniotic fluid
        Dale, 1980; Dale et al., 1981
    rapidly migrating amniotic fluid acetylcholinesterase isoenzyme on gel electrophoresis
        Wald and Cuckle, 1981; Milunsky and Saperstein, 1982; Polanska et al., 1983; Raymond and Simpson, 1988
        Comments: In fetuses with Turner syndrome who have a cystic hygroma, cystic hygroma fluid rather than amniotic fluid inadvertently may be collected at the time of amniocentesis. When this occurs, acetylcholinesterase isozyme may be detected in the fluid, giving the false impression that there is a surface breakdown in the fetus. Brock and associates (1985a) have demonstrated that cystic hygroma fluid actually was collected with four fetuses with Turner syndrome.
Alpha-fetoprotein[c]: elevated in amniotic fluid
        Hunter et al., 1976; Seller, 1977; Milunsky and Sapirstein, 1982; Polanska et al., 1983
        Comments: Elevation of AFP may be present because cystic hygroma fluid was collected rather than amniotic fluid at the time of amniocentesis. This

has been shown to be the case with four fetuses with Turner syndrome (Brock et al., 1985a).
    elevated in maternal serum
        Brock, 1982; Holmes-Siedle et al., 1987; Cervetti et al., 1995
    low level in maternal serum
        Holliday et al., 1988; Redwine et al., 1988; Shah et al., 1989; Koeberl et al., 1995
Amniocentesis: karyotype from cells in the fluid aspirated from the cystic hygroma
        Barry et al., 1985; Patil et al., 1987; Al Saadi, 1989
    decreased levels of gamma-glutamyltranspeptidase activity in amniotic fluid[c]
        Brock et al., 1984a; Aitken et al., 1985; Macek et al., 1987
    decreased levels of aminopeptidase M activity in amniotic fluid[c]
        Brock et al., 1984a
    increased percentage of phenylalanine-resistant alkaline phosphatase in amniotic fluid[c]
        Brock et al., 1984a; Aitken et al., 1985
    decreased percentage of homoarginine-resistant alkaline phosphatase in amniotic fluid[c]
        Brock et al., 1984a; Aitken et al., 1985
    decreased levels of activity of amniotic fluid disaccharidases, maltase, and sucrase[c]
        Kleijer et al., 1985
    fluid contained meconium or the amniotic fluid was green in color[c]
        Allen, 1985
Amniography[c]: cystic hygroma
        Frigoletto et al., 1980
Chorionic villus sampling[g]: 45,X karyotype of chorionic villi
        Nicolaides et al., 1986b; Reuss et al., 1987a; Bovicelli et al., 1988
Echocardiography[c]: coarctation of the aorta
        Allan et al., 1981
Embryoscopy[c,g]: omphalocele
        Cullen et al., 1988
Maternal blood sampling[c]: elevated levels of hCG in maternal serum
        Bogart et al., 1987
Preimplantation embryo biopsy[g]: FISH demonstrated only one X chromosome
        Weier et al., 1993
Ultrasound[c]: hydrops fetalis
        Allan et al., 1981b; Curry et al., 1983; Marchese et al., 1985a; Palmer et al., 1987; Yu and Stephens, 1987; Cosper et al., 1988; Nyberg et al., 1989; Verp et al., 1989b; Bradley et al., 1994; Koeberl et al., 1995
    encephalocele[d]
        Palmer et al., 1987
    ventriculomegaly
        Drugan et al., 1989a
    microcephaly[h]
        Eydoux et al., 1989

cystic hygroma, edema of the head, lower thorax, and/or abdomen
> Leonard et al., 1979; Frigoletto et al., 1980; Tabor et al., 1981; Hunter et al., 1982; Chervenak et al., 1983c; Toftager-Larsen et al., 1983; Redford et al., 1984; Carr et al., 1986; Barsel-Bowers and Abuelo, 1986; Nicolaides et al., 1986a; Palmer et al., 1987; Palumbos et al., 1987

cystic hygroma
> Polanska et al., 1983; Marchese et al., 1985a; Marchese et al., 1985b; Palmer et al., 1987; Chodirker et al., 1988; Cullen et al., 1988; Wladimiroff et al., 1988a; Abramowicz et al., 1989; Eydoux et al., 1989; Hentemann et al., 1989; Nyberg et al., 1989; Verp et al., 1989b; Wolstenholme et al., 1989; Neu et al., 1993; Bradley et al., 1994

> *Comments:* Chodirker and associates (1988) reported on a fetus with Turner syndrome and a large cystic hygroma detected at 16 weeks' gestation. The hygroma resolved with time and was undetectable by 33 weeks, suggesting that normal communication between the jugular vein and lymph sac had been established.

> The diagnosis of Turner syndrome has be made by aspirating fluid from cystic hygromas, and culturing and karyotyping the cells that are within the fluid (Barry et al., 1985; Patil et al., 1987; Al Saadi, 1989).

cystic hygroma with hydrops fetalis[g]
> Abramowicz et al., 1989; Vats et al., 1989; Bradley et al., 1994

symmetrical, smooth-walled, echo-free, cystic structure (cystic hygroma) in the nuchal region; abnormality found at 12 weeks and the diagnosis established by CVS
> Reuss et al., 1987a

multinucleated cystic mass arising from the posterior aspect of the neck
> Spirt et al., 1987

hydrothorax
> Marchese et al., 1985a; Verp et al., 1989b; Nicolaides and Azar, 1990

hypoplastic aortic arch associated with a small left ventricle and dilated right ventricle
> Allan et al., 1981a; Allan et al., 1981b

diaphragmatic hernia[d]
> Palmer et al., 1987

omphalocele
> Eydoux et al., 1989; Nyberg et al., 1989

increased echogenicity of fetal bowel
> Strasberg et al., 1995

ascites
> Allan et al., 1981b; Marchese et al., 1985a; Palmer et al., 1987; Eydoux et al., 1989; Hentemann et al., 1989

male genitalia in fetuses with 45,X/46XY mosaicism
> Wheeler et al., 1988

hydronephrosis
> Marchese et al., 1985a

hexadactyly[d]
>Hentemann et al., 1989
hydramnios[d]
>Palmer et al., 1987
oligohydramnios
>Marchese et al., 1985a; Palmer et al., 1987; Hentemann et al., 1989; Nyberg et al., 1989; Verp et al., 1989b
intrauterine growth retardation
>Wheeler et al., 1988; Hentemann et al., 1989
decreased fetal movement
>Hentemann et al., 1989

45,X/46,XY/47,XYY MOSAICISM

Ultrasound[c,h]: IUGR, oligohydramnios
>Chang et al., 1990

PD 105250 TURNER SYNDROME, ISOCHROMOSOME Xp {46,X,i(Xp)}[b] (McKusick No. None)

Alpha-fetoprotein[c]: elevated in maternal serum
>Koontz et al., 1983
Doppler ultrasound[c]: decreased umbilical arterial blood flow
>Reuwer et al., 1987
Ultrasound[c]: oligohydramnios
>Kontz et al., 1983

PD 105260 TURNER SYNDROME, ISOCHROMOSOME Xq[b] (McKusick No. None)

Alpha-fetoprotein[c]: low levels in maternal serum
>Ben-Yishay et al., 1988

PD 105265 UNIPARENTAL ISODISOMY OF CHROMOSOME 14, PATERNAL {Chromosome 14 uniparental disomy, Paternal; Paternal uniparental disomy, chromosome 14; Paternal UPD, chromosome 14; UPD chromosomal 14, paternal; 45,XX,t(14q14q)}[b] (McKusick No. None)

Ultrasound[c,d]: fetal abdominal distention, hydramnios
>Papenhausen et al., 1995
>*Comments*: In the above case reported by Papenhausen and associates (1995), paternal uniparental isodisomy was shown by absence of maternal VNTR polymorphism and homozygosity of paternal polymorphism using chromosome 14–specific probes. The translocation in the fetus was de novo.

PD 105275 WOLF–HIRSCHHORN SYNDROME {Deletion chromosome 4p;46,XX,del(4)(p14), 46,XX,del(4)(p15); 46,XX,del(4)(p15.3); 46,XY,del(4)(p15); 46,XY,del(4)(p16)}[b] (McKusick No. None)

Ultrasound[c]: cleft lip and palate
>Tachdjian et al., 1992
>structural abnormalities of the kidneys[h,i]
>>Eydoux et al., 1989

hypoplastic kidneys
Tachdjian et al., 1992
left diaphragmatic hernia
Tachdjian et al., 1992
single umbilical artery
Tachdjian et al., 1992
intrauterine growth retardation
Eydoux et al., 1989; Tachdjian et al., 1992; Leonard et al., 1995
oligohydramnios
Leonard et al., 1995
Chorionic villus sampling[g,i]: DNA analysis from chorionic villi indicated absence of maternal alleles for various DNA probes
Goodship et al., 1992
Comments: In the family reported by Goodship and co-authors (1992), the mother carried a submicroscopic balanced translocation between chromosomes 4 and 10 {46,XX,t(4;10) (p16.3;p15)} that gave rise to the deletion in the fetus.

PD 105300 X;Y TRANSLOCATION {46,X,t(X;Y)(p11.2)}[b] (McKusick No. None)

Alpha-fetoprotein[c]: elevated in maternal serum
Roberts et al., 1987

PD 105330 XXYY SYNDROME (48,XXYY syndrome) (McKusick No. None)

Alpha-fetoprotein[c]: slightly elevated levels in maternal serum
Fejgin et al., 1990

PD 105335 45,X MALE (X;Y translocation male; Y; autosome male) (McKusick No. None)

Condition Note: Maleness in this condition comes about by the testis determining factor gene, which is normally present on the short arm of the Y chromosome, being translocated to an autosome or the X chromosome. The remaining portion of the Y chromosome is then lost. This situation then results in a 45,X karyotype. Because the testis determining factor gene is present, normal testes and male genitalia develop. These fetuses may or may not have hydrops fetalis, cystic hygroma, and cardiovascular anomalies that are often seen in fetuses with Turner syndrome.
Abuelo and Barsel-Bowers, 1988
Prenatal Diagnosis: The diagnosis should be suspected in any fetus possessing a 45,X karyotype with male external genitalia. The external genitalia should be evaluated in any fetus determined to have a 45,X chromosomal constitution. Both cytogenetic and DNA probe studies may be necessary to demonstrate the Y-autosome or Y–X translocation.
Differential Diagnosis: Turner syndrome (PD 10500); 45,X/46,XY mosaicism (PD 105000); 46,XX male. In one case, the mosaicism in a 45,X/46,XY fetus was not detected prenatally, and the infant had normal external genitalia at birth.
Abuelo and Barsel-Bowers, 1988
Alpha-fetoprotein[c]: low levels in maternal serum
Abuelo and Barsel-Bowers, 1988

Amniocentesis[c]: 45,X chromosomal constitution on karyotype of amniotic fluid cells
>   Abuelo and Barsel-Bowers, 1988
Ultrasound[c]: normal male external genitalia
>   Abuelo and Barsel-Bowers, 1988

PD 105337 45,X/46,XY PLACENTAL MOSAICISM[b] (McKusick No. None)

Chorionic villus sampling[g]: 45,X karyotype found in chorionic villus cells
>   Leschot et al., 1989
Comments: In the above case reported by Leschot and associates (1989), all nine chorionic villus cells examined had a 45,X chromosome constitution. After the termination of the pregnancy, the fetus was found to have a 46,XY complement. Two biopsies of the placental revealed two chromosomal makeups; one biopsy was 45,X/46,XY and the second was 46,XY.

PD 105340 45,X/48,XYYY/45,X MOSAICISM[b] (McKusick No. None)

Alpha-fetoprotein[c]: low level in maternal serum
>   DiMaio et al., 1988
Comment: The amniotic fluid AFP level was normal in the above case.

PD 105350 46,XX/46,XY CHIMERISM[b] (McKusick No. None)

Amniocentesis: 46,XX/46,XY chimerism from cultured amniotic fluid cells
>   Freiberg et al., 1988; Knops et al., 1989
Comments: The parents declined fetal blood sampling in the case published by Freiberg and associates (1988). In the case of Knops and co-workers (1989), study of parental cytogenetic polymorphisms indicated that the XY cell line was derived from both parents, whereas the XX cell line was of paternal origin. The fetus was delivered at 27 weeks of gestation and was found to have microcephaly, microglossia, omphalocele, enlarged kidneys, and asymmetrical hypertrophic toes. The infant died shortly after birth.
Ultrasound[c]: omphalocele, hydramnios
>   Knops et al., 1989

PD 105400 46,XY/47,XYY MOSAICISM[b] (McKusick No. None)

Alpha-fetoprotein[c]: elevated in maternal serum
>   Wheeler et al., 1987

Chapter 2

Congenital Malformations, Deformations, Disruptions, and Related Disorders[a]

THE CARDIOVASCULAR SYSTEM[a]

General Reference: Davis et al., 1990
General Comments: Congenital heart defects (CHDs) as a group are among the most commonly encountered birth defects. These defects lead to more than half of childhood deaths. The frequency of congenital heart defects is approximately 8 per 1000 pregnancies, of which half are serious. With the technological advances in ultrasonography and the routine evaluation of the fetal heart at the present time, about 50% of serious heart conditions are now being detected prenatally.

In a study published by Davis and associates (1990) of 1924 pregnancies referred for prenatal evaluation, 129 fetuses were found to have structural abnormalities of the heart. Of these 129 fetuses, the most common reason for referral (5%) was a suspected fetal heart abnormality detected on routine ultrasound scan (the four-chamber view). Sixty-nine of the 129 fetuses (53%) were found to have a single defect, while the rest (60, or 47%) had multiple cardiac problems. Chromosomal analyses were done either prenatally or postnatally on 51 of the 129 fetuses. Twenty-seven (53%) of these fetuses had abnormal karyotypes (11 with trisomy 21, 6 with trisomy 18, and 4 with Turner syndrome).

Of the 68 pregnancies that were less than 28 weeks of gestation at the time of diagnosis, 47 (69%) were terminated. Of the 82 pregnancies that were continued, 23 infants (27%) were stillborn, while 59 (72%) were born alive. Only 12 liveborns (16% of the original 129 fetuses, or 34% of those born alive), survived more than 11 months.

In 111 of the 129 fetuses determined to have a CHD, the exact condition was correctly diagnosed in 90 (81%), partially correctly diagnosed in 17 (15%), and incorrectly diagnosed in 4 (4%). On the other hand in the original 1924 pregnancies evaluated, 26 fetal CHDs were not diagnosed. These problems included 15 minor defects and 11 major ones. The sensitivity and specificity of CHDs in this study were 83.6% and 99.9%, respectively; the positive and the negative predictive values were 98.8% and 98.6%, respectively.

PD 106000 AORTA, ENLARGED ASCENDING (McKusick No. None)

Ultrasound[d]: enlarged ascending aorta
Hackeloer, 1979

PD 106250 AORTIC VALVE ATRESIA (McKusick No. None)

Doppler color flow mapping[d]: absence of forward flow in hypoplastic ascending aorta, reverse flow from the ductus arteriosus into a severely hypoplastic ascending aorta in late systole, pansystolic mitral valve regurgitation, absent flow across the foramen ovale
> Gembruch et al., 1990a

Pulsed-wave Doppler insonation: no aortic root signal was recorded
> Silverman et al., 1984
>> mitral regurgitation
>> Gembruch et al., 1990a

Ultrasound: hydrops fetalis with fetal ascites, pleural effusion and subcutaneous edema, absent aortic valve cusps
> Silverman et al., 1984

Comments: In the fetus reported by Silverman and associates (1984), the mitral valve and left ventricle could not be identified and the left atrium was hypoplastic.
> cardiomegaly[c,d]
> Gembruch et al., 1990a

marked dilatation of the left atrium[c,d]
> Gembruch et al., 1990a

hydramnios[c,d]
> Gembruch et al., 1990a

left ventricular hypertrophy with hyperechogenicity of the left ventricular wall
> Gembruch et al., 1990a

hypoplastic mitral valve and aortic annulus
> Gembruch et al., 1990a

hypoplastic ascending aorta
> Silverman et al., 1984; Gembruch et al., 1990a

PD 106350 AORTIC VALVULAR STENOSIS (Valvular aortic stenosis) (McKusick No. None)

Condition Note: Aortic valvular stenosis has multiple etiologies. When stenosis occurs, there is usually an increase in the left ventricular pressure, which in turn may cause left ventricular enlargement, mitral insufficiency, and mitral regurgitation. The latter in turn causes premature closure of the foramen ovale with resulting enlargement of the right atrium. If the heart condition is severe enough, congestive heart failure ensues, hydrops fetalis develops, and death results (Olson et al., 1987).

The term aortic stenosis is used in this catalog to mean immediate preaortic or postaortic valve narrowing. Coarctation of the aorta refers to narrowing elsewhere in the aorta.

Prenatal Diagnosis: The diagnosis should be considered whenever there is either enlargement or hypoplasia of the left ventricle or ascending aorta. Mitral regurgitation, if present, may be detected by Doppler echocardiography; the turbulent flow in the ascending aorta probably cannot be seen by this technique.
> Romero et al., 1988, pp. 175–176

Differential Diagnosis: Other conditions involving the aorta should be considered, including Supravalvar aortic stenosis, Subaortic stenosis, Idiopathic hypertrophic subaortic stenosis (Ventricular hypertrophy, hereditary [PD 117130]) and Coarctation of the aorta (PD 108500).

Doppler color and pulse echocardiography[d]: turbulent blood flow pattern in the dilated ascending aorta behind the aortic valve
Hata et al., 1990

Echocardiography[d]: thickened and abnormal aortic valve, poststenotic dilatation of the ascending aorta
Hata et al., 1990

Magnetic resonance imaging[d]: poststenotic dilatation of the ascending aorta
Hata et al., 1990

Ultrasound[c,d]: aortic valve appeared abnormal and stenotic, postvalvular aortic dilation, hypoplastic aortic valve annulus, enlargement of both ventricular chambers, increased echodensity of the mitral papillary muscles
Huhta et al., 1987a

enlargement of the right and left atria and the left ventricle
Olson et al., 1987

fetal abdominal wall edema, ascites, enlarged placenta, hydrops fetalis, decreased fetal movements, hydramnios, fetal demise
Olson et al., 1987

PD 106750 ARTERIOVENOUS FISTULA, BRAIN (Arteriovenous malformation, brain; AV fistula, brain; Varix of the vein of Galen; Vein of Galen aneurysm) (McKusick No. None)

Condition Note: The vein of Galen is the major venous drainage system of the cerebrum, running from a superior position posteriorly to the thalami, where it joins the inferior sagittal sinus. When aneurysms of the vein of Galen occur, they usually are found in association with cerebral arteriovenous communications of either the carotid or vertebrobasilar systems. The severity of clinical presentations in this condition depends on the size of the aneurysm and the extent of the arteriovenous fistulas. When there is extensive communication, much of the cardiac output (up to 80%) may be diverted through the shunt, which in turn may lead to high-output cardiac failure and death. Associated findings may include hydrocephalus, porencephaly, and nonimmune hydrops fetalis.
Romero et al., 1988, pp. 77–79

Prenatal Diagnosis: The condition should be suspected whenever there is a cyst-like lesion extending posteriorly from above the thalami to the straight sinus. Doppler ultrasound may be helpful in demonstrating increased blood flow in the lesion.

Differential Diagnosis: Arachnoid cyst (PD 118500); Dandy–Walker syndrome (PD 121000); Encephalocele (PD 122000); Iniencephaly (PD 126000)

Ultrasound: well-defined midline cerebral cystic lesions that were nonpulsatile[c,d]
Mao and Adams, 1983

Comments: Postnatal angiography showed that posterior cerebral and pericallosal posterior communicating arteries had formed a fistula with the vein of Galen in the patient reported by Mao and Adams (1983).

midline cystic supratentorial lesion located posterior to the third ventricle but not communicating with it[c]
Mendelsohn et al., 1984

large midline cystic mass that was contiguous with a normal-appearing

lateral ventricle and surrounded by an abnormal heterogeneous zone of increased echogenicity
> Mizejewski et al., 1987

Comments: After the child reported by Mizejewski and co-workers (1987) was born, high-output congestive heart failure developed and she died. At autopsy, there was a vein of Galen aneurysm with a fistula to an unstated artery. The maternal serum alpha-fetoprotein (AFP) was also elevated to 2.3 multiples of median (MOMs). This level of AFP is generally not considered to be significantly elevated above normal, and thus, an elevation in the maternal serum AFP has not been included under this category.

a large interhemispheric cystic mass[c]
> Romero et al., 1988, p. 78

cardiomegaly[c]
> Mendelsohn et al., 1984

PD 106880 ATRIAL BIGEMINAL RHYTHM (McKusick No. None)

Echocardiography: atrial rate twice that of the ventricular rate
> Steinfeld et al., 1986

Gated pulsed Doppler: left ventricular ejection occurred only after every other ventricular contraction; ventricular filling occurred only after each effective ventricular beat
> Steinfeld et al., 1986

Ultrasound[c]: bradycardia
> Steinfeld et al., 1986

PD 106950 ATRIAL FIBRILLATION (McKusick No. None)

External fetal electrocardiogram[d]: irregular rate of 120–160 beats per minute
> Gleicher and Elkayam, 1982b

PD 107000 ATRIAL FLUTTER (McKusick No. None)

Condition Note: Atrial flutter is a cardiac arrhythmia in which the atrial contraction rate is between 200 and 460 per minute, and is regular. Because the ventricles usually are unable to respond to this rapid of an atrial rate, there often is partial atrial-ventricular block with a regular or irregular ventricular rate of between 60 and 200 beats per minute. If the ventricular rate is regular, the antenatal diagnosis of this condition may not be made.
> Shenker, 1979

Auscultation[d]: fetal tachycardia
> Herin and Thoren, 1973; Shenker, 1979; Kleinman et al., 1983

Echocardiography[d]: atrial rate of 220 beats or more per minute
> Kleinman et al., 1980; Crawford, 1982; Kleinman and Santulli, 1983; Mao and Adams, 1983; Agarwala, 1985; Steinfeld et al., 1986

2:1 to 6:1 atrial-ventricular block
> Crawford, 1982; Kleinman and Santulli, 1983; Kleinman et al., 1983; Nagashima et al., 1986

regular fetal heart rate of 320–420 beats per minute
> Blumenthal et al., 1968; Shenker, 1979

2 : 1 to 4 : 1 block with ventricular rates between 104 and 220 beats per minute or ventricular fibrillation
Blumenthal et al., 1968; Herin and Thoren, 1973
Ultrasound[d]: pericardial effusion
Kleinman et al., 1983; Stewart et al., 1983a
hydrops fetalis
Kleinman and Santulli, 1983; Kleinman et al., 1983; Stewart et al., 1983a; Nagashima et al., 1986
fetal ascites
Kleinman et al., 1983; Stewart et al., 1983a; Nagashima et al., 1986
pleural effusion
Nagashima et al., 1986
hydramnios
Kleinman and Santulli, 1983; Kleinman et al., 1983; Stewart et al., 1983a

PD 107500 ATRIAL SEPTAL DEFECT (ASD) (McKusick No. Unknown; see 108800, 108900, 209400)

Echocardiography: no echoes from the atrial septum
Allan et al., 1981a

PD 107600 ATRIAL TACHYCARDIA, TYPE UNSPECIFIED (McKusick No. None)

Condition Note: According to the classification of Wildemeersch and Raven (1975), atrial tachycardia includes all forms of rapid heart action resulting from an increased atrial rate. Included in this category would be atrial fibrillation (PD 106950), atrial flutter (PD 107000), nodal tachycardia, and atrial tachycardia.
Ultrasound[c,d]: very irregular fetal heart rate pattern
Wildemeersch and Raven, 1975
Comments: Wildemeersch and Raven (1975) did not specify which type of atrial tachycardia the fetus they reported had. Postnatally, the atrial rate was between 300 and 400 beats per minute and irregular, while there was a 2 : 1 to a complete ventricular block.

PD 107700 ATRIOVENTRICULAR HEART BLOCK, PARTIAL (AV block, partial) (McKusick No. Unknown; see 140400, 234700)

Electrocardiography[d]: irregular fetal heart rate with a 2 : 1 or 3 : 2 atrioventricular heart block
Komaromy et al., 1977

PD 108000 ATRIOVENTRICULAR CANAL (AV Canal; Complete atrioventricular septal defect) (McKusick No. None)

Echocardiography[d]: large echo-free space above the crest of the interventricular septum
Kleinman et al., 1983
dilated right atrium; bradycardia with complete heart block
Kleinman et al., 1982
defect in the inflow portion of the interventricular septum
Kleinman and Santulli, 1983

single atrioventricular valve leaflet with valve insertion over both ventricles at the same horizontal plane
>Kleinman and Santulli, 1983
Ultrasound[d]: sinus or irregular bradycardia
>Wladimiroff et al., 1988b
hydrops fetalis
>Chiba et al., 1990

PD 108120 ATRIOVENTRICULAR NODE, ABSENCE OF (McKusick No. Unknown; see 140400)

Ultrasound[c,d]: third-degree heart block, right heart dilation
>Wladimiroff et al., 1988b

PD 108250 BRADYCARDIA, SINUS (McKusick No. None)

Condition Note: The normal fetal heart rate is between 120 and 160 beats per minute. The diagnosis of fetal sinus bradycardia is made when the fetal heart rate drops below 100 beats per minute for 1 minute or longer.
>Gleicher and Elkayam, 1982a

Prenatal Diagnosis: Diagnosis is made when the fetal heart rate is below 100 beats per minutes for 1 minute or more. The cause for the bradycardia needs to be sought; in other words bradycardia per se is not a diagnosis.

Differential Diagnosis: See Bradycardia in the Index.

Echocardiography[d]: bradycardia, dilated left atrium and ventricle
>Kleinman et al., 1983
Ultrasound[c,d]: hydramnios, hydrops fetalis
>Kleinman et al., 1983; Stewart et al., 1983a

PD 108300 BRADYCARDIA, SINUS-NODE ARREST WITH JUNCTIONAL BRADYCARDIA (McKusick No. Unknown; see 140400)

Echocardiography[c,d]: bradycardia (50–60 beats per minutes) of both the atria and ventricles with synchronous movements of the atrial wall, atrioventricular valves, and ventricular wall; congestive heart failure
>Minagawa et al., 1987

PD 108400 CARDIAC ARREST (McKusick No. None)

Condition Note: Fetal cardiac arrest has been reported on several occasions in association with various fetal conditions and/or with treatment of these condi-tions. This situation is included here because cardiac resuscitation has been successful in some cases.

Prenatal Diagnosis: The situation is diagnosed by finding no cardiac beat with ultrasound, or no fetal heart beats on fetal electrocardiogram.

Differential Diagnosis: Acardia (PD 182000); Fetal demise (PD 260000)

Prenatal Treatment: Too few cases have been reported to draw any conclusions with regards to efficacy of treatment.

Treatment Modality: Intracardiac injection of epinephrine
>Elliott et al., 1994; Rodeck and Roberts, 1994

Comments: The 20-week fetus reported by Elliott and co-workers (1994) had hydrops fetalis, anemia, and absent spontaneous fetal movements. At the time of cordocentesis, cardiac arrest occurred. Following injection of 50 μg of epinephrine directly into a ventricle, regular systolic activity

resumed almost immediately. However, 12 hours later, after intracardiac blood transfusion had been accomplished, the fetus died. No autopsy was done.
Intracardiac injection of sodium bicarbonate
    Rodeck and Roberts, 1944
Intracardiac exchange transfusion with normal saline[c]
    Rodeck and Roberts, 1994
    Comments: The period of asystole in the situation reported by Rodeck and Roberts (1994) lasted approximately 5 minutes. The episode occurred following an intravascular platelet transfusion at 28 weeks of gestation. A healthy infant was born at 36 weeks who was developing normally at age 2 years.
Methods and Findings: Ultrasound: asystole
    Elliott et al., 1994; Rodeck and Roberts, 1994

PD 108500 COARCTATION, AORTA (McKusick No. Unknown; see 120000)

Condition Note: The term aortic stenosis is used in this catalog as meaning immediate preaortic or postaortic valve narrowing. Coarctation of the aorta refers to narrowing elsewhere in the aorta.
Echocardiography: failure to demonstrate a segment of the aortic arch
    Allan et al., 1981a
Ultrasound[c,d]: enlarged left atrium, right ventricle, and left ventricle; ascites; hydrops fetalis; enlarged homogeneous placenta; hydramnios; fetal demise
    Olson et al., 1987
    Comments: At autopsy the fetus described by Olson and colleagues (1987) was found to have severe aortic stenosis, an incompetent mitral valve, and a nearly closed foramen ovale. In this case the aortic stenosis probably resulted in increased left ventricular end diastolic pressure that led to mitral regurgitation and increased left atrial pressure. The latter would then have produced functional closure of the foramen ovale, right-side overload, heart failure, venous congestion, hydrops, and death.

PD 109000 COMPLETE HEART BLOCK (Complete atrioventricular block) (McKusick No. Unknown; see 234700)

Condition Note: Complete heart block occurs when there is complete atrioventricular block. The condition is well tolerated by the fetus unless the ventricular rate becomes extremely slow or is associated with cardiac defects that result in mitral or tricuspid valve regurgitation. If fetal heart failure occurs, hydrops fetalis may develop. If the failure is severe, the fetus may die. Perinatal mortality even when treated remains in excess of 80%.
    Carpenter et al., 1986
Prenatal Diagnosis: The diagnosis is established by demonstration of complete dissociation of the atrial and ventricular beats detected either by echocardiography or ultrasound.
Differential Diagnosis: Atrioventricular node, absence of (PD 108120); Bilateral left-sidedness sequence (PD 187230); Lupus erythematosus (PD 267450); Sjogren syndrome (PD 198450)
Prenatal Treatment: Terbutaline has been used to increase the fetal ventricular rate. Transuterine transthoracic fetal ventricular pacing has also been successful on a short-term basis.

Treatment Modality: Maternal ingestion of terbutaline
Carpenter et al., 1986
Transuterine transthoracic fetal ventricular pacing
Carpenter et al., 1986
Comments: In the case reported by Carpenter and associates (1986), the method was only effective in increasing the heart rate for a few hours. Problems arose when the leads became detached.
Methods and Findings: Auscultation[d]: fetal bradycardia
Plant and Steven, 1945; Dunn, 1960; Smith et al., 1960; Teteris et al., 1968; Armstrong et al., 1976; Webster et al., 1977; Platt et al., 1979b; Kleinman et al., 1980; Kleinman et al., 1983
Echocardiography[d]: fetal bradycardia
Reid et al., 1979; Kleinman et al., 1983; Abrams et al., 1985a
atrioventricular beat dissociation
Crowley, 1980; Steinfeld et al., 1986
Electrocardiography[d]: fetal bradycardia
Plant and Steven, 1945; Dunn, 1960; Teteris et al., 1968
Phonocardiogram[d]: fetal bradycardia
Armstrong et al., 1976; Webster et al., 1977
Ultrasound: atrioventricular beat dissociation, bradycardia
Armstong et al., 1976; Kleinman et al., 1980; Herreman et al., 1982; Abrams et al., 1985a; Singsen et al., 1985
hydrops fetalis
Altenburger et al., 1977; Abrams et al., 1985a
"halo" around the fetal head
Altenburger et al., 1977
thickened placenta; scalp and skin edema, pericardial and pleural effusions, massive ascites
Abrams et al., 1985a
Method not stated[c,d]: fetal bradycardia
Altenburger et al., 1977

PD 109100 CONGENITAL INTRAVENTRICULAR TRIFASCICULAR BLOCK (McKusick No. None; see 113900)

Condition Note: Congenital intraventricular trifascicular block differs from the usual form of congenital heart block in that there is complete or intermittent block, or hemiblock of the right bundle-branch, or the left anterior and posterior bundles.
Chan et al., 1973
Prenatal Diagnosis: Not established.
Differential Diagnosis: Complete heart block (PD 109000) and other causes of fetal bradycardia (see Bradycardia in the Index).
Auscultation[c,d]: transient period of fetal bradycardia of about 40 beats per minute
Chan et al., 1973

PD 109250 DUCTUS ARTERIOSUS, CONSTRICTION OF (McKusick No. None)

Condition Note: Constriction of the ductus arteriosus during fetal life will produce pulmonary hypertension in the fetus. The administration of prostaglandin inhibitors in late gestation has been associated with persistent neonatal pulmonary hypertension. With the advent of Doppler echocardiography, it has been possible to assess the flow velocities in the fetal ductus, to detect ductal constrictions, and to determine pressure gradients across the ductus.

Huhta et al., 1987b

Prenatal Diagnosis: The systolic flow velocity through the fetal ductus arteriosus is the highest detectable velocity in the normal fetal cardiovascular system, and ranges from 50 to 140 cm/sec with a mean of 80 cm/sec. In constriction of the ductus, velocities normally exceed these upper limits as determined by Doppler echocardiographic studies.

Huhta et al., 1987b

Doppler echocardiograph[d]: increased systolic and diastolic velocities across the ductus arteriosus

Huhta et al., 1987b

Comments: Constriction of the ductus arteriosus was inducted in three fetuses when indomethacin was taken by their mothers. The changes disappeared after withdrawal of the drug (Huhta et al., 1987b).

PD 109260 DUCTUS VENOSUS, ABSENCE OF (McKusick No. None)

Condition Note: During embryonic and fetal life, the ductus venosus connects the umbilical vein to the inferior vena cava allowing blood to bypass the liver. Postnatally, this structure is no longer functional and becomes obliterated to form the ligamentum venosum. Absence of the ductus venosus prenatally means that the blood from the umbilical vein circulates through the liver or elsewhere, and as reported by Jorgensen and Andolf (1994), may lead to medical problems for the fetus. The pathogenesis of these medical problems may be related to aberrant oxygenation caused by the abnormal circulation.

Jorgensen and Andolf, 1994

Maternal Report[c]: no observed, or poor or no perceived fetal movements

Jorgensen and Andolf, 1994

Ultrasound[c]: hydrothorax, hydrops fetalis, fetal demise, hydramnios

Jorgensen and Andolf, 1994

Comments: Four fetuses with absence of the ductus venosus were reported by Jorgenson and Andolf (1994). Two were sibs (sex not stated) both of whom had absent ductus venosus, pulmonary hypoplasia, hypoplastic heart, hydrothorax, and hydrops fetalis at autopsy. The third fetus, who was unrelated to the first two, had the same findings plus a cystic hygroma. The fourth case had other multiple congenital anomalies and is listed under Microcephaly–arthrogryposis–absent ductus venosus (PD 355000).

PD 109500 EBSTEIN ANOMALY (McKusick No. Unknown; see 224700)

Echocardiography: tricuspid valve displacement, right atrial enlargement, pulmonary valve atresia, supraventricular tachycardia

Allan et al., 1982; Sharf et al., 1983

Ultrasound[d]: cardiomegaly

Sharf et al., 1983

PD 109600 ECTOPIA CORDIS (Ectopic heart; Cantrell's pentalogy; Pentalogy of Cantrell) (McKusick No. None)

PENTALOGY OF CANTRELL

Maternal history[c,d]: decreased fetal movement

Haynor et al., 1984

Ultrasound[d]: fetal heart, liver, and intestine identified outside the anterior chest and abdominal wall, membrane covering ectopic structures
> Mercer et al., 1983; Seeds et al., 1984; Spirt et al., 1987

beating heart outside of fetal chest[d]
> Haynor et al., 1984

omphalocele, ascites
> Spirt et al., 1987

multiple loops of bowel protruding outside of the fetus[d]
> Haynor et al., 1984

hydramnios[c,d]
> Haynor et al., 1984

ISOLATED ECTOPIA CORDIS

Ultrasound: pulsating fetal heart adjacent to the fetal face and exterior to the fetal chest[h]
> Hill et al., 1988b

beating extrathoracic heart[c]
> Haynor et al., 1984

hydramnios[c,d]
> Haynor et al., 1984

> *Comment:* The fetus reported by Haynor and associates (1984) also had craniofacial abnormalities though to be secondary to amniotic bands.

PD 109650 ECTOPIC BEAT (Bigeminal beats; Fetal ectopic beat; Premature atrial contraction; Trigenimal beats; Premature ventricular contraction) (McKusick No. None; see 115080)

Condition Note: The finding of ectopic beats is apparently benign because it is not usually associated with structural or functional cardiac abnormalities (Steinfeld et al., 1986).

Auscultation[c,d]: fetal cardiac irregularities
> Webster et al., 1977; Sugarman et al., 1978

bradycardia
> Webster et al., 1977

bigeminal beats
> Komaromy et al., 1977

trigeminal beats
> Komaromy et al., 1977

Echocardiography: recurrent and isolated atrial or ventricular ectopic beats
> Komaromy et al., 1977; Steinfeld et al., 1986

bigeminal beats
> Komaromy et al., 1977

trigeminal beats
> Komaromy et al., 1977

PD 109700 ENDOCARDIAL FIBROELASTOSIS (EFE) (McKusick No. Unknown; see 226000, 305300)

Condition Note: Endocardial fibroelastosis is characterized by diffuse thickening of the left ventricular endocardium. The condition may be familial in some cases. The pathogenetic mechanism producing the thickened endocardium is not known. Endocardial fibroelastosis occurs in about 1% of all congenital heart diseases. Clinically, the chief manifestation is heart failure. Treatment is directed toward treating this latter problem. The prognosis for an affected fetus is poor with most dying in utero or during infancy.

Aortic stenosis, coarctation of the aorta, and anomalous origin of the left coronary artery from the left trunk may be found in association with this condition.

Ben-Ami et al., 1986; Achiron et al., 1988

Prenatal Diagnosis: This condition should be suspected when the following abnormalities are found: ventricular diameters twice normal size; signs of congestive heart failure, such as pericardial effusion, pleural effusion, and ascites; an increased echogenic endocardial surface; and lack of congenital heart disease of the left obstructive type, such as aortic stenosis or coarctation of the aorta.

Ben-Ami et al., 1986

Differential Diagnosis: Isolated aortic valve stenosis (PD 106350); Hypoplastic left ventricle (PD 110500); Coarctation of the aorta (PD 108500); Congestive cardiomyopathy; Glycogen storage disease of the heart; Myocarditis

Echocardiography[c,d]: dilated left atrium, hypoplastic aortic root

Allan et al., 1981a

very echodense left ventricular myocardium, decreased contractility of both ventricles

Wiggins et al., 1986

Ultrasound: dilated right and left ventricles,[d] thickened endocardium,[d] hydrothorax,[d] oligohydramnios,[d] growth deficiency[d]

Bovicelli et al., 1984; Wiggins et al., 1986

enlarged heart[c]

Ben-Ami et al., 1986; Achiron et al., 1988

enlarged and globular left ventricle

Achiron et al., 1988

endocardial surface of the left ventricle very echogenic[d]

Ben-Ami et al., 1986

pericardial effusion[c]

Achiron et al. 1988

reduced motion of the left ventricular wall[c]

Achiron et al., 1988

mitral and tricuspid valvular thickening[d]

Ben-Ami et al., 1986

thickened and irregular left ventricular endocardium[c]

Achiron et al., 1988

interventricular septum thickened[d]

Ben-Ami et al., 1986

aortic valve stenosis[c]

Allan et al., 1981a; Achiron et al., 1988

ascites[c]

Ben-Ami et al., 1986; Achiron et al., 1988

hydrops fetalis[c]

Bovicelli et al., 1984; Wiggins et al., 1986; Chiba et al., 1990

hydramnios[c]

Ben-Ami et al., 1986; Wiggins et al., 1986; Achiron et al., 1988

PD 109720 FETAL AKINESIA/HYPOKINESIA SEQUENCE SECONDARY TO TWIN-TO-TWIN ANASTOMESES (McKusick No. None)

Ultrasound: monochorionic, diamniotic twins with a shared placenta[c]
> Perlman et al., 1995
>> cerebellar hypoplasia, fixed flexion of the upper extremities, fixed hyperextension of lower extremities, club feet, fisting, no fetal movements, no fetal breathing, intrauterine growth retardation (IUGR)
>>> Perlman et al., 1995
>>> *Comments*: Both twins reported by Perlman and associates (1995) had fetal akinesia/hypokinesia sequence at birth, and subsequently died. Autopsy revealed vascular anastomoses on the surface of the placenta, marked atrophy of both brains and long-standing cystic encephalomalacia, the latter of which was not detected prenatally. The authors postulated that an ischemic event secondary to the placental anastomoses caused the encephalomalacia that in turn lead to the fetal akinesia.

PD 109750 FETOMATERNAL TRANSFUSION (Fetomaternal hemorrhage) (McKusick No. None)

Condition Note: Fetal blood that passes into the maternal circulation from whatever cause is considered to be a fetomaternal transfusion. The three methods used to determine the presence of fetal blood in the maternal blood include the Kleihauer–Betke test, elevated levels of AFP in the maternal serum, and direct quantification of fetal hemoglobin (HbF). The latter test appears to be the most sensitive. Alpha-fetoprotein levels, at least following chorionic villus sampling (CVS), do not correlate well with the other two tests (Clark and Bissonnette, 1989).

Fetomaternal transfusions appear to be common following CVS. This notion comes from the work of Clark and Bissonnette (1989), who report that 78% of women who underwent CVS had HbF in their blood following the procedure.

Prenatal Diagnosis: The detection of fetal red blood cells in the maternal blood by the Kleihauer–Betke test, or the detection of HbF in the maternal blood by direct quantification of HbF levels appear to be adequate for making the diagnosis.

Differential Diagnosis: Fetomaternal transfusion, massive (PD 109775); Fetomaternal transfusion, massive, chronic, and bidirectional (PD 109800); Umbilical vein thrombosis (PD 271970)

> Maternal blood sampling followed by direct quantification of HbF as determined by radioimmunodiffusion[g]: elevated levels in maternal blood following CVS
>> Clark and Bissonnnette, 1989

PD 109775 FETOMATERNAL TRANSFUSION, MASSIVE (Fetomaternal hemorrhage, massive) (McKusick No. None)

Condition Note: During the second and third trimesters, a small fetomaternal transfusion (blood entering the maternal circulation) is relatively common in uncomplicated pregnancies (8% second and 12% third trimesters). Massive fetomaternal hemorrhage, defined as greater than 150 mL fetal blood transferred, is less common, and may be associated with unexpected fetal demise. If the hemorrhage is of a chronic nature, nonimmune hydrops fetalis secondary to fetal anemia and heart failure may occur.

Elliott, 1991

Prenatal Diagnosis: By the use of the Kleihauer–Betke test, demonstration of more than 150 mL of fetal blood transfused into the maternal circulation. Decreased fetal movements and a sinusoidal fetal heart rate pattern are also associated with this condition.

Elliot, 1991

Differential Diagnosis: Fetomaternal transfusion (PD 109750); Fetomaternal transfusion, massive, chronic, and bideirectional (PD 109800); Umbilical vein thrombosis (PD 271970)

Treatment Modality: Intravascular transfusion by cordocentosis

Elliott, 1991

Comments: In both fetuses reported by Elliott (1991), bradycardia developed within 5 minutes of the transfusion and both were delivered by emergency cesarean sections. The infants survived, with the second one having moderate to severe hearing loss.

Methods and Findings: Cordocentesis (percutaneous umbilical blood sampling, or PUBS)[c]: severe anemia

Elliott, 1991

Comments: The fetuses reported by Elliott (1991) had hemoglobins and hematocrits of 3.7 g/dL and 2.4 g/dL, and 12.1% and 7%, respectively.

Continuous wave Doppler: no umbilical flow velocity wave form

Ash et al., 1988

Comments: Following transplacental cordocentesis, fetal heart rate of the fetus reported by Ash and co-authors (1988) dropped to 50 beats per minute with no indication of intraamniotic hemorrhage, or cord or retroplacental hematoma; the umbilical cord appeared uniformly echogenic; umbilical veins and arteries appeared empty; and there were weak-appearing contractility and empty appearance of the heart.

Ash et al., 1988

Fetal electrocardiography[c]: sinusoidal fetal heart rate

Elliott, 1991

late decelerations

Elliott, 1991

Maternal blood sampling: Kleihauer–Betke test indicated massive fetal transfusion

Ash et al., 1988; Elliott, 1991

strongly positive Coombs reaction

Ash et al., 1988

Maternal perception[c]: decreased or no fetal movement

Ash et al., 1988; Elliott, 1991

Ultrasound[c]: no respiratory effort

Elliott, 1991

PD 109800 FETOMATERNAL TRANSFUSION, MASSIVE, CHRONIC, AND BIDIRECTIONAL (Transplacental hemorrhage, massive, chronic, and bidirectional) (McKusick No. None)

Condition Note: Massive fetal-to-maternal transplacental hemorrhage is probably rare. When present on a long-term basis, severe progressive anemia, extreme hepatic erythropoiesis, portal hypertension, ascites, hepatocellular damage, hypoalbuminemia, and hydrops fetalis may develop in the fetus. Occasionally, the bleeding is bidirectional and the fetus is not anemic but may experience congestive heart failure with resulting hepatomegaly and hydrops fetalis.

Bowman et al., 1984

Prenatal Diagnosis: This condition should be considered whenever hydrops fetalis is detected. A relatively high percentage of circulating fetal red cells in the maternal circulation is positive evidence for the diagnosis.

Differential Diagnosis: Other conditions associated with hydrops fetalis (see the Index, under Hydrops fetalis). Fetomaternal transfusion (PD 109750); Fetomaternal transfusion, massive (PD 109775); Umbilical vein thrombosis (PD 271970)

Ultrasound[d]: ascites, hepatosplenomegaly, placental edema, hydrops fetalis

Bowman et al., 1984

Maternal blood sampling[d]: 5.4% of the maternal circulating red blood cells were of fetal origin as determined by the Kleihauer acid elution test (Kleihauer–Betke test)

Bowman et al., 1984

Comments: The above fetus was delivered by cesarean section at 32 weeks' gestation. She was plethoric and cyanotic, and required immediate intubation and positive-pressure ventilation with 100% oxygen. Initial hemoglobin concentration and hematocrit were 20.5 g/dL and 63%, respectively. Normal total serum protein and albumin concentrations from cord and preexchange blood samples were within normal limits (5.8 g/dL and 3.3 g/dL, respectively). Ninety percent of the red cells in cord and preexchange transfusion blood sampled were Kleihaur–Betke negative, indicating a maternal origin for these cells.

The neonate was given a total-blood-volume exchange transfusion, treated with digoxin and furosemide, and maintained on positive-pressure ventilation. She responded rapidly and has been a healthy child on follow-up.

PD 109850 FORAMEN OVALE, PREMATURE CLOSURE (Parachute mitral valve) (McKusick No. None)

Auscultation[c,d]: fetal tachycardia

Buis-Liem et al., 1987

Echocardiography[d]: hydrops fetalis, absent foramen ovale, thickened interatrial septum that bulged toward the right atrium, cardiomegaly, pericardial effusion, irregular movements of the atrioventricular valves, hydramnios, ascites

Pesonen et al., 1983

atrial flutter with ventricular rates of more than 400 beats per minute

Buis-Liem et al., 1987

Ultrasound[c,d]: dilation of the right heart, obstructed foramen ovale detected by 36 weeks' gestation

Buis-Liem et al., 1987

PD 110500 HYPOPLASTIC LEFT VENTRICLE (McKusick No. 241550)

Echocardiography[d]: pericardial and pleural effusion, hypoplastic left ventricle, dilated right ventricle

DeVore et al., 1982b

Comment: The above fetus was found to have trisomy 13 after birth.

Ultrasound[c]: hydrops fetalis
>Chiba et al., 1990

External fetal monitoring[c,d]: alternating episodes of mild tachycardia and bradycardia
>Katz et al., 1986a

PD 111000 HYPOPLASTIC RIGHT VENTRICLE (McKusick No. 277200)

Echocardiography[d]: small right ventricular cavity, thickened ventricular wall, larger than normal left ventricular cavity, hydrops fetalis
>Kleinman and Santulli, 1983

PD 111500 ILIOFEMORAL ARTERIAL THROMBOSIS (McKusick No. None)

Ultrasound[h]: hydrops fetalis
>Curry et al., 1983

PD 111750 PAROXYSMAL ATRIAL TACHYCARDIA (Bouver syndrome) (McKusick No. None; see 108950)

Condition Note: This disorder is marked by atrial tachycardia with sudden onset and equally rapid cessation.

Auscultation[d]: heart rates of 240–250 beats per minutes with spontaneous conversion to 150 beats per minute
>Silber and Durnin, 1969; Hedvall, 1973; Herin and Thoren, 1973

PD 112000 PERICARDIAL EFFUSION (McKusick No. Unknown; see 260900)

Condition Note: Pericardial effusion is excessive fluid accumulation within the pericardial sac. It has been found in a number of fetal conditions (see Pericardial effusion in the Index). If the fluid collection is extensive enough, venous return to the heart may be compromised, and hydrops fetalis will ensue.

Prenatal Diagnosis: The detection of excessive pericardial fluid or fluid surrounding the heart is sufficient evidence to make the diagnosis. Cardiac and other malformations, prenatal infections, fetal anemia, cardiac tumors, and fetal chromosomal problems need to be ruled out.

Prenatal Treatment: Treatment of the underlying problem producing the pericardial effusion, such as fetal transfusion when fetal anemia is present, may be the most effective treatment modality. Pericardioamniotic shunting has also been effective.

Treatment Modality: Pericardioamniotic shunting
>Nicolaides and Azar, 1990

Pericardiocentesis
>Nicolaides and Azar, 1990

>*Comments:* In the case reported by Nicolaides and Azar (1990), pericardiocentesis was effective in removing the excessive pericardial fluid. However, the fluid reaccumulated and the problem was treated with a pericardioamniotic shunt which apparently prevented reaccumulation of fluid. A healthy neonate was born at term. No cause for the pericardial fluid accumulation was found after postnatal investigation.

Methods and Findings: Ultrasound: cystic mass surrounding the fetal heart
>Morgan et al., 1978; Nicolaides and Azar, 1990

compression of both lungs due to a large pericardial effusion
Nicolaides and Azar, 1990

PD 112100 PREMATURE ATRIAL CONTRACTION (Atrial premature beats; PAC; Premature atrial beat; Premature atrial contracture) (McKusick No. None)

Auscultation[c,d]: irregular fetal heart rate varying from 120 to 160 beats per minute
Itskovitz et al., 1979
Ultrasound[c,d]: irregular fetal heart rate varying between 110 and 170 beats per minute
Itskovitz et al., 1979

PD 112150 PREMATURE VENTRICULAR CONTRACTION, BENIGN (Premature ventricular beat, benign) (McKusick No. None)

Condition Note: Occasionally with fetal electrocardiogram (ECG) recordings, premature ventricular contractions are seen which appear to be benign in nature. These contractures seem to be benign because when the child is born, there are normally no cardiac problems.
Nielsen and Moestrup, 1968
Prenatal Diagnosis: Detection of premature beats on occasion by fetal ECG.
Differential Diagnosis: Ectopic beat (PD 109650); Premature atrial contracture (PD 112100); Rhabdomyoma, heart (PD 280500)
Auscultation[c,d]: irregular heart sound with the loss of approximately every fourth beat
Nielsen and Moestrup, 1968
Fetal electrocardiogram: premature ventricular contractions
Nielsen and Moestrup, 1968

PD 112250 PULMONARY STENOSIS (McKusick No. Unknown; see 265500)

Ultrasound[c,d]: sinus bradycardia
Wladimiroff et al., 1988b

PD 112380 PULMONARY-VALVE ATRESIA (Absent pulmonary valve syndrome) (McKusick No. None)

Condition Note: Pulmonary-valve atresia is the congenital lack of development and patency of the pulmonary valve. When pulmonary-valve atresia occurs with a ventricular septal defect, the prognosis may be good. When there is an intact ventricular septum, the prognosis is usually poor. In the latter situation, when the right atrium and ventricle are enlarged, there may be compression of the fetal lung, which may further compromise the chance for survival.
Prenatal Diagnosis: The diagnosis should be considered whenever there is enlargement of the right atrium and ventricle and the tricuspid valve is normal. Further evidence for the diagnosis is the lack of blood flow through the pulmonary artery on Doppler studies.
Differential Diagnosis: Ebstein anomaly (PD 109500); Pulmonary stenosis (PD 112250); Tricuspid atresia (PD 115000)
Alpha-fetoprotein[c,h]: elevated in maternal serum
Hajdu et al., 1995

Doppler flow studies: no forward blood flow through the pulmonary artery, tricuspid regurgitation
Allan et al., 1986
Echocardiography: lack of opening of the pulmonary valve or membrane or dense echo where the main pulmonary artery and pulmonary valve should have been, smaller-than-normal diameter of the pulmonary artery, heart occupying more than half of the fetal thorax
Allan et al., 1986
right atrial and right ventricular enlargement
Kleinman et al., 1982; Allan et al., 1986
displaced ascending aorta[c,d]
Kleinman et al., 1982
hydrops fetalis
Chiba et al., 1990
Ultrasound[c]: cardiac enlargement, hydrops fetal
Allan et al., 1986
hydramnios, placental edema[d]
Kleinman et al., 1982

PD 112360 SICK SINUS SYNDROME (McKusick No. None)
Ultrasound[c,d]: irregular bradycardia
Wladimiroff et al., 1988b

PD 112500 SUPRAVENTRICULAR ECTOPIC BEATS (McKusick No. None)

Auscultation[c,d]: arrhythmia
Kleinman et al., 1983
Echocardiography[d]: arrhythmia
Kleinman et al., 1983
Ultrasound[d]: arrhythmia
Stewart et al., 1983a

PD 113000 TACHYCARDIA, SUPRAVENTRICULAR (Supraventricular tachycardia) (McKusick No. None)

Condition Note: Fetal tachycardia is relatively common, occurring in an estimated 0.4 to 0.6% of all pregnancies. The most common of the fetal tachycardias is supraventricular tachycardia (SVT). The latter condition is part of a group of disorders called supraventricular tachyarrhythmias that includes SVT, paroxysmal atrial tachycardia, atrial flutter, and atrial fibrillation. This group of disorders is characterized by atrial frequencies of 180–400 beats per minute, and atrial to ventricular conduction of 1:1 to 1:2 (Romero et al., 1988). Fetal heart rates of 200–240 beats per minute are common in SVT. When the fetal tachycardia is sustained, congestive heart failure may develop in the fetus (Killeen and Bowers, 1987), and if prolonged enough may lead to hydrops fetalis and fetal death (Hallak et al, 1991). The normal fetal heart rate is between 120 and 160 beats per minute (Gleicher and Elkayam, 1982a).

Prenatal Diagnosis: The diagnosis is indicated when there is sustained SVT of 180 beats per minute or greater, with synchronous auricular and ventricular contractions in an anatomically normal heart.

Differential Diagnosis: See Tachycardia in the Index.

Prenatal Treatment: Although a variety of antidysrhythmic agents have been used for the treatment of supraventricular tachycardia, digoxin has been the one most commonly selected (Hallak et al., 1991). Several articles, however, have been published reporting decreased or minimal transplacental transfer of digoxin when the drug has been administered to the mother, and as a result, little or no therapeutic effect to the fetus has occurred. In these cases, digoxin may be given to the fetus intramuscularly or other agents utilized with success (Hallak et al., 1991).

Treatment Modality: Maternal medications
> digoxin
>> Kerenyi et al., 1980; Kovats-Szabo et al., 1990; Hallak et al., 1991
>> *Comments:* For the patient reported by Hallak and co-workers (1991), treatment with digoxin was started intravenously (loading dose 0.5 mg every 6 hours for 24 hours) and followed by an oral route (1.5–2.25 mg/d). After 2 weeks of oral digoxin treatment, the maternal digoxin level was 2.5 ng/mL, while umbilical venous level at the same time was 0.5 ng/mL. At this fetal level, the fetus was in sunus rhythm only half the time. Subsequently, procainamide was administered to the mother. The sinus rhythm increased to 90% with eventual resolution of the hydrops fetalis present in the fetus.
> procainamide, 1 g every 4 hours, orally
>> Hallak et al., 1991
> propranol
>> Kovats-Szabo et al., 1990

Intramuscular fetal injections of digoxin (20 μg in 3 divided doses over 24 hours based on a neonatal loading dose of 10–20 μg/kg body weight)
> Hallak et al., 1991
> *Comments:* Hallak and associates (1991) selected this route of administration because they suspected poor placental transfer of digoxin, and because the fetus was in precarious physical condition.

Methods and Findings: Alpha-fetoprotein[c,d]: elevated level in amniotic fluid
> Kerenyi et al., 1980

Auscultation[d]: fetal tachycardia
> Hedvall, 1973; Newburger and Keane, 1979; Chitkara et al., 1980;
> Dumesic et al., 1982; Kleinman et al., 1983; Buis-Liem et al., 1987

Echocardiography[d]: supraventricular flutter
> Ramzin and Napflin, 1982; Steinfeld et al., 1986; Buis-Liem et al., 1987
> supraventricular tachycardia
>> Kerenyi et al., 1980; Nagashima et al., 1986; Kovats-Szabo et al., 1990; Hallak et al., 1991
> paroxysmal tachycardia
>> DeVore et al., 1982b; Agarwala, 1985
> paradoxical ventricular wall movement
>> DeVore et al., 1982b
> supraventricular tachycardia of 240 beats per minute or greater with synchronous auricular and ventricular contractions in an anatomically normal heart
>> Dumesic et al., 1982; Rey et al., 1985; Steinfeld et al., 1986; Killeen and Bowers, 1987; Hallak et al., 1991

fetal heart failure manifesting by enlarged left atrium
>   Gleicher and Elkayam, 1982b

Electrocardiography: 2:1 block with ventricular rates up to 230 beats per minute
>   Herin and Thoren, 1973

Maternal history: decrease in fetal movements as perceived by the mother
>   Kerenyi et al., 1980; Nagashima et al., 1986; Hallak et al., 1991

Ultrasound[c,d]: fetal hydrops
>   Newburger and Keane, 1979; Kerenyi et al., 1980; Crawford, 1982; Ramzin and Napflin, 1982; Campbell and Pearce, 1983; Kleinman and Santulli, 1983; Kleinman et al., 1983; Stewart et al., 1983a; Wester et al., 1984; Dennis et al., 1985; Guntheroth et al., 1985; Rey et al., 1985; Nagashima et al., 1986; Rein et al., 1986; Wiggins et al., 1986; Kovats-Szabo et al., 1990; Hallak et al; 1991

scalp edema
>   Chitkara et al., 1980; Kerenyi et al., 1980

enlarged heart
>   Chitkara et al., 1980

fetal heart rate over 200 beats per minute
>   Chitkara et al., 1980; Kerenyi et al., 1980; Dennis et al., 1985; Guntheroth et al., 1985; Nagashima et al. 1986; Rein et al., 1986; Wiggins et al., 1986; Killeen and Bowers, 1987

obstruction of the foramen ovale with dilation of right atrium
>   Buis-Liem et al., 1987

enlarged left atrium
>   Kerenyi et al., 1980

congestive heart failure with enlargement of the cardiac chambers and inadequate heart contractility
>   Bertrand et al., 1986

pericardial effusion
>   DeVore et al., 1982b

pleural effusion
>   Guntheroth et al., 1985; Rey et al., 1985; Nagashima et al., 1986; Kovats-Szabo et al., 1990

fetal ascites
>   Chitkara et al, 1980; Kerenyi et al., 1980; Crawford, 1982; Ramzin and Napflin, 1982; Dennis et al., 1985; Guntheroth et al., 1985; Rey et al., 1985; Bertrand et al., 1986; Nagashima et al., 1986; Rein et al., 1986; Wiggins et al., 1986; Kovats-Szabo et al., 1990

hepatomegaly
>   Rein et al., 1986

hydramnios
>   Chitkara et al., 1980; Kerenyi et al., 1980; Kleinman et al., 1983; Stewart et al., 1983a; Dennis et al., 1985

thickened placenta, placental edema
>   Guntheroth et al., 1985; Bertrand et al., 1986

marked edema of the umbilical cord
>   Guntheroth et al., 1985; Rein et al., 1986

biophysical profile 2 out of 10
Hallak et al., 1991

PD 114000 TETRALOGY OF FALLOT (McKusick No. 187500)

Alpha-fetoprotein[c,d]: elevated in amniotic fluid
Seppala, 1975
Doppler flow analysis[c,d]: turbulent flow, to-and-fro pattern of blood in the dilated right ventricle outflow area through the pulmonary trunk
Sameshima et al., 1993
Echocardiography[d]: chaotic rhythm
Kleinman et al., 1982; Kleinman et al., 1983
single ventricle, hypoplastic left atrium and atrioventricular valve, oligo-hydramnios, IUGR
Stewart et al., 1983b
enlarged right ventricle
Sameshima et al., 1993
ventricular septal defect
Sameshima et al., 1993
overriding of the aorta
Sameshima et al., 1993
aneurysmal dilatation of the pulmonary artery and both branches
Sameshima et al., 1993
absence of the pulmonary valves
Sameshima et al., 1993
no visualization of the ductus arteriosus
Sameshima et al., 1993
Ultrasound[c,d]: hydrops fetalis
Kleinman et al., 1982; Kleinman et al., 1983; Sameshima et al., 1993
no stomach echo
Sameshima et al., 1993
intrauterine growth retardation
Stewart et al., 1983b
hydramnios
Kleinman et al., 1982; Kleinman et al., 1983; Sameshima et al., 1993
oligohydramnios
Stewart et al., 1983b
Method not stated[c,d]: fetal tachycardia
Pearl, 1977

PD 114500 TOTAL ANOMALOUS PULMONARY VENOUS RETURN
(Anomalous pulmonary venous return) (McKusick No. 106700)

Alpha-fetoprotein[c,h]: decreased in maternal serum
Hajdu et al., 1995

PD 114700 TRANSPOSITION OF THE GREAT VESSELS (TGV) (McKusick No. None)

Alpha-fetoprotein[c,h]: elevated in maternal serum
Hajdu et al., 1995

PD 115000 TRICUSPID ATRESIA (McKusick No. None)

Alpha-fetoprotein[c,h]: decreased levels in maternal serum
  Hajdu et al., 1995
Echocardiography[d]
  DeVore and Hobbins, 1979

PD 115100 TRICUSPID INCOMPETENCE (McKusick No. None)

Ultrasound[c,d]: cardiomegaly, cardiothoracic ratio decreased (51/91), enlarged atrium, no identifiable atrial septum
  Brown et al., 1986
  Comments: The fetus reported by Brown and associates (1986) was born alive at term with no congenital defects other than those in the heart. A cardiac catheterization demonstrated severe tricuspid regurgitation. At autopsy the tricuspid valve was dysplastic and incompetent with enlargement of the right side of the heart. No other defects were found.

PD 115250 TRUNCUS ARTERIOSUS, PERSISTENT (McKusick No. None)

Ultrasound: ventricular septal defect[c], single umbilical artery[c], IUGR[c]
  Herrmann and Sidiropoulos, 1988
  hydrops fetalis [c,d]
  Aughton et al., 1990
  Comments: In the report by Aughton and colleagues (1990), twins were diagnosed at 15 weeks by ultrasound. By 31 weeks of gestation, hydrops fetalis had developed in both twins; it was thought not to be due to infection or immunologic problems. At birth, both female twins were hydropic, had a systolic murmur, and were in congestive heart failure. Subsequent evaluation revealed that both neonates had isolated persistent truncus arteriosus. The first twin underwent successful cardiac repair and was doing well; the other twin died while undergoing cardiac catheterization. They were dizygotic twins.

PD 115500 TWIN TRANSFUSION SYNDROME (Fetofetal transfusion syndrome; Twin-to-twin transfusion) (McKusick No. None)

Syndrome Note: When monozygotic twins share a common placenta, arteriovenous anastomoses frequently develop and blood may be pumped from one twin (donor) to the co-twin (recipient). This situation may lead to hypervolemia, hypertrophy of the heart, heart failure, excessive urination resulting in hydramnios, and hydropic changes indicated by scalp edema, pleural and pericardial effusions, and ascites in the recipient twin. As a result of pumping to the recipient twin, the donor twin may develop anemia, growth failure, and oligohydramnios. The size of the shunt directly determines the severity of the condition, the disparity of growth between the twins, and the amniotic fluid volume in each sac. The mortality rate in this condition can be as high as 70%.
  Brennan et al., 1982; Feingold et al., 1986
Prenatal Diagnosis: The ultrasound criteria for the prenatal diagnosis of this condition have been delineated by Brennan and associates (1982) and include: (1) significant disparity in size of like-sexed twins; (2) disparity in size between the two amniotic sacs; (3) two separate umbilical cords with significant differences in the size or number of vessels; (4) a single placenta with areas of disparity in echogenicity of the cotyledons supplying the two cords; and (5) evidence of

hydrops in either fetus, or finding of congestive cardiac failure in the recipient twin. Urig and his associates (1990) used the combination of severely discordant growth of the twins, acute hydramnios in the larger twin, and profound oligohydramnios in the undergrown twin as their criteria for diagnosis.

Differential Diagnosis: Acardia (PD 182000); Conjoined twins (PD 255000)

Prenatal Treatment: When the diagnosis of twin transfusion syndrome is clearly established, the parents have several options. First, they can continue the pregnancy to determine the natural progress of the condition, which usually leads to death of both twins. Second, they can elect termination of the pregnancy or early induction of labor. Last, they may select feticide by clipping, clamping, or ligation of the umbilical cord of the donor twin, by delivery of one fetus via a hysterotomy (sectio parva), or by inducing cardiac arrest in the donor twin using one of several methods. The selection of the most appropriate options will need to be made by the parents and the medical team involved with the case (Wittmann et al., 1986). Urig and associates (1990) and Mahony and co-workers (1990) have shown that aggressive and repeated amniocenteses removing 1–5-1/2 liters of fluid each time from the twin with hydramnios leads to a 60–69% survival rate.

Methods and Findings: Cordocentesis (PUBS)[c]: low hematocrit (anemia)
> Murotsuki et al., 1992

Maternal examination[c]: rapid increase in fundal height
> Urig et al., 1990

Ultrasound: scalp edema and ascites present in the larger twin[c,d]
> Wittmann et al., 1981a
> *Comment:* Arteriovenous anastomoses between the twins' umbilical cords were detected only after birth.

hydrocephalus[c,d]
> Chervenak et al., 1983b

significant discrepancy in the biparietal diameters between the twins
> Wittmann et al., 1986

pericardial effusion; enlargement of the right atrium, inferior vena cava, and liver; calcification of one or more cotyledons
> Brennan et al., 1982

significant growth disparity between twins
> Wittmann et al., 1981a; Brennan et al., 1982; Wittmann et al., 1986; Feingold et al., 1986; Urig et al., 1990

ascites
> Holzgreve et al., 1985c

"stuck" to the uterine wall appearance of the smaller twin
> Mahony et al., 1990; Urig et al., 1990; Wax et al., 1991
> *Comments:* This phenomenon is probably the result of hydramnios of the other twin compressing the "stuck" twin, plus the effects of oligohydramnios of the latter twin (Urig et al., 1990; Wax et al., 1991).

hydrops fetalis[c,d]
> Chiba et al., 1990

hydramnios in larger twin
> Wittmann et al., 1981a; Brennen et al., 1982; Holzgreve et al., 1985c; Wittmann et al., 1986; Feingold et al., 1986; Mahony et al., 1990; Urig et al., 1990; Wax et al., 1991

oligohydramnios in the smaller twin
> Wittmann et al., 1986; Mahony et al., 1990; Urig et al., 1990; Wax et al., 1991

enlarged umbilical vein(s)
>Brennan et al., 1982; Feingold et al., 1986

PD 115900 UMBILICAL VEIN ANEURYSM (McKusick No. None)

Doppler flow analysis[c,d]: no documented flow of blood within the mass
>Babay et al., 1996

Ultrasound[c,d]: tubular translucent, cystic mass located within the umbilical cord and extending through the abdominal wall for approximately 1 cm, elongation of the mass with time
>Babay et al., 1996

Comments: The fetus reported by Babay and associates (1996) was born at 39 weeks of gestation after an otherwise uneventful pregnancy. The neonate was physically normal. Histopathology of the umbilical cord demonstrated an aneurysmal dilatation of the umbilical vein.

PD 116000 UNIVENTRICULAR HEART (Single ventricle) (McKusick No. None)

Echocardiography[d]: large posterior ventricular septal defect, common ventricular chamber
>Kleinman et al., 1980

>side-to-side great vessels, single ventricle, one large atrioventricular valve, IUGR
>>Stewart et al., 1983a

Ultrasound[d]: supraventricular ectopic beats, IUGR, coarctation of the aorta
>Stewart et al., 1983a

>pleural fluid
>>Blott et al., 1988a; Nicolaides and Azar, 1990

>hydramnios
>>Nicolaides and Azar, 1990

>hydrops fetalis
>>Chiba et al., 1990; Nicolaides and Azar, 1990

PD 116500 VENTRICULAR ANEURYSM (McKusick No. None)

Ultrasound[d]: large, thin-walled aneurysm located at the apex of the left ventricle, hypokinetic wall motion,[c] subaortic myocardial hypertrophy,[c] extrasystolic ventricular beats,[c] hydramnios[c]
>Gembruch et al., 1990b

Comments: After the birth of the fetus reported by Gembruch and coworkers (1990b), the neonate was evaluated by left ventricular angiogram, and was found to have an apical aneurysm extending nearly to the sternum anteriorly and to the left lateral wall laterally.

PD 117000 VENTRICULAR ENLARGEMENT, HEART (McKusick No. None)

Ultrasound[d]: enlarged ventricle
>Hackeloer, 1979

>right ventricular dilation and hypertrophy, hydramnios, fetal ascites
>>Allan et al., 1982

PD 117130 VENTRICULAR HYPERTROPHY, HEREDITARY (Asymmetric septal hypertrophy [ASH]; Hypertrophic cardiomyopathy; Idiopathic hypertrophic subaortic stenosis [IHSS]) (McKusick No. 192600)

> Echocardiography[c]: generalized hypertrophy of the myocardium with markedly thickened interventricular septum in a fetus at risk
>> Stewart et al., 1986

PD 117250 VENTRICULAR PAUSE (McKusick No. None)

> Fetal electrocardiogram: periodic absence of ventricular contraction
>> Crawford, 1982

PD 117400 VENTRICULAR SEPTAL DEFECT (VSD) (McKusick No. None; see 121000, 178370)

> Alpha-fetoprotein[c,h]: elevated in maternal serum
>> Hajdu et al., 1995

PD 117450 VENTRICULAR TACHYCARDIA (McKusick No. None; see 192605)

Condition Note: This condition is defined by the presence of three or more consecutive ventricular premature systoles with a heart rate in excess of 160 beats per minute.
>> Shenker, 1979

Differential Diagnosis: Atrial fibrillation (PD 106950); Atrial flutter (PD 10700); Tachycardia, supraventricular (PD 113000); Ventricular tachycardia, familial; Wolff–Parkinson–White syndrome (PD 117500).

> Auscultation[c,d]: irregular fetal heart rate
>> Shenker, 1979

> Electrocardiogram[d]: ventricular premature contractions, runs of ventricular tachycardia
>> Shenker, 1979

PD 117500 WOLFF–PARKINSON–WHITE SYNDROME (McKusick No. 194200)

> Auscultation[c,d]: fetal cardiac tachyarrhythmia
>> Belhassen et al., 1982

> Echocardiography[c,d]: irregular ventricular tachyarrhythmia associated with atrial fibrillation, cardiac enlargement
>> Belhassen et al., 1982
>> supraventricular tachycardia
>>> Wiggins et al., 1986
>> conducted and blocked supraventricular extra systoles
>>> Kleinman and Santulli, 1983

> Ultrasound[c,d]: hydrops fetalis, hydramnios
>> Wiggins et al., 1986

THE CENTRAL NERVOUS SYSTEM[a]

General References: Seppala, 1975; Brock, 1976; Campbell, 1977; Kimball et al., 1977; Wald et al., 1977; U.K. Collaborative Study, 1979; Fiske and Filly, 1982; Campbell and Pearce, 1983; Laurence et al., 1983; Fuhrmann, 1985

PD 118000 ANENCEPHALY (Exencephaly) (McKusick No. 182940; see also 206500, 301410)

Acetylcholinesterase[c]: elevated in amniotic fluid, increased ratio of acetylcholinesterase activity to percentage of total cholinesterase activity, and/or fast-migrating amniotic fluid isozyme activity

Chubb et al., 1979; Smith et al., 1979; Buamah et al., 1980; Dale, 1980; Seller and Cole, 1980; Dale et al., 1981; Hullin et al., 1981; Lawton, 1981; Voigtlander et al., 1981; Wald and Cuckle, 1981; Webb et al., 1981a; Crandall et al., 1982; Milunsky and Sapirstein, 1982; Read et al., 1982a; Aitken et al., 1984b; Albrechtsen et al., 1984; Crandall and Matsumoto, 1984a; Crandall and Matsumoto, 1984b; Sindic et al., 1984; Toftager-Larsen et al., 1984; Wyvill et al., 1984; Holbrook et al., 1987b; Raymond and Simpson, 1988

acetylcholinesterase to cholinesterase isozyme density ratio greater than 0.13

Lawton, 1981; Goldfine et al., 1983; Burton, 1986

Comments: For Gastroschisis (PD 137000) and Omphalocele (PD 144000), the ratio of acetylcholinesterase to cholinesterase is normally less than 0.075. This is not a definitive test to differentiate between neural tube defects and ventral wall defects because there are a number of other conditions that will cause acetylcholinesterase to be present in the amniotic fluid (see Acetylcholinesterase in the Index) (Burton, 1986).

elevated in amniotic fluid as determined by an immunoassay method (monoclonal antibody, AE-2)

Brock et al., 1985c

fast-migrating amniotic fluid isozyme

Anneren et al., 1988; Schnatterly and Hogge, 1988; Boogert et al., 1989; Crandall et al., 1989

Alpha-fetoprotein[c]: elevated in maternal serum and amniotic fluid

Brock and Sutcliffe, 1972; Brock et al., 1973; Leighton et al., 1975; Wald and Cuckle, 1977; Crandall et al., 1978; U.K. Collaborative Study, 1979; Brock, 1981; Macri et al., 1981; Ward, 1982; Burton et al., 1983; Freeman and Harbison, 1983; Haddow et al., 1983; Aitken et al., 1984b; Albrechtsen et al., 1984; Crandall and Matsumoto, 1984a; Crandall and Matsumoto, 1984b; Schnittger and Kjessler, 1984; Sindic et al., 1984; Toftager-Larsen et al., 1984; Wyvill et al., 1984; Laurence et al., 1985; Ghosh et al., 1986; Papp et al., 1986; Holbrook et al., 1987b; Kaffe et al., 1987; Winsor et al., 1987

Comments: Diamniotic, monochorionic twins, one of whom had anencephaly, were reported by Holbrook and associates (1987b). The AFP concentration was elevated and an acetylcholinesterase isozyme was present in the amniotic fluids from both twins, even though they were in separate sacs.

Four sets of diamniotic and dichorionic twins who were discordant for either anencephaly (2) or spina bifida cystica (2) have each been reported to have normal amniotic fluid AFP levels with no acetylcholinesterase isozyme in the amniotic fluids from the normal twins, but elevated AFP levels and acetylcholinesterase isozyme in the fluids of the affected twins

(Schnatterly and Hogge, 1988). Schnatterly and Hogge (1988) suggest that four membranes present between the diamniotic, dichorionic twins prevents the diffusion of AFP and acetylcholinesterase between sacs, whereas two membranes, found in the diamniotic, monochorionic twins, do not.

elevated in maternal serum

> Macri et al., 1986; Anneren et al., 1988; Milunsky et al., 1988; Crandall et al., 1989; Evans et al., 1995a

elevated in amniotic fluid

> Macri et al., 1986; Schnatterly and Hogge, 1988; Boogert et al., 1989

Amniocentesis: rapidly adhering cells in 20-hour culture of amniotic fluid cells, percentage ranging from 9–100% (normal being 6% or less),[c] presence of glial fibrillary acid protein in some of these cells (astrocytes)[c]

> Gosden and Brock, 1977; Gosden and Brock, 1978a; Cremer et al., 1981; von Koskull et al., 1981; Medina-Gomez and Bard, 1983; Medina-Gomez and McBride, 1986

Comment: Adhering cell types include long bipolar, filamentous pseudopodial, large vacuolated, and multinucleated cells.

increased number of amniotic fluid cells attached in 20–24 hours[c]

> Bryant and Hoehn, 1977

identification of uncultured glial cell (one type of rapidly adhering cells) in amniotic fluid by use of glial fibrillary acidic protein-specific antibodies[c]

> von Koskull, 1984

increased number of nonsquamous amniotic fluid cells[c]

> Medina-Gomez and McBride, 1986

increased phagocytic index (phagocytic cell number/adherent cells × 100) in amniotic fluid cells[c]

> Medina-Gomez and McBride, 1986

increased number of macrophages in uncultured cytologic preparations

> Papp et al., 1986

increased number of amniotic fluid cells that stained or did not stain for nonspecific acid esterase[c]

> Medina-Gomez and McBride, 1986

increased proportion of macrophages and elongated cells on smears of uncultured amniotic fluid cells[c]

> Papp and Bell, 1979

presence of macrophages and neural cells in cultured amniotic fluid cells[c]

> Medina-Gomez and Bard, 1983

increased number of amniocytes that take up neutral red dye (2700 cells/mL)[c]

> Polgar et al., 1984

lowered glucose levels in amniotic fluid[c]

> Pettit et al., 1977; Guibaud et al., 1978; Weiss et al., 1984; Weiss et al., 1985

elevated fibrin/fibrinogen degradation products in amniotic fluid[c]

> Weiss et al., 1976; Legge, 1983

decreased amniotic fluid levels of 17-hydroxyprogesterone, 17-hydroxy-pregnenolone, and androstenedione (females only)[c]

    Pang et al., 1986

presence of beta-trace protein in amniotic fluid[c]

    Macri et al., 1974

elevated amniotic fluid levels of D2-protein[c]

    Jorgensen and Norgaard-Pedersen, 1981; Jorgensen, 1982

decreased percentage of amniotic fluid AFP that does not react with concanavalin A[c]

    Toftager-Larsen et al., 1980; Albrechtsen et al., 1984; Toftager-Larsen et al., 1984

decreased level of amniotic fluid trypsin inhibitor[c]

    Kolho, 1986

elevated levels of alpha-2-macroglobulin in amniotic fluid[c]

    Legge, 1983; Toftager-Larsen et al., 1984

elevated levels of plasmin in amniotic fluid[c]

    Legge, 1983

decreased levels of plasminogen in amniotic fluid[c]

    Legge, 1983

elevated levels of T4, T3, and TSH in the amniotic fluid[c]

    Hollingsworth and Alexander, 1983

decreased percentage of lens culinaris agglutinin reacting to AFP in amniotic fluid[c]

    Toftager-Larsen et al., 1984

decreased levels of gamma-glutamyltranspeptidase activity in amniotic fluid[c]

    Brock et al., 1984a

increased levels of S-100 protein in amniotic fluid[c]

    Sindic et al., 1984; Anneren et al., 1988

decreased level of activity of the amniotic fluid disaccharidases, maltase, sucrase, trehalase, and lactase[c]

    Kleijer et al., 1985b

increased concentration of glial fibrillary acidic protein in amniotic fluid[c]

    Albrechtsen et al., 1984

increased levels of neuron-specific enolase activity in amniotic fluids

    Anneren et al., 1988

Amniography[d]: hydramnios, absent skull, flat facial bones

    Queenan and Gadow, 1970; Weiss et al., 1978; Balsam and Weiss, 1981

Cholinesterase[c]: elevated in amniotic fluid

    Milunsky et al., 1979; Simpson et al., 1982

Fetoscopy: yellow-gray lesion that was devoid of hair and contained superficial network of small blood vessels

    Rodeck and Campbell, 1978

Maternal blood sampling: decreased levels of human chorionic gonadotropin (hCG) in maternal serum[c]

    Canick et al., 1989

decreased levels of unconjugated estriol in maternal serum[c]

    Canick et al., 1989

Ultrasound: absence of the typical spherical outline of the fetal head, decreased ratio of the fetal-head-to-trunk measurement, absence of or diminished fetal forehead, hydramnios

> Campbell et al., 1972; Campbell, 1977; Hobbins et al., 1979; Sarti et al., 1980; Schmidt and Kubli, 1982; Zamah et al., 1982; Hill et al., 1983a; Quinlan et al., 1983; de Elejalde and Elejalde, 1984; Holbrook et al., 1987b; Hill et al., 1988b

failure to visualize the fetal head or calvarium

> Nisani et al., 1981; Carrasco et al., 1985; Rutledge et al., 1986; Spirt et al., 1987

in fetuses with exencephaly, floating extracranial mass protruding through the incompletely formed calvarium

> Papp et al. 1986

buphthalmos, absence of the roof of the orbits[c]

> de Elejalde and Elejalde, 1984

micrognathia[c,d]

> Pilu et al., 1986

single umbilical artery[c]

> Tortora et al., 1984

abnormal or sluggish fetal movements[c]

> Ianniruberto and Tajani, 1981

hydramnios[c]

> Tortora et al., 1984

PD 118250 AQUEDUCTAL STENOSIS, ETIOLOGY UNDETERMINED
(McKusick No. Unknown; see 307000)

Ultrasound: massive dilatation of the lateral ventricles (hydrocephalus)[c]

> Spirt et al., 1987

increased lateral ventricular to hemispheric width ratio[c]

> Drugan et al., 1989a

PD 119000 ARNOLD–CHIARI MALFORMATION (Arnold–Chiari syndrome; Chiari II malformation) (McKusick No. 207950)

Ultrasound[c,d]: enlarged skull, gross hydrocephalus, enlarged lateral ventricles, posteriorly located skull lesion

> Johnson et al., 1980a; Williams and Barth, 1985; Spirt et al., 1987

absent cerebellum, ventriculomegaly, meningomyelocele

> Drugan et al., 1989a

PD 119250 ATELENCEPHALIC MICROCEPHALY (Telecephalic hypophasia) (McKusick No. None)

Condition Note: Embryologically, the telencephalons are paired cerebral vesicles that arise as anterolateral evaginations of the prosencephalon. They ultimately form the cerebral hemispheres. In atelencephalic microcephaly, the telencephalons are missing or dysplastic. The condition normally is not inherited.

> Siebert et al., 1986; Tick et al., 1990

Prenatal Diagnosis: The diagnosis should be considered whenever there is severe fetal microcephaly with an intact calvarium.

Ultrasound: small, malformed head with overlapping sutures[c]

> Siebert et al., 1986

severe microcephaly, abnormal head shape, intact osseous calvarium, severe underdevelopment of the brain especially in the anterior portion
> Tick et al., 1990

PD 119380 CEREBELLAR LOBE HYPOPLASIA (McKusick No. None; see however 213000)

Condition Note: The fetus reported by Daffos and associates (1988b) apparently had an isolated hypoplasia of the cerebellar lobe with dilated subtentorial cisternae. The child's neurologic development was normal at 12 months of age.

Prenatal Diagnosis: The diagnosis should be considered when atrophy of the cerebellar hemisphere is detected by magnetic resonance imaging (MRI).

Differential Diagnosis: Dandy–Walker syndrome (PD 121000); Joubert syndrome (Familial agenesis of the cerebellar vermis) (PD 126140)

Magnetic resonance imaging[c,d]: dilation of the subtentorial cisternae
> Daffos et al., 1988b

Comments: Imaging by this technique was made possible by intraumbilical vein injection of vecuronium to prevent fetal movements. The fetus had a normal third ventricle, frontal horns, and corpus collosum. The diagnosis of the infant's condition was established by computerized tomography (CT scan) after birth (Daffos et al., 1988b).

Ultrasound[c,d]: an anechogenic area with wide separation of the cerebellar lobes extending up to the cerebellar peduncles in the region of the vermis
> Daffos et al., 1988b

PD 119500 CEREBROVENTRICULAR HEMORRHAGE (McKusick No. None)

Ultrasound: dilated lateral and third ventricles filled with echogenic material (intraventricular blood), intracerebral hematoma
> Kim and Elyaderani, 1982; Spirt et al., 1987

subependymal, parietal and occipital parachymal hemorrhages
> Sibony et al., 1993

parenchymal intracerebral hemorrhage
> Leidig et al., 1988

enlarged fetal head, enlargement of the lateral ventricles, large echogenic complex mass within the right hemisphere, deviation of falx cerebri and apparent fluid level near the dependent ventricle, fetal demise
> Donn et al., 1984; Mintz et al., 1985; Spirt et al., 1987

enlarged ventricles
> Leidig et al., 1988

enlarging head size (head circumference)
> Leidig et al., 1988

hydrocephalus
> Spirt et al., 1987; Leidig et al., 1988

fetal demise[c]
> Kim and Elyaderani, 1982

hydramnios[c,d]
> Leidig et al., 1988

oligohydramnios
> Leidig et al., 1988

PD 119700 CORPUS CALLOSUM, AGENESIS OF THE (Absence of the corpus callosum; Callosal agenesis) (McKusick No. 217990)

Condition Note: Agenesis of the corpus callosum is the congenital absence of the white matter structure that connects the cerebral hemispheres. There may be complete or partial absence of the structure.

The absence of the corpus callosum is not life threatening, and in fact, in isolated situations, it may be completely asymptomatic. Normally, however, when the corpus callosum is absent, there are neurologic problems such as seizures, intellectual deficiency, and psychoses, and the defect may be associated with a number of syndromes.

Romero et al., 1988, pp. 67–70

Prenatal Diagnosis: The prenatal diagnosis of agenesis of the corpus callosum can be made either by CT or ultrasound with the demonstration of (1) increased separation of the lateral ventricles, (2) enlargement of the occipital horns and atria, and (3) upward displacement of the third ventricle.

Romero et al., 1988, p. 68

Differential Diagnosis: A number of different conditions may be associated with agenesis of the corpus callosum some of which include Aicardi syndrome (seizures, chorioretinal lacunae, mental retardation, microcephaly, vertebral anomalies, and X-linked dominant inheritance); Acrocallosal syndrome (mental retardation, macrocephaly, polydactyly, and autosomal recessive inheritance); Andermann syndrome (mental retardation, progressive motor neuropathy, and autosomal recessive inheritance); FG syndrome (mental retardation, macrocephaly, and hypotonia); Trisomy 13 syndrome (PD 103000), and Trisomy 18 syndrome (PD 104000).

Romero et al., 1988, p. 67

Ultrasound[d]: dilatation of the occipital horns of both lateral ventricles

Amato et al., 1986

normal-sized lateral ventricles that are markedly separated, enlarged atria, abnormal convulsional pattern between lateral ventricles, enlarged and upward displacement of the third ventricle

Romero et al., 1988, p. 68

dilatation of lateral ventricles

Birnholz and Frigoletto, 1981; Amato et al., 1986

inability to visualize the corpus callosum

Birnholz and Frigoletto, 1981

PD 119750 CORPUS CALLOSUM, PARTIAL AGENESIS (McKusick No. Unknown; see 304100)

Condition Note: Partial agenesis of the corpus callosum is not uncommon and usually benign. The condition is associated with ventriculomegaly, and thus, it is important to make this diagnosis to avoid undue apprehension in the parents of the fetus with this condition.

Lockwood et al., 1988

Prenatal Diagnosis: The condition should be suspected when there is discrete enlargement of the posterior horns and atria of the lateral ventricles, and the frontal horns, third ventricle, and choroid plexuses are normal in size and location. Diagnosis of complete absence of the corpus callosum is made on transverse scan by finding superior displacement and enlargement of the third ventricle, lateral displacement of the frontal horns, and dilation of the posterior horns of the lateral ventricles (Lockwood et al., 1988).

Differential Diagnosis: Partial or complete absence of the corpus callosum may be associated with other central nervous system abnormalities including Arnold–Chiari malformation (PD 119000); Dandy–Walker syndrome (PD 121000); Encephalocele (PD 122000); Interhemispheric cysts, and Neurofibromas, which in themselves may lead to other significant problems.

Ultrasound[d]: discrete enlargement of the posterior horns and atria of the lateral ventricles; increased lateral ventricular wall to hemispheric width ratio at the level of the posterior horn; normal frontal horns, third ventricle, and choroid plexuses; and normal diameter of the cerebellum
> Lockwood et al., 1988

Comments: The fetus reported by Lockwood and associates (1988) was confirmed to have partial agenesis of the corpus callosum after birth by computerized tomography. Neurologically the child was normal.

PD 120000 CRANIORACHISCHISIS (Rachischisis) (McKusick No. None; see 182940)

Acetylcholinesterase[c]: elevated in amniotic fluid, presence of fast-migrating amniotic fluid isozyme
> Webb et al., 1981a; Streit et al., 1989

Alpha-fetoprotein[c]: elevated in amniotic fluid
> Rodeck and Campbell, 1978; Holzgreve, 1985; Streit et al., 1989
> elevated in maternal serum
> Streit et al., 1989

Amniocentesis: increased number of amniocytes that take up neutral red dye (2700 cells/mL)[c]
> Polgar et al., 1984

Auscultation[c]: no fetal heart sounds
> Case, 1917

Cholinesterase[c]: elevated in amniotic fluid
> Webb et al., 1981a

Fetoscopy: yellow-gray lesion that was devoid of hair and contained a superficial network of small blood vessels
> Rodeck and Campbell, 1978

Maternal perception[c,d]: no fetal movements
> Case, 1917

Maternal examination[c]: large-for-gestation age, hydramnios
> Case, 1917

Radiograph[c,d]: conspicuous absence of the cranial bones, unusually prominent bones of the face and base of the skull
> Case, 1917

Comments: In the fetus reported by Case (1917), intrauterine death occurred. Postnatal analysis revealed anencephaly as well as rachischisis of the upper cervical vertebrae.

Ultrasound: no caput with spina bifida extending down to the upper thoracic region
> Rodeck and Campbell, 1978; Holzgreve, 1985
> absence of bony calvarium and brain
> Ardinger et al., 1987; Spirt et al., 1987

open cervical spine with U-shaped posterior ossification centers
Spirt et al., 1987
hydramnios
Ardinger et al., 1987; Spirt et al., 1987

PD 121000 DANDY–WALKER SYNDROME (Dandy–Walker cyst; Dandy–Walker malformation; Posterior fossa arachnoid cyst) (McKusick No. 220200)

Syndrome Note: The major features of the Dandy–Walker syndrome result from a primary maldevelopment of the rostral part of the roof of the fourth ventricle of the brain, and include hypoplasia of the cerebellar vermis, a posterior fossa cyst, and variable degrees of hydrocephalus. The cause of the condition is unknown, although it may be part of number of syndromes of various etiologies (Romero et al., 1988, p. 31). Associated anomalies may occur in as many as 68% of cases.
Dempsey and Koch, 1981; Romero et al., 1988, pp. 30–34

Prenatal Diagnosis: The diagnosis of this syndrome should be considered whenever there is a posterior fossa cyst detected in the fetus. A defect in the vermis, through which a cyst communicates with the fourth ventricle, is stated to be pathognomonic for Dandy–Walker syndrome. However, detection of hypoplasia of the vermis alone appears not to be diagnostic because this finding may disappear in the third trimester and in some cases vermis hypoplasia represents a transient situation with no major clinical implications (Toi et al., 1993).
Romero et al., 1988, pp. 32–33

Differential Diagnosis: Arachnoid cyst (PD 118500); Enlarged cisterna magna; Joubert syndrome (PD 126140); Posterior fossa cyst (PD 279000)

Alpha-fetoprotein[c]: elevated in amniotic fluid
Crandall and Matsumoto, 1984b
elevated in the maternal serum
Burton, 1987
Computerized axial tomography[d]: large posterior fossa cyst, supratentorial ventriculomegaly
Filly et al., 1984
Ultrasound: posterior fossa cystic mass that may be herniated through the tentorial notch[d]
Johnson et al., 1980a; Kirkinen et al., 1982; Newman et al., 1982; Fileni et al., 1983; Filly et al., 1984
posterior fossa cyst that communicated with the fourth ventricle
Dempsey and Koch, 1981; Spirt et al., 1987
hypoplastic cerebellar hemispheres
Dempsey and Koch, 1981; Spirt et al., 1987
dilated aqueduct
Spirt et al., 1987
increased fetal biparietal diameter, mild hydrocephalus with poorly visualized temporal horns of the lateral ventricles[d]
Kirkinen et al., 1982
minimal degree of hydrocephalus with the lateral ventricular width/hemispheric width ratio reduced[d]
Dempsy and Koch, 1981

dilated lateral ventricles
    Simpson et al., 1988
displaced tentorium
    Simpson et al., 1988
ventriculomegaly
    Nyberg et al., 1987; Simpson et al., 1988
hydrops fetalis
    Simpson et al., 1988
ascites
    Simpson et al., 1988
scalp edema
    Simpson et al., 1988
skin thickening
    Simpson et al., 1988
hydramnios[c]
    Newman et al., 1982; Simpson et al., 1988

PD 121500 DIASTEMATOMYELIA (McKusick No. 222500)

Condition Note: Diastematomyelia describes an equal or unequal division of the spinal cord in the anteroposterior plane by a fibrous or bony septum. The condition may be associated with occult spinal dysraphism or meningomyelocele. Furthermore, this abnormality is occasionally reported in siblings, probably being inherited in an autosomal recessive mode.
    Williams and Barth, 1985; McKusick, 1986

Prenatal Diagnosis: Other than in exceptional situations in which the condition is inherited, the diagnosis probably cannot be established prenatally. It should be suspected, however, whenever an abnormal widening of the posterior spinal ossification centers is detected on ultrasound.

Alpha-fetoprotein[c]: elevated in maternal serum
    Williams and Barth, 1985
Ultrasound: abnormal widening of the posterior ossification centers of the fetal spine associated with a central, bright linear echo within the canal at the level of the lesion
    Williams and Barth, 1985

PD 122000 ENCEPHALOCELE (McKusick No. None)

Acetylcholinesterase[c]: elevated in amniotic fluid, and/or fast-migrating amniotic fluid isozyme
    Voigtlander et al., 1981; Crandall et al., 1982; Read et al., 1982a; Aitken et al., 1984b; Albrechtsen et al., 1984; Crandall and Matsumoto, 1984a; Crandall and Matsumoto, 1984b; Raymond and Simpson, 1988; Boogert et al., 1989; Crandall et al., 1989
Alpha-fetoprotein[c]: elevated in amniotic fluid
    Crandall et al., 1978; U.K. Collaborative Study, 1979; Albrechtsen et al., 1984; Crandall and Matsumoto, 1984a; Crandall and Matsumoto, 1984b; Boogert et al., 1989; Crandall et al., 1989
    elevated in maternal serum
    Wald et al., 1977; Brock, 1982; Read et al., 1982a; Aitken et al., 1984b; Dyer et al., 1986

Amniocentesis: elevated amniotic fluid levels of D2-protein[c]
> Jorgensen and Norgaard-Pedersen, 1981

increased concentration of glial fibrillary acidic protein in amniotic fluid[c]
> Albrechtsen et al., 1984

less than 40% intestinal fraction of total alkaline phosphatase activity in amniotic fluid, normal being 78.7% ± 21.8% (±2 SD)[c]
> Beaudet et al., 1985

rapidly adhering cells in 20-hour culture of amniotic fluid cells, presence of glial fibrillary acid protein in some of these cells (astrocytes)[c]
> Harrod et al., 1979; Cremer et al., 1981

increased number of nonsquamous amniotic fluid cells
> Medina-Gomez and McBride, 1986

Amniography: lucent shadow associated with the fetal head
> Miskin et al., 1978

microcephaly,[c] hydramnios[c]
> Queenan and Gadow, 1970

Ultrasound: bulge or gap in the skull, saclike structure in close proximity to the head and neck regions
> Campbell, 1977; Hood and Robinson, 1978; Hill et al., 1983a; Carrasco et al., 1985; Spirt et al., 1987; Boogert et al., 1989

protrusion of brain parenchyma through skull defect
> Chervenak et al., 1984d; Carrasco et al., 1985

macrocephaly[c]
> Chervenak et al., 1984d

hydrocephalus[c]
> Chervenak et al., 1984d; Nyberg et al., 1987; Spirt et al., 1987

ventriculomegaly[c]
> Boogert et al., 1989

microcephaly[c]
> Chervenak et al., 1984d; Chervenak et al., 1987; Spirt et al., 1987

oligohydramnios[c]
> Dyer et al., 1986

PD 122250 ERDL SYNDROME (McKusick No. None; see 208150)

Syndrome Note: Erdl and associates described in 1989 a central nervous system (CNS) malformation syndrome that resulted in the Pena–Shokeir phenotype. They reported two opposite-sex siblings who were affected and had severe arthrogryposis, hydrops fetalis, seizures, microcephaly, very small and severely disrupted brain with reduced number of neurons and missing nuclei, and numerous other minor anomalies. Death occurred in both during the first 3 months after birth. Chromosomal and biochemical studies were normal.

Prenatal Diagnosis: The presence of hydrops fetalis, hydramnios, and reduced fetal movements should be sufficient to make the diagnosis in fetuses at risk.

Differential Diagnosis: Herva arthrogryposis fetal hydrops syndrome (PD 191280); Pena–Shokeir phenotype (PD 192880); and other disorders associated with arthrogryposis (see Arthrogryposis in the Index) should be considered.

Ultrasound[i]: microcephaly, hydrops fetalis, fetal tachycardia, IUGR,[c] lack of fetal movement,[c] thin umbilical cord,[c] small stomach,[c] abnormal configuration and positioning of limbs,[c] partially overlapping fingers,[c] short neck,[c] ocular hypertelorism,[c] retrognathia,[c] small mouth with ballooned-out cheeks
> Erdl et al., 1989

PD 122500 FETAL BRAIN DISRUPTION SEQUENCE (McKusick No. None)

Sequence Note: Russell and her associates described this sequence in 1984. It appears that if the brain is partially destroyed in the second half of pregnancy, the fetal skull can collapse leading to microcephaly, overriding sutures, prominence of the occiput, and rugation of the scalp. The condition has been produced by intrauterine infections and in utero death of a twin. In severe cases, death may occur postnatally. In those that survive, there is usually severe neurologic deficiency.

Prenatal Diagnosis: The sequence should be suspected in any fetus who has suffered a CNS insult resulting in severe microcephaly. Alternatively, if severe microcephaly develops in the second half of pregnancy in a fetus who previously had normal results on ultrasonic evaluation of the head, this condition should be considered.

Differential Diagnosis: Hydranencephaly (PD 124000); Hydrocephalus (PD 125500); and the various conditions resulting in microcephaly (see Microcephaly in the Index) should be considered.

Maternal history[c,h]: intermittent vaginal bleeding, decreased fetal movements
Ultrasound[c,d]: severe microcephaly
        Russell et al., 1984
    intrauterine growth retardation
        Moore et al., 1990
    hydramnios
        Moore et al., 1990

PD 123000 HOLOPROSENCEPHALY (Includes Aprosencephaly; Cebocephaly; Cheilognathopalatoschisis; Cyclopia; Ethmocephaly) (McKusick No. Unknown; see 157170, 236100)

ALOBAR TYPE

General Comments: Pilu and associates (1987) have presented criteria for diagnosis of alobar holoprosencephaly and distinguishing alobar type from the semilobar type.

Ultrasound: microcephaly (biparietal diameter and head area greater than 3 SD below mean, head-to-upper-abdominal diameter ratio less than 1) or macrocephaly, fetal head growth rate below normal, ventricular dilation or single large cerebral ventricle, boomerang-shaped rostrally displaced cerebral cortex, no midline fetal brain echo indicating absence of falx cerebri, septum pellucidum and interhemispheric fissure, irregular cortical mantle, hydrocephalus, large for gestational age, small for gestational age
        Kurtz et al., 1980; Blackwell et al., 1982; Mayden et al., 1982; Chervenak et al., 1983b; Hill et al., 1983a; Chervenak et al., 1984c; Filly et al., 1984; Carrasco et al., 1985; Chervenak et al., 1985c; Harsanyi et al., 1985; Spirt et al., 1987
large intracranial cystic structure filling most of the cranial vault and no indication of midline structures[d]
        Simpson et al., 1988
dorsal cyst connecting to a single ventricle
        Pilu et al., 1987; Spirt et al., 1987

fused thalami
> Spirt et al., 1987; Simpson et al., 1988

orbital hypotelorism[d]
> Blackwell et al., 1982; Mayden et al., 1982; Carrasco et al., 1985; Chervenak et al., 1985c

macrocephaly[c,d]
> Pilu et al., 1987; Simpson et al., 1988

microcephaly[d]
> Pilu et al., 1987

increased biparietal diameter[c,d]
> Simpson et al., 1988

monoventricle (holoventricle) of the brain
> Pilu et al., 1987; Simpson et al., 1988

absence of the third ventricle
> Pilu et al., 1987

anophthalmia[d]
> Pilu et al., 1987

hypotelorism
> Pilu et al., 1987

absence of the nasal bridge[d]
> Pilu et al., 1987

median cleft lip[d]
> Pilu et al., 1987

midline cleft palate[d]
> Pilu et al., 1987

oligohydramnios[c]
> Chervenak et al., 1983b

hydramnios[c]
> Mayden et al., 1982; Chervenak et al., 1984c; Filly et al., 1984; Chervenak et al., 1985c

APROSENCEPHALY

Condition Note: This type of holoprosencephaly appears to represent the most severe end of this CNS sequence.

> Ultrasound[c,d]: anterior encephalocele
>> Reynolds and Waldstein, 1989

Comments: The infant reported by Reynolds and Waldstein (1989) had microcephalus, a bony defect of the calvarium in the center of the forehead, a diamond-shaped opening in midface, a single fused ocular structure, absence of the nose, small philtrum and mouth, and absence of the premaxilla. At autopsy the cerebral hemispheres were absent and replaced by separate cystic structures, the prosencephalon was represented by an ovoid mass, and there was absence of the crista galli, cribriform plate, and the first, second, fourth, and sixth cranial nerves.

CEBOCEPHALY

Condition Note: Cebocephaly is a form of holoprosencephaly in which the nose has formed a single, usually rounded, nostril. The nose is present in its normal location on the face.

Ultrasound[h]: absence of the falx and other midline structures
> Nyberg et al., 1987

centrally fused thalami
> Nyberg et al., 1987

monoventricle (fused lateral ventricles)
> Nyberg et al., 1987

unusual and protuberant nose seen on coronal scan of the face
> Nyberg et al., 1987

CYCLOPIA

Ultrasound: absence of nose and presence of a supraorbital proboscis, fused orbits separated by a midline septum, abnormally shaped sphenoid and ethmoid bones, only one orbit, fused thalamus, large single ventricle
> Filly et al., 1984; de Elejalde and Elejalde, 1984; de Elejalde and Elejalde, 1985a

SEMILOBAR TYPE

Ultrasound: anterior interhemispheric fissure, large central cavity communicating with a dorsal cyst, partially formed lateral ventricles
> Spirt et al., 1987

dilated single cerebral ventricle[d]
> Cayea et al., 1984

hypotelorism as determined by decreased interorbital distances[d]
> Cayea et al., 1984

hydrops fetalis[c,d]
> Cayea et al., 1984

fetal demise[c,d]
> Cayea et al., 1984

hydramnios[c,d]
> Cayea et al., 1984

LOBAR TYPE

Ultrasound[d]: single cerebral ventricle
> Schoene and Holmes, 1989

TYPE NOT STATED

Ultrasound: increased lateral ventricular width to hemispheric width ratio[c,d]
> Drugan et al., 1989a

microcephaly
> Pilu et al., 1986

increased biparietal diameter[c,d]
> Simpson et al., 1988

absence of paired lateral ventricles
> Hill et al., 1988b

large intracranial fluid-filled structure surrounded by a thin cerebral mantle[d]
> Simpson et al., 1988

enlarged third ventricle that communicated directly with a large median ventricle and was flanked by brain tissue
> Fiske and Filly, 1982

ocular hypotelorism
    Pilu et al., 1986; Berry et al., 1990
anophthalmia
    Pilu et al., 1986
proboscis
    Berry et al., 1990
median cleft lip and palate
    Pilu et al., 1986
facial cleft
    Berry et al., 1990
absent nasal bridge[d]
    Pilu et al., 1986
single median opening of nose[d]
    Pilu et al., 1986
absence of the nose[d]
    Pilu et al., 1986
hydronephrosis
    Berry et al., 1990
prominent heel
    Berry et al., 1990
clubfoot
    Berry et al., 1990

PD 124000 HYDRANENCEPHALY (McKusick No. None)
    Ultrasound[d]: fluid-filled fetal head (no cortex visualized), increased biparietal diameter; normal, incomplete, or absent falx formation
        Lee and Warren, 1977b; Regec and Bernstine, 1979; Campbell and Pearce, 1983; Chervenak et al., 1983b; Carrasco et al., 1985
    absence of most of the telencephalon
        Fiske and Filly, 1982
    preservation of third ventricle, basal ganglia, aqueduct of Sylvius, and hippocanthal and parahippocampal gyri
        Fiske and Filly, 1982
    presence of posterior fossa contents concurrent with deficiency of cerebrum
        Carrasco et al., 1985
    no identifiable falx
        Fiske and Filly, 1982
    multiple episodes of rapid jerking motions of the upper extremities and head thought to represent intrauterine seizures
        Conover et al., 1986
    hydramnios
        Quinlan et al., 1983; Conover et al., 1986

PD 125000 HYDROCEPHALUS (McKusick No. 236600)

Condition Note: Fetal or congenital hydrocephalus is the presence of increased ventricular size in the fetus as determined by an increase in the lateral ventricular/hemisphere diameter ratio (Johnson et al., 1980a). The etiology of ventriculomegaly is diverse (see Hydrocephalus and Ventriculomegaly of the brain in the Index), and when present the abnormality is frequently associated with other intracranial and extracranial abnormalities (70–83%) (Drugan et al., 1989a). The prognosis associated with ventriculomegaly varies according to the associated anomalies, the severity of the hydrocephalus, and etiology. Borderline isolated ventricular enlargement that is not progressive usually results in a child with normal neurologic function. Isolated ventriculomegaly is usually associated with aqueductal stenosis (PD 118250) and the outcome for neurologic function is mixed, ranging from normal to severe developmental delay. Neurologic impairment is usually greater when the hydrocephalus is extensive and there are other anomalies present (Drugan et al., 1989a).

Ventriculomegaly may be detected as early as 16 weeks of gestation but head enlargement usually does not occur until 20 weeks of gestation or later.

Prenatal Diagnosis: The presence of enlarged ventricles as determined by standard nomograms of lateral ventricular size and lateral ventricular width to hemispheric width are the usual criteria for making the diagnosis.

Johnson et al., 1980a; Romero et al., 1988, pp. 3–11, 21–24

Differential Diagnosis: See Hydrocephalus and Ventriculomegaly of the brain in the Index.

Prenatal Treatment: The results of intrauterine ventricular shunting of hydrocephalus has been disappointing when compared to the results of standard neonatal treatment. As a consequence, the practice has largely been abandoned. Therefore, treatment is deferred until after birth and is based on the diagnosis, presenting problems, and condition of the neonate.

Drugan et al., 1989a

Methods and Findings: Alpha-fetoprotein[c,d]: elevated in amniotic fluid

Seppala, 1975

elevated in maternal serum

Seppala and Unnerus, 1974; Seppala, 1975; Burton, 1987

Amniocentesis: reduced levels of glucose in amniotic fluid[c]

Weiss et al., 1984

Computerized axial tomography[d]: increased biparietal diameter, absence of cortical mantle, fluid replacement of cortex, dilated ventricles, pulsating falx

Patterson et al., 1981; Hill et al., 1983a; Olund et al., 1983

Continuous wave Doppler evaluation[c,d]: increased peripheral arterial resistance

Meizner et al., 1987

Maternal history or examination[c]: size–date discrepancy, large for gestational age

Palumbos and Stierman, 1989

Radiograph[d]: increased fetal head size

Freeman et al., 1977

Ultrasound: dilated lateral and third ventricles, increased biparietal diameter, increased lateral ventricular width to hemispheric dimension ratio, dilation of occipital horns of the ventricles, absence of midline structures, microcephaly, orbital hypotelorism, dilation of the posterior horn of the ventricles with normal anterior ones

Hobbins et al., 1979; Johnson et al., 1980a; Cochrane and Myles, 1982; Campbell and Pearce, 1983; Chervenak et al., 1983b; Hill et al., 1983a; Chervenak et al., 1985d

increased lateral ventricular width to hemispheric dimension ratio

Drugan et al., 1989a; Palumbos and Stierman, 1989

markedly enlarged fetal head
>Kovnar et al., 1984

bilateral cystic intracranial structures with an intact skull and midline interhemispheric fissure, decreased cortical thickness
>Carrasco et al., 1985

dilation of the frontal and occipital horns
>Fiske and Filly, 1982

dilation of the third ventricle
>Fiske and Filly, 1982

enlargement of all ventricles except for the aqueduct of Sylvius
>de Elejalde and Elejalde, 1985b

dilated ventricle with compression of the choroid plexus
>Hill et al., 1988b

bilaterally dilated ventricles with a ventricle-to-hemisphere ratio greater than 80%
>Leikin and Randall, 1987

visibility of the medial ventricular wall
>Fiske and Filly, 1982

spina bifida
>de Elejalde and Elejalde, 1985b

abnormal or reduced fetal movements, permanent extension and scissoring of lower limbs[c]
>Ianniruberto and Tajani, 1981

hydramnios[d]
>Chervenak et al., 1983b; Quinlan et al., 1983; Meizner et al., 1987

oligohydramnios[d]
>Chervenak et al., 1983b

PD 126000 INIENCEPHALY (McKusick No. None)

Condition Note: Iniencephaly is characterized by bony defects of the occiput; malformed cervical and thoracic vertebrae, or spina bifida or rachischisis of the cervical spine; and retroflexion of the head. The condition has been classified into two types: *iniencephalus apertus* (membrane-covered lesion) and *iniencephalus clausus* (presence of an encephalocele in the cervical region). The condition is normally lethal, resulting in stillbirth or in death within hours after birth. Ninety percent of the cases occur in females. The postpartum diagnostic criteria for iniencephaly include (1) variable deficiency of the occipital bones, resulting in an enlarged foramen magnum, (2) partial or total absence of cervical and thoracic vertebrae, with irregular fusion of those present, accompanied by incomplete closure of the vertebral arches and/or bodies, (3) significant shortening of the spinal column due to marked lordosis and hyperextension of the malformed cervical–thoracic spine, and (4) upward-turned face with mandibular skin directly continuous with that of the chest, probably due to a shortened neck and lack of neck movement. Additional anomalies may be present and may include anencephaly, various forms of spina bifida, omphalocele, diaphragmatic hernia, congenital heart defects, and renal anomalies. Hydramnios is also frequently present.
>Morocz et al., 1986

Prenatal Diagnosis: The diagnosis should be suspected whenever spina bifida in the cervical–thoracic spine region is detected by ultrasound in the presence of elevated levels of maternal serum and/or amniotic fluid, rapidly adhering amniotic fluid cells, and/or hydramnios. Elevated AFP levels, presence of amniotic acetylcholinesterase isozyme, and rapidly adhering amniotic fluid cells may not be present if the spinal defect is skin covered; that is, an encephalocele is not present.

Differential Diagnosis: Anencephaly with spinal retroflexion (PD 118000); Craniorachischisis (PD 120000); Klippel–Feil anomaly; Thoracic spina bifida cystica (PD 129000)

Acetylcholinesterase[c]: elevated in amniotic fluid
      Chubb et al., 1979; Smith et al., 1979
Alpha-fetoprotein[c]: elevated in amniotic fluid
      U.K. Collaborative Study, 1979
   elevated in maternal serum
      Wald et al., 1977; Evans et al., 1995a
Amniocentesis: rapidly adhering cells in 20-hour culture of amniotic fluid cells[c]
      Gosden and Brock, 1978a; Morocz et al., 1986
   increased number of amniocytes that take up neutral red dye (900 cells/mL in one case)[c]
      Polgar et al., 1984
Ultrasound: malformation of the fetal neck[c,d]
      Santos-Ramos and Duenhoelter, 1975
   spina bifida cystica or encephalocele in the cervical spine region
      Morocz et al., 1986; Hill et al., 1988b
   direct continuation of the skin of the chin with that of the anterior chest, contour defect of the occiput, retroflexion of the head
      Morocz et al., 1986
   splaying of the ossification centers of the cervical spine
      Hill et al., 1988b
   hydramnios[c,d]
      Santos-Ramos and Duenhoelter, 1975; Morocz et al., 1986

PD 126140 JOUBERT SYNDROME (Familial agenesis of the cerebellar vermis) (McKusick No. 213300)

Ultrasound: single large cavity in the posterior fossa of a fetus at risk
      Campbell et al., 1984

PD 126150 JOUBERT SYNDROME WITH BILATERAL CHORIORETINAL COLOBOMA (Chorioretinal coloboma with cerebellar vermis aplasia; Joubert syndrome associated with Leber amaurosis and multicystic kidneys) (McKusick No. 243910)

Syndrome Note: A number of families have been reported with the combination of cerebellar vermis aplasia, chorioretinal colobomas, and retinal dystrophy. In addition, there may be meningocele, micrognathia, congenital heart defects, multiple cortical renal cysts, nystagmus, poor vision, ataxia, and mental retardation. The condition appears to be an autosomal recessive disorder.
      McKusick, 1995
Ultrasound[i]: meningocele, multiple renal cysts
      Ivarsson et al., 1993

PD 126250 LIPOMYELOMENINGOCELE (Intraspinal lipoma; Lipomyeloschisis) (McKusick No. None)

Condition Note: Lipomyelomeningocele is a fatty tumor of the lumbosacral spine that occurs in conjunction with spina bifida occulta. It often originates from the spinal cord or cauda equina. The disorder presents itself in the newborn period as a benign-appearing subcutaneous lumbosacral mass. Serious neurologic damage can result as the child grows if tethering of the spinal cord by the tumor occurs. The prognosis is good if the diagnosis is made early and successful neonatal tumor resection is accomplished.

> Seeds and Jones, 1986

Prenatal Diagnosis: Method of diagnosis is as noted below under Ultrasound.

Acetylcholinesterase[c]: presence of a rapidly migrating amniotic fluid isozyme on gel electrophoresis

> Raymond and Simpson, 1988

Ultrasound: splaying of the lateral posterior lower spine, identification of a distinct, echogenic soft-tissue mass immediately posterior to the dysraphic fetal spine; the mass was diffusely echogenic except for a small, spherical echo-free space within the most caudal part of the mass

> Seeds and Jones, 1986

PD 126300 LISSENCEPHALY, TYPE I (McKusick No. None; see 247200, 257320)

Condition Note: Type I lissencephaly is associated with microcephaly, a thickened cortex, and a thin inner white-matter region. The cortex has four rather than six layers. Miller–Dieker (PD 101510) and Norman–Roberts syndromes are two syndromes associated with type I lissencephaly; the former is produced by a deletion at 17p13, the latter by autosomal recessive inheritance.

Prenatal Diagnosis: The data reported by Okamura and co-workers (1993) indicate that lissencephaly can be reliably diagnosed by MRI of the fetal brain during pregnancy.

Differential Diagnosis: Miller–Dieker syndrome (PD 101510); Norman–Roberts syndrome; Walker–Warburg syndrome (PD 130750); see also Microcephaly in the Index.

Magnetic resonance imaging: smooth surface of the cortex, remarkably large sylvian fissures, lateral ventriculogmegaly

> Okamura et al., 1993

Comments: Okamura and associates (1993) reported the diagnosis of two fetuses with apparent isolated lissencephaly. The lissencephaly was not diagnosed in either fetus by ultrasound, but was clearly detected by MRI. Prenatal chromosomal analysis on fetal blood was normal in both cases, but it does not appear that the DNA probe for detection of 17p13 deletion was utilized in either fetus. Autopsy in both cases demonstrated lissencephaly.

Ultrasound[c]: microcephaly which became worse with advancing gestational age (−4 standard deviations [SD] at 41 weeks)

> Baggot et al., 1995

Comments: The fetus reported by Baggot and colleagues (1995) had microcephaly prenatally, and microencephaly, type I lissencephaly with enlarged ventricles, agenesis of the corpus callosum, overlapping sutures, linear scalp creases, epicanthal folds, and micrognathia postnatally. Chromosomal analysis was normal, and no 17p13 deletion was found.

bilateral ventriculomegaly[c]

> Okamura et al., 1993

PD 127000 MASA SYNDROME (Adducted thumb with mental retardation, Gareis–Mason syndrome, clasped thumb and mental retardation) (McKusick No. 303350)

Syndrome Note: This condition is caused by a mutation in the gene for L1 cell adhesion molecule (L1CAM). The gene is an X-linked recessive one, and located at Xq28. MASA stands for mental retardation, aphasia, shuffling gait, and adducted thumbs; other features include hydrocephalus and agenesis of the corpus callosum.

Timor-Tritsch et al., 1996

Ultrasound[i]: absence of the corpus callosum, small cavum septi pellucidi, dilated posterior horn of the lateral ventricles (colpocephaly), short pericallosal artery, adducted and completely fixed (clasped) thumbs

Timor-Tritsch et al., 1996

Comments: In the fetus cited by Timor-Tritsch and associates (1996), the ventricular sizes and head size were normal at 20 weeks. By 22 weeks, the ventricles were enlarged, and the structural abnormalities of the fetus were found.

PD 128150 MICROCEPHALY, AUTOSOMAL DOMINANT (McKusick No. 156580)

Ultrasound[d,i]: fetal head size 4 SD below the mean for gestational age

Persutte et al., 1990

Comments: The fetus reported by Persutte and co-authors (1990) had a head circumference at term birth of 25.7 cm that was approximately 8 SD below the mean for age and sex. By MRI, the child had hypoplasia of most brain structures, and pachygyria. His mother had a head circumference of 44.5 cm, which is also nearly 8 SD below the mean. Other than the microcephaly in both individuals, mild hypotonia and hyperreflexia in the infant, and mild mental retardation in the mother, both were normal.

PD 128250 MICROCEPHALY, AUTOSOMAL RECESSIVE ISOLATED (True microcephaly) (McKusick No. 251200)

Ultrasound[d]: biparietal diameter greater than 2 SD below the mean; relative head size decreases with gestational age; femur length was normal for gestational age

Pescia et al., 1983; Schinzel and Litschgi, 1984; Nguyen The et al., 1985

PD 128300 MICROCEPHALY, UNSPECIFIED TYPE (McKusick No. Unknown; see 156580, 156590, 251250, 251270, 251280, 311400)

Condition Note: Microcephaly means a small head, as usually determined by the occipitofrontal circumference (OFC), postnatally, and being less than -2 SD (greater than 2 SD below the mean) for age and sex of the child. Prenatally, the same criteria would apply; the head size is greater than 2 SD below the mean for gestational age. However, in addition to the fetal head perimeter (OFC), the biparietal diameter, occipitofrontal diameter, and the fetal chest and abdominal diameters to biparietal diameters are also used for determining the size of the head. Microencephaly means a small brain, and because the head size is generally determined by the brain size when one is discussing microcephaly, microencephaly is implied. Frequently with microcephaly, even though the head is small, there is relative enlargement of the ventricles. In other words, there is increased ventricular diameter to thickness of the brain. This alteration is usually a reflection of undergrowth of the brain and decreased thickness of the cortex itself.

Microcephaly is associated with many genetic disorders, chromosomal aberrations, and environmental insults. The etiology is not established in most cases, and thus, if the disorder happens to be inherited, say in an autosomal recessive fashion, the parents would be at increased risk for recurrence of the disorder in subsequent pregnancies.

The entry here (microcephaly, unspecified type [PD 128300]) includes reported cases of prenatal detection of microcephaly in which the diagnoses (or etiologies) were not stated or were not known to the authors. If the diagnoses were known, then the finding of microcephaly would be included under the appropriate condition category.

Prenatal Diagnosis: The prenatal diagnosis of microcephaly is fraught with problems. The most significant one is that the head and brain growth during the initial half or more of the pregnancy may be normal. Subsequently, growth will slow and the microcephaly will be recognized. It is, therefore, imperative that fetuses at risk for developing microcephaly be followed by serial ultrasound evaluations when a normal fetal head size is initially found. On the other hand, if the head size is significantly less than normal, that is, if there is an occipitofrontal diameter, a head perimeter, and a head perimeter/abdominal perimeter ratio equal to or greater than 4 SD, 5 SD, and 3 SD, respectively, below the predicted mean for fetal age and a femur length/head perimeter ratio larger than the predicted mean of 3 SD, the fetus will most likely have significant microcephaly after birth (Chervenak et al., 1987). Standards for head size measurements during gestation can be found in several sources (Chervanak et al., 1984e; Romero et al., 1988, pp. 56–58).

Differential Diagnosis: See Microcephaly in the Index.

Alpha-fetoprotein[c]: elevated in maternal serum
        Macri et al., 1981; Freeman and Harbison, 1983
    elevated in amniotic fluid
        Macri et al., 1981

Radiograph[d]: reduced cranial volume, craniolacunae
        Russell, 1973

Ultrasound: abnormally slow fetal head growth rate, fetal chest and abdominal diameters greater than biparietal diameter, head circumference greater than 2 SD below the mean, no midline fetal brain echo, relative hydrocephalus, oligohydramnios
        Gottesfeld, 1978; Kurtz et al., 1980; Rodeck et al., 1982b; Campbell and Pearce, 1983; Chervenak et al., 1983b
    fetal head growth rate as measured by the biparietal diameter, less than the fifth percentile after 24 weeks of gestation
        Tolmie et al., 1987e
    occipitofrontal diameter 4 SD below the predicted mean, a head perimeter 5 SD below the predicted mean, a head perimeter/abdominal perimeter ratio 3 SD below the predicted mean, a femur length/head perimeter ratio 3 SD larger than the predicted mean
        Chervenak et al., 1984e; Chervenak et al., 1987

PD 128400 MICROCEPHALY–LYMPHEDEMA SYNDROME, AUTOSOMAL RECESSIVE TYPE (McKusick No. None; see 152950)

Syndrome Note: An apparent autosomal dominant disorder of lymphedema, microcephaly, normal intelligence, and other features exists (see Lymphedema and microcephaly, No. 152950 [McKusick, 1995]). Kozma and associates (1996) reported a brother and sister with microcephaly, lymphedema of the hands and feet that resolved with time, and attention deficit hyperactivity disorder. The sister had normal intellectual abilities, whereas the brother had borderline function (IQ of 76 by The Stanford–Binet Intelligence Scale). Both the parents had normal head sizes and intelligence.

Prenatal Diagnosis: The presence of microcephaly in the at-risk fetus is presumptive evidence for this disorder.

Differential Diagnosis: See Microcephaly in the Index.

Ultrasound[h,i]: microcephaly, hydrothorax, nonimmune hydrops fetalis, hydramnios
  Kozma et al., 1996

PD 128500 PITUITARY AGENESIS (Congenital absence of pituitary gland; Primary pituitary dysgenesis) (McKusick No. None)

Amniocentesis: low level of amniotic fluid prolactin in the fetus at risk
  Stoll et al., 1978
  Comments: Prolactin level was measured by double antibody radioimmunoassay method (Stoll et al., 1978).

PD 128750 PORENCEPHALY (McKusick No. Unknown; see 175780)

Ultrasound[d]: decreased biparietal diameter, intracranial cystlike structures
  Hughes and Miskin, 1986
  Comments: At 30 weeks the surviving twin, whose co-twin had died at 21 weeks, was found to have a decreased biparietal diameter (microcephaly) and intracranial cysts. Prior to the 21st week of gestation, both twins had normal biparietal diameters and brain structures. The defects in the surviving twin were thought to be caused by a vascular disruption secondary to the death of the co-twin.
  increased lateral ventricular width to hemispheric width ratio
    Drugan et al., 1989a
  large unilateral posterior cerebral cystic structure that communicated with the lateral ventricle
    Simpson et al., 1988

PD 128880 RACHISCHISIS (McKusick No. None)

Acetylcholinesterase[c]: presence of a rapidly migrating amniotic fluid isozyme on gel electrophoresis
  Rodeck et al., 1982b; Raymond and Simpson, 1988
Alpha-fetoprotein[c]: elevated in amniotic fluid
  Rodeck et al., 1982b
Fetoscopy: direct visualization of an open spine
  Rodeck et al., 1982b
Ultrasound: most of the vertebral column open; scoliosis
  Rodeck et al., 1982b

PD 128890 SCHIZENCEPHALY (True porencephaly) (McKusick No. None)

Condition Note: Schizencephaly is a brain defect in which there is a full-thickness cleft within the cerebral hemisphere(s) such that the lateral ventricle(s) communicates directly with the subarachnoid space. This condition is differentiated from porencephaly by the presence of gray matter infolding along the cleft in schizencephaly. Some authors classify schizencephaly as a form of porencephaly (true porencephaly as opposed to pseudoporencephaly, the latter being a lesion within the brain produced by local necrosis of brain tissue) (Romero et al., 1988, p. 50).

Lituania et al., 1989

Prenatal Diagnosis: The diagnosis should be suspected whenever a communication between the lateral ventricle and the subarachnoid space is detected.

Differential Diagnosis: Cytomegalovirus (PD 199000); Hydranencephaly (PD 124000); Triploidy (PD 102000); and conditions producing hydrocephalus (see Hydrocephalus in the Index).

Ultrasound[d]: dilatation of the lateral ventricles, communication between the ventricle and subarachnoid space

Klingensmith and Cioffi-Ragan, 1986; Lituania et al., 1989

intrauterine growth retardation

Klingensmith and Cioffi-Ragan, 1986; Lituania et al., 1989

PD 129000 SPINA BIFIDA CYSTICA (Includes Meningocele, Meningomyelocele, Myelocele, and Spinal dysraphism) (McKusick No. 182940)

Condition Note: Spina bifida cystica is a midline defect of the spinal cord involving partial or complete deficiency of the posterior arch of one or more vertebrae. Occasionally, the defect is anterior, involving the vertebral bodies. The most frequent etiology of spina bifida cystica is thought to be multifactorial inheritance; the condition, however, may result from single mutant gene defects such as Jarcho-Levin syndrome (PD 160500); chromosomal defects such as Trisomy 18 syndrome (PD 104000); teratogen exposures, such as valproic acid (valproic acid embryopathy) (PD 271980); and maternal disorders such as maternal diabetes (Diabetic embryopathy [PD 243500]); and is seen in a number of syndromes of unknown etiology such as Exstrophy of the cloaca (PD 135500). The incidence of spina bifida cystica varies worldwide from a low of 0.3 per 1000 births in Japan to a high of 4.1 per 1000 births in Wales.

Romero et al., 1988, pp. 36–37

Prenatal Diagnosis: The diagnosis may be suspected with elevation in either maternal serum or amniotic fluid AFP. The disorder is more likely if the acetylcholinesterase isozyme is also present in amniotic fluid. Under the usual circumstances, the definitive diagnosis is made by detecting one or more ultrasonic findings, including absence of skin covering the spinal defect, a bulging posterior sac, interruption in the posterior processes and soft tissue on sagittal section, widening of the spinal processes on coronal section, and a defect in the posterior arch on transverse section.

Romero et al., 1988, pp. 39–40

Differential Diagnosis: Diabetic embryopathy (PD 243500); Exstrophy of the cloaca (PD 135500); Sacral dysgenesis (PD 169040); Sacral/spina bifida, familial (PD 169020); Sirenomelia (PD 194130); Spina bifida occulta (PD 130000)

Prenatal Treatment: No effective intrauterine treatment has been devised. However, affected fetuses have been followed for excessive ventricular enlargement and, if present, delivered by cesarean section at 32–34 weeks of gestation. If no excessive enlargement is present, the fetus is delivered by cesarean section at or near term.

Hogge et al., 1990

Acetylcholinesterase[c]: elevated in amniotic fluid, increased ratio of acetylcholinesterase activity to percentage of total cholinesterase activity, and/or fast-migrating amniotic fluid isozyme

Chubb et al., 1979; Smith et al., 1979; Buamah et al., 1980; Dale, 1980; Seller and Cole, 1980; Dale et al., 1981; Macri et al., 1981; Lawton, 1981; Voigtlander et al., 1981; Wald and Cuckle, 1981; Webb et al., 1981a; Crandall et al., 1982; Milunski and Sapirstein, 1982; Read et al., 1982a; Simpson et al., 1982; Aitken et al., 1984b; Albrechtsen et al., 1984; Schnittger and Kjessler, 1984; Sindic et al., 1984; Toftager-Larsen et al., 1984; Wyvill et al., 1984; de Elejalde and Elejalde, 1985b; Raymond and Simpson, 1988

acetylcholinesterase to cholinesterase isozyme density ratio greater than 0.13

Lawton, 1981; Goldfine et al., 1983; Burton, 1986

Comments: For Gastroschisis (PD 137000) and Omphalocele (PD 144000), the ratio of acetylcholinesterase to cholinesterase is normally less than 0.075. However, this is not a definitive test to differentiate between neural tube defects and ventral wall defects because there are a number of conditions that will cause acetylcholinesterase to be present in the amniotic fluid (see Acetylcholinesterase in the Index) (Burton, 1986).

elevated in amniotic fluid as determined by an immunoassay method using a monoclonal antibody

Brock et al., 1985c; Goldfine et al., 1989

fast-migrating amniotic fluid isozyme

Anneren et al., 1988; Schnatterly and Hogge, 1988; Boogert et al., 1989; Crandall et al., 1989; McDonnell et al., 1989

Alpha-fetoprotein[c]: elevated in maternal serum and amniotic fluid

Brock and Sutcliffe, 1972; Campbell et al., 1975; Leighton et al., 1975; Wright et al., 1975; Wald and Cuckle, 1977; Crandall et al., 1978; U.K. Collaborative Study, 1979; Brock, 1981; Macri et al., 1981; Wald and Cuckle, 1981; Ward, 1982; Burton et al., 1983; Freeman and Harbison, 1983; Haddow et al., 1983; Aitken et al., 1984b; Albrechtsen et al., 1984; Crandall and Matsumoto, 1984; Schnittger and Kjessler, 1984; Sindic et al., 1984; Toftager-Larsen et al., 1984; Wyvill et al., 1984; de Elejalde and Elejalde, 1985b; Ghosh et al., 1986

Comment: Diamniotic, monochorionic twins, one of whom had anencephaly, were reported by Holbrook and associates (1987b). The AFP concentration was elevated and an acetylcholinesterase isozyme was present in the amniotic fluids from both twins, even though they were in separate sacs. Four sets of diamniotic and dichorionic twins who were discordant for either anencephaly (2) or spina bifida cystica (2) have each been reported to have normal amniotic fluid AFP levels with no acetylcholinesterase isozyme in the amniotic fluids from the normal twins, but elevated

AFP levels and acetylcholinesterase isozyme in the fluids of the affected twins (Schnatterly and Hogge, 1988). Schnatterly and Hogge (1988) suggest that the four membranes present between the diamniotic, dichorionic twins prevent the diffusion of the AFP and acetylcholinesterase between sacs whereas the two membranes found in the diamniotic, monochorionic twins do not.

elevated in maternal serum

Milunsky et al., 1988; McDonnell et al., 1989; Van den Hof et al., 1990; Evans et al., 1995a

elevated in amniotic fluid

Anneren et al., 1988; Schnatterly and Hogge, 1988; Boogert et al., 1989; Crandall et al., 1989; McDonnell et al., 1989

Amniocentesis: rapidly adhering cells in 20-hour culture of amniotic fluid cells,[c] percentage ranging from 9–100%, normal being 6% or less

Gosden and Brock, 1977; Gosden and Brock, 1978a; Medina-Gomez and Bard, 1983

Comments: Rapidly adherent cell types include long bipolar, filamentous pseudopodial, large vacuolated, and multinucleate cells.

increased number of cells attached in 20 to 24 hours[c]

Bryant and Hoehn, 1977

identification of uncultured glial cells (one type of rapidly adhering cells) in amniotic fluid by use of glial fibrillary acidic protein-specific antibodies[c]

von Koskull, 1984

increased proportion of macrophages and elongated cells in smear of uncultured amniotic fluid cells[c]

Papp and Bell, 1979

presence of macrophages and neural cells in cultured amniotic fluid cells[c]

Medina-Gomez and Bard, 1983

increased number of amniocytes, which take up neutral red dye (2700 cells/mL)[c]

Polgar et al., 1984

increased activity of amniotic fluid disaccharidases prior to 21 weeks' gestation[c]

Morin et al., 1980

elevated fibrin/fibrinogen degradation products in the amniotic fluid[c]

Weiss et al., 1976; Legge, 1983

elevated amniotic fluid levels of D2-protein[c]

Jorgensen and Norgaard-Pedersen, 1981; Jorgensen, 1982

decreased percentage of amniotic fluid AFP that does not react with concanavalin A[c]

Toftager-Larsen et al., 1980; Toftager-Larsen et al., 1984

elevated levels of alpha-2-macroglobulin in amniotic fluid[c]

Legge, 1983; Toftager-Larsen et al., 1984

increased plasmin levels in the amniotic fluid[c]

Legge, 1983

decreased plasminogen levels in the amniotic fluid[c]

Legge, 1983

decreased percentage of lens culinaris agglutinin reacting to amniotic fluid AFP[c]

Toftager-Larsen et al., 1984

decreased level of gamma-glutamyltranspeptidase activity in amniotic fluid[c]

Brock et al., 1984a

elevated levels of S-100 protein in amniotic fluid[c]

Sindic et al., 1984; Anneren et al., 1988

decreased levels of amniotic fluid glucose[c]

Weiss et al., 1985

elevated levels of neuron-specific enolase activity in amniotic fluid

Anneren et al., 1988

increased concentrations of glial fibrillary acidic protein in amniotic fluid[c]

Albrechtsen et al., 1984

greater than 50% residual alkaline phosphatase activity in cell-free amniotic fluid expressed as a percentage of the total activity to residual activity after phenylalanine inhibition

Carey and Pollard, 1986

less than 50% residual alkaline phosphatase activity in cell-free amniotic fluid expressed as a percentage of the total activity to residual activity after l-homoarginine inhibition

Carey and Pollard, 1986

Amniography: bulging or depressed lesion in lumbosacral area

Weiss et al., 1978; Balsam and Weiss, 1981

displacement of opacified amniotic fluid by soft tissue malformation (the meningomyelocele)

Queenan and Gadow, 1970

Cholinesterase[c]: elevated in amniotic fluid

Milunsky et al., 1979; Hullin et al., 1981; Webb et al., 1981a; Simpson et al., 1982

Fetoscopy: yellow-gray lesion that was devoid of hair and contained a superficial network of small blood vessels

Rodeck and Campbell, 1978

Radiograph[c,d]: legs hyperextended on the thighs, and thighs flexed onto the abdomen

Epstein, 1961

Ultrasound: absence of posterior ossification centers of the spine producing a U-shaped or "open circle" deformity (sonolucent area) of the fetal spine

Michell and Bradley-Watson, 1973; Hobbins et al., 1979; Fiske and Filly, 1982; Platt et al., 1982; Campbell and Pearce, 1983; Hill et al., 1983a

widening of vertebral column and interpedicular distances in area of the spina bifida

Macri et al., 1981; Spirt et al., 1987; Hill et al., 1988b

V-shaped configuration or splaying of the posterior ossification centers when the lumbar spines were visualized on transverse scan

Nyberg et al., 1987; Spirt et al., 1987

soft tissue mass protruding posteriorly from spine (meningocele)

Nyberg et al., 1987; Spirt et al., 1987; Hill et al., 1988b

hydrocephalus[c]
>Fiske and Filly, 1982; Platt et al., 1982; Chervenak et al., 1983b; Quinlan et al., 1983; de Elejalde and Elejalde, 1985b

ventriculomegaly (increased lateral ventricular width to hemispheric width ratio)[c]
>Chervenak et al., 1984a; Nyberg et al., 1987; Drugan et al., 1989a; Dungan et al., 1989; Hogge et al., 1990; Van der Hof et al., 1990

Comment: Dungan and co-workers (1989) defined ventriculomegaly as a cortical/mantle thickness of less than 10 mm as measured by ultrasound.

progressive enlargement of the ventricles[c]
>Hogge et al., 1990

lemon sign
>Van den Hof et al., 1990

Comment: The lemon sign, or lemon-shaped skull, is an ultrasonic finding associated with open spina bifida, and is produced by frontal bone scalloping (Van den Hof et al., 1990). In a prospective study, Van den Hof and associates (1990) found the lemon sign present in 98% of fetuses with spina bifida cystica when the gestational ages of the fetuses were less than or at 24 weeks, but in only 13% of those at greater than 24 weeks.

banana sign
>Van den Hof et al., 1990

Comments: The banana sign is an ultrasonic finding found in many fetuses with spina bifida cystica, caused by an abnormal anterior curvature of the cerebellar hemispheres (Van den Hof et al., 1990). In a prospective study, Van den Hof and associates (1990) found the banana sign in 69% of affected fetuses who were at 24 weeks gestational age or less, and in only 19% after that gestational age. Failure to detect the cerebellum by ultrasound in these fetuses was also common, and this failure was present in 27% before or at 24 weeks of gestation, and 81% after this age.

failure to detect the cerebellum
>Van den Hof et al., 1990

decreased biparietal diameter[c]
>Roberts and Campbell, 1980; Wald et al., 1980

no movement and/or functional impairment of lower limbs movement in association with spina bifida cystica
>de Elejalde and Elejalde, 1985b

abnormal fetal movements and/or positioning of limbs[c]
>Ianniruberto and Tajani, 1981

oligohydramnios[c]
>Chervenak et al., 1983b

intrauterine growth retardation
>Nyberg et al., 1987

PD 130000 SPINA BIFIDA OCCULTA (McKusick No. 182940)

Differential Diagnosis: Diabetic embryopathy (PD 243500); Exstrophy of the cloaca (PD 135500); Sacral agenesis (PD 169000); Sacral agenesis/spina bifida, familial (PD 169020); Sirenomelia (PD 194130); Spina bifida cystica (PD 129000)

Ultrasound: low spinal defect
Hood and Robinson, 1978

PD 130250 SPINAL CORD NECROSIS (McKusick No. None)

Maternal history[c]: decreased fetal movement
Young et al., 1983
Physical examination of the mother[c]: breech position
Young et al., 1983
Comments: Postmortem examination of the case reported by Young and associates (1983) revealed a softened, discolored spinal cord in the cervical region that on microscopic examination showed loss of neurons and axons. These findings were consistent with necrosis of the cord.

PD 130750 WALKER–WARBURG SYNDROME (Chemke syndrome; HARD ± E syndrome; Hydrocephalus, agyria and retinal dysplasia syndrome; Pagon syndrome; Walker lissencephaly; Warburg syndrome) (McKusick No. 236670)

Syndrome Note: An autosomal recessively inherited syndrome, the Walker–Warburg syndrome is a distinct malformation syndrome that includes congenital hydrocephalus or ventricular dilation, type 2 lissencephaly (agyria), microcephaly, encephalocele, microphthalmia, dysplastic and detached retina, cataracts, myopathy, and severe neonatal neurologic dysfunction. The acronym HARD ± E is defined as *h*ydrocephalus, *a*gyria, and *r*etinal *d*ysplasia with or without *e*ncephalocele.
Crowe et al., 1986
Prenatal Diagnosis: The presence of hydrocephalus, encephalocele, and/or microcephaly with abnormalities of the eye is suggestive of the diagnosis. With a family history, the diagnosis should be considered with any one of the above findings.
Differential Diagnosis: Cerebrooculomuscular syndrome; Fukuyama congenital muscular dystrophy; Hydrolethalus syndrome (PD 191330); Knobloch–Layer syndrome; Meckel syndrome (PD 192140)
Crowe et al., 1986
Maternal history: decreased fetal movements as perceived by the mother[i]
Crowe et al., 1986
Ultrasound: encephalocele[i]
Crowe et al., 1985; Crowe et al., 1986; Farrell et al., 1987
hydrocephalus
Ayme et al., 1990; Chitayat et al., 1995c
hydrocephalus with macrocephaly and ventriculomegaly[i]
Crowe et al., 1985; Crowe et al., 1986; Farrell et al., 1987
severe hydrocephalus with markedly dilated lateral and third ventricles, and almost no occipital parenchyma visible[d]
Chitayat et al., 1995c
cerebellar hemispheres separated by a fluid space[d,i]
Farrell et al., 1987
no identifiable vermis[d,i]
Farrell et al., 1987
usually small right eye with conical structure within which was thought to be retinal detachment,[d,i] no identifiable left orbit[d,i]
Farell et al., 1987

identification of a conical structure within the globe of one eye representing a retinal detachment[d]

Chitayat et al., 1995c

PD 131000 X-LINKED HYDROCEPHALUS (X-linked aqueductal stenosis) (McKusick No. 307000)

Condition Note: X-linked hydrocephalus is caused by a mutation in the gene that codes for L1 cell adhesion molecules (L1CAM). Mutations in this gene also can cause the MASA syndrome (PD 127000).

Prenatal Diagnosis: Demonstration of ventricular enlargement by 19 weeks of gestation, or later, in a fetus at risk should be diagnostic in most cases.

Radiography[c,d]: enlarged fetal head

Benke and Strassberg, 1980

Ultrasound[i]: enlargement of lateral ventricles, progressive increase in the ventricular width to head diameter ratio, reduced cerebral mantle thickness, hydrocephalus

Clewell et al., 1981; Sandlin et al., 1981; Rogers and Danks, 1983; Van Egmond-Linden et al., 1983; Friedman and Santos-Ramos, 1984; Horvath et al., 1985; Rawnsley et al., 1985; Nicolaides et al., 1986a; Varadi et al., 1987; Ko et al., 1994

Comments: Friedman and Santos-Ramos (1984) found no ventricular enlargement prior to 22 weeks of gestation. Rawnsley and associates (1985) reported enlargement of ventricles in each of a set of at-risk twins by the 19th week of gestation. Ko and co-workers (1994) reported a couple who had four consecutive males affected with X-linked hydrocephalus. In the third case, the lateral ventricles were mildly dilated by 17 weeks of gestation, and were moderately enlarged by 20 weeks. In the fourth pregnancy, the lateral ventriclar sizes in the fetus were normal at 16 and 20 weeks, but dilated by 24 weeks. It is apparent that dilation of the ventricles is variable in this condition even in the same family, and cannot be totally relied on for diagnosis before about 22 weeks of gestation.

THE GASTROINTESTINAL AND RELATED SYSTEMS[a]

PD 131250 ANNULAR PANCREAS (McKusick No. None)

Amniography[c,d]: no fetal swallowing, no contrast material in the intestinal tract

White and Stewart, 1973

Ultrasound[c]: distended loops of bowel, hydramnios

Jassani et al., 1982

cystic mass located in the midabdominal cavity close to the stomach and caudal to the liver

de Elejalde and Elejalde, 1985b

PD 131380 BILIARY DUCT ATRESIA, COMPLETE (McKusick No. None)

Amniocentesis[c]: low levels of gamma-glutamyltranspeptidase, aminopeptidase M, and total alkaline phosphatase in amniotic fluid

Muller et al., 1988

PD 131500 CHOLEDOCHAL CYST (McKusick No. None)

Condition Note: A choledochal cyst is a congenital cystic dilatation of the common bile duct. Clinical signs and symptoms may not develop until the second decade of life or later. The condition usually presents as an ascending cholangitis with pain and a subhepatic mass. If it is undiagnosed, biliary cirrhosis and death may result. Usually it is not inherited.

Elrad et al., 1985

Prenatal Diagnosis: Any cystlike structure in the right upper abdominal quadrant that is not attached to the kidney should cause one to consider this condition.

Ultrasound[d]: cystic structure in the right upper quadrant of the abdomen that is separate from the bladder and kidney, and attached to tubular structures at both ends, hydramnios

Dewbury et al., 1980; Elrad et al., 1985

PD 131750 CONGENITAL CHLORIDE DIARRHEA (McKusick No. 214700)

Disease Note: Congenital chloride diarrhea, which is a rare autosomal recessive disease, is a disturbance in chloride transport in the ileum. This defect leads to massive, watery diarrhea beginning in the neonatal period. Treatment involves providing adequate electrolyte replacement.

Kirkinen and Jouppila, 1984

Prenatal Diagnosis: distended, well-defined loops of intestine in at-risk fetuses

Amniocentesis[c,d]: elevated levels of chloride in amniotic fluid

Muller et al., 1988

elevated levels of gamma-glutamyltranspeptidase, aminopeptidase M, and total alkaline phosphatase activities in amniotic fluid[c,d]

Muller et al., 1988

Ultrasound[i]: increased abdominal circumference, hydramnios, ascites

Kirkinen and Jouppila, 1984

multiple well-defined distended loops of intestine

Kirkinen and Jouppila, 1984; Muller et al., 1988

PD 132000 DIAPHRAGMATIC HERNIA (McKusick No. 142340; see also 222400)

Condition Note: Diaphragmatic hernias are the protrusions of abdominal organs into the thoracic cavity through defects in the diaphragm. These hernias include posterolateral, anteromedial, and right-sided defects. The etiology is varied, with most being sporadic. Occasionally, the condition is familial. In about 50% of the cases, associated defects are found, with defects of the CNS being the most frequent, followed by those of the cardiovascular system. Diaphragmatic hernias are found in a number of syndromes, some of which involve chromosomal disorders.

The prognosis for congenital diaphragmatic hernia is not good. Even though the defect is usually corrected in the postnatal period, 20–80% of infants die of pulmonary insufficiency related to hypoplasia of the lungs. The survival rate is somewhat related to the occurrence of hydramnios. When hydramnios is present, only 11% of affected infants survive, whereas 55% of those without hydramnios live. This finding may be related to the fact that hydramnios is more likely to occur when larger volumes of viscera are present in the chest cavity, which in turn causes more lung compression and lung hypoplasia (Harrison et al., 1990a).

Postnatal treatment with extracorporeal membrane oxygenation (ECMO) has improved the outcome of these infants to some extent.

> Adzick et al, 1985; Harrison et al., 1985; Romero et al., 1988, pp. 211–219

Prenatal Diagnosis: The in utero diagnosis of diaphragmatic hernia has been made by a number of methods that basically rely on the demonstration of abdominal organs being present in the fetal thorax. Information about the prenatal diagnosis of diaphragmatic hernias is listed below under posterolateral, anteromedial, and right-side subsections reflecting the location of the hernias.

Differential Diagnosis: When a diaphragmatic hernia is detected prenatally, other congenital abnormalities should be sought in the fetus, and if found, a chromosomal analysis on fetal or chorionic villus tissue should be considered. Among the disorders that have been reported with diaphragmatic hernias are Beckwith–Wiedemann syndrome (PD 187000); Fryns syndrome (PD 191240); and VATER association (PD 194650). Everted diaphragm is seen in Eventration of the diaphragm (PD 135250); and Trisomy 18 syndrome (PD 104000). Tumors and cysts need to be considered, including Congenital bronchial cyst (PD 272380); Cystic adenomatoid malformation of lung (PD 272500); Hamartoma of the lung; Sequestration of lung (PD 193750); Teratoma, lung (PD 281750); Teratoma, mediastinal (PD 281770).

Prenatal Treatment: Successful in utero repair of a left-sided fetal diaphragmatic hernia has been reported by Harrison and colleagues (1990a). The repair was done at 24 weeks of gestation, and the child was delivered at 32 weeks. After ventilatory support for 4 weeks, the child did well and was normal at 8 months.

POSTEROLATERAL (DIAPHRAGMATIC HERNIA OF THE FORAMEN OF BOCHDALEK)

General Comments: The posterolateral diaphragmatic hernia is the more common type of diaphragmatic hernia and is a herniation of bowel and other abdominal viscera through the foramen of Bochdalek (pleuroperitoneal hernia).

Alpha-fetoprotein[c]: elevated in amniotic fluid
> Lazzarini et al., 1985

Amniography: displacement of the fetal gut into the thorax
> Boyd et al., 1969

Ultrasound: echo-spared area within fetal chest (intrathoracic cystic mass), intrathoracic solid mass representing herniated liver, shift of the mediastinum and heart to the right, peristalsis of the chest contents, reduced abdominal circumference, stomach not identified in the abdomen, hydramnios; with fetal breathing abdominal contents on the side of the defect moved superiorly while the rest of the bowel and liver descended
> Hobbins et al., 1979; Comstock, 1986; Meizner et al., 1986c; Spirt et al., 1987

large left-sided diaphragmatic hernia
> Narayan et al., 1993

dilated loops of bowel in the fetal chest
> Spirt et al., 1987; Harrison et al., 1990a

dilated stomach present in the left chest
> Spirt et al., 1987; Harrison et al., 1990a; Narayan et al, 1993

herniation of abdominal viscera into the fetal chest[c]
> Harrison et al., 1985; Simpson et al., 1988

abnormal upper abdominal anatomy
    Harrison et al., 1985
mediastinal shift away from the side of the herniation
    Harrison et al., 1985; Simpson et al., 1988; Harrison et al., 1990a
herniated abdominal viscera that moved in and out of the chest
    Harrison et al., 1985
hypoplastic lungs
    Narayan et al., 1993
little visible lung
    Harrison et al., 1990a
hydrothorax
    Narayan et al., 1993
displacement of the heart to the right
    Narayan et al., 1993
liver present in the thorax
    Narayan et al., 1993
ascites[c]
    Narayan et al., 1993
hydramnios[c]
    Harrison et al., 1985; Narayan et al., 1993

ANTEROMEDIAL (DIAPHRAGMATIC HERNIA OF MORGAGNI)

Ultrasound: heart found in the normal position but surrounded by excessive amounts of pericardial fluid, intrathoracic mass lateral to heart, compression of the lung posteriorly, normal abdominal circumference, stomach identified in abdomen
    Comstock, 1986

RIGHT-SIDED

Ultrasound: herniation of the bowel and liver into the right chest,[d] pleural effusion,[d] ascites,[d] skin edema,[d] hydrops fetalis[d]
    Benacerraf and Frigoletto, 1986
hydrothorax-like appearance[c,d]
    Whittle et al., 1989
hydramnios
    Benacerraf and Frigoletto, 1986; Blott et al., 1988a; Whittle et al., 1989

TYPE NOT STATED

Ultrasound[d]: pleural effusion
    Blott et al., 1988a
hydrops fetalis
    Blott et al., 1988a

PD 132050 DIAPHRAGMATIC HERNIA, FAMILIAL (Diaphragm, unilateral agenesis of; Familial congenital diaphragmatic defects) (McKusick No. 222400)

Condition Note: A few families have been reported where there has been recurrence of diaphragmatic hernias in sibs. At this time, it is not known if the recurrence is autosomal recessive or multifactorial.
    McKusick, 1995

Ultrasound[i]: dextroposition of the heart, enlargement of the thorax, disproportionate thoracic to abdominal diameter ratio
        Gualandri et al., 1983
     Comment: Gualandri and co-workers (1983) reported two sibs with dia-
phragmatic hernias.

PD 133000 DUODENAL ATRESIA (McKusick No. Unknown; see 223400)

Alpha-fetoprotein[c]: elevated in amniotic fluid
        Weinberg et al., 1975
Amniocentesis: lower levels of glucose in amniotic fluid[c]
        Weiss et al., 1984
     decreased activity of amniotic fluid disaccharidases prior to 21
     weeks' gestation[c]
        Morin et al., 1980
     elevated optical density at 450 nm of amniotic fluid[c,d]
        Sankaran et al., 1984
     elevated total bile acid concentration in the amniotic fluid cells[c]
        Legge and Rippon, 1982
     elevated levels of gamma-glutamyltranspeptidase, aminopeptidase M,
     and total alkaline phosphatase activities in amniotic fluid[c]
        Muller et al., 1988
        Comment: Where the above enzymes were found to be elevated, the
        atresia was below the sphincter of Oddi.
     bile-stained amniotic fluid[c,d]
        Nelson et al., 1982a
Amniography[d]: absence of fetal swallowing, absence of contrast material in
the fetal gastrointestinal tract, hydramnios
        White and Stewart, 1973; Houlton et al., 1974
Ultrasound[d,e]: two fluid-filled masses ("double bubble" sign) in the upper
fetal abdomen, dilated stomach, hydramnios, dilated proximal duodenum
        Hobbins et al., 1979; Morin et al., 1980; Canty et al., 1981; Legge
        and Rippon, 1982; Zamah et al., 1982; Campbell and Pearce,
        1983; Hill et al., 1983a; Filkins et al., 1985; Nicolaides et al., 1986a;
        Spirt et al., 1987
     two fluid-filled spaces or masses ("double bubble" sign)
        Nelson et al., 1982a; Sankaran et al., 1984; Hill et al., 1988b
     cystic mass found in the mid-abdominal cavity close to the stomach and
     located caudally to the liver over the posterior aspect of the abdomen
        de Elejalde and Elejalde, 1985b
     single umbilical artery[c]
        Tortora et al., 1984
     hydramnios[c]
        Nelson et al., 1982a; Tortora et al., 1984; Sankaran et al. 1984;
        Hill et al., 1988b
     no significant increase in maternal serum 17 beta-estradiol following
     injection of dehydroisoandrosterone sulfate into the amniotic cavity[c]
        Strecker and Jonatha, 1982

PD 134000 ECTOPIC FETAL LIVER (McKusick No. None)

Ultrasound[c]: mass adjacent to fetal abdomen
        Mack et al., 1978

PD 135000 ESOPHAGEAL ATRESIA (McKusick No. None)

Acetylcholinesterase[c,d]: elevated in amniotic fluid in the presence of normal AFP levels

> Holzgreve and Golbus, 1983; Holzgreve et al., 1983

> fast-migrating amniotic fluid isozyme

> Holzgreve and Golbus, 1983; Aitken et al., 1984b

Alpha-fetoprotein[c,d]: elevated in amniotic fluid

> Seppala, 1973

> elevated in maternal serum

> Aitken et al., 1984b

Amniocentesis: lower levels of glucose in amniotic fluid[c]

> Weiss et al., 1984

Amniography[d]: no fetal swallowing, no contrast material present in intestines, hydramnios

> Seppala, 1973; White and Stewart, 1973

Fetography[d]: lack of swallowing of opacified amniotic fluid

> Suzumori and Yagami, 1975

> *Comment:* Caution must be taken in the interpretation of this test because partial passage of the radiographic contrast medium into the fetal intestine in some cases of esophageal atresia has occurred, giving rise to a false negative diagnosis (Holzgreve and Golbus, 1983).

Maternal blood sampling: no significant increase in maternal serum 17-beta-estradiol following injection of dehydroisoandrosterone sulfate into the amniotic cavity[c]

> Strecker and Jonatha, 1982

Ultrasound[c,d]: increased swallowing activity, fetal regurgitation, hydramnios

> Bowie and Clair, 1982; Nelson et al., 1982b; Quinlan et al., 1983

> inability to detect stomach or loops of intestine, hydramnios

> Jassani et al., 1982

PD 135100 ESOPHAGEAL ATRESIA, FAMILIAL (Esophageal atresia with or without tracheoesophageal fistula, familial; Tracheoesophageal fistula with or without esophageal atresia, familial) (McKusick No. 189960)

> **Condition Note:** Although most cases of esophageal atresia with or without tracheoesophageal fistula (EA ± TEF) are isolated, nonfamilial anomalies, or associated with syndromes, the occasional EA ± TEF appears to be inherited in an autosomal dominant fashion. The empiric recurrence risk for parents with a single affected child appears to be between 0.5% and 2%. This risk rises to 20% if more than one sib is affected. If an affected parent reproduces, the risk of having an affected child is 3–4%.

> > Pletcher et al., 1991

> **Prenatal Diagnosis:** The diagnosis can be suspected in a fetus at risk whenever there is hydramnios present. Lack of swallowing of opacified amniotic fluid and no contrast material in the intestinal tract is further evidence for this condition. However, lack of these latter findings does not rule out the condition; a tracheoesophageal fistula may allow continuity of the alimentary tract.

> **Differential Diagnosis:** Bilateral left-sidedness sequence (PD 187230); Diabetic embryopathy (PD 243500); DiGeorge syndrome (PD 100995); Down syndrome (PD 101000); Esophageal atresia (PD 135000); Holt–Oram syndrome (PD

191310); Robin sequence (PD 136000); Trisomy 13 syndrome (PD 103000); Trisomy 18 syndrome (PD 104000); VATER association (PD 194650).

Ultrasound[d,i]: hydramnios
    Pletcher et al., 1991

PD 135250 EVENTRATION OF THE DIAPHRAGM (McKusick No. None)

Ultrasound[c,d]: displacement of the heart, right shift of the mediastinum, stomach identified in the chest, cystic mass in the thorax; postnatally, the infant was found to have trisomy 18
    Comstock, 1986

PD 135500 EXSTROPHY OF THE CLOACA (Exstrophia splanchnica; OEIS sequence) (McKusick No. None)

Acetylcholinesterase[c]: fast-migrating amniotic fluid isozyme
    Gosden and Brock, 1981
Alpha-fetoprotein[c]: elevated in maternal serum
    Gosden and Brock, 1981; Kutzner et al., 1988
    elevated in amniotic fluid
    Gosden and Brock, 1981
Amniocentesis: rapidly adhering amniotic fluid cells (types I and II fetal distress cells and exomphalos/omphalocele cells [peritoneal macrophages])[c]
    Gosden and Brock, 1981
Ultrasound: spina bifida cystica, dilated cerebral ventricles, multicystic kidney, hydronephrosis, ascites
    Gosden and Brock, 1981; McLaughlin et al., 1984
    shortening of the thoracic cage
    Meizner et al., 1986c
    narrow chest cage
    Meizner and Bar-Ziv, 1985
    ascites
    Kutzner et al., 1988
    spina bifida cystica (meningomyelocele)
    Meizner and Bar-Ziv, 1985; Kutzner et al., 1988
    enlarged liver
    Meizner and Bar-Ziv, 1985
    omphalocele that contained liver and bowel
    Kutzner et al., 1988
    omphalocele
    Meizner and Bar-Ziv, 1985
    multiple cervical and thoracic and/or lumbosacral vertebral defects
    Meizner and Bar-Ziv, 1985; Kutzner et al., 1988
    ventriculomegaly
    Kutzner et al., 1988
    clubfoot deformity
    Meizner and Bar-Ziv, 1985

PD 135750 GASTRIC DUPLICATION CYST (Duplication of the stomach; Stomach duplication) (McKusick No. None)

Condition Note: Duplication cysts of the gastrointestinal tract may occur anywhere along the length of the gut. Duplication of the stomach is the least commonly reported gastrointestinal tract duplications, but when present may lead to life-threatening complications such as bleeding from an ulcer, perforation, or fistula formation. The most common location for these cysts is the greater curvature of the stomach. Gastric duplications can be tubular or cystic, with the tubular type usually communicating with the lumen of the stomach while the cystic type usually does not. Because gastric duplication cysts may lead to life-threatening complications, it is important to suspect this condition prior to or shortly after birth.

Bidwell and Nelson, 1986

Prenatal Diagnosis: The diagnosis should be considered any time an intraabdominal cyst is located in the upper half of the abdomen. At present, there is no definitive method for diagnosing this malformation.

Differential Diagnosis: Congenital thoracic gastroenteric cyst (PD 272440); Choledochal cyst (PD 131500); Duodenal atresia (PD 133000); Enteric duplication cyst of the small intestine (PD 273500); Meconium pseudocyst (PD 276500); Mesenteric cyst; Urinary tract cysts

Duplication cysts of the small bowel are most commonly ileal and usually located in the lower abdomen. The "double bubble" sign is often indicative of duodenal atresia, but a communicating gastric duplication cyst may have a similar appearance. An abdominal cyst is more likely to be of gastrointestinal origin if the urinary tract system appears to be normal.

Bidwell and Nelson, 1986

Ultrasound[c,d]: multiple anechoic structures in the right upper quadrant of the fetal abdomen

Bidwell and Nelson, 1986

Comments: After delivery, the fetus cited by Bidwell and Nelson (1986) had a duplication cyst attached to the greater curvature of the stomach. The diagnosis of gastric duplication cyst was confirmed histopathologically.

PD 136000 GASTRIC OBSTRUCTION, ANTRAL DIAPHRAGM (McKusick No. None)

Ultrasound[c,d]: ovoid sonolucent area in the upper left abdomen

Zimmerman, 1978

PD 136500 GASTROINTESTINAL BLEEDING (McKusick No. Unknown)

Amniocentesis[d]: sterile brown amniotic fluid that contained more than 10,000 red blood cells/mm^3, elevated digestive enzymes gamma-glutamyltranspeptidase, leucine aminopeptidase and intestinal alkaline, phosphatase

Decoret et al., 1994

Comments: In the case reported by Decoret and associates (1994), a Kleihauer–Betke test performed on the amniotic fluid that was collected at the time of delivery showed that 98.8% of the red blood cells were of fetal origin. After birth the hemoglobin was low, but the hematocrit and hemostasis were normal. The child was discharged from the hospital at 25 days of age in good health; no source of bleeding was found although there were diffuse hemorrhagic esophagitis and gastritis detected by gastrofibroscopy.

Ultrasound[c,d]: small, floating echogenic particles present in the amniotic fluid, dilated bowel in the abdominal cavity, hydramnios

Decoret et al., 1994

PD 137000 GASTROSCHISIS (McKusick No. 230750)

Prenatal Treatment: None; however, the prenatal diagnosis of gastroschisis is associated with reduced neonatal morbidity and mortality when the fetus is delivered in a facility capable of handling the repair of the defect immediately and appropriately.

> Phelps-Sandall et al., 1989

Acetylcholinesterase[c]: fast-migrating amniotic fluid isozyme, acetylcholinesterase to cholinesterase isozyme density ratio less than 0.13

> Wald and Cuckle, 1981; Crandall et al., 1982; Goldfine et al., 1983; Aitken et al., 1984b; Nielsen et al., 1985

acetylcholinesterase to cholinesterase isozyme density ratio less than 0.13

> Burton, 1986

> *Comments:* For Anencephaly (PD 118000) and Spina bifida cystica (PD 129000), the ratio of acetylcholinesterase to cholinesterase is normally greater than 0.13. This is not a definitive test to differentiate between neural tube defects and ventral wall defects because there are a number of conditions that will cause acetylcholinesterase to be present in the amniotic fluid (see Acetylcholinesterase in the Index) (Burton, 1986).

Alpha-fetoprotein[c]: elevated in maternal serum and amniotic fluid

> Douglas, 1977; Fisher et al., 1980; Fisher et al., 1981; Gardner et al., 1981; Macri et al., 1981; Jassani et al., 1982; Holmgren and Sigurd, 1984; Mann et al., 1984; Toftager-Larsen et al., 1984; Nielsen et al., 1985; Knott and Colley, 1987; Rodriguez et al., 1987b

Comments: In the two patients reported on by Knott and Colley (1987), no gastroschises were identified by ultrasound during the second trimester, even though both fetuses were born with these defects.

elevated in maternal serum

> Evans et al., 1995a; McMahon et al., 1995

decreased percentage of AFP that reacts with concanavalin A

> Nielsen et al., 1985

Amniocentesis: decreased percentage of amniotic fluid AFP that does not react with concanavalin A[c]

> Toftager-Larsen et al., 1980; Toftager-Larsen et al., 1984

elevated level of alpha-2-macroglobulin in amniotic fluid[c]

> Toftager-Larsen et al., 1984

elevated amniotic fluid alkaline phosphatase activity[c,d]

> Jalanko et al., 1983

decreased percentage of lens culinaris agglutinin reacting to AFP in amniotic fluid

> Toftager-Larsen et al., 1984

Amniography: loops of intestine floating freely in the amniotic cavity, large defect in abdominal wall

> Balsam and Weiss, 1981; Holmgren and Sigurd, 1984

Ultrasound: sonolucent cystic structures (fetal bowel) outside fetal abdomen, thickened bowel wall, hydramnios

> Giulian and Alvear, 1978; Canty et al., 1981; Jassani et al., 1982; Davidson et al., 1984; Nielsen et al., 1985

multicystic mass that was in front of and attached to the abdominal wall and showed peristaltic movement, mass not membrane covered
Bjornstahl et al., 1983; Spirt et al., 1987
hyperperistaltic intraabdominal dilated loops of echogenic bowel
McMahon et al., 1995
extraabdominal bowel that remained hyperechoic and aperistatic
McMahon et al., 1995
Comments: The above finding was correlated with the presence of an extremely short but viable small intestine in the neonate after birth.
McMahon et al., 1995
umbilical cord insertion not seen[c,d]
Spirt et al., 1987
oligohydramnios[c,d]
Spirt et al., 1987
hydramnios
McMahon et al., 1995

PD 137500 HIRSCHSPRUNG DISEASE (Aganglionic megacolon; Congenital megacolon; Hirschsprung's disease) (McKusick No. 249200)

Disease Note: Hirschsprung disease is produced by a deficiency or absence of intestinal ganglia resulting in absence of peristalsis and functional intestinal obstruction. Different degrees of involvement, from small segments in the distal colon, to total colonic or total colonic plus partial small intestine, or in rare cases, to total intestinal involvement, occur. The latter condition is fatal. Short- or intermediate-segment Hirschsprung disease can be surgically treated, and the affected individuals can subsequently live near-normal or normal lives. The cause of this condition is heterogeneous, with most appearing to be multifactorial, 4% familial, and 2% associated with chromosomal abnormalities.
Jarmas et al., 1983
Prenatal Diagnosis: Definitive prenatal diagnosis of this condition has not been accomplished (Jarmas et al., 1983).
Differential Diagnosis: Cystic fibrosis (PD 256000); Duodenal atresia (PD 133000); Imperforate anus (PD 138000); Ileal atresia (PD 137750); Jejunal atresia (PD 139000); Meconium ileus (PD 140000); Multiple intestinal atresia (PD 142500); Multiple intestinal atresia, autosomal recessive type (PD 143000).
Ultrasound[c,d]: cystic areas in the fetal abdomen thought to represent distended loops of bowel, increased abdominal circumference, hydramnios
Vermesh et al., 1986
Comments: Jarmas and associates (1983) failed to diagnose total colonic Hirschsprung disease in a fetus at risk for the condition. Midtrimester prenatal diagnosis utilizing amniotic fluid disaccharidase analyses, ultrasound, and amniography all failed to indicate any abnormality in the fetus. Postnatally, the neonate was found to have aganglionosis of the entire colon and distal half of the ileum. Removal of the colon and distal ileum at 17 months of age was followed by an ileorectal anastomosis.

PD 137750 ILEAL ATRESIA (McKusick No. None)

Amniograph[c,d]: hydramnios, no contrast material in intestine
Queenan and Gadow, 1970
Comment: At birth the infant had terminal ileal atresia with meconium ileus.

Ultrasound[c,d]: dilated loops of bowel, hydramnios
>> Filkins et al., 1985
>> cystic mass in the lower right side of the fetal abdomen detected at 30 weeks' gestation; by 35 weeks, there were distended, large, fluid-filled loops of small intestine, which showed strong peristaltic movements, and distended stomach and abdomen.
>>> Kjoller et al., 1985
>> dilated loops of bowel
>>> Spirt et al., 1987
>> hydramnios
>>> Spirt et al., 1987

PD 138000 IMPERFORATE ANUS (Anal atresia) (McKusick No. Unknown; see 207500, 301800)

Alpha-fetoprotein[c]: low levels in maternal serum
>> van Rijn et al., 1995
Amniocentesis: decreased activity of amniotic fluid disaccharidases prior to 21 weeks' gestation[c]
>> Potier et al., 1977; Morin et al., 1980; Kleijer et al., 1985b
Ultrasound[d]: fluid-filled bowel in the lower fetal abdomen
>> Bean et al., 1978
>> rounded sonoreflective structures (calcified meconium) in the fetal abdomen[c]
>>> Shalev et al., 1983a

PD 138500 INTESTINAL PERFORATION (McKusick No. None)

Ultrasound[d]: fetal ascites, thickened visceral peritoneum[c]
>> Shalev et al., 1982
>> microcalcifications detected as linear, high-amplitude echoes on the liver surface, ascites, intraabdominal adhesions
>>> Glick et al., 1983
>> meconium pseudocyst appearing as a tubular mass surrounded by a thick calcified rim
>>> Foster et al., 1987

PD 139000 JEJUNAL ATRESIA (McKusick No. Unknown; see 243600)

Ultrasound[c,d]: multiple dilated fluid-filled bowel loops
>> Lee and Warren, 1977a; Canty et al., 1981; Campbell and Pearce, 1983; Filkins et al., 1985; Spirt et al., 1987
hydramnios
>> Canty et al., 1981; Zamah et al., 1982; Filkins et al., 1985; Spirt et al., 1987
evidence of intestinal perforation, (ie, microcalcifications on the surface of the liver, ascites, and intraabdominal adhesions)
>> Glick et al., 1983
hyperactive peristalsis
>> Filkins et al., 1985

PD 139250 JEJUNAL ATRESIA, "APPLE-PEEL" TYPE (McKusick No. 243600)

Condition Note: Apple-peel intestinal atresia is a distinct disorder that includes proximal intestinal atresia, absence of the distal superior mesenteric artery and dorsal mesentery, and retrograde blood supply to the viable small intestine via the right colic artery. Apple-peel jejunal atresia accounts for less than 5% of all intestinal atresias. Fifteen percent of affected children with the latter disorder have other anomalies. The condition may be an autosomal recessive disorder.

Seashore et al., 1987; Cook and Bennett, 1995

Prenatal Diagnosis: Although the intestinal obstruction may be noted by distended loops of bowel, there is no specific means of prenatally diagnosing this condition.

Ultrasound[c,d]: dilated loops of bowel, increased echogenicity of the abdomen

Cook and Bennett, 1995

hydramnios

Seashore et al., 1987; Farag et al., 1993; Cook and Bennett, 1995

PD 139500 JEJUNOILEAL ATRESIA WITH PERSISTENT OMPHALOMESENTERIC DUCT (McKusick No. None)

Condition Note: The combination of jejunoileal atresia with persistent omphalomesenteric duct apparently has been reported only by Petrikovsky and associates (1988). In the child on whom they reported, there was partial atresia of the jejunum and complete atresia of the ileum with a remnant of the omphalomesenteric duct. The authors postulated that the blood supply to the atretic segments of bowel became compromised by becoming entangled and strangulated with the omphalomesenteric duct.

Prenatal Diagnosis: The definitive diagnosis of this disorder cannot be made prenatally. However, bowel obstruction may be suspected by the presence of dilated loops of bowel.

Differential Diagnosis: Duodenal atresia (PD 133000); Hirschsprung disease (PD 137500); Ileal atresia (PD 137750); Jejunal atresia (PD 139000); Jejunal atresia, apple-peel type (PD 139250); Multiple intestinal atresia (PD 142500); Multiple intestinal atresia, autosomal recessive type (PD 143000).

Ultrasound[c,d]: markedly dilated multiple loops of bowel

Petrikovsky et al., 1988

PD 139700 LARYNGEAL ATRESIA (McKusick No. Unknown; see 150300)

Ultrasound[c]: massively enlarged lungs, compressed heart that appeared otherwise normal, ascites, scalp and placental edema, hydrops fetalis, oligohydramnios

Watson et al., 1990b

Comments: In the case reported by Watson and colleagues (1990b), delivery was induced, and at autopsy, laryngeal atresia, lung hyperplasia, extensive general edema, and duodenal atresia were found.

PD 140000 MECONIUM ILEUS (Meconium plug syndrome) (McKusick No. None)

Condition Note: Meconium is the stool in the fetal intestinal track that normally accumulates when the fetus stops defecation after about the 20th week of gestation. In meconium ileus, the meconium is abnormal in that it is excessively thick and tenacious. After birth in the neonatal period, the neonate frequently is unable to pass this meconium creating a functional bowel obstruction. Between 10 and 20% of meconium ileus cases have cystic fibrosis and have this finding probably as a result of pancreatic insufficiency. Meconium plug syndrome is a form of meconium ileus where a mass of meconium is formed above the anorectal area. This latter type of meconium ileus is often associated with Hirschsprung disease (PD 137500). Complications of meconium ileus include volvulus, gangrenous bowel, and perforation and meconium peritonitis. Postnatal treatment of uncomplicated cases normally consists of high Gastrografin enemas. Some cases may require surgical intervention.

Samuel et al., 1986

Prenatal Diagnosis: The condition should be suspected in any fetus with unexplained bowel distension.

Differential Diagnosis: Cystic fibrosis (PD 256000); Hirschsprung disease (PD 137500); Ileal atresia (PD 137750); Jejunal atresia (PD 139000); Jegunoileal atresia with persistent omphalomesenteric duct (PD 139500); Multiple intestinal atresia (PD 142500); Multiple intestinal atresia, autosomal recessive type (PD 143000).

Prenatal Treatment: The only prenatal treatment reported is that of intraamniotic injections of Urograffin (Samuel et al., 1986).

Treatment Modality: Intraamniotic injection of Urograffin (third trimester only)

Samuel et al., 1986

Comments: In the two cases reported by Samuel and associates (1986), the first was treated at 34 weeks' gestation, the other at 35 weeks. Both were treated after their intestinal dilatation had worsened. At birth each neonate had meconium stained amniotic fluid, and passed copious amounts of watery meconium. Both were otherwise healthy and required no further treatment.

Methods and Findings: Radiograph[d]: calcification in fetal abdomen

Russell, 1973

Ultrasound[d]: multiple loops of distended bowel

Hobbins et al., 1979; Shalev et al., 1983b; Szabo et al., 1985b; Samuel et al., 1986

hydramnios[c]

Shalev et al., 1983b; Samuel et al., 1986

highly echogenic intraabdominal mass

Muller et al., 1984a

highly echogenic meconium

Van Allen et al., 1992

Comments: Van Allen and associates (1992), in a study of 18 pregnancies with fetuses having highly echogenic meconium (HEM) on fetal ultrasound, found ten with isolated HEM, seven with associated anomalies, and one with cystic fibrosis.

PD 141000 MECONIUM PERITONITIS (McKusick No. None)

Condition Note: Meconium peritonitis is a sterile chemical reaction to intraabdominal meconium, resulting from in utero small bowel perforation and meconium spillage. The etiology of the bowel perforation is varied and includes small bowel atresia, meconium ileus, volvulus, internal bowel hernia, intussusception, congenital bands, Meckel diverticulum, and vascular insufficiency. In many cases the cause is unknown, the exception being cystic fibrosis, which accounts for 15–40% of neonatal meconium ileus. The peritonitis resulting from spilled meconium frequently results in abdominal calcifications, or echogenic masses, and fetal ascites, all of which can be detected by prenatal ultrasound. Hydramnios also is present frequently.

The detection of meconium peritonitis should alert one to the possibility of bowel pathology that will need further evaluation and perhaps will lead to treatment in the neonatal period. When not detected until after birth, the associated mortality rate is 10–55% (Chitayat et al., 1995b).

> Foster et al., 1987

Prenatal Diagnosis: The detection of intraabdominal fetal calcification, masses, and/or ascites should raise the suspicion of this condition.

Differential Diagnosis: Intestinal perforation (PD 138500); Intraabdominal tumors; Congenital infections; McKusick–Kaufman syndrome (PD 192250); Meconium pseudocyst (PD 276500); and Teratoma, sacrococcygeal (PD 284000) are conditions frequently associated with intraabdominal masses or calcification.

Ultrasound: fetal abdominal mass[c]

> Brugman et al., 1979

intraperitoneal calcification[d]

> Foster et al., 1987

abnormal fluid collection within the fetal abdomen; the fluid was encapsulated and showed fluid–debris level

> Clair et al., 1983

microcalcifications on the liver surface intraabdominal adhesions[d]

> Glick et al., 1983

hepatosplenomegaly[c]

> Nancarrow et al., 1985

ascites[c]

> Glick et al., 1983; Foster et al., 1987; Chitayat et al., 1995b

meconium pseudocyst[c]

> Chitayat et al., 1995b

echogenic bowel[c]

> Chitayat et al., 1995b

matted small bowel[c]

> Chitayat et al., 1995b

echogenic material in the fetal stomach[c]

> Chitayat et al., 1995b

complex scrotal mass that was shown postnatally to represent abdominal fluid, bowel, and calcified meconium in the scrotum (meconium hydrocele)

> Spirt et al., 1987

coarse calcifications adjacent to the urinary bladder[d]

> Foster et al., 1987

hydramnios[c,d]

> Foster et al., 1987; Spirt et al., 1987

PD 142000 MEGACYSTIS–MICROCOLON–INTESTINAL HYPOPERISTALSIS SYNDROME (Berdon syndrome; Intestinal hypoperistalsis–megacystis–microcolon syndrome; MMIHS) (McKusick No. 155310)

Syndrome Note: The features of this rare disorder include massive abdominal enlargement from distention of the bladder (megacystitis), intestinal hypoperistalsis with malrotation and/or malfixation of a small microcolon, dilation of the

small intestine, and shortened intestinal–colon length. No anatomic cause for the intestinal and bladder obstruction is known. Death usually occurs within the first years of life. The condition is more common in females, with a 6:1 ratio. Hydramnios is present in 25% of patients; the rest usually have oligohydramnios.
> Wiswell et al., 1979; Hartsfield, 1990

Prenatal Diagnosis: The diagnosis should be considered in any fetus with distention of the bladder and renal pelvis, and hydramnios, and is diagnostic in a fetus at risk for the condition. Distention of the renal pelvis has been reported to have occurred by 21 weeks' gestation while the enlargement of the bladder did not occur until after 25 weeks. Thus, caution must be stated when a fetus at risk appears to be normal prior to 21 weeks of gestation (Garber et al., 1990).

Ultrasound[c,d]: dilated bladder with or without hydronephrosis, hydramnios
> Vezina et al., 1979; Hadlock et al., 1981; Nelson and Reiff, 1982

dilated bladder[i]
> Farrell, 1988; Young et al., 1989; Garber et al., 1990

no heartbeat and fetal demise[c,d]
> Farrell, 1988

dilated renal pelvises[i]
> Farrell, 1988; Garber et al., 1990

ascites
> Young et al., 1989

oligohydramnios
> Young et al., 1989

PD 142500 MULTIPLE INTESTINAL ATRESIA (McKusick No. None; see 243150)

Acetylcholinesterase[c]: fast-migrating isozyme present in amniotic fluid
> Shih et al., 1984

Alpha-fetoprotein[c]: minimally elevated in amniotic fluid
> Shih et al., 1984

PD 143000 MULTIPLE INTESTINAL ATRESIA, AUTOSOMAL RECESSIVE TYPE (McKusick No. 243150)

Amniocentesis: decreased activity of amniotic fluid disaccharidases prior to 21 weeks' gestation[c]
> Morin et al., 1980

PD 144000 OMPHALOCELE (Amniocele; Exomphalos; Hepatoomphalocele) (McKusick No. Unknown; see 164750, 310980)

Condition Note: An omphalocele is a defect in the ventral wall of the abdomen with herniation of the intraabdominal contents into the base of the umbilical cord. The herniation is a normal developmental process, and part of the small intestine is normally present in the umbilical cord (body stock) from the 6th week after conception through the 10th week. After the 10th week, the abdominal cavity is large enough for the intestines to return. An omphalocele is produced by failure of the intestines to return to the abdominal cavity, either because the cavity is too small or because the abdominal space is occupied by a mass or enlarged visceral organs. Alternatively, an omphalocele may be the failure of one or more of the body folds (cephalic, caudal, or two laterals) to meet and close to form the umbilicus and umbilical cord (see Incomplete embryonic body folding [PD 191450]). Whenever an omphalocele is detected, other fetal defects need to be sought. If found, a chromosomal analysis should be considered. Six percent of fetuses with omphalocele have trisomy 18 syndrome (PD 104000) (Moore et al., 1988).

Jones, 1988

Prenatal Diagnosis: The diagnosis is made by the detection of a mass attached to the abdominal wall that contains viscera and is surrounded by a membrane that itself is continuous with the umbilical cord. On occasion, the membrane covering the omphalocele may be ruptured and may not be seen to cover the defect. The herniated bowels will be echogenic. In most cases of omphalocele, the abdominal circumference will be smaller than normal. The liver may or may not be protruding into the omphalocele.

Differential Diagnosis: Allantoic cyst (PD 272000); Beckwith–Wiedemann syndrome (PD 187000); Ectopia cordis (pentalogy of Cantrell) (PD 109600); Exstrophy of the cloaca (PD 135500); Gastroschisis (PD 137000); Incomplete embryonic body folding (PD 191450); Triploidy (PD 102000); Trisomy 18 syndrome (PD 104000)

Gastroschisis is usually devoid of a surrounding membrane and lacks the attachment of the umbilical cord. Pentalogy of Cantrell can be suspected if the heart is displaced outside of the chest cavity and the liver is included within the omphalocele. Beckwith–Wiedemann syndrome (PD 187000) should be a consideration when there is visceromegaly and macroglossia.

Ardinger et al., 1987; Romero et al., 1988; Nyberg et al., 1989

Acetylcholinesterase[c]: increased level in amniotic fluid, increased ratio of acetylcholinesterase activity to percentage of total cholinesterase activity, fast-migrating amniotic fluid isozyme, acetylcholinesterase to cholinesterase isozyme density ratio of less than 0.13

Davis et al., 1979; Buamah et al., 1980; Dale, 1980; Dale et al., 1981; Hullin et al., 1981; Lawton, 1981; Macri et al., 1981; Voigtlander et al., 1981; Wald and Cuckle, 1981; Crandall et al., 1982; Goldfine et al., 1983; Aitken et al., 1984b; Crandall and Matsumoto, 1984b; Toftager-Larsen et al., 1984; Wyvill et al., 1984; Leschot et al., 1985; Nielsen et al., 1985; Ardinger et al., 1987

acetylcholinesterase to cholinesterase isozyme density ratio in amniotic fluid of less than 0.13

Burton, 1986

Comments: For Anencephaly (PD 118000) and Spina bifida cystica (PD 129000) the ratio of acetylcholinesterase to cholinesterase is normally greater than 0.13. However, this is not a definitive test to differentiate between neural tube defects and ventral wall defects because there are a number of conditions that will cause acetylcholinesterase to be present in the amniotic fluid (see Acetylcholinesterase in the Index) (Burton, 1986).

Alpha-fetoprotein[c]: elevated in maternal serum and amniotic fluid

Campbell et al., 1978; Fisher et al., 1980; Fisher et al., 1981; Macri et al., 1981; Read et al., 1982a; Ward, 1982; Freeman and Harbison, 1983; Crandall and Matsumoto, 1984b; Mann et al.; 1984; Toftager-Larsen et al., 1984; Wyvill et al., 1984; Nielsen et al., 1985; Ardinger et al., 1987; Rodriguez et al., 1987b; Spirt et al., 1987 elevated in amniotic fluid

   Macri et al., 1986; Grange et al., 1987

elevated in maternal serum

   Evans et al., 1995a

Amniocentesis: rapidly adhering peritoneal cells in 20-hour culture of amniotic fluid cells[c]

   Gosden and Brock, 1978a

increased number of nonsquamous cells in amniotic fluid[c]

   Medina-Gomez and McBride, 1986

increased number of amniotic cells that did not stain for nonspecific acid esterase[c]

   Medina-Gomez and McBride, 1986

increased activity of amniotic fluid disaccharidases before 21 weeks' gestation[c]

   Morin et al., 1980

decreased levels of activity of amniotic fluid disaccharidases, maltase, sucrase, and trehalase[c]

   Kleijer et al., 1985b

decreased percentage of amniotic fluid AFP not reacting with concanavalin A[c]

   Toftager-Larsen et al., 1980; Toftager-Larsen et al., 1984; Nielsen et al., 1985

elevated amniotic fluid alkaline phosphatase activity[c,d]

   Jalanko et al., 1983

elevated level of alpha-2-macroglobulin in amniotic fluid[c]

   Toftager-Larsen et al., 1984

decreased percentage of lens culinaris agglutinin reacting to AFP in amniotic fluid[c]

   Toftager-Larsen et al., 1984

reduced levels of amniotic fluid glucose[c]

   Weiss et al., 1984; Weiss et al., 1985

elevated levels of pseudocholinesterase in amniotic fluid[c,d]

   Grange et al., 1987

increased percentage of phenylalanine-resistant alkaline activity in amniotic fluid[c]

   Carey and Pollard, 1986

decreased percentage of homoarginine-resistant alkaline phosphatase activity in amniotic fluid[c]

   Carey and Pollard, 1986

Amniography: loops of bowel outside the fetal abdomen, bulging anterior abdominal wall of the fetus

   Roberts, 1978; Balsam and Weiss, 1981

Cholinesterase[c]: increased level in amniotic fluid

   Hullin et al., 1981; Lawton, 1981; Webb et al., 1981a

Continuous-wave Doppler evaluation[c,d]: increased peripheral arterial resistance

   Meizner et al., 1987

Ultrasound: loops of bowel outside of the fetal abdomen (echogenic mass anterior to fetal abdominal wall) that are membrane-covered, umbilical cord inserting into apex of mass, small abdominal circumference

Campbell et al., 1978; Canty et al., 1981; Sabbagha et al., 1981; Nelson et al., 1982b; Davidson et al., 1984; Meizner et al., 1987; Spirt et al., 1987

large, membrane-covered, solid mass (liver) protruding from fetal abdomen with the umbilical vein coursing through the lower margin of the mass

Didolkar et al., 1981; Hill et al., 1988b; Nyberg et al., 1989

Comment: If the omphalocele is ruptured, a membrane covering the herniated abdominal contents usually will not be seen.

liver anterior to abdominal wall

Ardinger et al., 1987, Spirt et al., 1987

ascites

Ardinger et al., 1987

umbilical cord allantoic cyst

Fink and Filly, 1983

hydramnios

Quinlan et al., 1983; Ardinger et al., 1987; Meizner et al., 1987; Hill et al., 1988b

PD 144200 PYLORIC ATRESIA, FAMILIAL (Familial congenital pyloric atresia; Pyloric atresia) (McKusick No. 265950)

Condition Note: Isolated pyloric atresia may be an autosomal recessive disorder where the normal pylorus is reduced to a fibrous band or replaced by a diaphragm. The condition can be surgically repaired postnatally.

Peled et al., 1992; McKusick, 1996

Ultrasound[d,i]: dilated stomach, hydramnios

Peled et al., 1992

Comment: In the fetus reported by Peled and associates (1992), neither a double bubble sign nor other anomalies were found prenatally.

PD 144225 PYLORIC DUPLICATION CYST (Duplication cyst of the pylorus) (McKusick No. None)

Differential Diagnosis: Choledochal cyst (PD 131500); Congenital thoracic gastroenteric cyst (PD 272440); Gastric duplication cyst (PD 135750)

Ultrasound[c]: unilocular mass arising immediately inferior to the liver, and medial to the gallbladder, 1×2 mm echogenic focus present within the mass

Goyert et al., 1991

PD 144250 PYLORIC STENOSIS (Infantile pyloric stenosis) (McKusick No. 179010)

Ultrasound[c,h]: increased echogenicity of fetal bowel

Strasberg et al., 1995

PD 144500 VOLVULUS OF SMALL BOWEL (McKusick No. Unknown; see 193250)

Maternal history: marked decrease in fetal movements as perceived by the mother[c,d]

Witter and Molteni, 1986

Oxytocin challenge test[c,d]: positive test with nonreactive fetal heart pattern that was without fetal tachycardia but with variability in the pattern
  Witter and Molteni, 1986
  Comments: After birth the neonate reported by Witter and Molteni (1986) was found to have a distended abdomen, anemia, hemoperitoneum, and a volvulus involving the distal jejunum and proximal ileum. Following corrective surgery for the latter condition, the infant did well.
Ultrasound[c,d]: a cystic loculation (pseudocyst) in the right hypochondrium associated with ascites, hydramnios, and IUGR
  Baxi et al., 1983
  Comment: Perforation of the small bowel was detected after the delivery of the child in the above case.
  hydrops fetalis
    Curry et al., 1983

THE SKELETAL SYSTEM[a]

General Comments: Bone or skeletal dysplasias constitute a relatively large group of disorders with diverse presentations and varying degrees of severity. Most are inherited or represent new mutations. For instance, thanatophoric dysplasia, normally a neonatal lethal, has been found to be caused by a mutation in the fibroblast growth factor receptor III gene. The discovery of the etiology of bone dysplasias is rapidly evolving, and insights to the pathogenesis and biochemistry of these disorders is fast being elucidated.

However, until there is a genetic or biochemical test for most bone dysplasias, the prenatal diagnosis of these conditions will be problematic. For example, in one study of bone dysplasias Rasmussen and co-investigators (1996) found that in 73% of fetuses with bone dysplasias, the diagnosis was suspected but could not be confirmed prenatally. The incidence of all bone dysplasias in their study was 2.14 cases per 10,000 births.

In a similar study, Sharony and associates (1993) analyzed in detail 226 fetuses and stillborns suspected to have skeletal dysplasias. The ultrasonic diagnosis was only made in a minority of cases. Interestingly, 15 of the fetuses they studied turned out to be "probably normal." Suspected "short limbs" in this latter group most likely was related to inaccurate gestational aging. Ninety percent of the cases had no previously affected relatives. Fetal radiographs were helpful in some cases in establishing the diagnosis, particularly in those fetuses with lethal disorders.

General References: Filly and Golbus, 1982; Hobbins and Mahoney, 1985; Donnenfeld and Mennuti, 1987; Thomas et al., 1987; Escobar et al., 1990; Sharony et al., 1993; Rasmussen et al., 1996

PD 145000 ACHONDROGENESIS, TYPE I (Achondrogenesis, type IA [Houston–Harris]; Achondrogenesis, type IB [Fraccaro]; Parenti–Fraccaro type of achondrogenesis) (McKusick No. 200600)

Syndrome Note: Achondrogenesis is a lethal autosomal recessive bone dysplasia with marked shortening of limbs, alteration in the shapes of long bones, and decreased calcification of all bones. In addition, there usually is severe IUGR.

The condition is always either a lethal disorder in neonates, primarily because of the small chest size, or results in a stillborn birth.

Achondrogenesis has been divided into types I and II based on radiographic, histologic, and biochemical findings. Achondrogenesis type I has been further subdivided into type IA (Houston–Harris) and type IB (Fraccaro) on radiographic and histologic grounds. Type IA has no ossification of the pubis, talus, calcaneus, and vertebrae. In addition, rib fractures and characteristic shapes of the pelvis and certain long bones are found. Type IB does not involve fractured ribs, but does involve ossification of the posterior pedicles of the vertebrae and characteristic shapes of the pelvis and certain long bones. The chondro-osseous morphology on histologic section is also distinct for each type. At present, types IA and IB cannot be differentiated on prenatal evaluation. Thus, they are included together under the category of achondrogenesis, type I.

Borochowitz et al., 1988

Prenatal Diagnosis: The presence of short long bones in a fetus at risk should be adequate information for the diagnosis. The diagnosis should be considered in any fetus with quite short limbs and IUGR.

Differential Diagnosis: Achondrogenesis, type II (PD 145500); Achondroplasia, homozygous type (PD 147000); Diastrophic dysplasia (PD 154000); Greenberg dysplasia (PD 160130); Graff–Laxova lethal skeletal dysplasia (PD 160120); Osteogenesis imperfecta, type II (PD 164000)

Amniography[i]: shortened limbs, small thorax
> Golbus et al., 1977

Radiograph[i]: poor fetal bone calcification especially in the lower spine, relatively large head, extremely misshapened and shortened long bones
> Golbus et al., 1977; Smith et al., 1981b

Ultrasound[i]: cleft palate
> Weldner et al., 1985

very short limbs
> Smith et al., 1981b; Johnson et al., 1984b; Weldner et al., 1985; Donnenfeld and Mennuti, 1987; Thomas et al., 1987; Meizner & Bar-Ziv, 1993

shortening and deformity of the long bones
> Kurtz and Wapner, 1983

very short humeri
> Johnson et al., 1984b

very short femora
> Filly and Golbus, 1982; Johnson et al., 1984b

reduced echogenicity of fetal vertebrae
> Johnson et al., 1984b

absence of ossification of the vertebral bodies
> Meizner and Bar-Ziv, 1993

reduced echogenicity of the spine and head
> Filly and Golbus, 1982; Kurtz and Wapner, 1983; Weldner et al., 1985; Donnenfeld and Mennuti, 1987; Thomas et al., 1987

limbs held in flexed positions
> Johnson et al., 1984b

soft skull as indicated by deformation of the skull with external pressure from the transducer
> Meizner and Bar-Ziv, 1993

narrow thorax
  Johnson et al., 1984b; Weldner et al., 1985
disproportion between the size of the thorax and abdomen with the
thorax being smaller
  Johnson et al., 1984b
protuberant abdomen
  Johnson et al., 1984b; Donnenfeld and Mennuti, 1987
bilateral hydronephrosis[c]
  Thomas et al., 1987
hydramnios[i]
  Thomas et al., 1987; Borochowitz et al., 1988

PD 145500 ACHONDROGENESIS, TYPE II (Achondrogenesis,
Langer–Saldino type; Langer–Saldino type of achondrogenesis) (McKusick No.
200610)

  Ultrasound: markedly shortened limbs[i]
      Bingol et al., 1987; McGuire et al., 1987; Thomas et al., 1987;
      Wenstrom et al.,1989; Rittler and Orioli, 1995
  extremely short femora with broad metaphyses
      Meizner and Bar-Ziv, 1993
  enlargement of the head in respect to body
      Meizner and Bar-Ziv, 1993
  decreased mineralization of the spine[i]
      McGuire et al., 1987; Wenstrom et al., 1989
  spine is not identified
      Meizner and Bar-Ziv, 1993
  decreased mineralization of the rib[c]
      Wenstrom et al., 1989
  excessive subcutaneous tissue around the skull and neck
      Meizner and Bar-Ziv, 1993
  small chest size and chest circumference[c]
      Wenstrom et al., 1989
  hydronephrosis with bilateral pelviureteric stenosis[c]
      McGuire et al., 1987
  small iliac bones
      Meizner and Bar-Ziv, 1993
  cystic hygroma[c]
      Wenstrom et al., 1989; Rittler and Orioli, 1995
  hydrops fetalis[c]
      Wenstrom et al., 1989; Rittler and Orioli, 1995
  hydramnios[i]
      Bingol et al., 1987; Thomas et al., 1987; Rittler and Orioli, 1995

PD 146000 ACHONDROPLASIA, HETEROZYGOUS TYPE (McKusick No.
100800)

Condition Note: Achondroplasia, an autosomal dominant condition, is characterized by rhizomelic short stature, macrocephaly with midfacial hypoplasia, brachydactyly, trident configuration of the fingers, and normal intelligence. The condition is produced by a mutation in the fibroblast growth factor receptor III gene
(FGFR3) located on the short arm of chromosome 4. In most individuals with

achondroplasia, the mutation is located at nucleotide 1138 which results in a glycine or arginine substitution at codon 380 (Bellus et al., 1994).

Chorionic villus sampling[g,i]: detection of both the mutant and normal pattern in DNA sample using polymerase chain reaction (PCR) and appropriate polymorphic markers

Bellus et al., 1994

Radiograph[d,i]: squared pelvis, flattened vertebral bodies

Russell, 1973

Ultrasound[i]: abnormal head to body ratio

Leonard et al., 1979

shortened and bowed femora

Filly et al., 1981; Hill et al., 1983a; Kurtz and Wapner, 1983; Kurtz et al., 1986

Comments: The femora are often normal in length prior to 20 weeks of gestation but may fail to maintain normal growth rates in affected fetuses during the last half of the pregnancy.

short limbs

Weldner et al., 1985

shortened base of the skull

Meizner and Bar-Ziv, 1993

depressed nasal bridge

Meizner and Bar-Ziv, 1993

PD 147000 ACHONDROPLASIA, HOMOZYGOUS TYPE (McKusick No. 100800)

Radiograph[d,i]: flattened vertebral bodies, femoral flaring

Omenn et al., 1977

Ultrasound[i]: shortened femora before 20 weeks' gestation

Filly and Golbus, 1982

shortened long bones of the extremities

Hummel et al., 1989

PD 147500 AMELIA/HEMIMELIA SYNDROME (McKusick No None; see also 104400)

Condition Note: Michaud and associates (1995) have described a family where three full fetuses from normal parents had amelia of the arms, hemimelia to amelia of the legs, and unusual facial features. The facial findings included depressed nasal bridge, epicanthal folds, prominent cheeks, V-shaped philtrum, and micrognathia. All fetuses were terminated during the second trimester.

Prenatal Diagnosis: Detection of upper limb amelia and amelia or hemimelia in the lower ones in at-risk fetuses is sufficient evidence for making the diagnosis.

Differential Diagnosis: Amniotic band disruption sequence (PD 185000); Amelia and terminal transverse hemimelia (McKusick No. 104400); Ohdo syndrome (PD 192780); Tetraamelia, isolated (PD 173550); Tetraamelia syndrome (PD 194180); Tetraamelia with pulmonary hypoplasia (McKusick No. 273395)

Ultrasound[i]: absense of both upper extremities, absence to normal length of the femora with amelic to hemimelic shortening of the lower extremities

Michaud et al., 1995

PD 148000 ANHALT DYSPLASIA (Spinal dysplasia, Anhalt type) (McKusick No. 601344)

Dysplasia Note: Anhalt and co-workers (1995) described an apparently new bone dysplasia in a father and his son. The father was strikingly short (131.6 cm tall; −7.5 SD). In addition he had a decrease of the anteroposterior dimension of the vertebral bodies, other multiple abnormalities of the vertebral bodies, scoliosis, arthritic changes of the interphalangeal and metacarpal–phalangeal joints, and bilateral coxa vara with overgrowth of the greater trochanters, and overtubulation. The son at age 2 8/12 years also had short stature, platyspondyly with underdevelopment and sagittal clefting of the vertebral arches, narrowed anterior–posterior vertebral body diameters, absence of the normal spinous processes of the lower thoracic and lumber spines, and widely disparate shapes of vertebral arches. Because of father–son transmission, the condition is assumed to be an autosomal dominant disorder.

Ultrasound[c,d]: abnormal lumbar spine
> Anhalt et al., 1995

PD 148500 APERT SYNDROME (Acrocephalosyndactyly, type I) (McKusick No. 101200)

Fetoscopy[i]: syndactyly of fingers, no separate motion of the fingers
> Leonard et al., 1982

Ultrasound[c,d]: hydrocephalus with increased biparietal diameter, enlarged ventricles, cloverleaf shape of the skull, frontal bone bossing
> Kim et al., 1986b

PD 149000 ASPHYXIATING THORACIC DYSTROPHY (Jeune syndrome) (McKusick No. 208500)

Physical examination of the mother[c,d]: uterus large for dates
> Rawnsley et al., 1986

Radiograph[d,i]: short ribs
> Russell, 1973

Ultrasound[i]: shortened femora, humeri, and tibiae; shortened limbs; thorax abnormally flattened, small, and narrow in anterior/posterior diameter; or thorax bell-shaped; hypoplastic ribs
> Lipson et al., 1984; Elejalde et al., 1985c; Schinzel and Savoldelli, 1985; Rawnsley et al., 1986; Donnenfeld and Mennuti, 1987

narrow, bell-shaped thorax
> Meizner and Bar-Ziv, 1993

abnormally flattened thorax
> Schinzel et al., 1985

shortened humeri, femora, and tibiae
> Schinzel et al., 1985

bowed femur[c]
> Donnenfeld and Mennuti, 1987

bilateral clubfoot[c]
> Elejalde et al., 1985c

hydramnios[c,d]
> Rawnsley et al., 1986

PD 149200 ATELOSTEOGENESIS, TYPE I (Giant cell chondrodysplasia; Spondylohumerofemoral hypoplasia) (McKusick No. 108720)

Condition Note: Atelosteogenesis is a lethal chondrodysplasia. The main characteristics are hypoplasia of the mid-thoracic spine, occasional complete lack of ossification of single hand bones, distal hypoplasia of the hemeri and femora, and on histologic examination of the cartilage, multiple degenerated chondrocytes that are encapsulated in fibrous tissue.
McKusick, 1996
Ultrasound[c]: decreased ossification of the skull, no ossification of the fetal spine, marked shortening of the fetal long bones, hydramnios
Herzberg et al., 1988

PD 149400 BALLER–GEROLD SYNDROME (Craniosynostosis with radial defects) (McKusick No. 218600)

Syndrome Note: The Baller–Gerold syndrome is an autosomal recessive disorder characterized by craniosynostosis, leading to turrocephaly, ocular hypotelorism, conductive hearing loss, absent radius, absent or hypoplastic thumbs, vertebral defects, short stature, imperforate anus, congenital heart defect, and mental retardation. This syndrome shares a number of features in common with the VATER association (PD 194650) but is inherited in an autosomal recessive fashion.
McKusick, 1995
Prenatal Diagnosis: The prenatal diagnosis of this condition has not been established. Presence of skull abnormalities or absence of the radius in an at-risk fetus would be presumptive evidence for the diagnosis, however.
Differential Diagnosis: Holt–Oram syndrome (PD 191310); Roberts syndrome (PD 193570); Thrombocytopenia–absent radius syndrome (PD 175000); VATER association (PD 194650)
Ultrasound[c,h]: hydrocephalus
Rossbach et al., 1996
Comment: The child reported by Rossbach and co-workers (1996) also had features consistent with the VATER association (PD 194650) and Fanconi anemia (PD 205000).

PD 149450 BOOMERANG DYSPLASIA (McKusick No. 112310)

Dysplasia Note: Boomerang dysplasia is a lethal neonatal bone dysplasia with a unique pattern of features including normal head size; marked shortening and deformity of all limbs; partial or complete syndactyly of fingers and toes; and radiographically absent, hypoplasia, or abnormally modeled long bones that may resemble a boomerang; ossification of the phalanges restricted to the terminal phalanges; hypoplastic ilia; absent pubic bones; and well-developed ischia. Inheritance is thought to be autosomal dominant.
Winship et al., 1990; McKusick, 1996
Radiograph[c,d]: short limbs
Winship et al., 1990
Examination of mother[c,d]: hydramnios
Winship et al., 1990

PD 149500 BRACHYDACTYLY, TYPE B (Brachydactyly B) (McKusick No. 113000)

Condition Note: This type of brachydactyly is associated with middle phalangeal shortening, rudimentary or absent terminal phalanges, deformed thumbs and big toes, and symphalangism. Both the hands and feet are affected in the condition. As with many other types of brachydactyly, the disorder is inherited in an autosomal dominant fashion.

Glendon et al., 1993; McKusick, 1995

Ultrasound[i]: deficient distal phalanges and shortened middle phalanges of the second to the fifth fingers, normal thumbs and feet

Glendon et al, 1993

PD 149600 CAFFEY DISEASE (Infantile cortical hyperostosis) (McKusick No. 114000)

Disease Note: Caffey disease is an unusual disorder in that it rarely ever appears after 5 months of age, and normally resolves by the age of 3. Occasionally onset is prenatally. Characteristics of the disease include inflammation of multiple bones such as the mandible and ribs, tenderness and swelling of the involved bone, thickened periosteum, infiltration of the periosteum with round cells, congenital bowing of the legs, and cortical hyperostosis. The condition often is inherited in an autosomal dominant fashion. Infants often are irritable, sleep and feed poorly, are pale, and have a mild fever.

Prenatal Diagnosis: The presence of curved long bones of the legs and hydramnios in an at-risk fetus probably is adequate evidence to make the diagnosis. The diagnosis may be suspected but cannot be made prenatally in isolated cases.

Differential Diagnosis: Campomelic dysplasia, short-limb type (PD 150000); Osteogenesis imperfecta, type II (PD 164000); Osteogenesis imperfecta, type III (PD 164500)

Radiograph[d]: angulation of long bones

Lecolier et al., 1992

Ultrasound[i]: micrognathia

Turnpenny et al., 1993; de Jong and Muller, 1995

short arms and legs

Turnpenny et al., 1993; de Jong and Muller, 1995; Drinkwater et al., 1995

diaphyses of long bones appeared thickened with irregular echodensities and angulations

de Jong and Muller, 1995

small thorax

Lecolier et al., 1992; de Jong and Muller 1995; Drinkwater et al., 1995

thickened ribs

de Jong and Muller, 1995

closed lumbosacral neural tube defect

Drinkwater et al., 1995

short femur

Turnpenny et al., 1993

bowing of the humeri, femora, ulna, tibiae, and fibulae

Lecolier et al., 1992

unilateral bowed femur

Turnpenny et al, 1993; Drinkwater et al., 1995

hydrops fetalis[c,d]

Lecolier et al, 1992; Turnpenny et al., 1993

abnormal fetal movements in that there was no apparent flexion or extension

> de Jong and Muller, 1995

hydramnios

> Lecolier et al., 1992; Turnpenny et al., 1993; de Jong and Muller, 1995; Drinkwater et al., 1995

fetal demise[c,d]

> Turnpenny et al., 1993

PD 149800 CAMPOMELIC DYSPLASIA, AUTOSOMAL DOMINANT TYPE (McKusick No. 114290)

Dysplasia Note: Campomelic dysplasia, autosomal dominant type is characterized by bowing of the long bones of both the upper and lower limbs, skin dimpling over the tibia, dolichocephaly, flattened supraorbital ridges and nasal bridge, hypoplastic scapula, 11 pairs of ribs, poor or absent ossification of the pelvis, and talipes equinovarus. Cleft palate in both sexes and sex reversal in males are often present. Death may occur from respiratory distress. The autosomal dominant form of this disease is distinguished from the classic autosomal recessive form by milder tibial bowing and significant shortening of first and fifth phalanges of the hands and feet.

> Lynch et al., 1994; McKusick, 1995

Prenatal Diagnosis: Shortening and bowing of long bones in an at-risk fetus would be presumptive evidence for the diagnosis.

Differential Diagnosis: Campomelic dysplasia, long-limb type; Campomelic dysplasia, short-limb type (PD 150000); Osteogenesis imperfecta, types II and III (PD 164000 and 164500, respectively); Kyphomelic dysplasia; Moore dysplasia (McKusick No. 211350); Prenatal bowing (McKusick No. 264050)

Ultrasound[i]: short femora, hydramnios

> Lynch et al., 1993

PD 150000 CAMPOMELIC DYSPLASIA, SHORT-LIMB TYPE (Campomelic syndrome, short-bone variety; Camptomelic dwarfism; Camptomelic dysplasia) (McKusick No. 211970)

Dysplasia Note: Campomelic dysplasia, autosomal recessive type, is divided into two main types: Campomelic dysplasia long-bone variety in which there are bent, long bones of normal width that are only slightly shortened and which rarely involves the upper extremities, and campomelic dysplasia short-bone variety in which the bowed bones are short and wide. A milder autosomal dominant form has also been described (Lynch et al., 1993). Additional features found in the long-bone variety include a large calvarium, low-set ears, ocular hypertelorism, depressed nasal bridge, flat facies, cleft palate, scoliosis, shortening and anterior bowing of the femora and tibiae, and clubfeet. Respiratory distress produced by a small thorax, a narrow larynx, and tracheomalacia usually leads to death in the first few weeks of life. In contrast, campomelic dysplasia short-bone variety has short and wide bones with smooth metaphyses involving both the upper and lower extremities, kleeblatschadel (clover leaf skull), craniostenosis with hydrocephalus, posterior encephalocele, hypoplastic facial bones, micrognathia, slender ribs, and radiohumeral synostosis. This latter variety is divided into a craniosynostosis type and normocephalic type (Khajavi et al., 1976; McKusick, 1995). Mutations in SOX9, an SRY-related gene that is located at 17q24.1-q25.1, have been found to cause both the condition, and the sex reveal seen in this disorder (Foster et al., 1994; Kwok et al., 1995).

Both the long- and short-bone type have been thought to be inherited in an autosomal recessive fashion (Khajavi et al., 1976; McKusick, 1995), but recent evidence indicates that these conditions may be autosomally dominant, genetically lethal with recurrence representing germline mosaicism (McKusick, 1995).

Prenatal Diagnosis: The diagnosis of this type of campomelic dysplasia cannot be made with certainty in the isolated case; detection of shortened long bones, and/or hydrocephalus in the at-risk fetus would be sufficient presumptive evidence to make the diagnosis.

Differential Diagnosis: Campomelic dysplasia, autosomal dominant type (PD 149800); Campomelic dysplasia, long-bone type; Osteogenesis imperfecta, types II and III (PD 164000 and 164500, respectively); Kyphomelic dysplasia; Moore dysplasia (McKusick No. 211350); Prenatal bowing (McKusick No 254050)

Ultrasound: massive hydrocephalus[i]
> Fryns et al., 1981

shortened femora and humeri, hydrocephalus, poor ossification of long tubular bones
> Hobbins et al., 1979; Fryns et al., 1981; Hobbins et al., 1982; Winter et al., 1985

abnormal curvature of the femora and tibiae, absence of the fibulae
> Winter et al., 1985

shortened extremities
> Fryns et al., 1981; Foster et al., 1994

severe shortening, thickening, and bowing of the humeri, ulnae, and radii
> Hobbins and Mahoney, 1985

marked shortening of lower limbs with bowing of femora and tibiae, moderate shortening of upper limbs and long bones
> Penchaszadeh et al., 1987

bowing of the lower limbs[c]
> Kwok et al., 1995

bowed femur
> Spirt et al., 1987

shortened fibula
> Spirt et al., 1987

hydramnios[c,d]
> Wong and Filly, 1983

normal female genitalia in the presence of a normal male chromosome constitution (46,XY)[c]
> Kwok et al., 1995

cystic hygroma
> Foster et al., 1994

PD 150250 CAREY DYSPLASIA (McKusick No. None)

Condition Note: Carey and associates (1979) reported a 19-month-old female with what appears to be a previously undescribed bone dysplasia. The characteristics of the child included marked short stature, prominent forehead, blue sclerae, flat nasal bridge, a short and upturned nose with a long philtrum, mid-facial flattening micrognathia, rhizomelic shortening of the extremities, broad thumbs and index fingers with radial deviation of these fingers, genu valgum, left club foot, and short halluces with marked fibular deviation. Radiographic findings included normally shaped vertebrae with coronal clefts in the thoracic and lumbar regions, an extra triangular-shaped bone just distal to both second metacarpal bones, squared ilia, and shortened femora and humeri with broad metaphyses.

A full fetus to the proband at 18 weeks of gestation was found to have similar findings, and the pregnancy was terminated. A postnatal examination showed similar findings to the proband plus a cleft of the soft palate.

Fetogram[i]: femoral shortening
      Carey et al., 1979
Fetoscopy[i]: unusual radial deviation of the index finger
      Carey et al., 1979
Ultrasound[i]: shortened humeri and femora
      Carey et al., 1979

PD 150300 CARTILAGE-HAIR HYPOPLASIA SYNDROME (Metaphyseal chondrodysplasia, McKusick type) (McKusick No. 250250)

Syndrome Note: The cartilage-hair hypoplasia syndrome is an autosomal recessive disorder characterized by short stature recognized during childhood; fine and sparse hair; hypopigmented skin; short hands, finger nails, and toe nails; anemia; immunodeficiency; metaphyseal dysplasia, excessive distal fibular growth; and platyspondyly.
      McKusick, 1995
Chorionic villus sampling[g,i]: linkage of the gene for cartilage-hair hypoplasia syndrome with closely linked DNA markers
      Sulisalo et al., 1995
Ultrasound[i]: shortened and bowed femora, flaring of the rib cage
      Emerson et al., 1993
   shortened bones
      Sulisalo et al., 1995

PD 150490 CHONDRODYSPLASIA PUNCTATA, AUTOSOMAL DOMINANT TYPE (Chondrodystrophia calcificans; Conradi–Hunermann syndrome) (McKusick No. 118650)

Syndrome Note: This form of chondrodysplasia punctata is inherited in an autosomal dominant mode and has a relatively good prognosis. The condition is primarily an epiphyseal disorder with punctate epiphyseal calcifications early in life, asymmetric limb shortening, low nasal bridge with flat facies, downslanting palpebral fissures, variable joint contractures, large skin pores, and sparse hair. Ichthyosis (27%) and cataracts (17%), short neck, and mild to moderate mental retardation also may be present.
      Smith, 1982; McKusick, 1990
Prenatal Diagnosis: The presence of asymmetry of limb length in a fetus at risk is probably sufficient evidence to conclude that the fetus is affected. It has not been established how often the asymmetry will be present in an affected fetus, however. The diagnosis has not been made in a sporadic situation (e.g., when both parents were unaffected and there is no family history of the condition).
Differential Diagnosis: Chondrodysplasia rhizomelic type (PD 150500); Chondrodysplasia punctata, X-linked recessive form (PD 150750); Warfarin embryopathy; Zellweger syndrome (PD 234500)

   Ultrasound[i]: asymmetry between the right and left femora, and the right and left humeri
      Tuck et al., 1990

PD 150500 CHONDRODYSPLASIA PUNCTATA, RHIZOMELIC TYPE
(Rhizomelic chondrodysplasia punctata) (McKusick No. 215100)

Syndrome Note: Chondrodysplasia punctata is the term used to describe punctate epiphyseal and extra epiphyseal calcifications seen on radiographs of affected infants. These lesions are seen in at least 22 different conditions including Zellweger syndrome (PD 234500), warfarin embryopathy, and four types of chondrodysplasia punctata. The latter disorders are inherited in autosomal dominant (Conradi–Hunermann form); autosomal recessive (the rhizomelic form); X-linked recessive (PD 150750); and X-linked dominant modes. In addition to the punctata calcifications, the rhizomelic type is characterized by psychomotor retardation, cataracts, flat facies with low nasal bridge, rhizomelic shortening of the extremities, coronal cleft of the vertebrae, severe growth deficiency, and death usually before the age of 2 years.

Recently, the biochemical defect in this condition has been elucidated. There is a defect in the postribosomal processing of peroxisomal 3-oxoacylcoenzyme A thiolase, which leads to an impairment of plasmalogen biosynthesis and defective phytanic acid oxidation.

Hoefler et al., 1988; Jones, 1988

Prenatal Diagnosis: Since the discovery of the biochemical defect in this condition, the definitive method of prenatal diagnosis would appear to be the demonstration of defective plasmalogen biosynthesis and lack of phytanic acid oxidation in tissue from a fetus at risk.

Differential Diagnosis: The autosomal dominant (PD 150490), X-linked recessive (PD 150750), and X-linked dominant forms of Chondrodysplasia punctata; Warfarin embryopathy; Zellweger syndrome (PD 234500)

Chorionic villus sampling[g,i]: reduction in plasmalogen biosynthesis and phytanic acid oxidation in cultured chorionic villus cells in which there is normal beta-oxidation of very-long-chain fatty acids in these cells

Hoefler et al., 1988

Ultrasound[i]: decreased growth rates of the femur and humerus in a fetus at risk.

Harrod et al., 1985

Radiograph[i]: apparent shortening of humerus

Harrod et al., 1985

PD 150600 CHONDRODYSPLASIA PUNCTATA, TIBIA–METACARPAL
TYPE (McKusick No. 118651)

Condition Note: This type of chondrodysplasia punctata is noted by flat midface and nose, short limbs, calcific stippling in the epiphyses, coronal clefts of the vertebral bodies, shortened third and fourth metacarpals, shortened tibiae, and normal development otherwise. Inheritance is autosomal dominant.

Rittler et al., 1990; McKusick, 1996

Ultrasound[h]: hydramnios

Rittler et al., 1990

PD 150750 CHONDRODYSPLASIA PUNCTATA, X-LINKED RECESSIVE
FORM (McKusick No. 302950)

Condition Note: Bick and associates (1989) reported a fetus and his brother who each had chondrodysplasia punctata, X-linked recessive form; X-linked ichthyosis; and Kallmann syndrome. These conditions were produced by a terminal deletion of the p arm of the X chromosome transmitted to them by their mother who was a carrier of the chromosome deletion.

After termination of the 18-week pregnancy, the fetus was found to have the abnormal physical and radiographic features consistent with chondrodysplasia punctata.

Prenatal Diagnosis: A karyotype of appropriate fetal tissue is the most definitive method of diagnosing the deletion when the condition is produced by an X-chromosome deletion.

Differential Diagnosis: Chondrodysplasia punctata, autosomal dominant type (PD 150490); Chondrodysplasia punctata, rhizomelic type (PD 150500); Warfarin embryopathy; Zellweger syndrome (PD 234500)

Ultrasound[c]: nasal hypoplasia
Bick et al., 1989

PD 151000 CLEIDOCRANIAL DYSPLASIA (McKusick No. 119600)

Radiograph[d,i]: absent clavicles
Noonan, 1974

PD 151500 CLUBFOOT DEFORMITY (McKusick No. 119800)

Ultrasound[d,i]: marked equinovarus deformity of the foot with no change in position with time
Chervenak et al., 1985a

PD 151750 CONGENITAL BOWED LONG BONES, ISOLATED (McKusick No. None)

Condition Note: Kapur and Van Vloten (1986) reported on a mother and her daughter with this condition. The disorder resulted in prenatal bowing of the humeri and femora in both the daughter and the mother, and congenitally dislocated hips in the mother. The bowing disappeared with time; both individuals had normal stature.

Prenatal Diagnosis: congenital bowing of long bones in fetuses at risk

Ultrasound[i]: bowing of long bones in an otherwise normal fetus
Kapur and Van Vloten, 1986

PD 152000 CONGENITAL COXA VARA (Proximal femoral dysplasia; Golding deformity) (McKusick No. None)

Radiograph[d]: underdeveloped proximal femur, varus angulation of shaft
Russell, 1973

PD 152900 CRANIOECTODERMAL DYSPLASIA (Levin syndrome I; Sensenbrenner syndrome) (McKusick No. 218330)

Dysplasia Note: Cranioectodermal dysplasia consists of sagittal suture synostosis with resulting dolichocephaly, epicanthal folds with ocular hypertelorism, hypodontia and/or microdontia, taurodontia, narrow thorax, brachydactyly, clinodactyly, syndactyly, rhizomelic limb shortening, and sparse, slow-growing and fine hair. The condition is inherited in an autosomal recessive mode.
McKusick, 1995

Prenatal Diagnosis: Probably shortening of the humeri and femora in the third trimester is sufficient for the diagnosis in the at-risk fetus.

Differential Diagnosis: Cartilage-hair hypoplasia syndrome (PD 150300); Ellis–van Creveld syndrome (PD 158000); GAPO syndrome; Trichodentoosseous syndrome

Ultrasound[d,i]: development with time of short humeri and femora for gestational age and in comparison to head size
Lang and Young, 1991

PD 153000 CRANIOSYNOSTOSIS, SAGITTAL SUTURE (Premature closure of the sagittal suture, Scaphocephaly) (McKusick No. Unknown; see 123100, 218500)

Ultrasound: unusual oval-shaped head, biparietal diameter more than 3 SD below the mean, cephalic index decreased (i.e., 60 [normal = 70–80])
Kurtz et al., 1980; Campbell and Pearce, 1983
Radiograph[d]: scaphocephalic fetal head shape, fusion of the sagittal suture
Russell, 1973

PD 153200 CROUZON SYNDROME (Craniofacial dysostosis; Pseudo-Crouzon disease) (McKusick No. 123500)

Ultrasound[d]: exophthalmos
Menashe et al., 1989

PD 153500 DE LA CHAPELLE DYSPLASIA (Atelosteogenesis type II; Neonatal osseous dysplasia I) (McKusick No. 256050)

Syndrome Note: de la Chapelle dysplasia is a rare neonatal, lethal skeletal dysplasia characterized by cleft palate, short limbs, small hands and chest, and equinovarus deformity. The long bones are short with the ulnae and fibulae reduced to almost triangular bony remnants. The other long bones are bowed. Death results from respiratory insufficiency. The disorder is probably inherited in an autosomal recessive mode. There is debate in the literature if de la Chapelle dysplasia and atelosteogenesis type II are one or separate entities (McKusick, 1995). They are listed together here until the issue is resolved.
Whitley et al., 1986
Alpha-fetoprotein[c]: decreased level in maternal serum
Nores et al., 1992
Physical examination of the mother[c,d]: hydramnios
Whitley et al., 1986
Ultrasound[i]: shortened limbs
Nores et al., 1992
shortened long bones
Nores et al., 1992
reduced femor-to-head size ratio
Nores et al., 1992
abnormal femor-to-abdominal circumference ratio
Nores et al., 1992
protuberant abdomen
Nores et al., 1992
increase nuchal skin thickness
Nores et al., 1992
shortened ribs
Nores et al., 1992

lumbosacral hyperlordosis with a horizontal sacrum
  Nores et al., 1992
coronal clefts of vertebral bodies L2–L5
  Nores et al., 1992
widened proximal humeral metaphysis and epiphysis
  Nores et al., 1992
hypoplastic and narrow distal humerus
  Nores et al., 1992
ulnar deviation of the fingers
  Nores et al., 1992
radial deviation of the thumbs (hitchhiker thumb)
  Nores et al., 1992
curved inward femurs with rounded proximal metaphyses
  Nores et al., 1992
club feet (talipes equinovarus)
  Nores et al., 1992
wide separation between the first and second toes
  Nores et al., 1992

PD 153750 DESBUQUOIS SYNDROME (Micromelic dwarfism with vertebral and metaphyseal abnormalities and advanced carpotarsal ossification) (McKusick No. 2514500)

Syndrome Note: The Desbuquois syndrome is a micromelic bone dysplasia with a narrow chest, vertebral anomalies, patellar and hip dislocations, supernumerary metacarpals resulting in deviation of fingers, advanced carpotarsal ossification, glaucoma, and mental retardation. The disorder appears to be inherited in an autosomal recessive fashion.
  McKusick, 1995
Prenatal Diagnosis: Shortened limbs in an at-risk fetus would be presumptive evidence for the diagnosis.
Differential Diagnosis: Larsen syndrome, autosomal dominant form (PD 161245); Larsen syndrome, autosomal recessive form (PD 161250)
  Ultrasound: severe rhizomelic shortening of limbs[i]
    Shohat et al., 1994
  hydramnios[c]
    Shohat et al., 1994; Rasmussen et al., 1996

PD 154000 DIASTROPHIC DYSPLASIA (Diastrophic dwarfism) (McKusick No. 222600)

Condition Note: Diastrophic dysplasia is a bone dysplasia characterized by moderate to severe shortening of all tubular bones (with the first metacarpals being most markedly affected), scoliosis with or without kyphosis, progressive limitation to joint movement leading to severe clubfoot deformities, stiffness of the fingers and other joint problems, proximally placed thumbs ("hitchhiker" thumbs), ulnar deviation of the hands, hypertrophied auricular cartilage, and in some cases cleft palate, micrognathia, and congenital heart defects. The chest size is either normal or slightly smaller than normal, and affected individuals normally do not have respiratory distress after birth. Death has been associated with airway obstruction secondary to posterior placement of the tongue, as a result of the micrognathia, laryngeal stenosis or tracheomalacia, and congenital heart disease. The condition is inherited in an autosomal recessive mode, and appears to be associated with inflammation of the cartilage following minimal trauma.

Jones, 1988; Gembruch et al., 1988; McKusick, 1988

Prenatal Diagnosis: The diagnosis can be made by demonstrating shortening of the long bones in a fetus at risk, or can be suspected in a fetus with moderate to severe shortening of the long bones, a near-normal-sized chest, and abducted thumbs when there is a negative family history.

Differential Diagnosis: Achondrogenesis, type I (PD 145000); Achondrogenesis, type II (PD 145500); Achondroplasia, homozygous type (PD 147000); Hypochondrogenesis (PD 160370); and the Short rib–polydactyly syndromes (PD 169250, PD 169500, PD 170000, and PD 171000)

Fetoscopy[i]: shortened proximal and middle upper extremity and fingers

O'Brien et al., 1980a

curved limbs

O'Brien et al., 1980a

micrognathia, cleft palate

O'Brien et al., 1980a

Ultrasound[i]: micrognathia

Gembruch et al., 1988

Comments: Gembruch and associates (1988) made the diagnosis of diastrophic dysplasia during the 31 weeks of gestation in a fetus who did not have affected siblings. The diagnosis was confirmed postnatally.

cervical kyphosis

Gembruch et al., 1988

rhizomelic and acromelic shortening of all limbs

Mantagos et al., 1981; Gollop and Eigier, 1987

shortening of the humerus, radius/ulna, femur, and tibia/fibula, thickened humerus and femur, flexed and medially deviated fingers, lateral projection of the thumb

O'Brien et al., 1980a; Hobbins et al., 1982; Kaitila et al., 1983; Wladimiroff et al., 1984; Hobbins and Mahoney, 1985; Gollop and Eigier, 1987

marked shortening of all tubular bones

Kaitila et al., 1983; Gembruch et al., 1988

bowing or curving of all long bones

Wladimiroff et al., 1984; Qureshi et al., 1995

short limbs

Qureshi et al., 1995

elbows and knees fixed in extension positions[d]

Gembruch et al., 1988

decreased crown-to-rump length

O'Brien et al., 1980a

ulnar deviation of the hands[d]

Gembruch et al., 1988

abducted and proximally inserted (hitchhiker) toes and/or thumbs

Kaitila et al., 1983; Gembruch et al., 1988; Meizner and Bar-Ziv, 1993; Qureshi et al., 1995

proximal location of the ovoid first metacarpal

Meizner and Bar-Ziv, 1993

bilateral clubfoot deformities
> Gembruch et al., 1988; Qureshi et al., 1995

curved and thickened right femur and left tibia
> Qureshi et al., 1995

PD 155000 DISLOCATED KNEE (McKusick No. None)

Radiograph[c,d]: hyperextended leg
> McFarland, 1929

PD 155500 DYSSEGMENTAL DYSPLASIA, SILVERMAN–HANDMAKER TYPE (McKusick No. 224410)

Ultrasound[i]: deformed contour and angulation of the spine, irregular width of the spinal canal, poor mineralization of the ossification centers of the vertebral bodies, poor mineralization of the tubular bones, shortening of all extremities
> Kim et al., 1986a

grossly disorganized vertebrae, varying in size
> Izquierdo et al., 1990

extreme shortening of all long bones
> Izquierdo et al., 1990

hydramnios
> Izquierdo et al., 1990

PD 156000 ECTRODACTYLY (Lobster claw deformity; Split hand/foot deformity) (McKusick No. 183600)

Fetoscopy[i]: syndactyly
> Henrion et al., 1980; Mieler and Weise, 1985

observation of ectrodactyly of one hand
> Tolarova and Zwinger, 1981

Ultrasound[i]: lobster claw deformity, syndactyly
> Henrion et al., 1980

PD 157000 ECTROMELIA (Phocomelia) (McKusick No. None)

Radiograph[d]: absence or abnormality of one or more long bones of the extremities
> Russell, 1969

PD 158000 ELLIS–VAN CREVELD SYNDROME (Chondroectodermal dysplasia) (McKusick No. 225500)

Syndrome Note: Ellis–van Creveld syndrome is an autosomal recessive bone dysplasia with moderate shortening of limbs, postaxial polydactyly, dysplastic nails and teeth, broad and persistent upper-lip frenula, congenital heart defects, and in some cases, restricted chest cage. The latter feature may lead to significant respiratory insufficiency and death. There is a higher incidence of this disorder among the old-order Amish.
> Gollop and Eigier, 1986a

Prenatal Diagnosis: shortened long bones in a fetus at risk
> Gollop and Eigier, 1986a

Fetoscopy[i]: polydactyly (hexadactyly)
> Mahoney and Hobbins, 1977; Hobbins et al., 1982; Bui et al., 1984

Ultrasound[i]: fetal scalp edema indicated by double contour of the scalp
> Gollop and Eigier, 1986a

atrial septal defect
> Meizner and Bar-Ziv, 1993

narrow and long thorax
    Meizner and Bar-Ziv, 1993
normal thorax and echogenicity of the spine and limbs
    Weldner et al., 1985
shortened humeri and femora
    Mahoney and Hobbins, 1977; Gollop and Eigier, 1986a
shortened fetal limbs
    Gollop and Eigier, 1986a
hexadactyly
    Filly and Golbus, 1982

PD 158300 FEMORAL–FACIAL SYNDROME (Femoral hypoplasia–unusual facies syndrome) (McKusick No. 134780)

Syndrome Note: The femoral–facial syndrome, which in the past has been called the femoral hypoplasia–unusual facies syndrome, is characterized by absence or hypoplasia of the femora, and a typical facial appearance consisting of upslanting palpebral fissures, short nose, long philtrum, thin upper lip, micrognathia, and cleft palate. The condition usually is sporadic.
    McKusick, 1995
Prenatal Diagnosis: Criteria for the diagnosis of this condition prenatally have not been established. The diagnosis should be included in the differential of femoral hypoplasia.
Differential Diagnosis: See Femur, absent and Femur, shortened in the Index.
    Ultrasound[c,d]: micrognathia
        Robinow et al., 1995
    cleft palate
        Tadmor et al., 1993
    short humeri
        Tadmor et al., 1993

PD 158500 FETAL FRACTURE SECONDARY TO MATERNAL ABDOMINAL TRAUMA (McKusick No. None)

Radiograph[d]
    Bucholz and Mauldin, 1978

PD 159000 FETAL RICKETS (Vitamin D deficient rickets) (McKusick No. None)

Radiograph[d,i]: poor bone mineralization, widened and irregular metaphyses, penciled outlines of vertebral bodies
    Russell and Hill, 1974

PD 159175 FIBROCHONDROGENESIS (McKusick No. 228520)

Syndrome Note: Fibrochondrogenesis is a neonatal lethal chondrodysplasia, the features of which include rhizomelic shortening of the limbs, broad metaphyses of the long bones, pear-shaped vertebral bodies, and on bone histology, distinctive interwoven fibrous septa and dysplasia of the chondrocytes. The disorder is inherited in an autosomal recessive fashion.
    Bankier et al., 1991; McKusick, 1996
Ultrasound[i]: short limbs
    Bankier et al., 1991

PD 159250 FUHRMANN SYNDROME (Fibular aplasia or hypoplasia-femoral bowing-poly-,syn-, and oligodactyly) (McKusick No. 228930)

Syndrome Note: The syndrome that Fuhrmann and co-workers (1982) reported consists of hypoplasia of the fingers and finger nails, postaxial polydactyly, clinodactyly of the fifth fingers, oligodactyly of the hands and feet, marked angulation of the femora, aplasia or hypoplasia of the fibulae, hypoplasia of the pelvis, congenital dislocation of the hips, hypoplasia of the patellae, absence or coalescence of the tarsal bones, and absence of various metatarsal bones. There were four affected sibs in the family reported by Fuhrmann and associates (1982), three males and one female. The fourth affected sib was diagnosed prenatally and the pregnancy was terminated at about 19 weeks of gestation. The first affected child, the only survivor, had normal intellectual function. The condition appears to be inherited in an autosomal recessive fashion.

> McKusick, 1995

Fetoscopy[i]: thin and bowed leg, shortened leg, clubfoot deformatiy, oligodactyly of the foot, thick toes

> Fuhrmann et al., 1982

Ultrasound[i]: cystic enlargement of the posterior fossa, dilation of the lateral ventricles

> Pfeiffer et al., 1988

shortened and bowed leg

> Fuhrmann et al., 1982

shortened femora and tibiae

> Pfeiffer et al., 1988

absence of the fibulae

> Pfeiffer et al., 1988

clubfoot deformity

> Pfeiffer et al., 1988

increased bone density

> Pfeiffer et al., 1988

oligohydramnios

> Fuhrmann et al., 1982

PD 159500 GELEOPHYSIC DYSPLASIA (Geleophysic dwarfism) (McKusick No. 231050)

Dysplasia Note: Geleophysic dysplasia is characterized by short stature, brachydactyly, and a happy facial appearance for which the condition is named. In addition, there are short palpebral fissures; long upper lip; full cheeks; infiltration of the cardiac valves, trachea, and liver with a mucopolysaccharide-like substance; limitation of joint movement that results in inability to make a fist and a tiptoe gait; mild developmental delay; and reduced hearing that leads to speech delay. The condition appears to be inherited as an autosomal recessive disorder.

> Rosser et al., 1995

Prenatal Diagnosis: Not established; the condition most likely would be present if an at-risk fetus were found to have short limbs.

Ultrasound[d]: short radius, ulna, humerus, femur, tibia, and fibula

> Rosser et al., 1995

PD 160120 GRAFF–LAXOVA LETHAL SKELETAL DYSPLASIA (Lethal platyspondylic short-limbed dwarfism) (McKusick No. None; see 151210)

Syndrome Note: This condition was first described by Graff and colleagues (1972) and Laxova and associates (1973) as thanatophoric dysplasia and achondrogenesis, respectively. The condition has been classified as a distinct and separate entity by Knowles co-authors (1986), using both radiographic and histologic features. The disorder is characterized by short-limbed bone dysplasia with straight long bones, widened cupped metaphyses, minute round-appearing vertebral bodies, highly curved short ribs, precocious ossification of the tarsal bones, and lack of macrocephaly. Histologically, the bone pattern is different from that seen in either thanatophoric dysplasia or achondrogenesis.

> Graff et al., 1972; Laxova et al., 1973; Knowles et al., 1986

Physical examination of the mother[c,d]: hydramnios

> Graff et al., 1972; Laxova et al., 1973

> lack of fetal movement

>> Laxova et al., 1973

Radiograph[c,d]: large fetus with shortened long bones

> Graff et al., 1972

PD 160130 GREENBERG DYSPLASIA (Chondrodystrophy, hydrops and prenatal lethal type; Greenberg hydrops–ectopic calcification–moth-eaten skeletal dysplasia; Hydrops–ectopic calcification–moth-eaten skeletal dysplasia; Lethal chondrodysplasia, Greenberg–Rimoin type) (McKusick No. 215140)

Condition Note: This bone dysplasia is an apparent autosomal recessive, lethal disorder with a characteristic pattern of defects including very short limbs and long bones, irregular pattern of calcification of some long bones giving a moth-eaten appearance radiographically, delayed calcification of other long bones, thin and irregular ribs, marked platyspondyly, polydactyly, hydrops fetalis, cystic hygroma, extensive extra medullary erythropoiesis, and hydramnions. Chondroosseous histology is depicted by marked disorganization of bone interspersed with pieces of cartilage, bone, and mesenchymal tissue. Intrauterine death occurred at 30 weeks' gestation in one case.

> Greenberg et al., 1988c; Chitayat et al., 1993a

Prenatal Diagnosis: The diagnosis should be made in an at-risk fetus who has short limbs/long bones and hydrops fetalis. The diagnosis should be considered seriously in any fetus who has short limbs, hydrops fetalis, and irregular calcification of the long bones.

Differential Diagnosis: Achondrogenesis, type I (PD 145000); Achondrogenesis, type II (PD 145500); Diastrophic dysplasia (PD 154000); Dyssegmental dysplasia, Silverman–Handmaker type (PD 155500); Graff–Laxova lethal skeletal dysplasia (PD 160120); Osteogenesis imperfecta, type II (PD 164000)

Radiographic[i]: defective skeletal mineralization

> Greenberg et al., 1988c

Ultrasound[i]: very short limbs

> Greenberg et al., 1988c; Chitayat et al., 1993a

> defective skeletal mineralization

>> Greenberg et al., 1988c

> severe hydrops fetalis

>> Greenberg et al., 1988c; Chitayat et al., 1993a

> cystic hygroma

>> Chitayat et al., 1993a

> hexadactyly of both hands

>> Chitayat et al., 1993a

> intrauterine fetal death

>> Greenberg et al., 1988c

short femora
> Tadmor et al., 1993

> *Comments*: The case reported by Tadmor and co-workers (1993) had normal femoral length at 19 and 23 weeks of gestation. Evaluation at 32 weeks, however, revealed almost no femoral growth since the 23rd week. Strangely, there was catch-up growth of the femora during the ensuing 5 weeks.

short and bowed femora with normal humeral lengths
> Robinow et al., 1995

PD 160150 HOLMGREN SEMILETHAL CHONDRODYSPLASIA (Bone dysplasia, lethal, Holmgren type; Lethal chondrodysplasia, round femoral, inferior epiphyses type; Semilethal chondrodysplasia, Holmgren–Forsell type) (McKusick No. 211120)

Condition Note: Holmgren and associates (1984b) described this condition in three Finnish siblings (one girl and two boys) who were either stillborn or died by the age of 3 months. Physical characteristics included very short arms and legs particularly in the proximal part of the limbs, bowed femora, and small chest. Radiographic findings included short long bones with broad metaphyseal ends of the humora, bowed radii, femora and tibiae with knobby, rounded ends of the femora, and short ribs. The two liveborn sibs died from pneumonia and respiratory arrest.

Ultrasound[i]: shortened femora
> Holmgren et al., 1984b

PD 160180 HYDROCEPHALUS–SHORT LIMBS–THORACIC DYSPLASIA SYNDROME (Thoracic dysplasia–hydrocephalus syndrome) (McKusick No. 273740)

Syndrome Note: This syndrome is characterized by communicating hydrocephalus, mild rhizomelic shortening of all limbs, short ribs, narrow chest, and developmental delay. The disorder was reported in opposite-sexed offspring of normal but consanguineous Pakistani parents by Winter and co-workers in 1987.

Ultrasound[i]: lateral ventricular dilation of the brain, decreased chest and abdominal circumferences, shortened long bones, with the most significant reduction involving the radii and ulnae
> Winter et al., 1987

PD 160250 HYPOCHONDROPLASIA (McKusick No. 146000)

Ultrasound[i]: shortening of the femur, tibia, radius, and humerus by 22 weeks of gestation in a fetus at risk
> Stoll et al., 1985

PD 160370 HYPOCHONDROGENESIS (McKusick No. None; see 200600)

Ultrasound[c]: short, straight limbs with normal bone density and no fractures, micrognathia, small chest diameter with normal head size
> Donnenfeld et al., 1986

hydramnios[c]
> Maroteaux et al., 1983; Donnenfeld et al., 1986; Potocki et al., 1995

PD 160500 JARCHO–LEVIN SYNDROME (Costovertebral dysplasia; Occipitofaciocervicothoracoabdominodigital dysplasia; OFCTAD dysplasia; Spondylothoracic dysostosis) (McKusick No. 277300)

Syndrome Note: This condition is a rare autosomal recessive disorder characterized by a short neck and trunk, and by a constricted thorax, the result of multiple rib and vertebral defects. Most affected infants die from respiratory failure during infancy. The condition should be distinguished from similar but less severe autosomal dominant and recessive spondylocostal dysostosis disorders.

Apuzzio et al., 1987; Tolmie et al., 1987b

Prenatal Diagnosis: Like many skeletal dysplasias, the prenatal physical findings of this condition are not specific enough to establish the diagnosis with reasonable certainty unless there has been a previously affected and diagnosed sibling with the condition. However, the diagnosis should be suspected in any fetus with a small or contracted chest, but normal or near-normal extremity lengths.

Radiograph: abnormal thorax
Comas and Castro, 1979
irregularly spaced ribs
Poor et al., 1983
Ultrasound[i]: abnormal spine, particularly in the thoracic region, and chest in a fetus at risk
Tolmie et al., 1987b
irregularly spaced vertebrae
Apuzzio et al., 1987
abnormally shaped chest with slight flattening of the ribs[d]
Apuzzio et al., 1987

PD 161000 KLEEBLATTSCHADEL SYNDROME (Cloverleaf skull syndrome) (McKusick No. 148800)

Syndrome Note: *Kleeblattschadel* is German for "cloverleaf skull," which describes the characteristic appearance of the skull in this syndrome. The cloverleaf skull deformity is produced by in utero synostosis of the coronal and lambdoid sutures. In addition to the trilobular configuration of the skull, there may be petrous ridges, hydrocephalus, low-set ears, flattened facies, and varying degrees of exophthalmos. The exophthalmos can be marked in some individuals and can lead to corneal ulcerations. In severe cases, death usually occurs shortly after birth; others may live into the second decade. The condition is usually sporadic

Kleeblattschadel is also occasionally seen in Apert syndrome (PD 148500), and thanatophoric dysplasia (PD 174000). A cloverleaf skull in the presence of shortened limbs is most likely thanatophoric dysplasia.

Brahman et al., 1979; Banna et al., 1980; Salvo, 1981; McKusick, 1986

Prenatal Diagnosis: A trilobed appearance of the skull by ultrasound is typical, but the condition should be considered in any fetus with a significantly abnormal calvarial shape.

Radiograph[d]: odd-shaped skull with craniolacunae
Russell, 1973
Ultrasound: decreased biparietal diameter and head–thorax diameter ratio, enlarged lateral ventricles, abnormal calvarial shape, cloverleaf appearance of the ventricular system[c,d]
Brahman et al., 1979; Banna et al., 1980

trilobate skull appearance
Salvo, 1981

PD 161120 KNIEST DYSPLASIA (Kniest syndrome; Metatropic dwarfism, type II) (McKusick No. 156550)

Alpha-fetoprotein[c]: elevated in maternal serum
Bofinger and Saldana, 1989
Ultrasound[c]: shortening of the long bones, which became proportionately shorter with advancing gestational age, hydramnios
Bofinger and Saldana, 1989

PD 161245 LARSEN SYNDROME, AUTOSOMAL DOMINANT TYPE (McKusick No. 150250)

Syndrome Note: The autosomal dominant form of this condition is usually present when adults are found to be affected. The condition tends to be milder than the autosomal recessive form. The features of this disorder are the same as those listed under Larsen syndrome, autosomal recessive type (PD 161250).
Petrella et al., 1993
Prenatal Diagnosis: The presumptive diagnosis of this condition can be made if there are joint dislocations in the fetus on ultrasound examination when one parent is known to have the diagnosis.
Differential Diagnosis: Dislocated knee (PD 155000); Larsen syndrome, autosomal recessive type (PD 161250); Larsen syndrome, lethal form (PD 161255)

Ultrasound[i]: clubfoot deformity
Petrella et al., 1993
Comments: In the family reported by Petrella and associates (1993), one of the two affected siblings gave birth to an affected child. Because the parents of the affected siblings were unaffected, Petrella and co-workers suggested autosomal dominant, germ-line mosaicism as an explanation of the inheritance in the family.

PD 161250 LARSEN SYNDROME, AUTOSOMAL RECESSIVE TYPE (McKusick No. 245600)

Syndrome Note: The major features of this condition include multiple congenital dislocations of joints (particularly anterior dislocation of the tibiae on the femora, dislocation of the hips, equinovarus or equinovalgus, and dislocation of the elbows), prominent forehead, ocular hypertelorism, depressed nasal bridge, spatulated thumbs, and short metacarpals with long and cylindrical fingers. The condition may be inherited either in an autosomal dominant or an autosomal recessive mode. The autosomal dominant form of this condition tends to be relatively mild, whereas the autosomal recessive form is normally more severe and may even be lethal in some patients. Sporadic cases of unknown etiology also occur.
Romero et al., 1988, p. 366; Mostello et al., 1989; Petrella et al., 1993
Prenatal Diagnosis: In a fetus at risk, the diagnosis should be made by detecting multiple joint dislocations. In the sporadic case, the diagnosis should be considered whenever there are present multiple joint dislocations with ocular hypertelorism and/or depressed nasal bridge.

Differential Diagnosis: Dislocated knee (PD 155000); Larsen syndrome, autosomal dominant (PD 161245); Larsen syndrome, lethal form (PD 161255)

Ultrasound[i]: genu recurvatum; bilateral clubfoot deformity; increased joint space (i.e., increased distance between the ends of long bones); oligohydramnios
Mostello et al., 1989

PD 161255 LARSEN SYNDROME, LETHAL FORM (Larsen-like syndrome, lethal type) (McKusick No. 245650)

Syndrome Note: The lethal form of the Larsen syndrome has all of the features seen in the autosomal dominant and recessive forms (see Larsen syndrome, autosomal recessive type [PD 161250]), but in addition has tracheomalacia, lung hypoplasia, and death during the neonatal period. The condition appears to be inherited in an autosomal recessive mode.

Alpha-fetoprotein[c]: elevated level in maternal serum
Mostello et al., 1991
Ultrasound[i]: hyperextension of the knee (genu recurvatum), large separation between bone and joint spaces, oligohydramnios
Mostello et al., 1991

PD 161500 LIMB/PELVIS HYPOPLASIA/APLASIA SYNDROME (Absence of ulna and fibula with severe limb deficiency) (McKusick No. 276820)

Syndrome Note: This disorder has been described in two families of Middle Eastern background and is characterized by major and symmetrical hypoplasia/aplasia of all extremities and the pelvis. In particular, there are shortened, bowed radii; absence of the ulnae; oligodactyly with absence of the carpal bones; hypoplasia/aplasia of the metacarpals, and phalanges; hypoplasia of the femurs and feet; absence of the fibulae with hypoplasia/aplasia of the tarsals, metatarsals and phalanges; upward displacement of the male genitalia; and normal intelligence. The condition most likely is inherited in an autosomal recessive mode.
Raas-Rothschild et al., 1988
Prenatal Diagnosis: Significant bone deficiency or absence of long bones in a fetus at risk should be sufficient for the diagnosis. The diagnosis should be considered in a fetus of Middle Eastern ancestry who has tetramelic limb deficiency.
Differential Diagnosis: Acheiropody; Achondrogenesis, type I and II (PD 145000 and PD 145500); Femoral–fibular–ulnar syndrome; Roberts syndrome, (PD 193570); Thrombocytopenia–absent radius syndrome (PD 175000)

Ultrasound[i]: short, single forearm bone; malformed, hypoplastic hand; shortened malformed bones of the lower extremities; oligohydramnios
Raas-Rothschild et al., 1988

PD 161900 MELNICK–NEEDLES SYNDROME (Melnick–Needles osteodysplasty; Osteodysplasty of Melnick and Needles) (McKusick No. 309350)

Syndrome Note: The Melnick–Needles syndrome is a osteochondrodysplasia of X-linked dominant inheritance. Features include exophthalmos, full cheeks, micrognathia, small chest, irregular constrictions in the ribs, metaphyseal flaring of the long bones, S-like curvature of the long bones of the legs, and sclerosis of the base of the skull.
McKusick, 1996

Ultrasound[i]: deficient mineralization of the calvarium, abdominal wall defects, intrauterine fetal death, oligohydramnios
> Donnenfeld et al., 1987
> *Comments*: The fetus reported by Donnenfeld and co-authors (1987) at autopsy had the prune belly syndrome in addition to the Melnick–Needles syndrome.

PD 162000 MESOMELIC DWARFISM, LANGER TYPE (Homozygous dyschondrosteosis; Langer type mesomelic dwarfism; Leri–Weill dyschondrosteosis; Mesomelic dwarfism of the hypoplastic ulna, fibula, and mandible type) (McKusick No. 249700)

Syndrome Note: Characteristics of this condition include aplasia or severe hypoplasia of the ulna and fibula, thickened and curved radius and tibia, displacement deformities of the hands and feet, micrognathia, and short stature. Radiographically, all bones are shorter than normal, and with the exception of the fibula, they have a thickened appearance. The distal portion of the ulna is hypoplastic and the epiphysis is absent. In addition, there is hypoplasia of the proximal portion of the fibula.

The condition appears to be the homozygous dominant state of dyschondrosteosis. The latter disorder features variable degrees of Madelung deformity and mesomelic shortening, and is inherited in an autosomal dominant mode.
> McKusick, 1986; Evans et al., 1988

Prenatal Diagnosis: The diagnosis should be suspected in any fetus with short limbs and a normal or near-normal chest circumference. It can be presumed to be present in a short-limbed fetus who has had a previously affected sibling with Langer-type mesomelic dwarfism or whose parents are each affected with dyschondrosteosis.

Differential Diagnosis: Other conditions that should be considered in the diagnosis include other forms of mesomelic dwarfism such as Nievergelt, Robinow, Rheinhardt–Pfeiffer, and Werner types; Achondrogenesis, types I and II (PD 145000, and PD 145500); and Diastrophic dysplasia (PD 154000).

Ultrasound[i]: short long bones of the extremities
> Quigg et al., 1985
> disproportionate shortening of the forearms and legs
> Evans et al., 1988

PD 162050 METATROPIC DYSPLASIA, TYPE I (Metatropic dwarfism) (McKusick No. 250600)

Dysplasia Note: Metatropic-dysplasia–affected neonates normally have short limbs at birth, and later develop shortened trunks secondary to severe kyphoscoliosis. Other findings include prominent joints, cervical vertebral subluxation, and respiratory distress. Radiographic features include short and broad dumbbell-shaped metaphyses, irregular epiphyses, and marked flattening of the vertebrae. The condition is inherited in an autosomal recessive fashion.
> Manouvrier-Hanu et al., 1995; McKusick, 1996

Radiograph[i]: severe shortening of the long bones with enlarged metaphyses giving a dumbbell appearance
> Manouvrier-Hanu et al., 1995

Ultrasound: short limbs, disproportionately long hands and feet, long and narrow thorax, increased biparietal diameter, hydramnios
> Manouvrier-Hanu et al., 1995.

PD 162100 MIEVIS SYNDROME (Familial short stature, Brussels type) (McKusick No. 601350)

Syndrome Note: Mievis and co-workers (1996) have described two brothers with severe intrauterine and postnatal growth deficiency affecting height, weight, and head size; unusual facial features; and skeletal changes. Facial features included a broad forehead, deep-set eyes, narrow palpebral fissures, wide mouth, thin upper lip, a pointed chin, and microretrognathia. The skeletal findings include delayed osseous maturation, narrow thorax with enlarged and in-curved anterior ends of the ribs, small iliac bones, narrow sciatic notch, and shortened long bones with unusual shaped humeral and femoral metaphyses. Histologic analysis of the cartilage and bone showed thick and dense islets of calcified growth-plate cartilage with irregularly organized rows and columns of chondrocytes. The disorder probably is inherited either as an autosomal recessive or as an X-linked recessive disorder.

Mievis et al., 1996

Prenatal Diagnosis: The diagnosis most likely is present in the at-risk fetus when IUGR is present.

Differential Diagnosis: Asphyxiating thoracic dystrophy (PD 149000); Metaphyseal chondrodysplasia, Sedaghatian congenital lethal type; Mulibrey nanism; Russell–Silver syndrome (PD 193610); Thoracic-pelvic dysostosis; Van Bieruliet syndrome

Ultrasound[i]: IUGR after 25 weeks

Mievis et al., 1996

Comments: Of the two children reported by Mievis and colleagues (1996), one was alive and well at 10-8/12 years. He had normal intellectual function, but had growth deficiency. The brother died immediately after birth from respiratory failure.

PD 162600 NANCE–SWEENEY SYNDOME (Chondrodystrophy with sensorineural deafness; Nance–Insley syndrome; Otospondylmegaepiphyseal dysplasia) (McKusick No. 215150)

Syndrome Note: The features that make up the Nance–Sweeney syndrome include severe and progressive sensorineural deafness, saddle-shaped nose, cleft palate, short stature with disproportionate short limbs, platyspondyly, carpal bone fusion, enlarged epiphyses, and subcutaneous calcifications. The condition appears to be a defect in collagen 11 and is inherited in an autosomal recessive mode.

McKusick, 1995; Rosser et al., 1996

Ultrasound[c,h]: increased nuchal-fold thickness

Rosser et al., 1996

PD 163000 OLIGODACTYLY (Absent toe) (McKusick No. None)

Radiograph[d]: only four metatarsals present

Russell, 1973

PD 163250 OPSISMODYSPLASIA (McKusick No. 258480)

Condition Note: Opsismodysplasia is a bone dysplasia that shows late bone maturation. Characteristics of the disorder include predominantly rhizomelic micromelia, macrocephaly, anterior large fontanel, prominent brow, depressed nasal bridge, small and anteverted nose, long philtrum, short hands and feet, sausage-like fingers, and hypotonia. Growth is slow. Death occurs frequently from pulmonary infections. Inheritance is autosomal recessive.

McKusick, 1994; Santos and Saraiva, 1995

Prenatal Diagnosis: In the at-risk fetus, any of the characteristics listed above, or described for the condition, and detected prenatally would be suggestive of the condition.

Ultrasound[c]: shortened limbs

Santos and Saraiva, 1995

PD 163500 OSTEOGENESIS IMPERFECTA, TYPE I (Osteogenesis imperfecta tarda) (McKusick No. 166200)

Amniocentesis: elevated amniotic fluid pyrophosphate[c]

Solomons and Gottesfeld, 1979

Ultrasound[i]: marked bowing and shortening of femora, reduced acoustic shadowing of the long bones by 32 weeks, shortened radius and ulna, upper extremities flipperlike in appearance

Chervenak et al., 1982; Hill et al., 1983a

overriding fracture of the femur

Hobbins and Mahoney, 1985

fractures of femur with movement at site of fracture (pseudoarthrosis) at 20 weeks' gestation; by 26 weeks the fracture had healed at an angle

Kurtz and Wapner, 1983

thinning, decreased echogenicity, and bowing of the femora

Hobbins and Mahoney, 1985

PD 164000 OSTEOGENESIS IMPERFECTA, TYPE II (Lethal perinatal osteogenesis imperfecta; Osteogenesis imperfecta congenita; OI, type II; Perinatally lethal osteogenesis imperfecta) (McKusick No. 259400)

Condition Note: Osteogenesis imperfecta, type II is a disorder characterized by short limbs with severe distortion of long bones, multiple fractures, decreased calcification of bones particularly marked in the skull, and in utero or early neonatal death. The condition is produced by a defect in type I collagen.

Prenatal Diagnosis: Munoz and associates (1990) have proposed a set of criteria for the prenatal diagnosis of osteogenesis imperfecta, type II that includes multiple fractures, demineralization of the calvarium, and femoral length more that 3 SD below the mean for gestational age. Six of eight fetuses with this condition met all three criteria. None of 25 other fetuses with other bone dysplasias possessed all three criteria. There were no false positives. In pregnancies at risk for recurrence of the condition, these authors reported that a normal sonogram after 17 weeks' gestation excluded this lethal condition.

Differential Diagnosis: Achondrogenesis, type I (PD 145000) and type II (PD 145500); Achondroplasia, homozygous type (PD 147000); Asphyxiating thoracic dystrophy (PD 149000); Campomelic dysplasia, short-limb type (PD 150000); Hypophosphatasia, congenital lethal form (PD 245000); Osteogenesis imperfecta, type III (PD 164500); Roberts syndrome (PD 193570); Thanatophoric dysplasia (PD 174000)

Amniocentesis: elevated amniotic fluid pyrophosphate[c]

Solomons and Gottesfeld, 1979

Chorionic villus sampling[g,i]: elevated alpha 1(I) : alpha 2(I) ratio, and reduced

electrophoretic mobility of alpha 1(I) procollagen after culture of chorionic villi in radioactive glycine
>Raghunath et al., 1994

Maternal history[c,d]: decreased fetal movement as perceived by the mother
>Shapiro et al., 1982a

Radiograph: poor fetal calcification of all bones, in some cases no calcification detected
>Lachman and Hall, 1979; Dinno et al., 1982; Shapiro et al., 1982a; Garver et al., 1984

total absence of visualization of the affected co-twin, the other twin was visualized well[d]
>Morin et al., 1991

absence of calvarial mineralization
>Shapiro et al., 1982a

decreased mineralization and multiple fractures of ribs
>McGuire et al., 1987

Ultrasound[i]: compression of the soft cranium with abnormal skull shape, distorted position of the limbs, poor visualization of the fetal spine, ribs (distally), and long bones; bell-shaped thorax, widened metaphyses and thin diaphyses of long bones; short, thickened, and bowed long bones; multiple fractures; abnormal fetal movements
>Dinno et al., 1982; Shapiro et al., 1982a; Elejalde and de Elejalde, 1983; Patel et al., 1983; Stephens et al., 1983; Garver et al., 1984; Ghosh et al., 1984; Hobbins and Mahoney, 1985; Weldner et al., 1985; Spirt et al., 1987

soft and easily deformed skull
>Raghunath et al., 1994

hydrocephalus
>Palumbos and Steirman, 1989

progressive ventriculomegaly[c]
>Shapiro et al., 1982a

easily identified intracranial structures
>Raghunath et al., 1994

decreased density or echogenicity of skull
>McGuire et al., 1987; Morin et al., 1991; Raghunath et al., 1994

exceptionally clearly visualized orbits
>McGuire et al., 1987

spine not found to be as echogenic as normal, that is, abnormal or absent shadowing due to delayed maturation and mineralization, abnormally shaped vertebrae
>de Elejalde and Elejalde, 1985b

narrow thorax, ribs with multiple irregular echos
>McGuire et al., 1987

decreased diameter or volume of the thorax
>Hill et al., 1988b; Knisely et al., 1988

abnormal angulation of the ribs
>Raghunath et al., 1994

inward bowing of fetal ribs
>Hill et al., 1988b

femoral length more than 3 SD below the mean for gestational age
    Munoz et al., 1990; Morin et al., 1991
short and bowed limbs
    Hill et al., 1988b; Kniseley et al., 1988; Raghunath et al., 1994
compressed and fractured femur and tibiae
    Raghunath et al., 1994
unusual angulation of foot
    Spirt et al., 1987
marked undermineralization of bones
    Munoz et al., 1990; Morin et al., 1991
multiple fractures as noted by more than one discontinuity along the
length of a single long bone
    Munoz et al., 1990
hydramnios[c]
    Rasmussen et al., 1996
intrauterine growth retardation[c,d]
    Morin et al., 1991

PD 164500 OSTEOGENESIS IMPERFECTA, TYPE III (Osteogenesis imperfecta, severe deforming type) (McKusick No. 259420)

Radiograph[i]: generalized diminished ossification of fetal skeleton
    Aylsworth et al., 1984
shortened and distorted femurs, fractures of the femora[d]
    Robinson et al., 1987
Ultrasound[i]
thin skull
    Chitayat et al., 1993b
abnormal rib angulation and fractures
    Chitayat et al., 1993b
bowed and shortened femora
    Aylsworth et al., 1984; Robinson et al., 1987
poor interval growth of long bones, shortening of the humerus, tibia, and fibula
    Robinson et al., 1987
bent and healing fractures of long bones
    Chitayat et al., 1993b
hydramnios[c,d]
    Rasmussen et al., 1996

PD 166000 OSTEOPETROSIS, AUTOSOMAL RECESSIVE, INFANTILE FORM (Albers–Schonberg disease; Marble bone) (McKusick No. 259700)

Syndrome Note: This form of osteopetrosis is inherited in an autosomal recessive mode in contrast to the milder autosomal dominant form (osteopetrosis, McKusick No. 166600). Manifestations of the disorder are most frequently discovered during the first few months of life with subsequent progression of the disease leading to increased bone density, anemia, hearing loss, optic atrophy, hepatosplenomegaly, thrombocytopenia, and severe infections. Death usually occurs in early childhood.
    Ogur et al., 1995; McKusick, 1997
Prenatal Diagnosis: No definite method has been established. Increased bone

density and metaphyseal splaying of the femora in an at-risk fetus is presumptive evidence for the diagnosis.

Differential Diagnosis: Osteogenesis imperfecta, type II (PD 164000) and type III (PD 1645000); Osteopetrosis, autosomal dominant form (McKusick No. 166600); Osteopetrosis, early lethal form (PD 166500); Osteopetrosis, mild autosomal recessive form (McKusick No. 259710)

Radiograph[i]: marked increase in bone density, metaphyseal splaying and clubbing of the femora, segmentation abnormality of a lumbar vertebra
Ogur et al., 1995

PD 166500 OSTEOPETROSIS, EARLY LETHAL FORM (Lethal osteopetrosis; Osteopetrosis, lethal) (McKusick No. 259720)

Condition Note: There is now recognized a number of different forms of osteopetrosis (see osteopetrosis in McKusick, 1996). The type cited here (osteopetrosis, early lethal form) appears to be inherited in an autosomal recessive fashion, is associated with severe osteopetrosis in utero, and results in intrauterine demise or infantile death. The condition may be severe enough to result in in utero fractures leading to the erroneous diagnosis of osteogenesis imperfecta, type II. The brain also may be abnormal in this disorder.
El Khazen et al., 1986; McKusick, 1995

Prenatal Diagnosis: No definite method has been established. The finding of increased bone density with lack of corticomedullary differentiation would be presumptive evidence for the diagnosis in the at-risk fetus.

Differential Diagnosis: Osteogenesis imperfecta, type II (PD 164000) and type III (PD 164500); Osteopetrosis, autosomal dominant form (McKusick No. 166600); Osteopetrosis, autosomal recessive, infantile form (PD 166000); Osteopetrosis, mild autosomal recessive form (McKusick No. 259710)

Radiograph: macrocephaly[i]
El Khazen et al., 1986
hydrocephalus[i]
El Khazen et al., 1986
generalized increased bone density with lack of corticomedullary differentiation of tubular bones[i]
Jenkinson et al., 1943; El Khazen et al., 1986
Comments: The case reported by Jenkinson and associates (1943) has radiographic findings similar to those found in Caffey disease (PD 149000), according to the assessment of de Jong and Muller (1995), and could have the latter condition. The fetus cited by Jenkinson and associates (1943) in our opinion appears to fit the early lethal form of osteopetrosis best because of the generalized increase of bone density in the fetal period, and because there was a decrease in the number of osteoclasts on bone histology.
sclerotic changes in the metacarpals, metatarsals, and phalanges of the hands and feet
Jenkinson et al., 1943
widening of the bones
Jenkinson et al., 1943
marble-like appearance of the bones
Jenkinson et al., 1943

multiple fractures of the long bones with hypertrophic bone callus formation
El Khazen et al., 1986
small dense vertebral bodies
El Khazen et al., 1986
Ultrasound[i]: dense skeleton, deformation of the humerus, fractures of the humerus and ribs associated with hypertrophic callus formation, hydrocephalus with macrocephaly, skin edema, hydramnios
El Khazen et al., 1986

PD 167000 OSTEOPOIKILOSIS (Osteopoikilie; Spotted bones) (McKusick No. Unknown; see 166700)

Radiograph: spotted bones
Martincic, 1952

PD 168000 PROXIMAL FEMORAL FOCAL DEFICIENCY (Congenital short femur; Femur–fibula–ulna syndrome; FFU) (McKusick No. 228200)

Ultrasound: femur length less than fifth percentile, with angulation deformity of the midshaft[d]
Graham, 1985
unilateral short femur in an otherwise normal fetus
Ashkenazy et al., 1990; Hadi and Wade, 1993
Comment: The fetus reported by Hadi and Wade (1993) was the product of an insulin-dependent diabetic mother.
clubfoot
Hadi and Wade, 1993

PD 168500 ROBINOW SYNDROME (Fetal face syndrome; Mesomelic dysplasia, Robinow type; Robinow–Silverman–Smith syndrome) (McKusick No. 180700)

Ultrasound[i]: shortened ulnae and radii, ulna/humerus ratio low (0.53) (normal, 0.92)
Loverro et al., 1990

PD 169020 SACRAL AGENESIS/SPINA BIFIDA, FAMILIAL (McKusick No. 182940)

Condition Note: Fellous and associates (1982) reported on a five-generation family with lower spinal defects ranging in severity from spina bifida occulta to complete agenesis of the sacrum, with or without spina bifida cystica. Seventeen of 28 descendents of the older affected family members had these defects. The condition appears to be inherited as an autosomal dominant disorder with variable expressivity.
Prenatal Diagnosis: The diagnosis is established in a fetus at risk whenever sacral agenesis or spina bifida is detected.
Differential Diagnosis: Diabetic embryopathy (PD 243500); Sacral dysgenesis (PD 169040); Sirenomelia (PD 194130); Spina bifida cystica (PD 129000); Spina bifida occulta (PD 130000)
Alpha-fetoprotein[c,i]: elevated levels in the amniotic fluid
Fellous et al., 1982

Ultrasound[i]: sacral agenesis indicated by absence of the sacrum between the two iliac bones, defect in the neural arch in the lumbar region
>> Fellous et al., 1982
>> absence of lumbosacral vertebrae
>>> Meizner and Bar-Ziv, 1993
>> abnormal flexion of the leg
>>> Meizner and Bar-Ziv, 1993
>> reduced crown-to-rump length[g]
>>> Tchobroutsky et al., 1985

PD 169040 SACRAL DYSGENESIS (Caudal regression syndrome; Sacral agenesis) (McKusick No. Unknown; see 182940)

Differential Diagnosis: Diabetic embryopathy (PD 243500); Sacral agenesis/spina bifida, familial (PD 169020); Sirenomelia (PD 194130); Spina bifida cystica (PD 129000); Spina bifida occulta (PD 130000)
>> Ultrasound: absence of the left side of the spine beginning at the level of the first lumbar vertebra, no pelvic bones present, severely shortened left lower limb attached to posterior aspect of the lumbar area
>>> de Elejalde and Elejalde, 1985b

PD 169100 SCHNECKENBECKEN DYSPLASIA (McKusick No. 269250)

Syndrome Note: *Schneckenbecken,* German for snail pelvis, is a distinctive feature of this lethal neonatal chrondrodysplasia. The condition is inherited as an autosomal recessive trait. Pregnancies are frequently complicated by third trimester hydramnios. The fetuses have short limbs, but their condition cannot be differentiated prenatally from many other lethal bone dysplasias per se. The fetus is usually stillborn or dies immediately after birth.

Besides the snail-like pelvis, the disorder is radiographically characterized by short ribs; flattened, hypoplastic vertebral bodies; short, broad long bones with dumbbell-like appearance; short, wide fibulae; and precocious ossification of the tarsi. Bone histology is also unique.
>> Borochowitz et al., 1986

Prenatal Diagnosis: Recurrence of a short-limb bone dysplasia in which the diagnosis previously has been made in an affected sibling is normally sufficient evidence for the diagnosis. Otherwise the diagnosis cannot be made prenatally with certainty.

Differential Diagnosis: Achondrogenesis, type I (PD 145000), and II (PD 145500); Neu–Laxova syndrome (PD 192700); Thanatophoric dysplasia (PD 174000)
>> Physical examination of mother[c]: hydramnios
>>> Borochowitz et al., 1986
>> Ultrasound[i]: shortened extremities and long bones
>>> Borochowitz et al., 1986

PD 169150 SELLER LETHAL CHONDRODYSPLASIA (McKusick No. None)

Dysplasia Note: Seller and associates (1996) have described a severe and lethal bone dysplasia characterized by absent ossification of the skull, and cervical and upper thoracic vertebral bodies; platyspondyly; short and angulated radii, ulnae, femora, and tibiae; trident-shaped acetabular roofs; sclerotic bands in the iliae wings and scapulae; hooked-shaped clavicles; and variable bone density.

Ultrasound[c]: short limbs, IUGR, oligohydramnios
Seller et al., 1996

PD 169200 SHEPHARD SYNDROME (McKusick No. None)

Syndrome Note: Shephard and associates (1995) reported male and female siblings who had a bone dysplasia characterized by deep-set facial creases, broad nasal bridge, small and dysmorphic ears, brachydactyly, clinodactyly of the index and fifth fingers, cystic hygroma, multicystic kidneys, narrow chest with shortened ribs, and shortening and bowing of the long bones. The male died shortly after birth. The authors concluded that the condition they reported was a previously unreported skeletal dysplasia syndrome.

Prenatal Diagnosis: No definitive method of diagnosis is available; the presence of cystic hygroma, and shortened and bowed long bones would be presumptive evident for the diagnosis in an at-risk fetus.

Differential Diagnosis: Achondrogenesis, type II (PD 145500); Asphyxiating thoracic dystrophy (PD 149000); Greenberg dysplasia (PD 160130)

Ultrasound[i]: cystic hygroma, multicystic kidney, shortened and bowed long bones, bowed femora and ulnae
Shephard et al., 1995

PD 169220 SHORT RIB–POLYDACTYLY SYNDROME,
BEEMER–LANGER TYPE (Short rib [polydactyly] syndrome, Beemer–Langer type; Short rib syndrome, Beemer type) (McKusick No. 269860)

Syndrome Note: Short rib–polydactyly syndrome, Beemer–Langer type, has as major features median cleft lip/palate, short ribs with a narrow chest, short and bowed limbs, renal cystic dysplasia, absence of internal genitalia, hydrops fetalis, and neonatal lethality from lung hypoplasia. Polydactyly in this condition has been reported by Yang and co-workers (1991). The disorder appears to be an autosomal recessive one.
McKusick, 1996

Physical examination of the mother[c,d]: increased fundal height[c,d]
Lin et al., 1991

Ultrasound: hydrocephaly[c,d]
Lin et al., 1991; Yang et al., 1991
cerebral abnormalities (not specified)[c,d]
Yang et al., 1991
hydrocephalus of the lateral ventricles[c,d]
Lin et al., 1991
posterior fossa cyst[c,d]
Lin et al., 1991
median cleft lip[c,d]
Lin et al., 1991
short ribs[c,d]
Lin et al., 1991
small thorax[i]
Balci et al., 1991; Lin et al., 1991
lung hypoplasia[c,d]
Lin et al., 1991

small heart[c,d]
  Yang et al., 1991
ascites[i]
  Balci et al., 1991
short limbs[c,d]
  Lin et al., 1991
short lower extremities[i]
  Balci et al, 1991
hydrops fetalis[c,d]
  Lin et al., 1991
hydramnios[c,d]
  Balci et al., 1991; Lin et al., 1991; Yang et al., 1991

PD 169250 SHORT RIB–POLYDACTYLY SYNDROME, MAJEWSKI TYPE
(Majewski dwarfism; Majewski syndrome; Polydactyly with neonatal chondrodystrophy, type II; Short rib–polydactyly syndrome, type II) (McKusick No. 263520)

Syndrome Note: The condition is characterized by a median cleft lip, pre- and postaxial polysyndactyly, short ribs, and defects of the limbs, genitalia, epiglottis, and viscera. The condition is lethal in the perinatal period.
  McKuskick, 1995

Differential Diagnosis: Alstrom syndrome (retinitis pigmentosa, obesity, diabetes mellitus, and perceptive deafness); Asphyxiating thoracic dystrophy (PD 149000); Bardet–Biedl syndrome (PD 186500); Biemond syndrome II (iris coloboma, hypogenitalism, obesity, polydactyly, and mental retardation); Ellis–van Creveld syndrome (PD 158000); Hydrolethalus syndrome (PD 191300); Laurence–Moon syndrome (mental retardation, pigmentary retinopathy, hypogenitalism, and spastic paraplegia); Meckel syndrome (PD 192140); Short rib–polydactyly syndromes (PD 169250, PD 169500, PD 170000, PD 171000); Smith–Lemli–Opitz syndrome (PD 194160); Trisomy 13 syndrome (PD 103000)
  Creech et al., 1988; McKusick et al., 1988
Fetoscopy[i]: polydactyly
  Tolarova and Zwinger, 1981; Toftager-Larson and Benzie, 1984
  median cleft lip
  Tolarova and Zwinger, 1981; Toftager-Larson and Benzie, 1984
  shortened tibia
  Toftager-Larson and Benzie, 1984
Radiograph[d,i]: short, upward-slanting ribs
  Thomson et al., 1982
  constricted chest
  Thomson et al., 1982
  femur shortened and bowed
  Thomson et al., 1982
Ultrasound: disproportionate head-to-body size,[c] quite short and broad extremities,[c] with marked shortening of the tibia and shortening of other long bones,[c] narrow thorax,[c] polydactyly[c]
  Gembruch et al., 1985
  ribs could not be identified[d,i]
  Thomson et al., 1982

upper limbs could not be identified[d,i]
  Thomson et al., 1982
shortened lower limbs[d,i]
  Thomson et al., 1982
large and protruberant abdomen[d,i]
  Thomson et al., 1982
hydramnios[d,i]
  Thomson et al., 1982

PD 169500 SHORT RIB–POLYDACTYLY SYNDROME, PIEPKORN TYPE

(Piepkorn dwarfism; Short rib–polydactyly syndrome, type IV) (McKusick No. Unknown)

Differential Diagnosis: Alstrom syndrome (retinitis pigmentosa, obesity, diabetes mellitus, and perceptive deafness); Bardet–Biedl syndrome (PD 186500); Biemond syndrome II (iris coloboma, hypogenitalism, obesity, polydactyly, and mental retardation); Hydrolethalus syndrome (PD 191300); Laurence–Moon syndrome (mental retardation, pigmentary retinopathy, hypogenitalism, and spastic paraplegia); Meckel syndrome (PD 192140); Short rib–polydactyly syndromes (PD 169250, PD 169500, PD 170000, PD 171000); Smith–Lemli–Opitz syndrome (PD 194260); Trisomy 13 syndrome (PD 103000)
  Creech et al., 1988; McKusick, 1988
Radiograph[c,d]: severe shortening of fetal limbs
  Piepkorn et al., 1977
Ultrasound[c,d]: severe shortening of fetal limbs, thickened fetal body, hydramnios
  Piepkorn et al., 1977

PD 170000 SHORT RIB–POLYDACTYLY SYNDROME,

SALDINO–NOONAN TYPE (Polydactyly with neonatal chondrodystrophy, type I; Saldino–Noonan dwarfism; Short rib–polydactyly syndrome, type I) (McKusick No. 263530)

Differential Diagnosis: Alstrom syndrome (retinitis pigmentosa, obesity, diabetes mellitus, and perceptive deafness); Bardet–Biedl syndrome (PD 186500); Biemond syndrome II (iris coloboma, hypogenitalism, obesity, polydactyly, and mental retardation); Hydrolethalus syndrome (PD 191300); Laurence–Moon syndrome (mental retardation, pigmentary retinopathy, hypogenitalism, and spastic paraplegia); Meckel syndrome (PD 192140); Short rib–polydactyly syndromes (PD 169250, PD 169500, PD 170000, PD 171000); Smith–Lemli–Opitz syndrome (PD 194160); Trisomy 13 syndrome (PD 103000)
  Creech et al., 1988; McKusick, 1988
Amniography[i]: oligohydramnios, shortened humeri and femora
  Johnson et al., 1982b
Radiograph[i]: poorly defined long bones
  Richardson et al., 1977
Ultrasound: decreased fetal movements, inability to identify fetal limbs[i]
  Johnson et al., 1982b
  oligohydramnios[c]
    Richardson et al., 1977; Johnson et al., 1982b

PD 171000 SHORT RIB–POLYDACTYLY SYNDROME, SPRANGER–VERMA TYPE (Polydactyly with neonatal chondrodystrophy, type III; Short rib–polydactyly syndrome, type III; Short rib–polydctyly syndrome, Verma–Naumoff type; Spranger–Verma dwarfism) (McKusick No. 263510)

> **Differential Diagnosis:** Alstrom syndrome (retinitis pigmentosa, obesity, diabetes mellitus, and perceptive deafness); Bardet–Biedl syndrome (PD 186500); Biemond syndrome II (iris coloboma, hypogenitalism, obesity, polydactyly, and mental retardation); Hydrolethalus syndrome (PD 191300); Laurence–Moon syndrome (mental retardation, pigmentary retinopathy, hypogenitalism, and spastic paraplegia); Meckel syndrome (PD 192140); Short rib–polydactyly syndromes (PD 169250, PD 169500, PD 170000, PD 171000); Smith–Lemli–Opitz syndrome (PD 194160); Trisomy 13 syndrome (PD 103000)
> > Creech et al., 1988; McKusick, 1988
> Radiograph[d]
> > Verma et al., 1975
> Ultrasound[d]: thoracic hypoplasia
> > de Sierra et al., 1992
> > reduced thoracic circumference to abdominal circumference ratio
> > > de Sierra et al., 1992
> > shortened long bones
> > > de Sierra et al., 1992
> > polydactyly
> > > de Sierra et al., 1992
> > complete situs inversus
> > > de Sierra et al., 1992

PD 171250 SHORT RIB–POLYDACTYLY SYNDROME, TYPE UNDETERMINED (McKusick No. None; see 263510)

> **Syndrome Note:** Wu and associates (1995) described four full siblings who had a form of short rib–polydactyly syndrome. Two of the sibs were thought by the authors to have short rib–polydactyly syndrome, Spranger–Verma type (PD 171000), while they concluded that the others had the condition described by Le Marec and co-authors (1973).
> Ultrasound[i]: short ribs with wide distal ends, narrow thorax, decreased chest circumference, progressively protuberant abdomen, increasing abdominal to thoracic circumference ratio, short long bones, marginal spurs of the femur and tibia, polydactyly
> > Wu et al., 1995

PD 172500 SKULL DEFORMATION SECONDARY TO UTERINE LEIOMYOMA (McKusick No. None)

> Ultrasound[d]: asymmetrical calvarial configuration produced by fetal skull compression from a uterine leiomyoma
> > Romero et al., 1981

PD 173000 SKULL FRACTURE (McKusick No. None)

> Radiograph[d]: head fixed in the inlet of the pelvis, marked depression of the left temporoparietal region against the promontory of the maternal sacrum
> > Alexander and Davis, 1969

PD 173430 SPONDYLOEPIMETAPHYSEAL DYSPLASIA, SHOHAT TYPE
(McKusick No. None)

Condition Note: This bone dysplasia is characterized by postnatal onset of severe short stature, severe lumbar lordosis, marked genu vara secondary to fibular overgrowth, platyspondyly, and probable autosomal recessive inheritance (Figuera et al., 1994).

Ultrasound[c,d]: short femora
Figuera et al., 1994

PD 173450 SPONDYLOEPIMETAPHYSEAL DYSPLASIA WITH JOINT LAXITY (McKusick No. 271640)

Dysplasia Note: Spondyloepimetaphyseal dysplasia with joint laxity is a unique bone dysplasia that has been mainly found in the Afrikaans-speaking population of South Africa. The condition is noted for prominent eyes with blue sclerae, long philtrum, cleft palate, micrognathia, congenital heart defect, severe kyphoscoliosis, joint laxity, dislocated hips, and clubfoot deformity. Radiographically, there are dumbbell-shaped long bones, flared metaphyse, and spatulate terminal phalanges. The disorder is inherited as an autosomal recessive condition.
McKusick, 1996; Pina-Neto et al., 1996

Ultrasound[c,d]: short long bones, oligohydramnios
Pina-Neto et al., 1996

PD 173500 SPONDYLOEPIPHYSEAL DYSPLASIA CONGENITA (SED congenita) (McKusick No. 183900)

Ultrasound: shortened femora, tibiae, fibulae, humeri, radii and ulnae[c]; micrognathia[c]; normal biparietal diameter[c]; small chest[c]
Donnenfeld and Mennuti, 1987

Comments: Although the long bones were short, they appeared ultrasonically to be straight and of normal density in the fetus reported by Donnenfeld and Mennuti (1987).

short limb[i]
Tiller et al., 1995

hydramnios
Donnenfeld and Mennuti, 1987; Rasmussen et al., 1996

PD 173515 SPONDYLOMETAPHYSEAL DYSPLASIA, SEDAGHATIAN TYPE (Metaphyseal chondrodysplasia, congenital lethal; Sedaghatian chondrodysplasia; Sedaghaian congenital lethal metaphyseal chondrodysplasia) (McKusick No. 250220)

Dysplasia Note: This bone dysplasia is a neonatal lethal disorder characterized by mild rhizomelic limb shortening, platyspondyly, "laciness" of the iliac wings, subacute myocarditis, cortical necrosis of the kidneys, and adrenal and pulmonary hemorrhage.
Peeden at al., 1992

Ultrasound[c,d]: mild short limbs
Peeden et al., 1992

PD 173525 TERMINAL TRANSVERSE LIMB DEFECTS (McKusick No. 102650)

Condition Note: Terminal transverse limb defects represent a spectrum of diminution or absence of digits of either the hands or feet, or both. Often the hand or foot of the affected extremity is reduced in size and occasionally the forearm or lower leg also may be deficient. The limb defect normally involves the terminal portion of the limb and the deficiency is at a right angle to the long axis of the limb. The incidence of terminal transverse limb defects is estimated to be 1.5 per 10,000 births. A vascular cause for this condition has been proposed.

> Harmon et al., 1995

Prenatal Diagnosis: The diagnosis should be considered when absent and/or shortened digits of the hand and/or feet are found by ultrasonic examination.

> Ultrasound: ascites, pleural effusion, terminal limb defects
>> Harmon et al., 1995

>> *Comments:* The parents of the fetus reported by Harmon and colleagues (1995) were thought to be carriers of alpha-thalassemia genes. The fetus probably had alpha-thalassemia. After termination of the pregnancy, the fetus was found to have terminal transverse limb defects of all extremities, the digits represented only by nubbin-like structures. Hydrops fetalis was also present.

PD 173550 TETRAAMELIA, ISOLATED (Amelia) (McKusick No. 104400)

Condition Note: Tetraamelia is absence of all four limbs with no other consistently associated anomalies. Usually this condition is sporadic.

Prenatal Diagnosis: Typically no identifiable limbs are noted in the affected fetus.

Differential Diagnosis: Tetraamelia syndrome (PD 194180)

> Radiograph[d]: absent limbs
>> Russell, 1973

PD 174000 THANATOPHORIC DYSPLASIA (Thanatophoric dwarfism)
(McKusick No. 187600; see also 151210, 187601, 273670)

> Amniocentesis[c,d]: lecithin/sphingomyelin (L/S) ratio low for 35 weeks
>> Goodlin and Lowe, 1974; Chervenak et al., 1983a; Hobbins and Mahoney, 1985

> Radiograph[c]: enlarged calvarium, small facial bones, poorly ossified spine, shortened and bowed long bones, shortened ribs, small iliac bones
>> Cremin and Shaff, 1977; Burrows et al., 1984; Camera et al., 1984

> Ultrasound: shortened limbs, small bell-shaped chest, thickened scalp, protuberant abdomen, shortened femora and humeri, bowed femura, hypoplastic vertebrae with rounded bodies, hypoplastic and abnormally shaped clavicles, decreased movement and range of movement of limbs, demineralization of all bones, flat facies with hypoplastic nose, hydramnios
>> Hobbins et al., 1979; Shaff et al., 1980; Chervenak et al., 1983a; Shih et al., 1983; Wong and Filly, 1983; Burrows et al., 1984; Elejalde and de Elejalde, 1985; Goodlin and Lowe, 1985; Weldner et al., 1985; Donnenfeld and Mennuti, 1987; Spirt et al., 1987

> hydrocephalus, macrocephaly, trilobed appearance of otherwise intact calvarium (cloverleaf skull), abnormally large subarachnoid space, enlarged superior sagittal sinus, narrow spinal canal
>> Chervenak et al., 1983a; Burrows et al., 1984; Elejalde and de Elejalde, 1985; Hobbins and Mahoney, 1985; Mahony et al., 1985a; Spirt et al., 1987

> cloverleaf-shaped skull[d]
>> McGuire et al., 1987

increased head circumference[d]
    McGuire et al., 1987
ventricular enlargement[d]
    McGuire et al., 1987
ocular hypertelorism,[d] saddle-shaped nose,[d] anteverted nares,[d] triangle-shaped mouth,[d] unusually mobile tongue[d]
    McGuire et al., 1987
short neck[d]
    McGuire et al., 1987
small chest[d]
    McGuire et al., 1987
shallow breathing[d]
    McGuire et al., 1987
protuberant abdomen[d]
    McGuire et al., 1987
shortened femoral length[d]
    McGuire et al., 1987
short, thick limbs[d]
    McGuire et al., 1987
prominent skin folds
    Donnenfeld and Mennuti, 1987
hydrops fetalis
    Hobbins and Mahoney, 1985
decreased fetal movement
    Burrows et al., 1984
hydramnios[d]
    McGuire et al., 1987; Rasmussen et al., 1996

PD 175000 THROMBOCYTOPENIA–ABSENT RADIUS SYNDROME
(TAR syndrome) (McKusick No. 274000)

Fetoscopy[i]: abnormal flexion of the hand
    Filkins and Russo, 1984
Radiograph[i]: absent radii and ulnae
    Luthy et al., 1979; Hobbins et al., 1982
Ultrasound: absent radii and radial deviation of the hands[i]
    Filkins and Russo, 1984
    bilateral symmetric rudimentary upper appendages with no identifiable humeri, radii, or ulnae (phocomelia)[d]
    Donnenfeld et al., 1990
    short or absent femora, short tibia
    Donnenfeld et al., 1990
Cordocentesis (PUBS)[d]: thrombocytopenia, anemia
    Donnenfeld et al., 1990

PD 175250 TRIGONOCEPHALY (McKusick Nos. 190440, 275600)

Condition Note: When the metopic suture closes prematurely, there are resulting lateral narrowness of the forehead, and often, a triangular shape to the skull when viewed from the top. The premature closure of the metopic suture may be part of a syndrome, found in association with other premature synostoses of other sutures, or an isolated finding either present at birth or occurring later in life. If the synostosis occurs prenatally, the closure may have been induced by fetal head constraint. Trigonocephaly may be inherited either as an autosomal dominant or autosomal recessive trait.

Prenatal Diagnosis: Narrowness of the fetal forehead should suggest this condition.

Differential Diagnosis: Autosomal dominant or recessive form of trigonocephaly; Fetal head constraint; Atelencephaly; C-syndrome; Lin–Gettig syndrome; Saethre–Chotzen syndrome; Sakati–Nyhan syndrome; Say–Meyer syndrome; VSR syndrome

> Ultrasound: egg-shaped appearance of the calvarium, narrow forehead
> > Meizner and Bar-Ziv, 1993

PD 175450 VERTEBRAL DEFECT, SINGLE (McKusick No. Unknown; see 277300)

> Ultrasound: abnormal ossification center representing a hemivertebra
> > Benacerraf et al., 1986a
> *Comment:* After birth the neonate was found to have by radiographic examination a single hemivertebra in the upper lumbar spine; no other defects were present.
> > Benacerraf et al., 1986a

PD 175500 VERTEBRAL DEFECTS, MULTIPLE (McKusick No. Unknown; see 277300)

> Ultrasound: absence of lateral processes of vertebral bodies, severe lordosis and kyphosis, missing ribs, no evidence of functional impairment
> > de Elejalde and Elejalde, 1985b
> > multiple irregular vertebral bodies that varied in both size and shape, malalignment of vertebral bodies
> > > Abrams and Filly, 1985
> > *Comments:* After birth the neonate reported by Abrams and Filly (1985) had multiple segmentation anomalies in the lower half of the thoracic spine from T5–T11 including hemivertebrae and butterfly vertebrae. No other defects were present.

THE UROGENITAL SYSTEM[a]

PD 176000 CONGENITAL NEPHROSIS, FINNISH TYPE (Congenital nephrotic syndrome; Finnish type of congenital nephrosis) (McKusick No. 256300)

Condition Note: Idiopathic nephrotic syndrome seldom has its onset before the age of 18 months, whereas congenital nephrosis, Finnish type, has the onset of clinical symptoms during the neonatal period. However, elevated levels of amniotic fluid AFP are normally found during the second trimester of pregnancy, indicating abnormal renal function at that time. Otherwise, the clinical, chemical, and pathologic findings are identical for the two conditions.
> > McKusick, 1994

Prenatal Diagnosis: The diagnosis is made by detecting an elevated level of amniotic fluid AFP, absence of amniotic fluid acetylcholinesterase, and no ultrasound abnormalities in an at-risk fetus (Livingston et al., 1995). Note should be made of fetuses with no family history of nephrosis but in whom the above findings have been reported, but who were completely normal at birth (Livingston et al., 1995).

Acetylcholinesterase activity: elevated in amniotic fluid[c]

Dale, 1980

Alpha-fetoprotein[c]: elevated in maternal serum and amniotic fluid

Seppala et al., 1976; Milunsky et al., 1977; Ryynanen et al., 1978; Ryynanen et al., 1983; Morin et al., 1984b

Amniocentesis: elevated amniotic fluid alkaline phosphatase activity[c]

Jalanko et al., 1983

elevated amniotic fluid trehalase activity and trehalase to palatinase activities ratio[c]

Morin et al., 1984b

decreased levels of amniotic fluid trypsin inhibitor[c]

Kolho, 1986

PD 176200 COWPER GLAND CYST (McKusick No. None)

Condition Note: Cowper glands are periurethal glands that function in the male during sexual activity producing a clear viscid mucoid substance that acts as a lubricant for spermatozoa. Ducts from these glands enter into the bulbar urethra. If one or more of these ducts becomes plugged or do not develop patency, a Cowper's gland cyst will develop. If sufficient in size, the cyst may cause urethral obstruction and retention of urine. Bartholin's glands in the female are analogous to Cowper's glands in the male.

Dhillon et al., 1993

Ultrasound[c]: bilateral hydronephrosis with a full bladder that failed to empty over time, hydroureters, thick-walled bladder, normal amniotic fluid volume

Dhillon et al., 1993

Comments: In the fetus reported by Dhillon and co-workers (1993), the urine retention decreased after 22 weeks of gestation, and by 33 weeks had totally resolved. After birth, the male infant was found to have a ruptured cyst that had drained into the bulbar urethra.

PD 176500 CROSSED RENAL ECTOPIA (McKusick No. None)

Ultrasound[d]: fused kidneys noted, contours of the fused kidneys and separate collecting systems could be discerned on the same side, no kidney in the opposite renal fossa

Greenblatt et al., 1985

PD 176550 DUPLICATED KIDNEY (Duplex kidney; Fetal duplex kidney; Obstructed duplex kidney) (McKusick No. None)

Condition Note: Duplication of the collecting system of the kidney is a common anomaly. Duplication of part or a whole kidney is uncommon. When the latter occurs, there is often concomitant obstruction of the collecting system.

Jeffrey et al., 1984

Prenatal Diagnosis: The condition should be suspected when there is asymmetric hydronephrosis with dilatation of the upper or lower kidney pole which would correspond to the location of the duplicated kidney.

Differential Diagnosis: Fanconi anemia (PD 205000); Ureteropelvic junction obstruction (PD 179500); see also Hydronephrosis in the Index
Ultrasound[d]: asymmetric hydronephrosis
Jeffrey et al., 1984
visualization of two separate collecting systems
Jeffrey et al., 1984

PD 176600 ECTOPIC KIDNEY (Pelvic kidney) (McKusick No. None)

Condition Note: An ectopic kidney is one in other than in its normal location. Although most are asymptomatic both prenatally and postnatally, they are important causes of urinary tract infections and morbidity (Colley and Hooker, 1989).
Prenatal Diagnosis: The condition can be suspected by the detection of a mass in the lower abdomen or pelvis, and no identifiable kidney, or kidneys, in the normal location(s).
Differential Diagnosis: Cross renal ectopia (PD 176500); McKusick–Kaufman syndrome (PD 192080); Radial-renal syndrome (PD 193520); Urethral obstruction malformation sequence (PD 180000); see also Ureteral obstruction and Caliectasis in the Index
Ultrasound[d]: echogenic area located above the bladder on the right side, normally located and appearing left kidney, no visualized right kidney
Colley and Hooker, 1989

PD 176750 EXSTROPHY OF THE BLADDER (Bladder exstrophy) (McKusick No. None)

Ultrasound[d]: Solid mass protruding from the ventral surface of the fetal bladder, no identifiable bladder or bladder filling; a scrotum was readily identified but a penis was not; after birth the neonate was found to have bladder exstrophy and epispadias
Mirk et al., 1986

PD 176850 GLOMERULOSCLEROSIS, DIFFUSE MESANGIAL (Familial mesangial sclerosis; Nephrotic syndrome, early-onset, with diffuse mesangial sclerosis) (McKusick No. 256370; see also 13l7960)

Disease Note: Diffuse mesangial glomerulosclerosis is an autosomal recessive disease characterized by onset of proteinuria, edema, and hematuria during the first month after birth. The full-blown nephrotic syndrome then ensues; the child then will die from renal failure during the first 3 years of life.
Ultrasound[i]: enlarged hyperechogenic kidneys with an uneven surface, slightly dilated renal pelvis
Hofstaetter et al., 1996
Comments: In the fetus reported by Hofstaetler and co-workers (1996), the maternal serum and amniotic fluid AFP levels were normal, as was amniotic fluid alpha-microglobulin levels.

PD 177000 HYDRONEPHROSIS (Cystic dysplasia kidney, Potter type IV) (McKusick No. Unknown; see 143400)

Ultrasound[d]: distention of renal pelvis, ureter, and/or bladder from urethral obstruction
Garrett et al., 1975b; Hobbins et al., 1979; Canty et al., 1981; Harrison et al., 1981; Diament et al., 1983

cystic mass replacing the right kidney; the left kidney was normal with normal bladder filling
Vintzileos et al., 1983

PD 177250 INFUNDIBULOPELVIC STENOSIS–MULTICYSTIC KIDNEY–CALIECTASIS DISORDER (Infundibulopelvic dysgenesis) (McKusick No. 600989)

Disorder Note: In this rare disorder, there is hydrocalycosis of a single or multiple calices that drain through a stenotic infundibula into a hypoplastic or stenosed renal pelvis. These defects may represent a spectrum of kidney problems ranging from cystic renal dysplasia to hydronephrosis. Kobayashi and co-authors (1995) have reported a family with such a spectrum with the condition appearing to be inherited as an autosomal dominant one with variable expression and reduced penetrance.
Kobayashi et al., 1995
Prenatal Diagnosis: The condition should be considered when obstructive renal lesions are found in the fetus with a family history of inherited obstructive renal problems.
Differential Diagnosis: See Caliceltasis, Hydronephrosis and Multicystic kidney disease in the Index.
Ultrasound[c,d]: multiple renal cysts
Kobayashi et al., 1995

PD 177400 MEGACYSTIS, FAMILIAL (Familial congenital megacystis) (McKusick No. None; see 155310)

Condition Note: Tomlinson and associates (1996) have reported sisters who had megacystis as fetuses, and who had tonic, nonfunctional bladders as infants and young children. Both were normal otherwise. Family history was significant in that a male first maternal cousin was born with "prune belly syndrome"; and a maternal great uncle had an enlarged bladder at birth.
Ultrasound[i]: normal bladder size until 21 weeks' gestation when the size progressively increased in the second of the affected fetuses of the parents
Tomlinson et al., 1996

PD 177500 MEGAURETER (Hydroureter; Megalourter; Primary megaureter) (McKusick No. None)

Ultrasound[d]: dilated ureter and renal pelvis with normal renal cortex, caliceal system, and bladder
Deter et al., 1980; Hadlock et al., 1981; Dunn and Glasier, 1985
hydramnios
Dunn and Glasier, 1985

PD 177540 PENOSCROTAL TRANSPOSTIION (McKusick No. None)

Condition Note: Penoscrotal transposition is an early development defect usually of unknown etiology that is characterized by posterior location of the penis on the perineum with the scrotum being completely or partially anterior to the penis. Renal abnormalities in the disorder are common, and vary from malpositioning to bilateral renal agenesis. Other associated defects include hypospadias, other genital and urinary anomalies, and abnormalities of the skeletal, gastrointestinal, and cardiac systems. The condition is occasionally inherited.
MacKenzie et al., 1994

Prenatal Diagnosis: None has been estalished.
Differential Diagnosis: Aarskog syndrome; Aarskog–Scott syndrome; Agenesis of the penis; Congenital adrenal hyperplasia, 11-beta-hydroxylase deficiency type (PD 240950); Congenital adrenal deficiency type, 21-hydroxylase deficiency type (PD 241000); Urorectal septum malformation sequence (PD 181000); VATER association (PD 194650)

> Ultrasound[c]: cystic dysplastic kidney, hydronephrosis, progressive oligohydramnios
> > MacKenzie et al., 1994

PD 177580 PERIRENAL URINIFEROUS PSEUDOCYST (Perinephric urinoma) (McKusick No. None)

Condition Note: Perirenal uriniferous pseudocyst is the extravasation of urine around a kidney, giving the appearance of a cyst. The extravasation of the urine in most cases is probably related to collection of urine in the paranephric space as a result of caliceal rupture, a secondary result of urinary tract obstruction that has caused high intracaliceal pressure. The urinary obstruction may be the result of a number of different problems.
> > Avni et al., 1987b
Prenatal Diagnosis: The condition should be suspected whenever there is fluid collection around a kidney. Differentiating paranephrotic urine collected from cysts of the kidney may be difficult, however.
Differential Diagnosis: Hydronephrosis (PD 177000); Polycystic kidney diseases (PD 177750, PD 178000, PD 178500, PD 178800); Ureteropelvic junction obstruction, bilateral (PD 179500); Ureterovesical junction obstruction (PD 179750); Urethral obstruction malformation sequence (PD 180000)

> Ultrasound: cystic mass attached to the kidney, cystic fluid collection around a markedly dilated fetal kidney
> > Avni et al., 1987b

PD 177620 PERSISTENT CLOACA (McKusick No. None)

> Alpha-fetoprotein[c]: elevated in maternal serum and amniotic fluid
> > Holzgreve, 1985
> Physical examination[c]: at 24 weeks' gestation the fundal height was equivalent to 32 weeks'
> > Holzgreve, 1985
> Ultrasound[c]: no caput detected, spina bifida extending into the thoracic vertebrae, intraabdominal cystic structures, oligohydramnios
> > Holzgreve, 1985
> *Comments*: At delivery, the fetus reported on by Holzgreve (1985) had anencephaly with craniorachischisis, upper-limb defects with absence of right thumb and radius, congenital heart defect, persistent cloaca with anal and urethral atresia, distended abdomen, right hydronephrosis, and left renal agenesis. The external genitalia were apparently normal male except than for undescended testes.

PD 177750 POLYCYSTIC KIDNEY DISEASE, AUTOSOMAL DOMINANT
(Polycystic kidney disease, Potter type III) (McKusick No. 173900)

Disease Note: The autosomal dominant form of polycystic kidney disease is one of the more common dominant conditions in humans with a frequency of 1 per

500 autopsied cases. Although the usual onset of symptoms of renal failure occurs in the third and fourth decades, renal cysts and enlargement of the kidney have been seen in the fetus.

Because of its frequency and its chronic nature, autosomal dominant polycystic kidney disease accounts for approximately 10% of the total requirement for chronic renal replacement therapy. Despite the importance of this one genetic disorder, nothing yet is known about its pathogenesis. It is now known that the gene for this condition (PKD1) is on the short arm of chromosome 16 (16p13.1-p13.3). The gene has been sequenced, and the predicted PKD1 protein, called polycystin, is a glycoprotein with multiple transmembrane domains and a cytoplasmic C-tail. Polycystin is thought to be involved in cell–cell/matrix interactions (McKusick, 1997).

The most significant additional abnormalities found in this disorder are cysts of other organs, particularly the liver. As a consequence, any individual with this disorder should have a careful evaluation of his or her other organs.

Reeders et al., 1986; Romero et al., 1988, pp. 268–270

Prenatal Diagnosis: Diagnosis may be established by detection of an enlarged kidney containing multiple cysts in a fetus at risk. The earliest diagnosis of this disorder has been at 14 weeks of gestation, but the condition may not be detected during gestation or it may develop any time after 14 weeks. The condition also may be detected by DNA linkage studies in informative families.

Reeders et al., 1986; Romero et al., 1988, p. 269

Differential Diagnosis: Meckel syndrome (PD 192140); Tuberous sclerosis (PD 271600); and Von Hippel–Lindau may have similar renal findings. Other forms of Polycystic kidney diseases (PD 178000, PD 178500, PD 178800) need to be considered when multiple cysts of the kidney are detected prenatally.

Chorionic villus sampling[g,i]: genetic linkage analysis on chorionic villi using appropriate DNA markers

Reeders et al., 1986; Ceccherini et al., 1989; Novelli et al., 1989; Waldherr et al., 1989; Melki et al., 1992; Michaud et al., 1993

Comments: At autopsy each of the kidneys of the three affected fetuses reported by Waldherr and associates (1989) showed numerous glomerular and tubular microcysts with diameters up to 300 μm. The tubular microcysts were noted to be lined by an increased number of tubular epithelial cells. Gestational ages of these fetuses were 12, 14, and 16 weeks, respectively.

Ultrasound: lung hypoplasia[c]

Ceccherini et al., 1989

enlarged fetal kidneys with centrally located cystic structure or increased echogenicity

Zerres et al., 1982; Zerres et al., 1984; Zerres et al., 1985

enlarged fetal kidneys with multiple cysts[i]

Main et al., 1983; Romero et al., 1988; Ceccherini et al., 1989; Gal et al., 1989

bilateral microcystic kidneys

Turco et al., 1993

enlarged kidneys without cysts[c]

Zerres et al., 1985

enlarged kidneys with increased echogenicity

Ceccherini et al., 1989; Gal et al., 1989

ascites[c]
> Zerres et al., 1982; Zerres et al., 1984

enlarged abdomen
> Ceccherini et al., 1989

hydrops fetalis[c]
> Zerres et al., 1985

oligohydramnios[c]
> Ceccherini et al., 1989; Gal et al., 1989

PD 178000 POLYCYSTIC KIDNEY DISEASE, AUTOSOMAL RECESSIVE
(ARPKD; Caroli disease; Congenital polycystic kidney disease; Cystic kidney, type I; Infantile polycystic kidney disease; Juvenile polycystic kidney disease; Multicystic kidney disease, Potter type I; Neonatal polycystic kidney disease; Renal–hepatic–pancreatic dysplasia) (McKusick No. 263200)

Disease Note: There are a number of causes of cystic disease of the kidney, some of which are inherited and primary to the kidney; others are secondary to obstructive uropathies. The etiology in many other cases is unknown.

Renal involvement in this category of polycystic kidney disease is usually bilateral and largely symmetrical with enlargement of both kidneys. On cut section of the kidney, diverticular, saccular, and cystic ectasia of the collecting system is seen. Invariably, this condition is associated with generalized and interlobular fibrosis of the liver.

The age of detection or onset of symptoms vary from the prenatal time to the adolescent period. The variation in onset is based on the proportion of dilated renal tubules present at the time of detection. In the congenital or perinatal type, 90% or more of the tubules are involved; in the neonatal type, about 60%; in the infantile group, about 25%; and in the juvenile type, less than 10%. The worst prognosis is in the congenital type, while the best is in the juvenile category. When oligohydramnios is present, the prognosis is usually poor.
> Zerres et al., 1988

Prenatal Diagnosis: The finding of enlarged kidneys, increased kidney circumference-to-abdominal circumference, increased echogenicity of the renal parenchyma or multiple abdominal cysts in a fetus at risk is highly suggestive of the diagnosis. Oligohydramnios is a variable finding in this condition. Kidney size may be normal in the second trimester but increased in the third (Zerres et al., 1988). In fetuses at risk, therefore, serial ultrasound studies are recommended. Enlargement of the kidney in fetuses with no family history of this disease cannot be assumed to be polycystic kidney disease and to have a poor prognosis (Case 5, Zerres et al., 1988). For an extensive review of the literature on the prenatal diagnosis of autosomal recessive polycystic kidney, the reader should consult the article by Zerres and associates (1988).

Differential Diagnosis: Hydronephrosis (PD 177000); Meckel syndrome (PD 192140); Polycystic kidney disease, autosomal dominant (PD 177750); Polycystic kidney disease, sporadic type (PD 178500); Sirenomelia (PD 194130); Triploidy (PD 102000); VATER association (PD 194650)

Alpha-fetoprotein[c]: elevated in maternal serum
> Koontz et al., 1983

Amniocentesis: elevated trehalase activity in amniotic fluid[c]
> Morin et al., 1981

Ultrasound[i]: increased kidney circumference to abdominal circumference (KC/AC ratio), multiple fluid-filled spaces in the abdomen, increased echogenicity of renal parenchyma, poor delineation of renal margin from surrounding tissues, poor caliceal definition, no bladder seen, oligohydramnios

> Bartley et al., 1977; Hobbins et al., 1979; Henderson et al., 1980; Hadlock 1981; Harrison et al., 1981; Koontz et al., 1983; Gruenewald et al., 1984; Zerres et al., 1984; Luthy and Hirsch, 1985; Spirt et al., 1987

increased echogenicity of renal parenchyma[d]

> Zerres et al., 1988

increase in kidney length[d]

> Zerres et al., 1988

enlarged kidneys that occupy most of the abdomen

> Hill et al., 1988b

cranial displacement of the diaphragm by enlarged kidneys

> Hill et al., 1988b

hydramnios[c]

> Henderson et al., 1980

oligohydramnios[c]

> Gembruch and Hansmann, 1988; Zerres et al., 1988; Hill et al., 1988b

PD 178500 POLYCYSTIC KIDNEY DISEASE, POTTER TYPE IIA

(Multicystic dysplastic kidney disease; Multicystic renal disease; Multicystic kidney disease, Potter type IIA) (McKusick No. None)

Prenatal Diagnosis: The diagnosis of polycystic kidneys normally can be made by ultrasonic visualization of large renal cysts after 21 weeks of gestation. Usually the volume of amniotic fluid is normal, but it may be decreased or increased. When hydramnios is present, other abnormalities that have led to the accumulation of the amniotic fluid are often present. Whenever polycystic kidneys and/or hydramnios are present, other fetal anomalies should be sought. If detected, a fetal chromosomal analysis should be considered.

> Rizzo et al., 1987b

Ultrasound: enlarged kidneys with one or multiple cysts of varying size within the kidney, little hyperechogenic tissue between the cysts, hydronephrosis, oligohydramnios

> Hadlock et al., 1981; Hill et al., 1983a; Zerres et al., 1984; Rizzo et al., 1987b; Spirt et al., 1987

oligohydramnios[c]

> Gembruch and Hansmann, 1988

PD 178600 POLYCYSTIC KIDNEY DISEASE, POTTER TYPE IIB

(Multicystic kidney disease, Potter type IIB) (McKusick No. None)

Ultrasound: No detectible kidneys, oligohydramnios

> Murphy et al., 1989

PD 178800 POLYCYSTIC KIDNEY DISEASE, UNILATERAL (Multicystic kidney disease, unilateral) (McKusick No. None)

Condition Note: Unilateral polycystic kidney disease is probably the result of multiple etiologies, but usually is sporadic in occurrence. The cysts seen in this condition tend to reach a maximum size sometime during the third trimester and then start to involute. In some cases, the kidney has completely disappeared or has involuted to a small echogenic mass. By birth most affected kidneys are nonfunctional.

Differential Diagnosis: Beckwith–Wiedemann syndrome (PD 187000); Hydronephrosis (PD 177000); Meckel syndrome (PD 192140); Polycystic kidney disease, autosomal dominant (PD 177750); Polycystic kidney disease, autosomal recessive (PD 178000); Roberts syndrome (PD 193570); Sirenomelia (PD 194130); Triploidy (PD 102000)

> Ultrasound[d]: multiple renal cysts of different sizes, septated cystic mass in kidney area, unilateral enlarged kidney or flank mass, hydramnios
>> Canty et al., 1981; Harrison et al., 1981; Gustavii and Edvall, 1984; Filion et al., 1985; Spirt et al., 1987
> unilateral multicystic and/or dysplastic kidney
>> Avni et al., 1987a; Nicolini et al., 1989b
> oligohydramnios[c]
>> Nicolini et al., 1989b

PD 179000 POTTER SEQUENCE (Bilateral renal agenesis, sporadic)
(McKusick No. Unknown; see 191830)

Condition Note: Potter sequence consists of bilateral renal agenesis, oligohydramnios, Potter facies, mild arthrogryposis, and hypoplastic lungs. Death usually occurs from the lung hypoplasia. Most cases of bilateral renal agenesis are sporadic and appear not to be genetically determined. In sporadic cases, the parents need to have an ultrasound evaluation of their kidneys to determine unilateral renal agenesis or cystic changes indicating the presence of autosomal dominant renal adysplasia (PD 179250), or other dominantly inherited disorders in the family.

Differential Diagnosis: See Renal agenesis in the Index for other conditions associated with renal agenesis.

Acetylcholinesterase[c]: rapidly migrating amniotic fluid isozyme
> Wald and Cuckle, 1981
Alpha-fetoprotein[c]: elevated in maternal serum
> Balfour and Laurence, 1980
> low levels (5–9 ng/mL) in maternal serum
>> Haddow et al., 1987
Fetal pyelography
> Miskin, 1979
Ultrasound: absent kidneys and bladder, oligohydramnios, intrauterine growth deficiency
> Kaffe et al., 1977a; Keirse and Meerman, 1978; Dubbins et al., 1981; Harrison et al., 1981; Schmidt et al., 1982b; Schmidt and Kubli, 1982; Helin et al., 1983; Hill et al., 1983a; Abramson et al., 1985; Nicolaides et al., 1986a; Spirt et al., 1987
> no kidneys visualized
>> Curry et al., 1984
> demonstration of bilateral renal agenesis after fetal intraperitoneal infusion of saline
>> Nicolini et al., 1989b

no fluid in the gastrointestinal tract
  Spirt et al., 1987
no filling of the urinary bladder after instillation of artificial amniotic
fluid into the amniotic cavity
  Gembruch and Hansmann, 1988
oligohydramnios[c]
  Curry et al., 1984; Gembruch and Hansmann, 1988; Murphy et
  al., 1989; Nicolini et al., 1989b
lack of response to fetal intravascular injection of furosemide
  Nicolaides et al., 1986a

PD 179200 PRUNE BELLY PHENOTYPE, FAMILIAL (Abdominal muscles, absence of, with urinary tract abnormality and cryptorchidism) (McKusick No. 100100)

Syndrome Note: Usually, prune belly syndrome (urethral obstruction malformation sequence [PD 180000]) is sporadic, and is the result of obstruction or partial obstruction of the urethra with retention of urine. Retention of the urine causes distention of the bladder, renal pelvis, and abdomen. Aylsworth and associates (1991), and others (McKusick, 1996) have reported familial occurrence of the prune belly phenotype where the urethras in the affected individuals were normal.
  Ultrasound: distended bladder, hydronephrosis
      Aylsworth et al., 1991
  Comments: In the family reported by Aylsworth and associates (1991), two sons were born with a flaccid abdomen, bilateral hydronephrosis with ureteral reflux, undescended testis(es), enlarged bladder, no spontaneous voiding, and normal urethra. Their mother at her birth had similar problems.

PD 179250 RENAL ADYSPLASIA (Hereditary renal adysplasia; Urogenital adysplasia) (McKusick No. 191830)

  Ultrasound[i]: no identifiable fetal kidneys or bladder, oligohydramnios
      Swinford et al., 1985

PD 179380 RENAL AGENESIS, BILATERAL, AUTOSOMAL RECESSIVE (McKusick No. Unknown; see 191830)

Condition Note: Bilateral renal agenesis is usually sporadic, that is, not inherited, or may represent a case of renal adysplasia (PD 179250), an autosomal dominant disorder. However, occasionally a family is encountered in which there is a recurrence of nonsyndromic bilateral renal agenesis in siblings, in which there is no other family history of the condition, and in which the parents and other relatives have no detectable renal defects. Autosomal recessive inheritance is likely in these situations.
Prenatal Diagnosis: No detectable kidneys, no filling of the bladder, and severe oligohydramnios in a fetus with a previously affected sib.
  Ultrasound[i]: no detectable kidneys or bladder, IUGR, oligohydramnios, disk-shaped adrenal glands
      Morse et al., 1987b

PD 179450 RENAL TUBULAR DYSGENESIS (Primitive renal tubule syndrome; Renotubular dysgenesis) (McKusick No. 267430)

Condition Note: Renal tubular dysgenesis is characterized by short and poorly formed proximal convoluted tubules, and results in oligohydramnios, Potter phenotype, lung hypoplasia, and death from neonatal respiratory failure. The condition is most likely inherited as an autosomal recessive disorder.

Prenatal Diagnosis: The diagnosis is most likely present if there is oligohydramnios in a fetus at risk. However, oligohydramnios may not be present until after 23 weeks of gestation (Swinford et al., 1989).

Differential Diagnosis: Bilateral renal agenesis seen in Potter sequence (PD 179000); Renal agenesis, bilateral, autosomal recessive (PD 179380); and Renal adysplasia (PD 179250), may be difficult to differentiate from Renal tubular dysgenesis prenatally because oligohydramnios may be present in all four conditions. The late onset of oligohydramnios and visualization of normal-sized kidneys in the fetus with Renal tubular dysgenesis helps with the differentiation. Chronic amniotic fluid leakage (Fetal membranes, premature rupture [PD 264100]) should be ruled out by checking for amniotic fluid in the vagina. Other causes of oligohydramnios should be considered (see Oligohydramnios in the Index).

Ultrasound[i] oligohydramnios, no visualization of the urinary bladder, increased echogenicity of normal sized kidneys
Swinford et al., 1989
Comments: In the two fetuses reported by Swinford and associates (1989), the first had oligohydramnios at 26 weeks of gestation, the first time that ultrasound evaluation was performed in that pregnancy. There were normal amniotic fluid volumes at 16 and 20 weeks of gestation, low-normal volumes at 23 weeks, and oligohydramnios shortly before delivery at 35 weeks in the next pregnancy of the same mother.

PD 179500 URETEROPELVIC JUNCTION OBSTRUCTION, BILATERAL (Pelvic–ureteric junction obstruction; UPJ obstruction) (McKusick No. None)

Condition Note: The condition is the result of partial or complete obstruction of the ureter at the junction of the renal pelvis and the ureter; thus, the name of the condition. In severe cases, progressive and massive hydronephrosis results, and if the pregnancy is continued to term or near term, irreversible renal damage invariably develops that subsequently may lead to the death of the child. Milder cases may not result in such damage, and the obstruction may then be relieved by pyeloplasty during infancy. The prognosis in these cases is frequently good.

Prenatal Diagnosis: The diagnosis should be considered when bilateral dilatation of the renal pelvis (calicectasis) with or without hydronephrosis in the presence of normal-sized ureters and bladder is detected. The diagnosis has been made as early as the 21st week of gestation.
Reuss et al., 1988

Differential Diagnosis: Infundibulopelvic stenosis–multicystic kidney–caliectasis disorder (PD 177250); Unilateral ureteropelvic junction obstruction; Ureterovesical junction obstruction (PD 179750); Urethral obstruction malformation sequence (PD 180000); Urorectal septum malformation sequence (PD 181000); Vesticoureteral reflex (PD 181500)

Maternal intravenous infusion of furosemide[c]: no change in the appearance of the bilateral hydronephrotic fetal kidneys
Callen et al., 1983

Ultrasound: large sonolucent mass in the region of the kidney, dilation of the pelvicaliceal system[d]

>Canty et al., 1981; Hadlock et al., 1981; Campbell and Pearce, 1983; Hill et al., 1983a; Gruenewald et al., 1984; Hobbins et al., 1984; Mandell et al., 1984; Hill et al., 1988b

pleural effusion[c,d]

>Callen et al., 1983
>
>*Comments:* In addition to ureteropelvic junction obstruction, one of the fetuses reported by Callen and co-workers (1983) had a left diaphragmatic hernia and bilateral perirenal pseudocyst (urinoma). These defects were not diagnosed prenatally.

hydronephrosis[c,d]

>Callen et al., 1983; Spirt et al., 1987; Reuss et al., 1988
>
>*Comments:* In the three cases reported by Callen and associates (1983) in addition to having ureteropelvic junction obstruction, each also had a perirenal pseudocyst (also known as paranephric pseudocyst or urinoma) diagnosed postnatally at the time of surgery or autopsy.

multicystic renal dysplasia

>Fryns et al., 1993
>
>*Comments:* In the fetus reported by Fryns and colleagues (1993), there was an apparent balanced, de novo translocation between chromosome 6 and 9 {46,XX,t(6;19)(p23.1;q13.4)}.

hydramnios

>Callen et al., 1983; Reuss et al., 1988
>
>*Comments:* Amniotic fluid volume may be normal, increased (Reuss et al., 1988), or decreased (Callen et al., 1983) in this condition. Decreased amniotic fluid probably is associated with bilateral involvement in most cases.

oligohydramnios[c]

>Callen et al., 1983; Fryns et al., 1993

PD 179750 URETEROVESICAL JUNCTION OBSTRUCTION (McKusick No. None)

>Ultrasound: hydroureter(s) with or without hydronephrosis, cystic dysplastic kidneys, inability to visualize bladder, oligohydramnios, hydramnios
>>Hobbins et al., 1984

PD 180000 URETHRAL OBSTRUCTION MALFORMATION SEQUENCE
(Bladder neck obstruction; Eagle–Barrett syndrome; Posterior urethral valves with obstruction; Prune belly syndrome; Triad syndrome) (McKusick No. 100100)

Sequence Note: When there is obstruction of the urethra prenatally (usually in males and usually from posterior urethral valves), there is build up of urine, distention of the bladder and abdomen, and if the obstruction is long standing, hydronephrosis and hydroureters. If the urethral obstruction is complete, oligohydramnios will be present; if partial obstruction, the amniotic fluid volume may be normal. Cystic changes in the kidneys and destruction of the kidneys with little or no renal function may also develop. Distention of the abdomen by seepage of urine through the distended bladder leads to hypoplasia of the abdominal musculature, stretching of the abdominal skin, and elevation of the diaphragm. The latter developments may contribute to the development of hypoplasia of the lungs. Death after birth is common, and is normally secondary to the lung hypoplasia.

Acetylcholinesterase[c]: fast-migrating amniotic fluid isozyme
>Nevin et al., 1983b

>*Comments*: The fetus reported by Nevin and associates (1983b) also had distention of the bladder, abdomen, and ureters, and hydronephrosis; diagnosis of trisomy 18 was made. After termination and an autopsy, the fetus was found to have double-outlet right ventricle with an overriding aorta, ventricular septal defect, and hypoplastic left atrium and ventricle. There was no neural tube defect present.

Alpha-fetoprotein[c]: elevated in amniotic fluid
>>Vinson et al., 1977; Nevin et al., 1978; Pescia et al., 1982; Read et al., 1982a; Nevin et al., 1983b; Curry et al., 1984

>elevated in maternal serum
>>Pescia et al., 1982; Koontz et al., 1983; Curry et al., 1984

Fetal bladder puncture (cystocentesis)[c]: fetal urine sodium greater than 100 mEq/L, chloride greater than 790 mEq/L, osmolality greater than 210 mosm/kg water[c]
>>Reuss et al., 1987b; Cullen et al., 1989

>amino acid concentration of urine greater than in the urine of normal newborns and similar to those found in the umbilical venous blood at birth[c]
>>Lenz et al., 1985

>increased vesicular pressure when compared to intraamniotic pressure
>>Cullen et al., 1989

Radiograph: fetal ascites, bladder injected with radiodense material showed megalocystis
>>Cooperberg et al., 1979

Ultrasound: distended bladder and urachus (urachal cysts), oligohydramnios, hydramnios,[h] hydroureter, hydronephrosis, cystic dysplastic kidneys (Potter type IV); ascites, pleural cavity effusion,[h] laxity of anterior abdominal wall[h]; dilated ureters that form loops, distended abdomen
>>Okulski, 1977; Hobbins et al., 1979; Bovicelli et al., 1980; Katz et al., 1980; Heller et al., 1981; Smythe, 1981; Berkowitz et al., 1982; Christopher et al., 1982; Gadziala et al., 1982; Pescia et al., 1982; Farrant, 1983; Hill et al., 1983a; Koontz et al., 1983; Nevin et al., 1983b; Shalev et al., 1983c; Gruenewald et al., 1984; Hobbins et al., 1984; Shalev et al., 1984; Zerres et al., 1984; Lenz et al., 1985; Mahony et al., 1985b; Wladimiroff et al., 1985a; Meizner et al., 1986; Spirt et al., 1987

>hydrops fetalis,[d] dilated umbilical vein,[d] hydropericardium[d]
>>Lenz et al., 1985

>distended bladder (megalocystis)
>>Callen et al., 1983; Curry et al., 1984; Reuss et al., 1987b; Gembruch and Hansmann, 1988; Hill et al., 1988b; Cullen et al., 1989; MacMahon et al., 1995

>dystrophic bladder wall, peritoneal calcification
>>Mahony et al., 1985b

hydroureter
> Callen et al., 1983; Curry et al., 1984; Reuss et al., 1987b; Hill et al., 1988b; Cullen et al., 1989; MacMahon et al., 1995

hydronephrosis
> Callen et al., 1983; Curry et al., 1984; Hill et al., 1988b; Cullen et al., 1989; MacMahon et al., 1995

multicystic renal dysplasia
> Fryns et al., 1992; MacMahon et al., 1995

echogenic to cystic appearance of kidneys
> Reuss et al., 1987b; Cullen et al., 1989; MacMahon et al., 1995

dilatation of the penile urethra
> Cullen et al., 1989

oligohydramnios[c]
> Callen et al., 1983; Curry et al., 1984; Cullen et al., 1989; MacMahon et al., 1995

PD 180500 URETHRAL OBSTRUCTION WITH HYDRONEPHNOSIS AND HYDROURETERS (McKusick No. 143400)

Condition Note: McCormack and associates (1981) reported a fetus with bilateral hydronephrosis, hydroureters, distended bladder, and urethral obstruction. The urethral obstruction must have been partial because neither a distended abdomen nor oligohydramnios was reported in the fetus. The father had a history of bilateral hydronephrosis with contracture of the bladder neck and narrowing of the prostatic urethra. Possible autosomal dominant inheritance was suggested by the authors.

Prenatal Diagnosis: Hydronephosis, hydroureters, bladder distention, and narrowing or obstruction of the urethra in an at-risk fetus would be suggestive of the diagnosis.

Differential Diagnosis: Hydronephrosis (PD 177000); Megaureter (PD 177500); Ureteropelvic junction obstruction, bilateral (PD 179500); Ureterovesical junction obstruction (PD 179750); Urethral obstruction malformation sequence (PD 180000)

> Ultrasound[c,d]: dilated urinary bladder with bilateral hydronephrosis, fetal demise with edema of the fetal scalp and abdomen
> > McCormack et al., 1981

PD 181000 URORECTAL SEPTUM MALFORMATION SEQUENCE
(Persistent cloaca) (McKusick No. None)

Sequence Note: This sequence consists of ambiguous genitalia with a phallus-like structure, no perineal openings (no urethral or vaginal openings and an imperforate anus), persistent cloaca with or without distended abdomen, and variable abnormalities of the vagina, uterus, and fallopian tubes. The condition has been reported in both males and females. No recurrence in families has been cited to date.
> Escobar et al., 1987

Amniocentesis[c,d]: cytology of aspirated cloacal fluid revealed squamous cells rather than the expected transitional cells of the normal bladder.
> Lande and Hamilton, 1986

Ultrasound[c]: small, funnel-shaped chest
> Murray et al., 1995

large omphalocele involving the liver and associated with a 90 degree lordosis
>Murray et al., 1995

hydronephrosis
>Lande and Hamilton, 1986; Murray et al., 1995

hydroureters
>Murray et al., 1995

septated cystic structure in the pelvis
>Lande and Hamilton, 1986

no detectable bladder
>Lande and Hamilton, 1986

clubbed feet
>Murray et al., 1995

oligohydramnios
>Lande and Hamilton, 1986; Harris et al., 1987; Hall, 1992; Murray et al., 1995

>*Comments*: At birth the infant reported by Lande and Hamilton (1986) was found to have persistence of the cloaca with imperforate anus, ambiguous genitalia, and apparent urethral atresia. At autopsy, the fetus reported by Murray and co-workers (1995), in addition to the above cited findings, had imperforate anus, a cloaca with the bowel and ureter emptying into this structure, ambiguous external genitalia, and a single umbilical artery. A chromosomal analysis show 46,XY.

PD 181500 VESICOURETERAL REFLUX (McKusick No. Unknown; see 193000, 314550)

Ultrasound[c,d]: hydronephrosis
>Reuter and Lebowitz, 1985; Spirt et al., 1987

dilated calyces
>Reuter and Lebowitz, 1985

no significant change in bladder size or shape over 8 hours
>Reuter and Lebowitz, 1985

OTHER MALFORMATIONS, DEFORMATIONS, DISRUPTIONS, AND RELATED DISORDERS[a]

PD 182000 ACARDIA (Acardius; Acephalus; Chorioangiopagus parasiticus; Holoacardium amorphous twin; TRAP sequence; Twin reversed arterial perfusion sequence) (McKusick No. None)

Condition Note: Acardia ranks high among the most dramatic congenital defects in humans. Although there is wide variation in the presentation of the condition, it is characterized by rudimentary development of the heart in the acardiac twin, arterial-to-arterial anastomosis between the umbilical arteries of the normal and the acardiac twin, reversed arterial perfusion to the acardiac twin, and a wide range of dysmorphic/amorphic development in the acardiac twin. Because the acardiac twin is totally dependent on the normal twin for its blood supply, the condition is always lethal in the acardiac twin, who is stillborn or dies immediately after delivery. It is not known at this time if there is some type of underlying disorder in the acardiac twin that produces the maldevelopment in that twin with the reversed arterial perfusion being a secondary phenomenon, or if the reversed umbilical arterial blood flow results in the arrest of the development of the acardiac twin. In some but not all acardiac twins, chromosomal abnormalities have been reported with normal chromosomal constitutions in the co-twins.

In contrast to recipient twins, the pump twins are usually morphologically normal. Nevertheless, there is an associated mortality rate of 50% in these twins as a result of in utero congestive heart failure and/or prematurity.

Robie et al., 1989

Prenatal Diagnosis: The disorder should be considered in twins or triplets whenever one fetus is amorphic/dysmorphic and hydropic, and has no detectable heart beat. Features of the acardiac twin in utero have been described as grotesque by some authors (Meizner and Bar-Ziv, 1993).

Differential Diagnosis: Conjoined twins (PD 255000); Twin transfusion syndrome (PD 135500)

Prenatal Treatment: Because of the high perinatal mortality rate of the normal twin in this condition, prenatal diagnosis is important; treatment of the condition has been effective. Four basic options are available, including continuation of the pregnancy with monitoring of the normal twin, termination of the pregnancy, selective delivery of the abnormal fetus by hysterotomy (sectio parva), and clamping, clipping, or ligation of the umbilical cord of the recipient twin. Four cases of sectio parva have been reported (Robie et al., 1989). The selection of the most appropriate option will need to be made by the parents and the medical team involved with the case.

Treatment Modalities: Selective delivery of the abnormal fetus by hysterotomy (sectio parva)

Robie et al., 1989

Methods and Findings: Acetylcholinesterase[c]: rapidly migrating amniotic fluid isozyme

Aitken et al., 1984a

Alpha-fetoprotein[c]: elevated in amniotic fluid

Harger et al., 1981; Aitken et al., 1984a; Thom et al., 1984
elevated in maternal serum

Harger et al., 1981; Thom et al., 1984; Robie et al., 1989
elevated in amniotic fluid with no fast-migrating acetylcholinesterase isozyme present in the amniotic fluid

Read et al., 1982c

Comment: A normal infant and a holoacardius amorphus twin were delivered at term.

elevated in maternal serum but not in amniotic fluid

Robie et al., 1989

Amniography[c]: single sac around the twins

Robie et al., 1989

Doppler analysis[g]: reversal of expected circulation pattern, that is, an arterial waver form was present in the vessel that brought blood toward the acardiac fetus

Martinez-Roman et al., 1995

Echocardiography: single ventricle heart in acardiac twin, cardiomegaly in the other twin

Gewolb et al., 1983

Transvaginal ultrasound[g]: in the second twin, absent heartbeat; no cranium, cervical spine, heart or thoracic organs; single umbilical artery

Martinez-Roman et al., 1995

Comment: The evaluation of the twin pregnancy by Martinez-Roman and co-workers (1995) was done at 10 weeks of gestation.

Ultrasound: absent head, no fetal movement or heartbeat, hydramnios, size/date discrepancy between twins, one twin with the appearance of being dead

Deacon et al., 1980; Thom et al., 1984

multiple pulsatile cystic structures in one twin who had poorly defined cranium, ribs, and limbs; edema of the placenta; dilated umbilical veins; and hydramnios.

Gewolb et al., 1983

Comments: The co-twin reported by Gewolb and co-workers (1983) had cardiomegaly and dilated umbilical veins. The twins at delivery were found to be dichorionic–diamnionic.

an amorphous mass with no discernible or rudimentary head, cardiac structure, and/or extremities, and a normal cotwin

Platt et al., 1983; Robie et al., 1989

remnant of the base of the skull

Meizner and Bar-Ziv, 1993

relatively well formed but short spine and ribs

Meizner and Bar-Ziv, 1993

missing leg

Meizner and Bar-Ziv, 1993

hydrops fetalis[c]

Curry et al., 1983; Gewolb et al., 1983; Payne and Robie, 1988; Robie et al., 1989

single placenta[c]

Platt et al., 1983

hydramnios[c]

Gewolb et al., 1983; Platt et al., 1983; Grange et al., 1987; Payne and Robie, 1988; Robie et al., 1989

PD 182500 ACROCALLOSAL SYNDROME (Schinzel acrocallosal syndrome) (McKusick No. 200990)

Syndrome Note: The acrocallosal syndrome is an autosomal recessive–multiple congenital anomalies–mental retardation syndrome characterized by macrocephaly, agenesis of the corpus callosum, cleft lip, cleft palate, pre- and postaxial polydactyly, mental retardation, seizures, and other neurologic problems.

Guion-Almeida and Richieri-Costa, 1992; McKusick, 1996

Ultrasound[c]: cleft lip, cleft palate, cystic hygroma

Guion-Almeida and Richieri-Costa, 1992

PD 182600 ADAMS–OLIVER SYNDROME (Absence defect of limbs, scalp, and skull) (McKusick No. 100300)

Syndrome Note: The delineating features of the Adams–Oliver syndrome include cutis aplasia of the scalp and terminal transverse limb deficiency of both the upper and lower extremities. Occasionally there are other defects including, most noticeably, congenital heart defects. The condition is inherited in an autosomal dominant fashion.

Bamforth et al., 1994; McKusick, 1996

Ultrasound[c]: two-vessel umbilical cord, IUGR, oligohydramnios
Bamforth et al., 1994

PD 183000 AGNATHIA–MICROSTOMIA–SYNOTIA SYNDROME

(Agnathia–holoprosencephaly; Astomia–agnathia–holoprosencephaly syndrome; Otocephaly) (McKusick No. Unknown; see 202650)

Syndrome Note: Agnathia–microstomia–synotia syndrome is a rare malformation syndrome characterized by extreme hypoplasia or absence of the mandible, microstomia, aglossia, and synotia. Holoprosencephaly may or may not be present. Associated findings include situs inversus totalis, renal defects, and multiple vertebral and rib abnormalities. The term synotia comes from the fact that the ears are usually partly fused in the anterior midfacial/neck region. The condition is thought to result from failure of development of the mandible, the etiology of which is unknown. The condition is lethal in the neonatal period.
Romero et al., 1988, pp. 110–112; Hersh et al., 1989

Prenatal Diagnosis: The condition should be considered when one is not able to visualize the mandible ultrasonographically, and when the ears are in an unusually low position. On the other hand, the jaw should be evaluated whenever holoprosencephaly, renal defects, or hydramnios are detected prenatally.
Romero et al., 1988, pp. 111–112

Differential Diagnosis: Esophageal atresia (PD 135000); Nager acrofacial dysostosis; RAG syndrome (PD 193540); Robin sequence (PD 193600); Treacher Collins syndrome (PD 194500)

Radiograph[d]: agnathia, hydramnios
Ursell, 1972; Scholl, 1977

Ultrasound[c,d]: poorly defined fetal cranium, no identifiable orbits or other facial structures, ears present in the midline of the midfacial region, protruding brain tissue in the forehead region
Ursell, 1972; Cayea et al., 1985

appendage arising from the forehead and superiorly located to the orbits
Romero et al., 1988 p. 111

Comments: In the above fetuses reported by Romero and associates (1988) and Rolland and co-workers (1991), holoprosencephaly in the form of cyclopia was also present and accounted for the placement of the nasal appendage.

cerebral ventricular abnormalities
Rolland et al., 1991

severe hypotelorism with eye balls almost contiguous
Rolland et al., 1991

well-defined ear located in the low face region
Rolland et al., 1991

absence of the chin
Rolland et al., 1991

unilateral cystic kidney
Hersh et al., 1989

intrauterine growth retardation
Rolland et al., 1991

hydramnios
Ursell, 1972; Cayea et al., 1985; Leech et al., 1988; Hersh and McChane, 1989; Hersh et al., 1989

PD 183500 AL-GAZALI SYNDROME (Hirschsprung disease with hypoplastic nails and dysmorphic facial features) (McKusick No. 235760)

Syndrome Note: Al-Gazali and associates (1988) have described three children—a male and two females—with Hirschsprung disease, renal abnormalities, unusual facial features, hypoplasia of the distal phalanges of both fingers and toes, and absent or hypoplastic fingers and toenails. The male and one female were from Sikh parents while the other female was an offspring of first-cousin Pakistani Muslims. All three children died between 1 week and 2 months of age.

Prenatal Diagnosis: No prenatal criteria have been established for the diagnosis of this condition, and no definitive method of diagnosing Hirschsprung disease prior to birth has been developed.

Differential Diagnosis: Isolated Hirschsprung disease (PD 137500), and other conditions in which Hirschsprung disease is a feature should be considered.

    Ultrasound[c]: bilateral hydronephrosis
        Al-Gazali et al., 1988

PD 184000 AMINOPTERIN SYNDROME (McKusick No. None)

    Radiograph[c,d]: delayed ossification of the calvarium, hydramnios
        Warkany et al., 1959

PD 185000 AMNIOTIC BAND DISRUPTION SEQUENCE (ADAM sequence; Amniotic adhesion malformation complex; Amniotic band syndrome; Streeter bands) (McKusick No. 217100)

Differential Diagnosis: Amniochorionic sheet (PD 252250); Blighted twin; Circumvallate placenta; Extrachorionic hemorrhage; Nonfusion of the amniotic and chorionic membranes; Septate uterus

    Alpha-fetoprotein[c]: elevated in amniotic fluid
        Herva et al., 1980; Burck et al., 1981; Macri et al., 1981; Burton et al., 1983; Aitken et al., 1984a; Borlum, 1984; Hughes and Benzie, 1984; Wallerstein et al., 1987
      elevated in maternal serum
        Macri et al., 1981; Burton et al., 1983; Aitken et al., 1984a; Borlum, 1984; Wallerstein et al., 1987

Ultrasound: fetal structural defects including total absence of fetal skull with appearance similar to that seen in anencephaly, focal absence of fetal skull, presence of fetal brain parenchyma in encephalocele, poorly calcified calvarium, microcephaly[d], occipital encephalocele, hydrocephaly, facial clefting, and cleft lip; amniotic bands entangling many parts of the body, relatively immobile fetus in close contact with the placenta, fetal head attached to placenta, hydramnios
        Herve et al., 1980; Worthen et al., 1980; Burck et al., 1981; Aitken et al., 1984a; Borlum, 1984; Hughes and Benzie, 1984; Carrasco et al., 1985; Donnenfeld et al., 1985; Stierman et al., 1985; Malinger et al., 1987
      non-midline encephalocele, ectopia cordis, abdominal wall defect, excessive spinal curvature, free-floating strands of tissue, tissue strands attached to fetus
        Stierman et al., 1985

abnormal fetus with deformed head, trunk, and limbs that defied anatomic classification
Spirt et al., 1987
complex fetal head structure with central anechogenic and peripheral
echogenic areas arising from the front of an abnormal fetal head, echogenic lines forming a V-shaped cleft-like appearance in the coronal
view of the craniofacial area
Chen and Gonzalez, 1987
micrognathia, presence of amniotic bands close to the fetus's mouth
Malinger et al., 1987
Comments: At birth, the infant was found to have lateral clefts of
the mouth, micrognathia, V-shaped cleft palate, and pressure scars
on each ear. In addition, there were amniotic bands attached to
the placenta.
partially amputated leg
Meizner and Bar-Ziv, 1993
amelia
Filly and Golbus, 1982; Stierman et al., 1985
multiple intrauterine adhesions
Meizner and Bar-Ziv, 1993
oligohydramnios[c]
Wallerstein et al., 1987

PD 185500 ANTLEY–BIXLER SYNDROME (McKusick No. 207410)

Syndrome Note: The Antley–Bixler syndrome is a rare dysmorphic disorder
consisting of craniosynostosis, choanal atresia or stenosis, radiohumeral synostosis, femoral bowing and fracture, and respiratory problems. If the choanal stenosis
is detected early and treated appropriately, and the child has not suffered brain
damåge form hypoxia, the intellectual function of the affected child usually
is normal.
Wolf et al., 1995
Prenatal Diagnosis: Fixed position of the elbows, and shortening and bowing of
the femora on ultrasonographic evaluation should be suggestive of the diagnosis
in the isolated case, and presumptive evidence for the diagnosis in the at-risk
fetus.
Ultrasound: brachycephaly[c]
Wolf et al., 1995
fixed elbow in flexion
Savoldelli and Schinzel, 1982; Wolf et al., 1995
lack of elbow movement
Savoldelli and Schinzel, 1982
humeroradial synostosis
Savoldelli and Schinzel, 1982
medial bowing of the ulnae leading to broad forearms
Savoldelli and Schinzel, 1982
relatively large hands
Savoldelli and Schinzel, 1982
short extremities
Wolf et al., 1995

femoral bowing
Wolf et al., 1995

PD 185750 ARTHROGRYPOSIS, AMYOPLASIA TYPE (Amyoplasia) (McKusick No. 108110)

Radiograph[c,d]: hyperextension of the legs and flexion of the thighs
Epstein, 1961

PD 185850 ARTHROGRYPOSIS, TYPE UNDETERMINED (McKusick No. Unknown; see 108110)

Continuous-wave Doppler evaluation[c,d]: increased peripheral arterial resistance
Meizner et al., 1987
Ultrasound[d]: severe clubhand deformity[h]
Meizner and Bar-Ziv, 1993
short limbs, lower limbs tightly flexed and crossed, elbows and wrists fixed in position
Goldberg et al., 1986
Comments: At birth the extremities of the fetus reported by Goldberg and colleagues (1986) were noted to be thin and the joints fixed in flexed positions with severe talipes equinovarus. In addition, there was generalized edema, bilateral cervical ribs, and inguinal hernias. Subsequently, the child died. At autopsy, the medulla contained normal lower motor neurons. The spinal cord was not available for examination. This case could be an example of Herva arthrogryposis–fetal hydrops syndrome (PD 191280).
pleural effusion[c]
Nicolaides and Azar, 1990
severe scoliosis[h]
Meizner and Bar-Ziv, 1993
extension of the knee[d]
Meizner and Bar-Ziv, 1993
dorsiflexion and lateral deviation of the foot[d]
Meizner and Bar-Ziv, 1993
plantar flexion of the feet[d]
Meizner and Bar-Ziv, 1993
severe joint contractures of the foot[d]
Meizner and Bar-Ziv, 1993
lack of fetal movement[c]
Rutledge et al., 1986
lack of normal limb movement
Goldberg et al., 1986
no change in positioning of limbs or limb flexion–extension[d]
Meizner and Bar-Ziv, 1993
hydrops fetalis
Goldberg et al., 1986; Nicolaides and Azar, 1990
hydramnios
Nicolaides and Azar, 1990

PD 186000 ARTHROGRYPOSIS MULTIPLEX CONGENITA (McKusick No. 108110; see also 208100)

> Radiograph[c,d]: long slender bones that were undermineralized
> > Miskin et al., 1979
> Ultrasound: absence of fetal movements, hydramnios
> > Miskin et al., 1979

PD 186250 ARTHROGRYPOSIS PRODUCED BY MUSCULAR DYSTROPHY (Muscular dystrophy, congenital, producing arthrogryposis) (McKusick No. 253900)

> **Condition Note:** This condition is an autosomal recessive disorder with congenital myopathy that produces arthrogryposis in fetuses and infants. Socol and coworkers (1986) reported two fetuses with this condition, one who went to term and who died 2 hours after birth, the other terminated during the second trimester. At autopsy, the neonate's skeletal muscle was replaced by adipose and connective tissue.
> > McKusick, 1993
> Ultrasound[i]: absence of fetal movements
> > Socol et al., 1985

PD 186500 BARDET–BIEDL SYNDROME (McKusick No. 209900)

> **Syndrome Note:** Bardet–Biedl syndrome, which has been incorrectly called Laurence–Moon–Bardet–Biedl syndrome is characterized by mental retardation, pigmentary retinopathy, polydactyly, obesity, hypogenitalism, and cystic renal disease with hepatic fibrosis. It is inherited as an autosomal recessive disorder. Most patients survive into later childhood or beyond.
> > Creech et al., 1988; McKusick, 1988
> **Prenatal Diagnosis:** In the fetus at risk, the presence of polydactyly and enlarged, echogenic kidneys in the absence of occipital encephalocele, and cleft lip and/ or palate should be sufficient to make the diagnosis.
> **Differential Diagnosis:** Alstrom syndrome (retinitis pigmentosa, obesity, diabetes mellitus, and perceptive deafness); Biemond syndrome II (iris coloboma, hypogenitalism, obesity, polydactyly, and mental retardation); Hydrolethalus syndrome (PD 191300); Laurence–Moon syndrome (mental retardation, pigmentary retinopathy, hypogenitalism, and spastic paraplegia); Meckel syndrome (PD 192140); Short rib–polydactyly syndromes (PD 169250, PD 169500, PD 170000, PD 171000); Smith–Lemli–Opitz syndrome (PD 194160); Trisomy 13 syndrome (PD 103000)
> > Creech et al., 1988; McKusick, 1988
> Ultrasound[c,h]: polydactyly, talipes equinovarus, large echogenic hydronephrotic kidneys
> > Creech et al., 1988;

PD 186800 BASAL CELL NEVUS SYNDROME (Basal cell carcinoma syndrome; Fifth phacomatosis; Gorlin syndrome; Gorlin–Goltz syndrome; Nevoid basal cell carcinoma syndrome) (McKusick No. 109400)

> **Syndrome Note:** The basal cell nevus syndrome has as features basal cell nevi, basal cell carcinoma and other tumors, broad facies with frontal bossing, ocular hypertelorism, cleft lip and palate, odontogenic keratocysts of the jaw, abnormal cervical vertebrae, bifid ribs, kyphoscoliosis, brachydactyly, pits in the skin of

the palms and soles, congenital lung cysts, and mild to moderate mental retardation. The disorder is inherited in an autosomal dominant fashion with full penetrance. The gene for the syndrome is located at 9q22.3-q31.

Amniocentesis[i]: linkage of the gene to polymoric DNA markers
> Bale et al., 1993; Bialer et al., 1994

Ultrasound[i]: hydrocephalus
> Bale et al., 1993; Bialer et al., 1994

> unilateral cleft lip
> > Bialer et al., 1994

PD 187000 BECKWITH–WIEDEMANN SYNDROME (EMG syndrome; Exomphalos–macroglossia–gigantism syndrome; Wiedemann–Beckwith syndrome) (McKusick No. 130650)

Syndrome Note: The major features of the Beckwith–Wiedemann syndrome include ear pits and creases, macroglossia, omphalocele, macrosomia with visceromegaly, adrenocortical cytomegaly, and dysplasia of the renal medulla. Hypoglycemia may occur in the first few days of life and if untreated may lead to brain damage and mental deficiency. Affected children are at increased risk for the development of tumors, particularly Wilms tumor, adrenocortical carcinoma, and neuroblastoma. Hemihypertrophy is found in about 12% of patients; when it is present, it increases the risk of neoplasms. Inheritance may be autosomal dominant in some families.

> McKusick, 1988; MacMillin et al., 1988

Prenatal Diagnosis: The diagnosis of Beckwith–Wiedemann syndrome should be considered in any fetus in which an omphalocele is detected. The diagnosis is likely if there is also an increased abdominal circumference, large and/or cystic kidneys, macrosomia in the fetus, and hydramnios. Couples who have given birth to a child with this condition should consider having any subsequent fetuses evaluated for the above physical findings, even though the parents appear unaffected; the condition may be inherited in an autosomal dominant fashion with no manifestation in the parent who carries the gene.

Differential Diagnosis: Allantoic cyst (PD 272000); Ectopia cordis (PD 109600); Incomplete embryonic body folding (PD 191450); Triploidy (PD 102000); Trisomy 13 syndrome (PD 103000); Trisomy 18 syndrome (PD 104000)

> Ultrasound: cystic kidneys, large fetus, omphalocele, increased abdominal circumference, hydramnios
> > Weinstein and Anderson, 1980; Nivelon-Chevallier et al., 1983; Winter et al., 1986

> large for gestational age
> > Cobellis et al., 1988; Meizner et al., 1989

> enlarged, protruding tongue (macroglossia)
> > Cobellis et al., 1988

> omphalocele (exomphalos)
> > MacMillin et al., 1988; Meizner et al., 1989; Nyberg et al., 1989; Stratakis and Garnica, 1995

> ascites
> > Nyberg et al., 1989

> enlarged liver
> > Meizner et al., 1989

unilateral multicystic dysplastic kidney[c]
  Avni et al., 1987
enlarged kidneys
  Meizner et al., 1989
hydramnios
  MacMillin et al., 1988; Meizner et al., 1989
oligohydramnios
  Nyberg et al., 1989

PD 187230 BILATERAL LEFT-SIDEDNESS SEQUENCE (Laterality sequence; Polysplenia syndrome) (McKusick No. 208530)

Sequence Note: The major features of this sequence include congenital heart defects and polysplenia. Other anomalies that may be present include bilateral bilobed lungs, both atria being left in type, drainage of the azygos vein into the inferior vena cava, anomalous pulmonary venous return, and right-sided stomach. The disorder is thought to be a failure in development of normal asymmetry during morphogenesis, which results in duplication of the left side on the right. The condition needs to be differentiated from bilateral right-sidedness sequence (PD 187250). Inheritance has not been clearly defined.
  Smith, 1982

Prenatal Diagnosis: In the presence of congenital heart defects and situs inversus, this sequence should be considered.

  Auscultation[c]: no fetal heart tones detected
    Sokol et al., 1974
  Comments: The fetus reported by Sokol and associates (1974) was found to have complete heart block on fetal electrocardiogram done during labor. The child died at 1 day of age. Autopsy revealed complex heart abnormalities, bilobed right lung, and polysplenia. Presumably the lack of audible heart sounds was secondary to the bradycardia.
  Echocardiography[c,d]: complete heart block, atrioventricular (AV)
    Kleinman et al., 1983
    canal defect
    Kleinman et al., 1983
  Ultrasound[c,d]: hydramnios, hydrops fetalis, levocardia, AV canal defect
    Kleinman et al., 1983

PD 187250 BILATERAL RIGHT-SIDEDNESS SEQUENCE (Asplenia syndrome; Asplenia with cardiovascular anomalies; Ivemark syndrome; Laterality sequence) (McKusick No. 208530)

Sequence Note: The triad that characterizes this sequence includes agenesis of the spleen, congenital heart defects, and situs inversus. In addition, there may be bilateral trilobed lungs, anomalous pulmonary venous return, transposition of the great vessels, bilateral inferior vena cava, bilateral liver, and incomplete rotation of the intestines. The disorder is believed to be a failure of normal asymmetry to occur during morphogenesis, resulting in duplication of the right side on the left. The condition needs to be distinguished from the polysplenia syndrome or bilateral left-sidedness sequence (PD 187230). The inheritance of bilateral right-sidedness sequence has not been clearly defined, although it appears in some cases to be familial.
  Smith, 1982; McKusick, 1986

Prenatal Diagnosis: Presence of congenital heart defect and situs inversus in a fetus at risk.

Ultrasound[c]: bradycardia, single ventricle, edema, ascites, displaced intestinal loops, liver in a midline position, decreased fetal movements
> Henrion and Aubry, 1979

hydrops fetalis, VSD
> Henrion and Aubry, 1979; Kleinman et al., 1982

hypoplastic left heart
> Wilson et al., 1989; Wilson et al., 1990

> *Comments:* The above fetus reported by Wilson and co-workers (1989, 1990) was ascertained by detecting a balanced 12;13 transloca-tion {[46,XX,+(12;13)(q13.1;p13)} in amniotic fluid cells. The mother also carried the same translocation. Subsequently, an ultrasound evaluation revealed the heart defect. Following termination, the fetus was found to have bilateral trilobar lungs, asplenia, and abdom-inal heterotaxia. The diagnosis of Ivemark syndrome was made.

PD 187500 BLAGOWIDOW SYNDROME (McKusick No. None)

Syndrome Note: Blagowidow syndrome is characterized by macrocephaly, lis-sencephaly, micropenis, and early death. It appears to be inherited as an X-linked recessive disorder.
> Blagowidow et al., 1986

Ultrasound[c]: enlarged lateral ventricles, macrocephaly
> Blagowidow et al., 1986

PD 188250 BRANCHIOOTORENAL SYNDROME (BO syndrome; BOR syn-drome; Branchiootic dysplasia; Branchiootorenal dysplasia) (McKusick No. 113650)

Syndrome Note: The branchiootorenal syndrome was first reported by Melnick and associates in 1975. This distinctive syndrome is characterized by mixed hearing loss in conjunction with hypoplasia of the cochlear apex (Mondini malfor-mation) and stapes fixation; cup-shaped, anteverted external ears; branchial cysts or fistulas; and renal defects. The renal abnormalities vary from bilateral renal agenesis to renal dysplasia of varying severity. Other findings reported include preauricular pits, lacrimal duct aplasia or stenosis, and myopia. The branchiooto-renal syndrome is inherited as autosomal dominant disorder with considerable variation in expressivity.
> Melnick et al., 1975; Greenberg et al., 1988b; McKusick, 1988

Prenatal Diagnosis: Until DNA testing is available, the only feasible method of diagnosing this syndrome is the detection of renal agenesis or dysplasia in a fetus at risk.

Differential Diagnosis: Isolated branchial cleft anomalies; Cat-eye syndrome (22q- syndrome); Renal adysplasia (PD 179250); Renal agenesis, bilateral, auto-somal recessive (PD 179380)

Ultrasound[i]: failure to demonstrate definite kidneys or fetal bladder, oligohy-dramnios
> Greenberg et al., 1988b

PD 188380 BRONCHIAL ATRESIA, MAIN-STEM (McKusick No. Unknown)

Condition Note: Atresia of the main-stem bronchi probably arises secondary to a vascular insult. In this disorder, bronchi distal to the atretic segment are usually normal in number. The atresia usually occurs in segmental or lobar bronchi and is not ordinarily fatal. The neonatal finding is a fluid-filled chest mass that is soon replaced by lucent areas as portions of lung distal to the atresia are aerated by collateral ventilation. Branching, dilated, and mucus-filled bronchi more distal to the atresia and congenital lobar emphysema may be associated with this congenital defect.

> McAlister et al., 1987

Prenatal Diagnosis: The diagnosis should be considered whenever there is a mass located in the thoracic cavity. However, there is no definitive method at this time to make the specific diagnosis.

Differential Diagnosis: Cystic adenomatoid malformation of the lung (PD 272500) and bronchial atresia cannot be differentiated from one another because both have echogenic lungs with anechoic areas within the lungs. Other conditions to consider are Diaphragmatic hernia (PD 132000), Bronchopulmonary foregut malformations, and Lobar emphysema.

Alpha-fetoprotein[c]: elevated level in maternal serum

> McAlister et al., 1987

elevated level in amniotic fluid

> McAlister et al., 1987

Ultrasound[c]: hyperechoic mass occupying two thirds of the hemithorax, depressed diaphragm, marked mediastinal shift, two small anechoic areas in the hyperechoic mass

> McAlister et al., 1987

Comments: During the pregnancy reported by McAlister and colleagues (1987), the anechoic areas became slightly larger, and there was less mediastinal shift and echogenicity of the lung. The child was delivered at 38 weeks and died from respiratory failure at 4 hours of age. At autopsy there was tracheal stenosis with circumferentially continuous cartilaginous rings and right main-stem bronchial atresia. The left main-stem bronchus and lung were normal.

PD 188400 CARDIOFACIOCUTANEOUS SYNDROME (CFC syndrome) (McKusick No. 115150)

Syndrome Note: The cardiofaciocutaneous syndrome, a sporadic condition, is characterized by a typical facial appearance consisting of a high forehead with bitemporal narrowing, hypoplastic supraorbital ridges, downslanting palpebral fissures, depressed nasal bridge, and posteriorly rotated ears with prominent helices; congenital heart defects usually being pulmonic stenosis and/or atrial septal defect; ectodermal changes normally being patchy hyperkeratosis, a generalized ichthyosis-like dermatosis and sparse, friable hair; growth deficiency; and mental retardation.

> McKusick, 1995; Leichtman, 1996

Prenatal Diagnosis: None has been established.

Differential Diagnosis: Costello syndrome; Noonan syndrome (PD 192750); Turner syndrome (PD 105000)

Ultrasound[c,h]: cystic hygroma, pleural effusion

> Leichtman, 1996

PD 188450 CARPENTER SYNDROME (ACPS II; Acrocephalopolysyndactyly, type II) (McKusick No. 201000)

Syndrome Note: Carpenter syndrome, an autosomal recessive disorder, is characterized by brachycephaly secondary to variable synostosis of the coronal, sagittal, and lambdoid sutures, brachydactyly and partial syndactyly of the fingers, pre-axial polydactyly and partial syndactyly of the toes, and obesity.

Smith, 1982, p. 308

Prenatal Diagnosis: No criteria have been established; the presence of brachy-cephaly and/or polydactyly of the toes, if these features can be detected in a fetus at risk, should be sufficient to make the diagnosis.

Differential Diagnosis: Apert syndrome (PD 148500); Pfeiffer syndrome (PD 192950); and other syndromes associated with craniosynostosis.

Ultrasound[c,h]: large for gestational age

Leonard, 1989

PD 188500 CEREBROCOSTOMANDIBULAR DYSPLASIA

(Cerebrocostomandibular syndrome; Rib-gap syndrome) (McKusick No. 117650)

Syndrome Note: Radiographic characteristics of this condition include very short ribs with apparent gaps (incomplete ossification) between the posterior ossified ribs and anterior cartilaginous ribs. In addition, there may be severe micro-gnathia, mental retardation, microcephaly, and either hydranencephaly or hydro-cephaly. Variability of inheritance has been reported, with apparent autosomal dominant inheritance with variable expressivity occurring in some families and autosomal recessive inheritance in other families.

Merlob et al., 1987

Prenatal Diagnosis: The presence of very short ribs and micrognathia in a fetus with an affected first-degree relative.

Ultrasound[d,i]: extremely short ribs, hydrocephalus, hydramnios

Merlob et al., 1987

PD 188600 CEREBROFACIOTHORACIC DYSPLASIA (McKusick No. 213980)

Dysplasia Note: Cerebrofaciothoracic dysplasia is a multiple congenital anomaly syndrome characterized by cerebral ventriculomegaly, enlargement of the sep-tum pellucidum, telecanthus, ocular hypertelorism, posteriorly rotated ears, short neck, multiple fused and bifid ribs, hemivertebrae, fusion of the posterior arches of the vertebrae, mental retardation, and affable personality. The disorder ap-pears to be inherited in an autosomal recessive fashion.

Philip et al., 1992; McKusick, 1995

Ultrasound[i]: dilation of the lateral ventricles,[d] enlarged septum pellu-cidum,[d] hydramnios

Philip et al., 1992

PD 188750 CEREBRORENODIGITAL SYNDROME (Meckel-like syndrome) (McKusick No. None)

Syndrome Note: Genuardi and co-authors (1993b) reported a male child with hepatic fibrosis, polycystic kidney disease, postaxial hexadactyly, genital abnor-malities and Dandy–Walker malformation without an occipital encephalocele. The child died at 43 months from progressive deterioration of kidney function.

Ultrasound[c,d]: agenesis of the cerebellar vermis

Genuardi et al., 1993b

PD 188900 CHITTY SYNDROME (Growth, retardation, deafness, femoral epiphyseal dysplasia, and lacrimal duct obstruction) (McKusick No. 601351)

Syndrome Note: Chitty and co-workers (1996) reported two brothers who appear to have a unique pattern of abnormalities. The brothers had unusual facies which consisted of prominent, triangular-shaped foreheads, microcephaly, and pointed chins; blocked lacrimal ducts; profound sensorineural deafness; umbilical and inguinal hernias; femoral epiphyseal dysplasia; short stature; and mental retardation. The condition probably is inherited as an autosomal recessive disorder because the parents of the boys were second cousins and unaffected.

Prenatal Diagnosis: Probably IUGR in a at-risk fetus would be sufficient for the diagnosis.

Differential Diagnosis: Cockayne syndrome (PD 254500); Epiphyseal dysplasia of femoral head, myopia, and deafness (McKusick No. 226950)

> Ultrasound[h,i]: IUGR
> > Chitty et al., 1996

PD 189000 CLEFT LIP (McKusick No. 119530)

Condition Note: If a cleft lip and/or palate is detected in a fetus, additional anomalies should be sought. In one series, other defects were recognized 83% of the time (Saltzman et al., 1986). If other defects are identified, a chromosomal analysis should be considered because autosomal trisomies have been found in as many as 33% of fetuses with a cleft lip and/or palate (Saltzman et al., 1986).

> Fetoscopy: direct visualization
> > Baraitser et al., 1982; Seeds and Cefalo, 1983
> Radiograph[d]: forward projection of maxilla
> > Russell, 1969
> Ultrasound: lack of continuity of the upper lip[d]
> > Meininger and Christ, 1982
> > in the frontal plane, disruption of normal midfacial architecture, absence of maxillary ridge, broadening of the nasal cavity
> > > Seeds and Cefalo, 1983
> > anterior projection of the midline nasal septum in sagittal view, central cleft of lip
> > > Seeds and Cefelo, 1983; Hobbins and Mahoney, 1985; Saltzman et al., 1986
> > separation of upper lip into two parts
> > > Benacerraf et al., 1984

PD 189500 CLEFT PALATE (McKusick No. 119540; see also 119570, 303400)

Condition Note: See Condition Note under Cleft lip (PD 189000).

> Ultrasound: upward displacement of the fetal tongue
> > Meininger and Christ, 1982; Seeds and Cefalo, 1983
> > nonvisualized fetal stomach[c,d]
> > > Bundy et al., 1986b
> > intrauterine growth retardation[c,d]
> > > Bundy et al., 1986b
> > hydramnios[c,d]
> > > Bundy et al., 1986b

PD 190000 CONGENITAL CHYLOTHORAX (McKusick No. None)

Condition Note: This condition results from the accumulation of chyle in the pleural cavity, usually as a result of direct drainage of the thoracic duct into this cavity. If the collection of fluid is extensive enough and the diagnosis is not made either prenatally or immediately after birth, death from pulmonary hypoplasia and respiratory insufficiency may occur postnatally.

Prenatal Diagnosis: The condition is more likely when the triad of pleural effusion, hydramnios, and male sex is present in the fetus (Lange and Manning, 1981). It is even more likely with the exclusion of other causes of pleural effusion. It may not be possible to differentiate congenital chylothorax from idiopathic hydrothorax (PD 191400) prenatally; if a high lymphocytic count is present in the pleural fluid, then congenital chylothorax is more likely.

Differential Diagnosis: See Pleural effusion in the Index.

Prenatal Treatment: Repeated thoracenteses to withdraw reaccumulation of pleural fluid has not been successful in preventing pulmonary hypoplasia and fetal death. Rather pleuroamniotic shunting appears to be the treatment of choice in these cases (Longaker et al., 1989). In addition, delivery of the fetus in a facility capable of handling difficult neonatal problems should be considered.

Treatment Modalities: Pleuroamniotic shunting
>Booth et al., 1987; Longaker et al., 1989
>Thoracocentesis
>Longaker et al., 1989

Methods and Findings: Continuous-wave Doppler evaluation[c,d]: increased peripheral arterial resistance
>Meizner et al., 1987

Ultrasound[c,d]: fluid-filled pleural cavity, hydrops fetalis, collapsed lungs, ascites, compression of the fetal heart, pericardial effusion, hydramnios
>Defoort and Thiery, 1978; Lange and Manning, 1981; Kleinman et al., 1982; Petres et al., 1982; Schmidt et al., 1985; Jaffa et al., 1985; Meizner et al., 1986a; Meizner et al., 1986c

pleural effusion[c]
>Booth et al., 1987; Reece et al., 1987; Longaker et al., 1989

hypoechoic area surrounding the lung
>Bruno et al., 1988

dextroposition of the heart with mediastinal shift
>Reece et al., 1987; Longaker et al., 1989

cystic hygroma
>Abramowicz et al., 1989

ascites
>Booth et al., 1987

hydrops fetalis
>Booth et al., 1987; Abramowicz et al., 1989; Longaker et al., 1989; Chiba et al., 1990

hydramnios[c]
>Booth et al., 1987; Reece et al., 1987; Bruno et al., 1988; Longaker et al., 1989

Thoracentesis[d]: marked lymphocytosis in pleural fluid
>Reece et al., 1987

PD 191000 CONGENITAL HYDROCELE (McKusick No. None)

Acetylcholinesterase[c]: presence of fast-migrating isozyme in amniotic fluid
>Verp et al., 1984

Alpha-fetoprotein[c]: elevated in amniotic fluid
>Verp et al., 1984

Ultrasound[d,e]: excess fluid in fetal scrotum
Vanesian et al., 1978; Hill et al., 1983a

PD 191015 CONGENITAL INTRAUTERINE INFECTION-LIKE SYNDROME (Intrauterine infection-like syndrome with microcephaly, intracranial calcification, and CNS disease; Pseudo-TORCH syndrome) (McKusick No. 600158)

Syndrome Note: Neonates with this condition appear to have a prenatal infection with congenital microcephaly, intracranial calcification, hepatosplenomegaly with abnormal liver function tests, thrombocytopenia, petechial rash, and seizures. However, the fundoscopic examination is normal, no infectious agent can be found, and in some families there has been a recurrence in siblings.
Reardon et al., 1994; McKusick, 1995

Ultrasound: microcephaly[c]
Reardon et al., 1994
intracranial calcification[c,d]
Reardon et al., 1994
ventriculomegaly[c,d]
Reardon et al., 1994
pericardial effusion[c,d]
Reardon et al., 1994
hepatomegaly[c,d]
Reardon et al., 1994
acites[c,d]
Reardon et al., 1994
intrauterine growth retardation[c,d]
Reardon et al., 1994
hydrops fetalis[c,d]
Reardon et al., 1994
oligohydramnios[c,d]
Reardon et al., 1994
fetal demise[c,d]
Reardon et al., 1994

PD 191050 CONGENITAL PULMONARY LYMPHANGIECTASIA (McKusick No. Unknown; see 265300)

Ultrasound: left pleural effusion
Kerr Wilson et al., 1985
hydramnios[c]
Kerr Wilson et al., 1985

PD 191060 COSTELLO SYNDROME (Faciocutaneoskeletal syndrome) (McKusick No. 218040)

Syndrome Note: Costello syndrome is characterized by loose skin of the neck, hands, and feet; coarse appearing face; papillomata around the mouth and nares; cardiomyopathy; dysrhythmia; curly hair; and mental retardation. The condition is inherited as an autosomal recessive disorder, and may represent an elastic fiber disorder because degeneration of elastic fiber has been observed.
McKusick, 1995; Mori et al., 1996

Prenatal Diagnosis: No method for the definitive diagnosis has been reported.

Differential Diagnosis: Cutis laxa; Cutis laxa with bone dysplasia (McKusick No. 219200)

Ultrasound[c,h]: hydramnios, fetal distress
>> Mori et al., 1996

PD 191075 CRANE–HEISE SYNDROME (McKusick No. 218090)

Syndrome Note: Crane and Heise (1981) described three siblings with a lethal multiple anomalies syndrome which included poorly mineralized calvarium, small face, depressed nasal bridge, short and upturned nose, ocular hypertelorism, low-set and posteriorly rotated ears, micrognathia, cleft lip and palate, absent cervical vertebrae form C1–C6, absent clavicles, talipes equinovarus, and syndactyly. The condition appears to be inherited as an autosomal recessive disorder.

Radiograph[d]: marked demineralization of the fetal calvarium
>> Crane and Heise, 1981

Ultrasound[i]: decreased calvarial mineralization with mineralization limited to the basal portions of the skull, disproportionately large head, micrognathia, upturned nose.
>> Crane and Heise, 1981

PD 191085 CRANIOMICROMELIC SYNDROME (McKusick No. None)

Syndrome Note: Barr and associates (1995) reported two sisters who had what they called the craniomicromelic syndrome, an assumed autosomal recessive disorder. Features present included IUGR, relative macrocephaly, turricephaly, absence of coronal sutures, irregular sutural margins, short palpebral fissures, pinched nose with anteverted nares, microstomia, micrognathia, U-shaped cleft palate in one sister, symmetrically short limbs, short hands with tapered fingers, absence of the middle phalanx of each index finger, and clubfeet. Internally, there were hypoplastic lungs, ventricular myocardial hyperplasia, hypoplastic ventricular myocardial hyperplasia, hypoplastic or absent gallbladder, and shortened midgut and colon with marked meconium distention of the mid-ileum. The long bones were short but otherwise normal. The first child died 30 minutes after birth; the second pregnancy was terminated at 24 weeks of gestation.

Prenatal Diagnosis: Abnormal head shape and short limbs in a fetus at risk probably is sufficient evidence for the diagnosis.

Differential Diagnosis: Campomelic syndrome with craniosynostosis; Carpenter syndrome (PD 188450); Cranioectodermal dysplasia (McKusick No. 218330), Ives–Houston microcephaly–micromelia syndrome (PD 191500); Thanatophoric dysplasia, type 2 (PD 174000)

Maternal examination[c]: small fundal height for gestation age.
>> Bar et al., 1995

Ultrasound[i]: abnormal skull shape, ventriculomegaly, small thorax, hydronephrosis, abnormally low head-to-abdominal circumference ratio, small abdomen, shortened long bones, mesomelic shortening of the arms
>> Barr et al., 1995

PD 191100 CRYPTOPHTHALMIA SYNDROME (Cryptophthalmos syndrome; Cryptophthalmos–syndactyly syndrome; Fraser syndrome) (McKusick No. 219000)

Syndrome Note: This condition, which is inherited as an autosomal recessive disorder, is noted by cryptophthalmos (hidden eye) frequently with hair growth onto the lateral forehead and extending to the lateral eyebrow, laryngeal stenosis resulting in an unusually high-pitched cry, ambiguous genitalia, separation of the pubic bones, syndactyly of the fingers and toes, and renal agenesis. Mental retardation and blindness are common in this condition. Many children are stillborn or die shortly after birth, in part due to the renal agenesis.

> Boyd et al., 1988

Prenatal Diagnosis: The findings of microphthalmia and/or renal agenesis in a fetus at risk should be adequate to make the diagnosis. The presence of ambiguous genitalia also might be detected by ultrasonic examination of the genitalia. **Differential Diagnosis:** Trisomy 13 syndrome (PD 103000); Trisomy 18 syndrome (PD 104000); and the conditions associated with renal agenesis (see Renal agenesis in the Index) should be considered.

Alpha-fetoprotein[c]: elevated in the amniotic fluid
> Boyd et al., 1988

Ultrasound: hydrocephalus[i]
> Feldman et al., 1985; Boyd et al., 1988

increased biparietal diameter, enlarged lateral ventricles[i]
> Feldman et al., 1985

decreased ocular diameter (microphthalmus)
> Feldman et al., 1985

ascites
> Comas et al., 1993

dysplastic cystic kidney[c]
> Boyd et al., 1988

dilation of calices[c,d]
> Boyd et al., 1988

renal agenesis
> Comas et al., 1993

hydronephrosis[c,d]
> Boyd et al., 1988

urinary bladder not visualized
> Comas et al., 1993

hydrops fetalis
> Comas et al., 1993

oligohydramnios
> Comas et al., 1993

PD 191200 DE LANGE SYNDROME (Brachmann–de Lange syndrome; Cornelia de Lange syndrome) (McKusick No. 122470)

Amniocentesis: absence of pregnancy-associated plasma protein A in maternal serum[c,d]
> Westergaard et al., 1983; Graham et al., 1988

Ultrasound[c]: single umbilical artery
> Herrmann and Sidiropoulos, 1988

intrauterine growth retardation
> Westergaard et al., 1983; Herrmann and Sidiropoulos, 1988

hydramnios
> Herrmann and Sidiropoulos, 1988

oligohydramnios
> Gembruch and Hansmann, 1988

PD 191203 DENYS–DRASH SYNDROME (Drash syndrome; Nephropathy–Wilms tumor–genital anomalies syndrome; Wilms tumor–pseudohermaphroditism) (McKusick No. 194080)

Syndrome Note: The Denys–Drash syndrome consists of ambiguous genitalia in males, Wilms tumor, and nephrotic syndrome. Renal failure usually developing before the age of three years. Other occasional features include gonadoblastoma, primary amenorrhea, and diaphragmatic hernia. The condition is caused by a mutation in the Wilms tumor gene, WT1, located at chromosomal region 11p13. WT1 is a tumor suppressor gene. Fifty percent of patients with Denys–Drash syndrome will develop a Wilms tumor; tumor formation appears to be associated with loss of heterozygosity, (loss of the normal WT1 allele).

Devriendt et al., 1995; McKusick, 1995

Prenatal Diagnosis: No definitive method has been published; detection of a mutation in the WT1 gene is feasible in the at-risk fetus, however.

Differential Diagnosis: Trisomy 3q (PD 102300)

Ultrasound[c]: diaphragmatic hernia

Devriendt et al., 1995

PD 191205 DEVI SYNDROME (HEC syndrome; Hydrocephalus–endocardial fibroelastosis–cataract syndrome) (McKusick No. None)

Syndrome Note: Devi and associates (1995) reported two unrelated male infants with similar findings and clinical courses. Hydramnios was present during both pregnancies. At birth both children were noted to have bilateral congenital nuclear cataracts. Between the ages 1 and 3 months, each child developed communicating hydrocephalus. Both children died at 4 months of age, one following an upper respiratory infection. The second died after the onset of congestive heart failure. At autopsy both infants had endocardial fibroelastosis. Neither child had any evidence of prenatal infection; they both were negative for galactosemia.

Ultrasound[c,d]: hydramnios

Devi et al., 1995

PD 191207 DISORGANIZATION MUTATION (Human homolog of the disorganization mutation in mice) (McKusick No. 223200)

Condition Note: This disorder is characterized by limb duplication defects that often involve excessive polydactyly, and limbs originating from unusual sites such as from the abdominal wall. The condition is thought to be a homolog to the mouse disorganization (Ds) mutation which produces similar abnormalities.

McKusick, 1994

Alpha-fetoprotein[c]: elevated in maternal serum

Donnai and Winter, 1989; Evans et al., 1995a

elevated levels in amniotic fluid

Donnai and Winter, 1989

Ultrasound[c]: severe distortion of the fetus

Donnai and Winter, 1989

hydrocephalus

Donnai and Winter, 1989

PD 191210 DISTAL ARTHROGRYPOSIS, KAWIRA–BENDER TYPE (McKusick No. None; see 108130)

Syndrome Note: First described by Kawira and Bender (1985), this form of distal arthrogryposis is characterized by unusual facial appearance, nuchal and axillary pterygia, cervical vertebral anomalies, scoliosis, contractures and ulnar deviation of the fingers, clubfoot deformities, and short stature. The condition appears to be inherited in an autosomal dominant fashion, although X-linked dominant inheritance has not been ruled out.

Prenatal Diagnosis: No definitive method has been described.

Maternal report: no fetal movement perceived by the mother[c]

Kawira and Bender, 1985

PD 191220 DISTAL ARTHROGRYPOSIS, TYPE I (McKusick No. 108120)

Condition Note: Distal arthrogryposis is congenital joint contractures limited to the hands and feet, and is inherited as an autosomal dominant trait. The hands are typically deviated to the ulnar side, held in a fisted position, and have overlapping fingers and adducted thumbs. The position and function of the hands usually improve with time, use of the hands and feet, and physical therapy. Foot deformities include calcaneovalgus, equinovarus, vertical talus, and planovalgus. When the feet are involved, surgical correction is usually required. The affected individual is usually normal otherwise with normal intellectual function.

Baty et al., 1988

Prenatal Diagnosis: Fixed contractures of the hands and/or feet with fisting of the hands or overlapping fingers in a fetus at risk is reasonable evidence for the diagnosis.

Differential Diagnosis: Distal arthrogryposis, Kawira–Bender type (PD 191210); Distal arthrogryposis, type II and other forms of arthrogryposis (see Arthrogryposis in the Index); Trisomy 18 syndrome (PD 104000)

Ultrasound[i]: flexed position of the fingers, extension of the right wrist, fisting of the hands, no extension of the fingers, no changing of the position of the hands in relationship to the arm, overriding of the thumb and fifth digit with flexion of the second, third, and fourth digits, dorsiflexed position of the wrists, inverted feet

Baty et al., 1988

PD 191223 DISTAL ARTHROGRYPOSIS, TYPE IIB (McKusick No. None; see 108130)

Syndrome Note: Distal arthrogryposis, type IIB is characterized by arthrogryposis of the hands and feet; ptosis with or without keratoconus; immobile face; large, prominent, dysmorphic ears; dislocated radial heads; and short stature. The disorder is inherited in an autosomal dominant mode.

Olney et al., 1989a

Prenatal Diagnosis: No criteria have been established for the diagnosis of this condition. Abnormal positioning of the hands and feet in a fetus at risk may be sufficient to make the diagnosis.

Differential Diagnosis: Distal arthrogryposis, Kawira–Bender type (PD 191210); Distal arthrogryposis, type I (PD 191220); Distal arthrogryposis, type IIA (Gordon syndrome); VSR syndrome

Maternal history[c,d]: reduced fetal movement

Olney et al., 1989a

PD 191226 ECTRODACTYLY–ECTODERMAL DYSPLASIA–CLEFT LIP/PALATE SYNDROME (EEC syndrome) (McKusick No. 129900)

Syndrome Note: The ectrodactyly–ectodermal dysplasia–cleft lip/syndrome is an autosomal dominant condition characterized by split-hand/split-foot anomaly (ectrodactyly), hypotrichosis and anadontia (ectodermal dysplasia), and clefting of the lip and palate. Other features include blepharitis, dacryocystitis, maxillary hypoplasia, choanal atresia, polysyndactyly without split-hand anomaly, and isolated growth hormone deficiency.

Anneren et al., 1991; McKusick, 1995

Ultrasound[i]: detection of cleft lip and palate

Anneren et al., 1991

PD 191228 ELEJALDE SYNDROME (Acrocephalo-polydactylyous dysplasia) (McKusick No. 200995)

Syndrome Note: The Elejalde syndrome is characterized by acrocephaly with closed anterior fontanel, short neck with excessive nuchal skin folds, lung hypoplasia, omphalocele, short limbs, postaxial polydactyly, pancreatic fibrosis, cystic dysplasia of the kidneys, marked generalized edema, and excessive birth weight. The condition is a neonatal lethal, and probably is inherited as an autosomal recessive disorder.

Nevin et al., 1994

Prenatal Diagnosis: Any abnormality found in the syndrome in an at-risk fetus is presumptive evidence for the diagnosis.

Ultrasound[c]: large cystic and loculated area at the base of the skull that extended around the neck, short limbs, pleural fluid, ascites

Nevin et al., 1994

PD 191230 FETAL AKINESIA SEQUENCE, TORIELLO TYPE
(Toriello–Bauserman–Higgins syndrome) (McKusick No. 208150)

Ultrasound[c,d]: hydramnios

Toriello et al., 1985

PD 191232 FETAL AKINESIA/HYPOKINESIA SEQUENCE (Pena–Shokeir phenotype; Pena–Shokeir syndrome, type I) (McKusick No. 208150)

Sequence Note: Fetal akinesia/hypokinesia sequence is produced by any factor or condition that results in absence of or severe reduction in fetal movement. Absent or decreased fetal movement leads to joint contractures with decreased range of motion; shortened, and abnormally shaped and positioned limbs; decreased bone calcification; hypoplastic lungs with respiratory distress after birth; short umbilical cord; short neck; micrognathia; and hydramnios from lack of or poor swallowing. Other features include IUGR and craniofacial anomalies. Death after birth from pulmonary hypoplasia is common. Various pathogenetic mechanisms of different etiology are known to cause the decrease in fetal movement.

Hall, 1986; Chen et al., 1995

Prenatal Diagnosis: This condition should be consistent in any fetus with absent or reduced movement and hydramnios. A chromosomal analysis either on the amniotic fluid cells or on the child postnatally should be considered to rule out a chromosome problem, particularly trisomy 18.

MacMillan et al., 1985; Muller and de Jong, 1986

Amniography[c,d]: impaired fetal swallowing

Lindhout et al., 1985

Ultrasound: overlapping cranial sutures[i]

MacMillan et al., 1985

scalp edema[i]
> Chen et al., 1983; Lindhout et al., 1985; Muller and de Jong, 1986
facial edema[i]
> Muller and de Jong, 1986
depressed nasal tip
> Shenker et al., 1985
micrognathia
> Chen et al., 1983; Lindhout et al., 1985; Shenker et al., 1985; Muller and de Jong, 1986; Ohlsson et al., 1988
deformed ear
> Shenker et al., 1985
small thorax
> Lindhout et al., 1985; Shenken et al., 1985; Muller and de Jong, 1986; Ohlsson et al., 1988
decreased chest movements with markedly diminished diaphragmatic excursions
> Ohlsson et al., 1988
absent fetal respiration
> Shenker et al., 1985
absent stomach echo
> Shenker et al., 1985
ascites[i]
> MacMillan et al., 1985
edema of the abdominal wall
> Muller and de Jong, 1986
fixed flexion deformities of elbows
> Ohlsson et al., 1988
fixed flexion deformities of the wrists and ankles[i]
> Muller and de Jong, 1986
ulnar deviation of a hand
> Shenker et al., 1985
claw-like hand, camptodactyly, raised index fingers
> Shenker et al., 1985; Muller and de Jong, 1986
small scrotum
> Ohlsson et al., 1988
decreased muscle mass
> Ohlsson et al., 1988
kyphosis of thoracic spine
> Ohlsson et al., 1988
decreased range of motion and flexion contractures of the fetal limbs, or limbs maintained in the same position and configuration[i]
> Chen et al., 1983; Shenker et al., 1985; Muller and de Jong, 1986; Ohlsson et al., 1988
bilateral ankle flexion with prominent heels
> Shenker et al., 1985; Muller and de Jong, 1986
clubfoot deformity
> Shenker et al., 1985; Ohlsson et al., 1988
absence of or decreased fetal movement[i]
> Lindhout et al., 1985; Muller and de Jong, 1986; Ohlsson et al., 1988

hydrops fetalis[i]
> Curry et al., 1983; MacMillan et al., 1985; Muller and de Jong, 1986
hydramnios[i]
> Chen et al., 1983; Lindhout et al., 1985; MacMillan et al., 1985; Shenker et al., 1985; Muller and de Jong, 1986; Ohlsson et al., 1988; Chen et al., 1995

PD 191234 FILIPPI SYNDROME (Syndactyly, type I with microcephaly and mental retardation) (McKusick No. 272440)

Syndrome Note: Filippi syndrome is an autosomal recessive condition characterized by low birth weight, congenital microcephaly, broad nasal bridge, thin alae nasi, thin upper lip, syndactyly of the three and fourth fingers, clinodactyly of the fifth fingers, syndactyly of toes 2, 3, and 4, pre- and postnatal short stature, and severe mental retardation.
> McKusick, 1994; Toriello and Higgins, 1995
Prenatal Diagnosis: None has been established.
Differential Diagnosis: Chitayat syndrome; Kelly syndrome; Scott craniodigital syndrome; Woods syndrome; Zerres syndrome
> Ultrasound[c,d]: IUGR
> > Toriello and Higgins, 1995; Fryer, 1996

PD 191236 FREEMAN–SHELDON SYNDROME (Craniocarpotarsal dystrophy; Whistling-face syndrome; Whistling face–windmill vane hand syndrome) (McKusick No. 193700)

Syndrome Note: The facial characteristics of the above syndrome include deep-sunken eyes, ocular hypertelorism, small nose and nostrils, long philtrum, and a small mouth. These features give an affected individual a whistling-facial appearance. The skeletal findings are ulnar deviation of the hands giving a windmill-vane appearance to the hand, camptodactyly, adducted thumbs, talipes equinovarus, and a steeply angulated anterior cerebral fossa. The condition is usually inherited in an autosomal dominant mode.
> McKusick, 1995
> Ultrasound[i]: abnormally appearing mouth with pursing of the lips, clenched hands with overlapping thumbs, bilateral equinovarus, abnormally positioned toes
> > Robbins-Furman et al., 1993

PD 191238 FRIEDMAN SYNDROME (Game-type multiple congenital anomalies with hydrocephalus; Hydrocephalus with associated malformations) (McKusick No. 236640)

Syndrome Note: This disorder, which was apparently first reported by Friedman and associates (1989), has as major features prenatal growth deficiency, hydrocephalus with patency of the aqueduct of Sylvius, micrognathia, hypoplastic multilobed lungs, omphalocele, intestinal malrotation, short limbs, bowed tibiae, and foot deformities. The condition was detected during the second trimester in three pregnancies, one of which had affected monozygotic twins. All three pregnancies occurred to the same parents and were terminated. The condition appears to be an autosomal recessive disorder.
> Friedman et al., 1989; Game et al., 1989
Prenatal Diagnosis: The diagnosis is most likely made when intrauterine growth

deficiency and hydrocephalus are detected in a fetus at risk, and it should be suspected in a fetus with these characteristics in which there is no family history of the disorder.

Differential Diagnosis: Aase–Smith syndrome; Atelosteogenesis; Campomelic dysplasia, short-limb type (PD 150000); Fullana syndrome; Hydrolethalis syndrome (PD 191330); Neu–Laxova syndrome (PD 192700); Smith-Lemli-Opitz syndrome (PD 194160); Triploidy (PD 102000); Trisomy 18 syndrome (PD 103000)

Ultrasound[i]: hydrocephalus, IUGR

Friedman et al., 1989; Game et al., 1989

PD 191240 FRYNS SYNDROME (McKusick No. 229850)

Syndrome Note: The major features of this disorder include early onset of hydramnios, premature delivery, perinatal mortality, and multiple birth defects. The latter consist of cloudy cornea, dysmorphic ears, cleft lip and palate, micrognathia, coarse face, diaphragmatic hernia, hypoplastic lungs with abnormal lobulations, congenital heart defects, distal limb hypoplasia, hypoplastic nails, shawl scrotum, dysplastic/cystic kidneys, and uterus bicornis. Other defects that may occur include Dandy–Walker anomaly, agenesis of the corpus callosum, intestinal malrotation, duodenal atresia, and short limbs. The condition is inherited in an autosomal recessive mode with an estimated incidence of 0.7 case per 10,000 births.

McKusick, 1986; Samueloff et al., 1987; Ayme et al., 1989; Fryns et al., 1990; Tsukahara et al., 1995

Prenatal Diagnosis: The disorder should be considered in any fetus detected to have a diaphragmatic hernia and hydramnios, particularly if there are other associated defects and/or there has been a previously affected sibling.

Differential Diagnosis: CHARGE association; Diaphragmatic hernia (PD 132000); Trisomy 22 (PD 104500); VATER association (PD 194650)

Alpha-fetoprotein[i]: elevated level in maternal serum

Samueloff et al., 1987; Bamforth et al., 1989; Bartsch et al., 1995

Ultrasound: sonolucent areas in the chest thought to represent dilated loops of bowel[i]

Samueloff et al., 1987; Ayme et al., 1989

fetal death, unilateral renal agenesis, polycystic kidneys, hydronephrosis

Ayme et al., 1989

hydrops fetalis[i]

Moerman et al., 1988

hydrocephalus[i]

Moerman et al., 1988; Ayme et al., 1989

dilation of the cerebral ventricles[i]

Moerman et al., 1988

cleft lip and palate[i]

Bamforth et al., 1989

short neck[c]

Bamforth et al., 1989

diaphragmatic hernia[i]

Samueloff et al., 1987; Moerman et al., 1988; Ayme et al., 1989; Bamforth et al., 1989

hypoplastic lungs[c,d]
    Tsukahara et al., 1995
omphalocele[i]
    Bamforth et al., 1989
single umbilical artery[c,d]
    Tsukahara et al., 1995
short humerus and femur
    Tsukahara et al., 1995
short limbs[c,d]
    Tsukahara et al., 1995
hydronephrosis
    Bartsch et al., 1995
abnormal finger positioning
    Bartsch et al., 1995
abnormal fetal movements
    Bartsch et al., 1995
hydramnios[i]
    Samueloff et al., 1987; Moerman et al., 1988; Ayme et al., 1989;
    Bamforth et al., 1989; Bartscht et al., 1995; Tsukahara et al., 1995

PD 191245 GALLOWAY–MOWAT SYNDROME (Microcephaly–hiatus hernia–nephrotic syndrome) (McKusick No. 251300)

Syndrome Note: The Galloway–Mowat syndrome, an autosomal recessive condition, consists of gyral abnormalities, microcephaly, and the nephrotic syndrome. The latter finding is caused by glomerulosclerosis. Other features include large and floppy ears; hiatal hernia, albuminuria; microcystic, dysplastic, and large kidneys; psychomotor retardation; hypotonia; and death from renal disease by age 5 years.
    McKusick, 1996; Hou and Wang, 1995
Prenatal Diagnosis: not established
    Alpha-fetoprotein[c]: elevated in maternal serum
        Silver et al., 1995
    Ultrasound[c]: dilation of the lateral and third ventricles, macrocephaly
        Silver et al., 1995
        intrauterine growth retardation, hydramnios
        Hou and Wang, 1995

PD 191255 HALLERMANN–STREIFF SYNDROME (Francois dyscephalic syndrome) (McKusick No. 234100)

Syndrome Note: The main features of Hallermann–Streiff syndrome are cataracts, deep-set eyes, microphthalmia, high forehead, pinched nose, proportionate short stature with slender bones, and hypotrichosis. Other features may include small nares, microstomia, natal teeth, hypodontia, malformed teeth, and normal mentation.
    Dennis et al., 1995; McKusick, 1995
Prenatal Diagnosis: None is established.
Differential Diagnosis: Absent eyebrows and eyelashes with mental retardation (McKusick No. 200130); Asymmetric short stature syndrome (McKusick No. 108450); Bird-headed dwarfism, Montreal type (McKusick No. 130070); Ehlers–

Danlos syndrome, progeroid form (McKusick No. 130070); Progeria (McKusick No. 176670)

Ultrasound[d,i]: deficient skull ossification, femoral fracture, short long bones
Dennis et al., 1995

Comments: The ultrasound evaluation of the fetus reported by Dennis and associates (1995) had what was considered to be normal ultrasound findings at 18 weeks of gestation; at 29 weeks, however, the above reported abnormalities were noted.

PD 191260 HERRMANN–OPITZ SYNDROME (McKusick No. None)

Syndrome Note: The delineation of this syndrome is based on only two patients; the first was reported by Herrmann and Opitz (1969) and the second by Anyane-Yeboa and co-workers (1987). Significant features include acrocephaly, hypertelorism, dysplastic ears, cleft palate, and oligosyndactyly. There was urethral atresia, oligohydramnios, and intrauterine death in one, and mental deficiency in the other individual.

Herrmann and Opitz, 1969; Anyane-Yeboa et al., 1987

Ultrasound[c,d]: severe growth retardation, bilateral hydronephrosis, and severe oligohydramnios
Anyane-Yeboa et al., 1987

PD 191280 HERVA ARTHROGRYPOSIS–FETAL HYDROPS SYNDROME
(LCCS; Lethal congenital contracture syndrome) (McKusick No. 253310)

Syndrome Note: The condition was reported by Herva and associates in 1985. Features include marked hydrops fetalis, micrognathia, and multiple joint contractures (arthrogryposis) as a result of loss of anterior horn motor neurons. The disorder is usually lethal in the third trimester. Fetal edema develops at around the 12th to 13th week of gestation and is progressive. It tends to be more severe in the trunk and less so in the scalp. Little or no fetal limb movement is detected after 16 weeks. The disorder is inherited in an autosomal recessive mode (Kirkinen et al., 1987), and appears to be one form of the fetal akinesia/hypokinesia sequence (PD 191232) (Ohlsson et al., 1988).

Prenatal Diagnosis: The condition can be diagnosed in a fetus at risk who develops hydrops fetalis and has limited or no limb movement.

Ultrasound: mild to severe hydrops fetalis, little or no fetal movement, ascites, hydrothorax, hydramnios
Herva et al., 1985; Kirkinen et al., 1987; Herva et al., 1988

PD 191290 HOLOPROSENCEPHALY–HYPOKINESIA SYNDROME
(Holoprosencephaly with fetal akinesia/hypokinesia sequence) (McKusick No. 306990)

Syndrome Note: The above syndrome appears to be a recently described unique dysmorphic syndrome of holoprosencephaly, hydranencephaly, fetal hypokinesia, multiple congenital contractures, and IUGR. Morse and his associates (1987a) first reported the disorder in two male fetuses who had the same parents. The pregnancies were interrupted at 19 and 24 weeks, respectively. There was no known consanguinity between the parents. Hockey and colleagues (1988) have reported a second pedigree with this condition, in which the inheritance clearly favors an X-linked recessive mode.

Prenatal Diagnosis: The presence of holoprosencephaly, microcephaly, and hypokinesia in a fetus at risk should be sufficient to establish the diagnosis.

Differential Diagnosis: Erdl syndrome (PD 122250); Fetal akinesia/hypokinesia sequence (PD 191232); and other disorders associated with arthrogryposis (see Arthrogryposis in the Index)

    Maternal history[i]: decreased fetal movements as perceived by the mother
            Morse et al., 1987a

    Ultrasound[i]: decreased biparietal diameter
            Morse et al., 1987a

      microcephaly with abnormal head shape
            Morse et al., 1987a; Hockey et al., 1988

      absent falx
            Hockey et al., 1988

      thickened skull
            Morse et al., 1987a

      small, narrow, and/or bell-shaped thorax
            Morse et al., 1987a; Hockey et al., 1988

      diminished or absent fetal movement
            Morse et al., 1987a; Hockey et al., 1988

      contractures of the hands
            Morse et al., 1987a

      extended and crossed legs
            Morse et al., 1987a

      intrauterine growth retardation
            Morse et al., 1987a; Hockey et al., 1988

      hydrops fetalis
            Hockey et al., 1988

PD 191310 HOLT–ORAM SYNDROME (Heart–hand syndromes; HOS) (McKusick No. 142900)

Syndrome Note: Holt–Oram syndrome, an autosomal dominantly inherited condition, is characterized by congenital heart defects and upper limb deformities. The skeletal abnormalities range in severity from minor defects of the carpal bones to phocomelia. The phenotypic expression may vary considerably from one individual to another and, in addition to the above findings, may include hypoplastic thenar eminences, triphalangeal thumbs, clinodactyly, syndactyly, absent first metacarpals, absent thumbs, short middle fifth phalanx, deformed or extra carpal bones, partial or complete absence of the radius and/or ulna, deformed head of the humerus, malformed scapula and/or clavicle, and sternal defects. In addition, there may be marked variation in the skeletal defects between the upper limbs.

    The cardiac abnormalities may include various combinations of atrial septal defect, ventricular septal defect, pulmonic stenosis, mitral valve prolapse, anomalous pulmonary venous return, and conduction defects; or there may be no cardiac defects.
            Brons et al., 1988

Prenatal Diagnosis: The detection of upper extremity skeletal and/or cardiac defects in a fetus at risk should be sufficient to make the diagnosis. However, because the abnormalities may be mild, caution needs to be taken in stating that the fetus is unaffected.

Differential Diagnosis: Aase syndrome; Fanconi anemia (PD 205000); Radial-renal syndrome (PD 193520); Thrombocytopenia–absent radius syndrome (PD 175000); VATER association (PD 194650)

Ultrasound[i]: unilateral cerebral ventriculomegaly
        Moola et al., 1995
    ventricular septal defect
        Muller et al., 1985d; Brons et al., 1988; Moola et al., 1995
    atrial septal defect
        Brons et al., 1988
    lack of ability to distinguish between forearm bones,[d] absence of one or two fingers, absence of radius, deviation of forearm, no movement at the elbow
        Muller et al., 1985d
    hypoplastic thumbs
        Moola et al., 1995
    clubbed hands
        Moola et al., 1995
    hydramnios[c,d]
        Muller et al., 1985d

PD 191320 HOLZGREVE–WAGNER–REHDER SYNDROME (McKusick No. None)

Syndrome Note: Holzgreve and associates in 1984 reported on a fetus with Potter sequence and other birth defects. Legius and co-authors (1988) have cited a second case of what appears to be a discrete disorder. Features of the condition include bilateral renal agenesis with resulting Potter phenotype, cleft palate with persistent buccopharyngeal membrane type II, cardiopathy, nonfixation of the intestine, postaxial polydactyly, and IUGR. Chromosomal analyses in both reported patients have been normal. The etiology of the disorder is not recognized.

Prenatal Diagnosis: The condition should be considered when renal agenesis is discovered in a fetus who, in addition, has IUGR and a cleft palate.

Differential Diagnosis: Other conditions associated with bilateral renal agenesis should be included in the differential diagnosis as listed under Renal agenesis in the Index. Conditions associated with IUGR also are listed under the latter title in the Index. The most frequent condition associated with renal agenesis appears to be Potter sequence (PD 179000), which usually is characterized by bilateral renal agenesis of undetermined etiology.

    Ultrasound[c,d]: cleft palate, no visualization of kidney or bladder filling, oligohydramnios, IUGR
        Legius et al., 1988

PD 191330 HYDROLETHALUS SYNDROME (McKusick No. 236680)

Syndrome Note: In 1981, Salonen and associates separated this disorder from Meckel syndrome (PD 192140), by reviewing a number of infants previously ascertained to have Meckel syndrome. Characteristics of the syndrome include absent pituitary gland, corpus callosum, and septum pellucidum; hydrocephalus; "keyhole"-shaped foramen magnum; microphthalmia or anophthalmia; malformed ears; micrognathia with a small tongue, cleft lip, and palate; abnormalities of the larynx, trachea, and/or bronchi; defective lung lobation; cardiac defects; and polydactyly. Although hydronephrosis may be present, polycystic kidney disease, a frequent feature of Meckel syndrome, is not. The disorder is inherited as an autosomal recessive condition, and affected individuals die shortly after birth or are stillborn.

Krassikoff et al., 1987

Prenatal Diagnosis: It can be assumed that the diagnosis is present when CNS abnormalities, hydrocephalus, and hydramnios are found in a fetus at risk for this disorder.

Differential Diagnosis: Alstrom syndrome (retinitis pigmentosa, obesity, diabetes mellitus, and perceptive deafness); Bardet–Biedl syndrome (PD 186500); Biemond syndrome II (iris coloboma, hypogenitalism, obesity, polydactyly, and mental retardation); Fryns syndrome (PD 191240); Laurence–Moon syndrome (mental retardation, pigmentary retinopathy, hypogenitalism and spastic paraplegia); Meckel syndrome (PD 192140); Septooptic dysplasia; Short rib–polydactyly syndromes (PD 169250, PD 169500, PD 170000, PD 171000); Smith–Lemli-Opitz syndrome (PD 194160); Trisomy 13 syndrome (PD 103000); Walker–Warburg syndrome (PD 130750)

Creech et al., 1988; McKusick, 1988

Ultrasound[i]: enlargement of the fetal head (hydrocephalus)

Salonen et al., 1981; Krassikoff et al., 1987

asymmetrical dilation of the lateral ventricles, excessive fetal head growth rate, no recognizable corpus callosum or choroid plexus, reduced or no recognizable cerebral cortex, abnormal floating structures within the cerebrospinal fluid

Hartikainen-Sorri et al., 1983

holoprosencephalic appearance to the brain, difficulty visualizing facial parts, widening of the posterior cervical spinal process[d]

Krassikoff et al., 1987

hydramnios[c,d]

Hartikainen-Sorri et al., 1983; Krassikoff et al., 1987

PD 191350 HYDROMETROCOLPOS (McKusick No. None)

Ultrasound[c,d]: homogeneous midline mass located posterior to the fetal bladder, tubular in shape, with smooth well-defined margins, and originating in the pelvic area with extension into the lower abdomen

Hill and Hirsch, 1985

5×7 cm cystic lesion that rose from the fetal pelvis and extended into the fetal abdomen, and was divided into four compartments by sagittal and transverse septations, hydronephrosis.

Russ et al., 1986

Comment: At birth the child was found to have a persistent urogenital sinus, septate vagina, and uterus didelphys.

PD 191400 HYDROTHORAX, IDIOPATHIC (Pleural effusion of unknown etiology; Primary fetal hydrothorax) (McKusick No. None)

Condition Note: An abnormal accumulation of pleural fluid of unknown etiology is defined as idiopathic hydrothorax. The accumulation may be either unilateral or bilateral, and if prenatally untreated is associated with lung hypoplasia in up to 90% of cases with a neonatal mortality rate that varies from 57–100%. Death usually occurs as a direct result of the respiratory insufficiency (Reece et al., 1987; Rodeck et al., 1988).

Hydrothorax is associated with many fetal conditions, such as, hydrops fetalis, and syndromes, such as, Turner syndrome (PD 105000). The cause of the hydrothorax should be sought anytime excessive pleural fluid is encountered. Often the etiology remains undetermined (Blott et al., 1988a; Nicolaides and Azar, 1990).

Prenatal Diagnosis: The diagnosis is established by the ultrasound detection of an abnormal fluid collection in the pleural cavity after other disorders have been excluded such as structural defects, chylothorax, tumors or cysts, and chromosomal abnormalities.

Differential Diagnosis: For conditions that have been associated with pleural effusion in the fetus, see Pleural effusion in the Index.

Prenatal Treatment: Fetuses with this condition have been treated successfully by either thoracocentesis and/or pleuroamniotic shunts (Rodeck et al., 1988). The preferred method of treatment is shunting, which is accomplished by utilizing ultrasound guidance to place a double-pigtail catheter through the chest wall and into the pleural space. The other end then lies in the amniotic cavity. Shunting usually has been done between the 21st and 35th week of gestation (Blott et al., 1988a; Thompson et al., 1993). On the other hand, in some cases of isolated bilateral hydrothorax, such as when there is no hydrops fetalis or other fetal anomalies, no treatment may be necessary. Pijpers and associates (1989b) have reported eight fetuses that met these criteria. In two, the pleural effusion resolved and in the other six the condition remained static. All eight survived after birth with only two requiring prolonged intubation (7 days).

Treatment Modalities: Pleuroamniotic shunting

Seeds and Bowes, 1986; Blott et al., 1988a; Rodeck et al., 1988a; Longaker et al., 1989; Nicolaides and Azar, 1990; Thompson et al., 1993

Comments: In the cases that were reported by Blott and associates (1988a), 7 of 11 had idiopathic hydrothorax. All of these seven cases had associated hydramnios, while four also had hydrops fetalis. Both the hydramnios and hydrops fetalis resolved within 1 week following the pleuroamniotic shunting in all four of the latter cases. The resolution of the fetal edema and hydramnios may be related to reducing intrathoracic pressure post shunting. An increased intrathoracic pressure in these situations probably leads to a decrease venous return to the heart (and increased intravenous pressure), and to compression of the esophagus. The latter situation probably leads to decreased swallowing, and the hydramnios. Once delivered, none of the treated fetuses had respiratory problems.

In a larger series that contained the 11 reported by Blott and co-workers (1988a); Nicolaides and Azar (1990) presented 47 fetuses with pleural effusion that were treated by shunting. In this series, 22 cases had unilateral effusions, all of whom had mediastinal shifts. Eight of these fetuses had fetal ascites and/or generalized skin edema (hydrops fetalis). These latter findings also were present in 22 of the 25 cases with bilateral effusions. Shunting resulted in rapid expansion of the lungs in 46 cases and a shift of the mediastinum back to a normal position in all unilateral cases. Hydramnios resolved in 20 of the 30 cases and 13 of 28 cases of fetal hydrops. Four pregnancies were terminated. Of the remaining 43 cases, all 15 of the fetuses without hydrops fetalis survived, while in those with hydrops fetalis, 2 in utero death occurred, 12 died in the neonatal period, and 14 neonates survived.

Thoracentesis
>Benacerraf et al., 1986c; Rodeck et al., 1988; Meizner, 1989; Longaker et al., 1989

>*Comments*: In general, repeated thoracocentosis to withdraw reaccumulation of pleural fluids has not been successful in preventing pulmonary hypoplasia, and most fetuses treated in this fashion have died (Longaker et al., (1989)

Methods and Findings: Ultrasound: scalp edema
>Seeds and Bowes, 1986

>echo-free area between the heart and chest wall (pleural fluid), hypoplastic lungs
>>Bovicelli et al., 1981

>unilateral or bilateral pleural effusion
>>Seeds and Bowes, 1986; Benacerraf et al., 1986c; Reece et al., 1987; Blott et al., 1988a; Rodeck et al., 1988; Longaker et al., 1989; Meizner, 1989; Pijpers et al., 1989b; Nicolaides and Azar, 1990

>dextroposition of the heart with mediastinal shift
>>Benacerraf et al., 1986c; Reece et al., 1987; Rodeck et al., 1988; Longaker et al., 1989

>hydrops fetalis
>>Blott et al., 1988a; Rodeck et al., 1988; Longaker et al., 1989; Nicolaides and Azar, 1990

>ascites
>>Benacerraf et al., 1986c; Seeds and Bowes, 1986; Blott et al., 1988a; Nicolaides and Azar, 1990;

>hydramnios
>>Seeds and Bowes, 1986; Blott et al., 1988a; Rodeck et al., 1988; Longaker et al., 1989; Pijpers et al., 1989b; Nicolaides and Azar, 1990

PD 191425 HYPOMANDIBULAR FACIOCRANIAL DYSPLASIA
(McKusick No. 241310)

Condition Note: Hypomandibular faciocranial dysplasia describes the major areas of involvement is this strikingly unique disorder. The major features include coronal synostosis; choanal stenosis; marked midfacial, orbital, maxillary and mandibular hypoplasia; pursed and protruding lips; minute oral aperture; persistent buccopharyngeal membrane; and atrial septal defect. The mandibular hypoplasia is quite severe. Most affected children die in the immediate neonatal period or shortly thereafter. The condition is an autosomal recessive disorder.
>Schimke et al., 1991; McKusick, 1996

Ultrasound[d,i]: upturned nose, pursed lips, hydramnios
>Schimke et al., 1991

PD 191450 INCOMPLETE EMBRYONIC BODY FOLDING
(Maldevelopment of embryonic body folding) (McKusick No. None)

Condition Note: At around the 22nd day postconception, the flat trilaminar embryo (the embryonic disk) begins a parallel set of body folds that eventually form the body walls and coeloms of the embryo. Defective folding may lead to such disorders as the pentalogy of Cantrell (Ectopia cordis, PD 109600), a defect in the cephalic folding; Omphalocele (PD 144000), a problem with the lateral folds; or Exstrophy of the cloaca (PD 135500), an error in caudal folding. Incomplete embryonic body folding as a condition per se, the result of maldevelopment in all four body folding processes, leads to the aberrant presence of intrathoracic and intraabdominal organs in the extraembryonic coelom, lack of umbilical cord formation, and the wide-based insertion of the amnioperitoneal membrane onto the placental chorionic plate.

Lockwood et al., 1986

Prenatal Diagnosis: The diagnosis should be considered whenever there is extensive evisceration of thoracic and abdominal organs, and lack of formation of the umbilicus in the fetus.

Differential Diagnosis: Ectopia cordis (PD 109690); Exstrophy of the cloaca (PD 135500); Gastroschisis (PD 136000); Limb–body wall complex (PD 191900); Omphalocele, (PD144000); Pentalogy of Cantrell (Ectopia cordis) (PD 109600); Trisomy 18 syndrome (PD 104000)

Ultrasound[c]: ventral wall defect that was covered by a cylindrical membrane; insertion of this membrane onto the placenta along a broad circular base and contiguous with the amniochorionic membrane; lack of umbilical cord; lack of spiraling of the umbilical vessels; no free loops of umbilical cord; short umbilical cords; constricted thorax; omphalocele containing liver, bowel, and left kidney; ectopia cordis; restricted fetal movement secondary to the intimate attachment to the placenta

Lockwood et al., 1986

small chest

Jauniaux et al., 1990

large abdominal hernia

Jauniaux et al., 1990

severe kyphoscoliosis

Lockwood et al., 1986; Jauniaux et al., 1990

no identifiable bladder or sacrum, and only one kidney

Jauniaux et al., 1990

hydramnios

Lockwood et al., 1986

oligohydramnios

Jauniaux et al., 1990

PD 191500 IVES–HOUSTON MICROCEPHALY–MICROMELIA SYNDROME (Microcephaly–micromelia syndrome) (McKusick No. 251230)

Syndrome Note: Ives and Houston (1980) reported 14 similarly malformed infants born to eight different mothers in the Cree Indians of northern Saskatchewan, Canada. Features of the disorder include IUGR, perinatal death, marked microcephaly, synostosis of the elbows, greatly shortened and malformed forearms that usually contain only a single bone, and oligodactyly of the hands. Examination of the brain has shown marked lack of myelin. The condition is inherited as an autosomal recessive disorder.

Prenatal Diagnosis: In fetuses at risk, the finding of either microcephaly or upper limb defects should be diagnostic. However, the diagnosis should be considered in any fetus with these features.

Physical examination of the mother[d,i]: no increase in uterine size during the third trimester

Ives and Houston, 1980

Radiograph[d]: microcephaly, absence or abnormalities of upper limbs
Ives and Houston, 1980

PD 191530 KLIPPEL–TRENAUNAY–WEBER SYNDROME (McKusick No. 149000)

Fetography[c,d]: multiple cystlike areas of the chest wall, abdominal wall, and lower limbs, hydramnios
Hatjis et al., 1981b
Ultrasound[c]: multiple echolucent (cystic) areas of the chest wall, abdominal wall, and lower limbs; hydramnios[d]
Hatjis et al., 1981b
large, solid, and cystic mass containing pulsating channels and a central pulsating vessel
Seoud et al., 1984

PD 191535 LACRIMOAURICULODENTODIGITAL SYNDROME (LADD syndrome; Levy–Hollister syndrome) (McKusick No. 149730)

Syndrome Note: The primary features of the lacrimoauriculodentodigital syndrome include aplasia or hypoplasia of the puncta resulting in nasal lacrimal duct obstruction, cup-shaped pinnas with or without mixed hearing loss, small and peg-shaped lateral maxillary incisors, mild enamel dysplasia, hypo- and anodontia, duplication of the distal phalanx of the thumb, triphalangeal thumb, and radial aplasia. The condition is inherited as an autosomal dominant disorder with considerable variation in expression.
Francannet et al., 1994; McKusick, 1995
Prenatal Diagnosis: Diagnosis can be made by the presence of radial aplasia in the at-risk fetus.
Ultrasound[i]: bilateral radial aplasia
Francannet et al., 1994

PD 191540 LEPRECHAUNISM (Donohue syndrome; Insulin receptor defect) (McKusick No. 246200)

Syndrome Note: The major features of leprechaunism consist prenatally of IUGR, and postnatally of failure to thrive, unusual facies, retarded bone age, sexual precocity, and hyperinsulinemia. The disorder is inherited in an autosomal recessive mode, and is caused by mutations in the insulin receptor gene located at 19p13.2. Numerous mutations have been found in this gene that give rise to various forms of leprechaunism.
Gorlin et al., 1990; Longo et al., 1993; McKusick, 1996
Prenatal Diagnosis: Detection of reduced insulin binding to the insulin receptor and detection of the mutation(s) in the insulin receptor gene has been successfully used to make the prenatal diagnosis of this condition.
Chorionic villus sampling[h]: failure of ^{125}I insulin to bind to the insulin receptor
Longo et al., 1993
detection of two mutations in the insulin receptor gene that produces the condition
Longo et al., 1993

PD 191550 LETHAL MULTIPLE PTERYGIUM SYNDROME (McKusick No. 253290)

Syndrome Note: There are two basic classes of multiple pterygium syndromes—one associated with intrauterine lethality and the other not. All of the syndromes in the multiple pterygium syndromes, both lethal and nonlethal ones, have cutaneous webs (pterygia) that extend across two or more joints. The lethal forms frequently have associated hydramnios, probably from little or no fetal swallowing, and hydrops fetalis.

The lethal multiple pterygium syndrome noted under this entry is not found to have congenital bone fusion or spinal fusion, and is inherited in an autosomal recessive mode. Death usually occurs in the late second or third trimester.

Prenatal Diagnosis: The finding of hydrops fetalis, hydramnios, and little or no fetal movement with fixation of limb position in a fetus at risk is probably diagnostic for this condition.

Differential Diagnosis: Other Lethal multiple pterygium syndromes (PD 191600, PD 191610, PD 191650, PD 191800); see also Hydrops fetalis and Hydramnios in the Index.

Ultrasound[c,i]: cystic hygroma[g]
> Martin et al., 1986; Rawnsley et al., 1988; Zeitune et al., 1988; Edwards et al., 1989a; Clementi et al., 1995

pterygium of the neck
> Clementi et al., 1995

edematous area from the back of the head to the coccyx
> Clementi et al., 1995

pleural effusion[d]
> Hogge et al., 1985

ascites[d]
> Hogge et al., 1985; Martin et al., 1986

camptodactyly
> Clementi et al., 1995

fixed, flexed, short limbs
> Zeitune et al., 1988

shortened femur length
> Martin et al., 1986

joint contractures (arthrogryposis)
> Clementi et al., 1995

no fetal movement
> Martin et al., 1986; Rawnsley et al., 1988; Zeitune et al., 1988; Edwards et al., 1989a

> *Comments:* Clementi and associates (1995) reported a fetus with the lethal multiple pterygium syndrome who had fetal movement at 15 weeks of gestation. An autopsy at 19 weeks was performed but the authors did not comment on whether or not pterygia were present in the fetus.

hydrops fetalis
> Hogge et al., 1985; Martin et al., 1986; Zeitune et al., 1988; Clementi et al., 1995

clubfoot deformities
> Zeitune et al., 1988; Clementi et al., 1995

fetal death[d]
> Hogge et al., 1985; Martin et al., 1986; Clementi et al., 1995

enlarged placental
> Martin et al., 1986

intrauterine growth retardation
    Clementi et al., 1995
hydramnios
    Hogge et al., 1985; Zeitune et al., 1988; Clementi et al., 1995

PD 191600 LETHAL MULTIPLE PTERYGIUM SYNDROME WITH CONGENITAL BONE FUSION (McKusick No. 253290)

Ultrasound[c]: absence of fetal limb or body movement, fetal demise, hydramnios, IUGR
    van Regemorter et al., 1984

PD 191610 LETHAL MULTIPLE PTERYGIUM SYNDROME WITH DYSGENETIC BRAIN (McKusick No. 253290)

Syndrome Note: Spearritt and co-authors (1993) reported a 22-gestational-week fetus with multiple pterygia, congenital contractures, muscle hypoplasia, cystic hygroma, hydrops fetalis, hypoplasia of the lungs and heart, and IUGR who had dysgenesis of the brain. The brain abnormality included microcephaly, immaturity of the cerebral cortex, cerebellar and pontine hypoplasia, absence of the pyramidal traits and hypoplasia of the white matter columns in the spinal cord. The affected fetus died in utero at 22 weeks of gestation.

Ultrasound[c]: cystic hygroma, hydrops fetalis, microcephaly, intrauterine demise
    Spearritt et al., 1993

PD 191620 LETHAL MULTIPLE PTERYGIUM SYNDROME WITH HYDRANENCEPHALY (McKusick No. 252390)

Syndrome Note: This type of lethal multiple pterygium syndrome was reported by Mbakop and associates (1986) in a fetus with multiple pterygia, congenital joint contractures, lung hypoplasia, hydranencephaly, abnormal facial features, and hydrops fetalis. Whether this condition represents a separate disorder or is part of the spectrum of the lethal multiple pterygium syndrome has not been determined.

Prenatal Diagnosis: Hydramnios, hydrops fetalis, and ventriculomegaly in a fetus at risk is probably adequate to make the diagnosis.

Differential Diagnosis: Herva arthrogryposis–fetal hydrops syndrome (PD 191280); other lethal multiple pterygium syndromes (PD 191550, PD 191600, PD 191610; PD 191650, PD 191800); lethal popliteal pterygium syndrome

Ultrasound[c]: hydrops fetalis, cystic hygroma, hydrocephalus, hydramnios
    Mbakop et al., 1986

Comments: The postnatal physical findings of the fetus reported by Mbakop and co-workers (1986) included cystic hygroma, cervical and bilateral axillary pterygia, multiple joint contractures with camptodactyly, cleft lip and palate, hypoplastic lungs, ulnar deviation of the hands, and talipes equinovarus. Hydranencephaly was described at autopsy.

PD 191650 LETHAL MULTIPLE PTERYGIUM SYNDROME WITH SPINAL FUSION (McKusick No. 253290)

Ultrasound[c,d]: hydramnios, hydrops fetalis, cystic hygroma of the posterior neck, ascites, enlarged and lobulated placenta
    Chen et al., 1984

PD 191800 LETHAL MULTIPLE PTERYGIUM SYNDROME WITH X-LINKED RECESSIVE INHERITANCE (McKusick No. Unknown)

Syndrome Note: There now have been a number of syndromes described that are characterized by multiple pterygia and fetal or neonatal death (Hall, 1984). The condition listed here is depicted by multiple pterygia, cystic hygroma, cleft palate, broad ribs and clavicles, lack of modeling of long bones, hypoplastic radii and ulnae, dislocated femoral heads, and fetal demise. Apparently it has an X-linked recessive mode of inheritance.

> Tolmie et al., 1987d

Prenatal Diagnosis: Findings noted below in a fetus at risk would be presumptive evidence for the diagnosis.

Maternal history[i]: diminished fetal movements as noted by the mother

> Tolmie et al., 1987d

Ultrasound[i]: cystic hygroma, ascites, hydrops fetalis, reduced fetal movement, fetal death

> Tolmie et al., 1987d

PD 191900 LIMB–BODY WALL COMPLEX (Body wall defects with reduction limb anomalies; Cyllosomus; Pleurosomus) (McKusick No. None)

Alpha-fetoprotein[c]: elevated in amniotic fluid and maternal serum

> Pagon et al., 1979; Haddow et al., 1983

elevated in maternal serum

> Evans et al., 1995a

Fetography[c,d]

> Pagon et al., 1979

Ultrasound[c,d]:

anencephaly[c]

> Patten et al., 1986

no calvarium seen

> Patten et al., 1986

hydrocephalus

> Patten et al., 1986

externalized meninges and brain[c]

> Patten et al., 1986

meningomyelocele[c]

> Patten et al., 1986

scoliosis

> Patten et al., 1986

spinal dysraphism

> Patten et al., 1986

thoracoabdominoschisis

> Patten et al., 1986

small thorax

> Patten et al., 1986

bradycardia

> Patten et al., 1986

abdominoschisis

> Patten et al., 1986

kidneys not visualized[c]

> Patten et al., 1986

amnion continuous with body wall
    Patten et al., 1986
short umbilical cord
    Patten et al., 1986
exstrophy of the bladder[c]
    Patten et al., 1986
malformed pelvis[c]
    Patten et al., 1986
only two extremities present
    Patten et al., 1986
absent lower extremity
    Patten et al., 1986
femoral lengths unequal
    Patten et al., 1986
bilateral clubfeet[c]
    Patten et al., 1986
amniotic bands adherent to fetus
    Patten et al., 1986
oligohydramnios
    Patten et al., 1986
hydramnios
    Patten et al., 1986; Grange et al., 1987
intrauterine growth retardation
    Grange et al., 1987

PD 191950 LOWE OCULOCEREBRORENAL (Lowe syndrome;
Oculocerebrorenal syndrome) (McKusick No. 309000)

Syndrome Note: The major features of Lowe oculocerebrorenal syndrome, an X-linked recessive condition, include cataract, hydrophthalmia, nystagmus, renal tubular acidosis, renal failure, generalized aminoaciduria and proteinuria, vitamin D-resistant rickets, and mental retardation. The gene for the condition is located at Xq26.1. Female carriers may have lens opacities and amnioaciduria.
    McKusick, 1996
Alpha-fetoprotein[c]: elevated in amniotic fluid
    Steele et al., 1993
    elevated in maternal serum
        Steele et al., 1993
Ultrasound[i]: bilateral cataracts
    Steele et al., 1993

PD 192000 LYMPHEDEMA (Atresia of lymphatic system) (McKusick No.
Unknown; see 153100)

Ultrasound: low-amplitude echoes surrounding the fetal head and trunk
    Adam et al., 1979

PD 192040 MARDEN–WALKER SYNDROME (McKusick No. 248700)

Syndrome Note: The Marden-Walker syndrome, an autosomal recessive condition, has as major features blepharophimosis, micrognathia, cleft palate, immobile facies, kyphoscoliosis, limb contractures, arachnodactyly, renal anomalies, and psychomotor retardation. Death usually occurs in the first year.

Ben-Neriah et al., 1995; McKusick, 1995

Prenatal Diagnosis: Discovery of renal abnormalities, IUGR, and/or other characteristics of the condition in an at-risk fetus is presumptive evidence for the diagnosis.

Differential Diagnosis: Blepharophimosis–epicanthus inversus–ptosis syndrome (McKusick No. 110100); Myotonia with skeletal abnormalities and mental retardation (McKusick No. 255710); Schwartz–Jampel syndrome (PD 271075); see also Intrauterine growth retardation in the Index.

Ultrasound[i]: unilateral multiple renal cysts, enlarged kidney

Ben-Neriah et al., 1995

intrauterine growth retardation

Ben-Neriah et al., 1995

Comments: After termination, the fetus reported by Ben-Neriah and associates (1995) was found to have micrognathia, apparent low-set and rotated ears, long and slender fingers, and left kidney hydronephrosis that contained cysts. The cysts on microscopic examination were secondary to focal cystic dysplasia.

PD 192080 McKUSICK–KAUFMAN SYNDROME
(Hydrometrocolpos–polydactyly syndrome; Kaufman–McKusick syndrome)
(McKusick No. 236700)

Syndrome Note: The cardinal features of this syndrome are hydrometrocolpos, postaxial polydactyly, and an autosomal recessive mode of inheritance. The hydrometrocolpos may produce obstruction of the bladder and urethra, and oligohydramnios. The dilation of the urinary tract may lead to renal damage. In addition there may be lung hypoplasia resulting from the oligohydramnios and/or perhaps lung compression by the diaphragm. Additional features may include eye defects; congenital heart anomalies; syndactyly; congenital dislocation of the hips; leg edema; vaginal septation, stenosis, or atresia; imperforate anus; vesicovaginal or rectovaginal fistulas; and Hirschsprung disease. Males may also be affected but usually have only polydactyly.

Chitayat et al., 1987

Prenatal Diagnosis: In the fetus at risk, the presence of a retrovesical mass or polydactyly should be sufficient to establish the diagnosis. In a fetus with no family history of the disorder, the diagnosis should be considered anytime there is a retrovesical or other pelvic mass.

Differential Diagnosis: Hydrometrocolpos (PD 191350); Fetal ovarian cyst (PD 274000); Mesenteric cysts; Anterior meningoceles, solid ovarian tumors, sacral tumors such as Chondroma, Chordoma, teratomas (Teratoma, sacrococcygeal [PD 284000]), Distended rectum

Romero et al., 1988, p. 307

Maternal history[c,d]: decreased fetal movements

Haspeslagh et al., 1981

Ultrasound[c,d]: pleural effusion, small thorax

Hutcheon et al., 1984; Chitayat et al., 1987

ascites

Hutcheon et al., 1984; Chitayat et al., 1987; Brady et al., 1989

large distended cystic mass in the lower abdomen or pelvis
>Haspeslagh et al., 1981; Brady et al., 1989

hydrops fetalis in the absence of a large pelvic mass
>Rosen and Bocian, 1989a; Rosen and Bocian, 1989b

hydronephrosis
>Hutcheon et al., 1984; Chitayat et al., 1987; Brady et al., 1989

hydrops fetalis
>Haspeslagh et al., 1981; Rosen and Bocian, 1989b

hydroureter
>Brady et al., 1989

ureteropelvic junction obstruction
>Rosen and Bocian, 1989a; Rosen and Bocian, 1989b

persistent visualization of the fetal bladder
>Rosen and Bocian, 1989b

distended bladder and urachus
>Hutcheon et al., 1984; Chitayah et al., 1987

intrauterine death
>Haspeslagh et al., 1981

hydramnios
>Rosen and Bocian, 1989a; Rosen and Bocian, 1989b

PD 192140 MECKEL SYNDROME (Dysencephalia splanchnocystica; Gruber syndrome; Meckel–Gruber syndrome) (McKusick No. 249000)

Syndrome Note: Meckel syndrome is a rare dysmorphic condition that is inherited in an autosomal recessive mode. The major features of the disorder include occipital encephalocele, postaxial polydactyly, multicystic kidneys, cleft lip and palate, portal fibrosis of the liver, and bile ductular proliferation. The phenotype is quite variable even within the same family.
>Shen-Schwarz and Dave, 1988

Prenatal Diagnosis: The finding of an encephalocele, enlarged and cystic kidneys, or cleft lip/cleft palate in a fetus at risk for this condition makes the diagnosis likely; finding two or more of these abnormalities makes the diagnosis highly probable.

Differential Diagnosis: Alstrom syndrome (retinitis pigmentosa, obesity, diabetes mellitus, and perceptive deafness); Bardet–Biedl syndrome (PD 186500); Biemond syndrome II (iris coloboma, hypogenitalism, obesity, polydactyly, and mental retardation); Cerebrorenodigital syndrome (PD 188750); Hydrolethalus syndrome (PD 191300); Laurence–Moon syndrome (mental retardation, pigmentary retinopathy, hypogenitalism, and spastic paraplegia); Short rib–polydactyly syndromes (PD 169250, PD 169500, PD 170000, PD 171000); Smith–Lemli–Opitz syndrome (PD 194160); Trisomy 13 syndrome, PD 103000
>Creech et al., 1988; McKusick, 1988

Acetylcholinesterase[c]: elevated in amniotic fluid, fast-migrating amniotic fluid isozyme
>Rehder and Labbe, 1981; Voigtlander et al., 1981; Schmidt and Kubli, 1982; Aitken et al., 1984b; Toftager-Larsen et al., 1984; Shen-Schwarz and Dave, 1988

Alpha-fetoprotein[c]: elevated in amniotic fluid
>Friedrich et al., 1979; Fryns et al., 1980; Verjaal et al., 1980; Karjalainen et al., 1981; Rehder and Labbe, 1981; Schmidt and Kubli, 1982; Shen-Schwarz and Dave, 1988

elevated in maternal serum
>   Rehder and Labbe, 1981; Aitken et al., 1984b

Amniocentesis: rapidly adhering cells in 20-hour culture of amniotic fluid cells[c]
>   Nevin et al., 1979; Fryns et al., 1980

identification of uncultured glial cells (one type of rapidly adhering cells) in amniotic fluid by use of glial fibrillary acidic protein-specific antibodies[c]
>   von Koskull, 1984

elevated pregnancy-specific beta$_1$-glycoprotein (SP1) in amniotic fluid[c]
>   Heikinheimo et al., 1982; Heikinheimo et al., 1984

elevated hCG in amniotic fluid[c]
>   Heikinheimo et al., 1982

elevated alkaline phosphatase activity in amniotic fluid[c]
>   Jalanko et al., 1983

decreased percentage of lens culinaris agglutinin reacting to amniotic fluid AFP[c]
>   Toftager-Larsen et al., 1984

elevated levels of alpha-2-macroglobulin in amniotic fluid[c]
>   Toftager-Larsen et al., 1984

decreased levels of amniotic fluid trypsin inhibitor[c]
>   Kolho, 1986

unable to perform amniocentesis because of oligohydramnios[c]
>   Verjaal et al., 1980

Amniography: encephalocele, amniotic bands
>   Kaffe et al., 1977b; Balsam and Weiss, 1981

Maternal examination[c]: fetal tachycardia, oligohydramnios
>   Summers and Donnenfeld, 1995

uterine size smaller than normal for gestational age
>   Verjaal et al., 1980

Ultrasound: encephalocele, microcephaly, enlarged ventricles, polycystic kidneys, enlarged kidneys, oligohydramnios, distended abdomen
>   Kaffe et al., 1977b; Seller, 1978; Fryns et al., 1980; Rehder and Labbe, 1981; Wapner et al., 1981; Schmidt and Kubli, 1982; Chervenak et al., 1983b; Gruenewald et al., 1984; Johnson and Holzwarth, 1984; Zerres et al., 1984

ventriculomegaly[c]
>   Drugan et al., 1989a

encephalocele
>   Gembruch and Hansmann, 1988; Shen-Schwarz and Dave, 1988

cerebellar vermis aplasia consistent with the Dandy-Walker malformation
>   Summers and Donnenfeld, 1995

posterior fossa cyst consistent with the Dandy–Walker malformation
>   Summers and Donnenfeld, 1995

abnormal anechoic intracranial cystic lesion[g,i]
>   Pachi et al., 1989

hydrocephalus
>   Summers and Donnenfeld, 1995

skull defect in the occipital region through which part of the brain and meninges was protruding into the amniotic cavity
>   Pachi et al., 1989

macrocephaly[c,h]
>Al-Gazali et al., 1996

interventricular septal defect[c]
>Chervenak et al., 1983b

cardiac wall thickening
>Summers and Donnenfeld, 1995

hexadactyly of hands and feet
>Gembruch and Hansmann, 1988

chest circumference less than the fifth percentile[c]
>Nimrod et al., 1986

distended fetal abdomen secondary to enlarged polycystic kidneys
>Hill et al., 1988b

cystic liver[c]
>Chervenak et al., 1983b

no filling of the urinary bladder after instillation of artificial amniotic fluid into the amniotic cavity[c]
>Gembruch and Hansmann, 1988

enlarged and/or polycystic kidneys
>Hill et al., 1988b; Shen-Schwarz and Dave, 1988; Murphy et al., 1989; Pachi et al., 1989; Summers and Donnenfeld, 1995

decreased fetal movements[c]
>Johnson and Holzwarth, 1984; Schmidt and Kubli, 1984

oligohydramnios[c]
>Verjaal et al., 1980; Nimrod et al., 1986; Gembruch and Hansmann et al., 1988; Hill et al., 1988b; Summers and Donnenfeld, 1995

intrauterine growth retardation[c]
>Nimrod et al., 1986

large for gestational age
>Leonard, 1989

PD 192500 MEDIAN CLEFT FACE SYNDROME (Frontonasal dysostosis; Frontonasal dysplasia) (McKusick No. 136760)

Syndrome Note: Median cleft face syndrome, a condition that normally is not inherited, is characterized by a widow's peak, anterior cranium bifidum occultum, ocular and orbital hypertelorism, broad nasal root, median facial clefts of the nose and/or lip, and in some cases malformations of the central nervous system and mental retardation
>Stevens and Qumsiyeh, 1995

Prenatal Diagnosis: The condition should be suspected when orbital hypertelorism with or without a cleft of the upper lip is discovered. Craniofacial measurements might be helpful in demonstrating the median facial clefting (Escobar et al., 1988).

Differential Diagnosis: Cleidocranial dysplasia (PD 151000)

Ultrasound[d]: orbital hypertelorism (increased inner and outer orbital distances), cleft lip (with protruding mass) without cleft palate, severe hydrocephalus, macrocephaly
>Chervenak et al., 1984b

hydramnios
>Stevens and Qumsiyeh, 1995

Comment: The patient reported by Stevens and Qumsiyeh (1995) appeared to have a balanced chromosome abnormality: 46,XY,t(7;3)(3;11)(7pter7q21.3::3q27;3qter;3pter3q23::11q21;11qter; 11pter11q21::3q23;3q27::7q21.3;7qter.

PD 192550 MICROCEPHALY–MICROGNATHIA–INTRAUTERINE GROWTH RETARDATION SYNDROME (McKusick No. None)

Syndrome Note: Majoor-Krakauer and co-workers (1987) described a female infant with a Seckel-like syndrome consisting of microcephaly; abnormal gyral development; small, dysplastic, low-set protruding ears; beak-like nose; extreme micrognathia; and neonatal death. The pregnancy was complicated by IUGR and oligohydramnios.

In a subsequent pregnancy by the same parents, a male fetus was found to be affected with the same condition. The pregnancy was terminated; in addition to the above features, he had malrotation of the large intestines, bifid scrotum, and hypospadias.

Prenatal Diagnosis: microcephaly, micrognathia, and IUGR in a fetus at risk

Ultrasound[i]: IUGR, microcephaly, reduced abdominal circumference, reduced femur and tibia–fibula lengths, extreme micrognathia, oligohydramnios

Majoor-Krakauer et al., 1987

PD 192600 MICROGASTRIA–LIMB REDUCTION ASSOCIATION

(Microgastria–limb reduction complex; Microgastria–limb reduction defects association) (McKusick No. 156810)

Association Note: This association, in addition to having microgastria, consists of limb deficiencies that include hypoplastic forearm, hand, and wrist; absent thumb; absent radius and ulna; absent arm with digital deficiency; or other combination limb-deficiency abnormalities; cardiovascular malformations; asplenia; dysplastic kidneys; ectopic kidney; and increased chromosome breakage. Less frequent anomalies include arhinencephaly, agenesis of the corpus callosum, microphthalmia, esophageal atresia, lung lobation defects, aplasic gall bladder, intestinal malrotation and anal atresia. There appears to be an increased frequency of this disorder in twins. The condition has not been recognized to be inherited.

McKusick, 1994; Lurie et al., 1995b

Prenatal Diagnosis: Has not been established.

Differential Diagnosis: VATER association (PD 194650)

Ultrasound[c,h]: cystic kidneys, IUGR, oligohydramnios

Lurie et al., 1995b

PD 192610 MIRROR IMAGE LIMB DUPLICATION DEFECTS (Fibula and ulna, duplication of, with absence of tibia and radius; Laurin-Sandrow syndrome; Mirror hands and feet with nasal defects; Mirror image duplication of the hands and feet; Sandrow syndrome) (McKusick No. 135750)

Condition Note: The condition presented here has a variable phenotype but basically consists of duplication and absence defects of the extremities. Characteristics described include bilateral cleft nares, grooved columella, dimelia of the ulna and fibula, hypoplasia or absence of the radius and tibia, and mirror image duplication of the hands and feet with both polydactyly and syndactyly being present. The disorder has been inherited in an autosomal dominant fashion in some families.

Hersh et al., 1995; McKusick, 1995

Prenatal Diagnosis: Polysyndactyly and duplication or absence of the long bones of the forearms and lower legs in an at-risk fetus would be evidence for the diagnosis. The diagnosis should be considered in any fetus with absence of a forearm and/or lower leg bone, or with polysyndactyly.

Differential Diagnosis: Weyer syndrome (PD 194700); see also Polydactyly; Radial aplasia, Syndactyly, and Tibia absent in the Index.

Ultrasound[c,d]: bilateral neck masses, short limbs, defects of the hands and foot
Hersh et al., 1995

PD 192620 MOHR SYNDROME (Orofaciodigital syndrome, type II)
(McKusick No. 252100)

Ultrasound[i]: hexadactyly, intraventricular septal defect, hydramnios in a fetus at risk
Iaccarino et al., 1985

PD 192660 MURCS ASSOCIATION (McKusick No. None)

Association Note: The MURCS association consists of the association of mullerian duct aplasia, renal agenesis or dysplasia, and cervicothoracic somite dysplasia. The disorder does not appear to be inherited.

McKusick, 1995; Lin et al., 1996

Prenatal Diagnosis: No method has been established, but the association should be considered whenever renal agenesis is detected.

Differential Diagnosis: Urorectal septum malformation sequence (PD 181000); see also Renal agenesis in the Index.

Ultrasound[c,d]: encephalocele
Lin et al., 1996

bilateral renal agenesis
Lin et al., 1996

> *Comments*: At autopsy, the fetus reported by Lin and associates (1996) in addition to the above findings had heterotopia of the brain cortex, hypoplastic right radius, bowed ulna, absent right thumb, Sprengel deformity, small bladder, absent right ovary, streaked left ovary, absence of the fallopian tubes and uterus, and normal vagina, clitoris and labia. Encephaloceles are not normally seen in the MURCS association.

PD 192700 NEU–LAXOVA SYNDROME (McKusick No. 256520)

Syndrome Note: The Neu–Laxova syndrome is an intrauterine or neonatal lethal autosomal recessive condition characterized by severe IUGR, microcephaly, severe CNS developmental deficiencies, prominent eyes, flexion contractures of the limbs, hypoplastic digits, apparent agenesis of the sacrum, edema, ichthyosis, and abnormal placentation.

Scott et al., 1981; Muller et al., 1987; Tolmie et al., 1987a

Prenatal Diagnosis: Ultrasound detection of two or more of the findings listed below in a fetus at risk should normally be adequate to establish the diagnosis.

Differential Diagnosis: Ichthyosis congenita (PD 197750); Lethal multiple pterygium syndromes (PD 191550, PD 191600, PD 191620, PD 191650, and PD 191800); Pena–Shokeir syndrome, type II (PD 192900)

Maternal urine sampling[c]: reduced excretion of the estriol and placental lactogen in maternal urine

        Scott et al., 1981

Ultrasound: lack of recognizable brain structures, receding forehead, prominent eyes

        Muller et al., 1987

    microcephaly, decreased biparietal diameter[i]

        Muller et al., 1987; Neidich et al., 1987; Tolmie et al., 1987a; Russo et al., 1989

    scalp edema[c]

        Scott et al., 1981; Muller et al., 1987

    bilateral hydrothorax[c]

        Scott et al., 1981

    head-to-abdomen ratio decreased[i]

        Tolmie et al., 1987a

    kyphosis

        Muller et al., 1987; Neidich et al., 1987

    flexion deformities of the fetal limbs[i]

        Scott et al., 1981; Muller et al., 1987; Tolmie et al., 1987a

    edema of the hands and/or feet[c]

        Muller et al., 1987; Neidich et al., 1987

    thickening of the skin[e]

        Russo et al., 1989

    hydrops fetalis[c]

        Curry et al., 1983

    arthrogryposis[c]

        Neidich et al., 1987

    no movements of the extremities[c]

        Muller et al., 1987

    feeble and jerking movements of the head and trunk, webbing at the knees and elbows[c]

        Scott et al., 1981; Muller et al., 1987

    intrauterine growth retardation[i]

        Scott et al., 1981; Muller et al., 1987; Tolmie et al., 1987a; Russo et al., 1989

    hydramnios[c]

        Scott et al., 1981; Muller et al., 1987; Russo et al., 1989

    oligohydramnios[c,i]

        Tolmie et al., 1987a

PD 192750 NOONAN SYNDROME (McKusick No. 163950)

Syndrome Note: Noonan syndrome's major features include short stature, facial anomalies, webbing of the neck, congenital heart defects, and mental retardation in some individuals. The condition is inherited as an autosomal dominant disorder in most families. Commonly, edema may be present at birth and is felt to be the pathogenesis of the phenotype in large part. Not uncommonly, hydramnios is present during pregnancy, but the cause for this problem is not known.

        Witt et al., 1987

Prenatal Diagnosis: Hydrops fetalis and hydramnios in a pregnancy of a fetus at risk is highly suggestive of the diagnosis. The diagnosis should be considered in any fetus with cystic hygroma and/or hydrops fetalis who is shown to be chromosomally normal. In suspected cases of Noonan syndrome, it may be helpful to examine the parents to determine if they have any features of the disorder.

Differential Diagnosis: Turner syndrome (PD 105000), is the primary other condition to consider when either cystic hygroma and/or hydrops fetalis is detected in the fetus. However, the differential should include the other conditions listed under Cystic hygroma and Hydrops fetalis in the Index.

Amniocentesis: reduced level of amniotic fluid glucose[c]
> Weiss et al., 1985

Ultrasound[i]: cystic hygroma, hydrops fetalis.
> Witt et al., 1984; Witt et al., 1987; Olney et al., 1989b
> *Comment:* Each affected fetus reported by Witt and associates (1984) had a parent who was recognized to have the condition.

scalp edema
> Witt et al., 1987; Olney et al., 1989

nuchal edema (nuchal translucency of greater than 3.5 cm)
> Brady et al., 1995

thickened subcutaneous tissue and folds of skin in the nuchal region[c,h]
> Donnai, 1989

pericardial effusion[c,d]
> Olney et al., 1989

pleural effusions[c,d]
> Bawle and Black, 1986; Witt et al., 1987

dilated inferior vena cava[c,h]
> Donnai, 1989

ascites
> Witt et al., 1987; Olney et al., 1989

marked dilation of the renal pelvis (calicectasis) bilaterally without detectable urinary tract obstruction postpartum
> Reuss et al., 1988

hydramnios[c,d]
> Bawle and Black, 1986; Witt et al., 1987

PD 192770 NORRIE DISEASE (Atrophia bulborum hereditaria; Microcephaly–vitreoretinal dysplasia; Vitreoretinal dysplasia, X-linked) (McKusick No. 310600)

Disease Note: Norrie disease is an X-linked recessive condition characterized by retinal dysplasia in hemizygous males and homozygous females, and leads to blindness at birth. Other abnormalities include microphthalmia, shallow anterior chamber, posterior synechia of the eye, hypoplastic iris, retinal folds, retinal detachment, cataract, microcephaly, mental retardation (25–40%), and severe sensorineural deafness (25–35%). The gene has been localized to the p11.3 region of the X chromosome.
> Ellsworth et al., 1990, pp. 1258–1259

Prenatal Diagnosis: The prenatal diagnosis of this condition has been made by linking the gene to a restriction-fragment-length polymorphism (RFLP) identified by the DNA probe L1.28 at DXS7.
> Curtis et al., 1989a

Differential Diagnosis: Encephaloretinal dysplasia; Oculopalatocerebral dwarfism; Retinal dysplasia; Trisomy 13 syndrome (PD 103000)
Chorionic villus sampling[g,i]: linkage of the gene to an RFLP identified by the DNA probe L1.28
Curtis et al., 1989a

PD 192775 OCULOAURICULOVERTEBRAL SPECTRUM
(Facioauriculovertebral spectrum; First and second branchial arch syndrome; Goldenhar syndrome; Goldenhar–Gorlin syndrome; Hemifacial microsomia; OAV; Oculoauriculovertebral dysplasia) (McKusick No. 257700)

Ultrasound[d]: asymmetric fetal face, absence of left eye, low-set and malformed left external ear, absence of left helix and antihelix
Tamas et al., 1986
hydrocephalus[c]
Saller et al., 1988
hydramnios[c,d]
Tamas et al., 1986

PD 192780 OHDO SYNDROME (Tetraamelia with ectodermal dysplasia and lacrimal duct abnormalities) (McKusick No. 273390)

Syndrome Note: Ohdo and associates (1987) described this condition in a male child and his aborted female sibling. The features noted included tetraamelia, upward slanting palpebral fissures, hypoplastic lacrimal ducts without openings, preauricular pits, prominent and bulbous nose, large and down-turned mouth, cryptorchidism, and mental retardation. The parents were second cousins, making autosomal recessive mode of inheritance likely.
Prenatal Diagnosis: The diagnosis is made by demonstrating amelia in a fetus at risk.
Differential Diagnosis: Tetraamelia, isolated (PD 173550); Tetraamelia syndrome (PD 194180)
Ultrasound[i]: no detectable limbs
Ohdo et al., 1987

PD 192790 OPITZ SYNDROME (BBB syndrome; Hypertelorism–hypospadias syndrome; Hypospadias–hypertelorism syndrome) (McKusick No. 313600)

Ultrasound[i]: orbital hypertelorism, penis very flexed toward scrotum
Hogdall et al., 1989

PD 192800 OPITZ–FRIAS SYNDROME (G syndrome; Hypertelorism–dysphagia syndrome; Oculogenitolaryngeal syndrome; Opitz-G syndrome) (McKusick No. 307100)

Syndrome Note: Opitz–Frias syndrome is a multiple congenital anomalies syndrome of hypertelorism, hypospadias, and laryngeal and tracheoesophageal defects. Brain abnormalities have included hypoplasia or agenesis of the corpus callosum, cerebellar vermal hypoplasia, cortical atrophy, and ventriculomegaly. The condition is considered to be inherited as an autosomal dominant disorder.
MacDonald et al., 1993
Fetoscopy with fetal blood drawing[c]: decreased serum albumin and total protein
Patton et al., 1986

Maternal report[c]: decreased fetal movement
>MacDonald et al., 1993

Ultrasound[c]: hydrops fetalis, pleural effusion, ascites
>Patton et al., 1986

>hydramnios
>>Patton et al., 1986; MacDonald et al., 1993

>oligohydramnios
>>Urioste et al., 1995

>*Comments*: The fetus reported by Urioste and associates (1995) had a terminal deletion of chromosome 13(q23.3qter). The fetus had oligohydramnios because of fetal membrane leakage. After birth, the child had physical abnormalities consistent with the Opitz–Frias syndrome. He also had deficiency of coagulation factors VII and X, genes which are located on 13q34.

PD 192840 OROFACIODIGITAL SYNDROME, TYPE IV (OFD syndrome, Baraitser–Burn type; OFD syndrome, type IV) (McKusick No. 258860)

Syndrome Note: There are now at least eight recognized variants of the orofaciodigital syndrome (OFD). Type IV OFD is characterized by mesomelic limb shortening, tibial dysplasia, hamartomas and lobulation of the tongue, cleft or high-arched palate, postaxial polydactyly of the feet, severe talipes equinovarus, delayed development, and conductive deafness. The disorder is inherited as an autosomal recessive condition.
>Nevin and Thomas, 1989

Prenatal Diagnosis: The identification of two or more of the features listed above in a fetus at risk is probably sufficient to establish the diagnosis.

Differential Diagnosis: The other forms of OFD should be considered (see Mohr syndrome [PD 192620]).
>Jones, 1988; McKusick, 1988

Physical examination[c,d]: hydramnios
>Nevin and Thomas, 1989

PD 192850 OTOPALATODIGITAL SYNDROME, TYPE II (Cranioorodigital syndrome; Faciopalatoosseous syndrome, OPD2) (McKusick No. 304120)

Syndrome Note: The characteristic features of the otopalatodigital syndrome, type II, include conductive deafness, frontal bossing, midfacial hypoplasia, ocular hypertelorism, micrognathia, overlapping deviated fingers, and splayed toes. The disorder is inherited in an X-linked recessive fashion with partial expression in some carrier females. Omphalocele has been reported as an occasional finding in this condition.
>Young et al., 1993; McKusick, 1996

Prenatal Diagnosis: Findings of features seen in the disorder in an at-risk fetus is presumptive evidence for the diagnosis.

Ultrasound: omphalocele[i]
>Young et al., 1993

>curvature of the long bones[c,d]
>>Young et al., 1993

>hydramnios[c]
>>Young et al., 1003

Method not stated[c]: hydramnios
Gendall and Kozlowski, 1992

PD 192860 PALLISTER–HALL SYNDROME (McKusick No. 146510)

Syndrome Note: The major features of Pallister–Hall syndrome include hypothalamic hamartoblastoma, hypopituitarism, postaxial polydactyly, and imperforate anus. Other features also reported include flat midface, dysplastic ears, micrognathia, cleft of the palate and larynx, abnormal lung lobation, endocardial cushion defect, renal agenesis or dysgenesis, microphallus, short fourth metacarpals, nail dysplasia, and IUGR. The anterior pituitary is absent and the hypothalamic tumor may have spread over the inferior surface of the cerebrum extending to the optic chiasma and the interpeduncular fossa. Most infants have died within hours after birth; most have been sporadic in occurrence.
Jones, 1988; McKusick, 1988

Prenatal Diagnosis: No reliable method is available for the prenatal diagnosis of sporadic cases. If there is a recurrence in a subsequent pregnancy, then the finding of any two features should be sufficient to make the diagnosis.

Differential Diagnosis: Cerebroacrovisceral-early lethal (CAVE) phenotype; Hydrolethalus syndrome (PD 191330); Orofaciodigital syndrome, type VI; Smith–Lemli–Opitz syndrome (PD 194160); Townes syndrome (auricular anomalies, duplicated or abnormal thumbs, imperforate anus)

Alpha-fetoprotein[c]: low level in maternal serum
Robinson et al., 1989
Ultrasound[i]: hydrocephalus, polydactyly
Robinson et al., 1989
multiple congenital anomalies that were not specified
Verloes et al., 1995

PD 192900 PENA–SHOKEIR SYNDROME, TYPE II
(Cerebrooculofacioskeletal syndrome; COFS syndrome) (McKusick No. 214150)

Syndrome Note: The Pena–Shokeir syndrome, type II is an autosomal recessive disorder consisting of microcephaly, cataracts, microphthalmia, blepharophimosis, prominent nasal root, large ears, micrognathia with the upper lip positioned over the lower one, kyphosis and/or scoliosis, flexion contractures, camptodactyly, prominent heels, vertical talus, and hypotonia. Death usually occurs within 5 years after birth following a downhill course with failure to thrive and CNS deterioration.
Preus et al., 1977

Prenatal Diagnosis: Recurrence of IUGR and decreased fetal movement in a fetus at risk for this condition should be sufficient evidence for the diagnosis.
Physical examination of the mother[c]: IUGR
Preus et al., 1977
Ultrasound[c,d]: clubfoot deformity
Gershoni-Baruch et al., 1991
Intrauterine growth retardation, no growth of the fetus over 2-week period during the third trimester
Preus et al., 1977

PD 192912 PERLMAN SYNDROME (Renal hamartomas, nephroblastomatosis, and fetal gigantism) (McKusick No. 267000)

Syndrome Note: The main characteristics of the Perlman syndrome include an unusual facies with a depressed nasal bridge, anteverted and inverted V-shaped upper lip, micrognathia, and round facial fullness; bilateral renal hamartomas with or without nephroblastomatosis; macrosomia; hypertrophy of the islets of Langerhans; and early lethality. The condition is inherited in an autosomal recessive mode.

        Greenberg et al., 1986; McKusick, 1996

Paracentesis of the fetal abdomen[c,d]: large cells of unknown origin

        Greenberg et al., 1986

Ultrasound[c,d]: macrocephaly

        Greenberg et al., 1988d

    diaphragmatic hernia

        Greenberg et al., 1988d

    nephromegaly with or without small cysts

        Greenberg et al., 1986; Greenberg et al., 1988d

    fetal ascites

        Greenberg et al., 1986

    macrosomia

        Greenberg et al., 1988d

    hydramnios

        Greenberg et al., 1986

PD 192925 PETERS–PLUS SYNDROME (Krause–Kivlin syndrome; Krause–van Schooneveld–Kivlin syndrome; Peters anomaly with short-limb dwarfism) (McKusick No. 261540)

Syndrome Note: The syndrome cited here has Peters anomaly, a specific anterior chamber cleavage defect of the eye resulting in corneal clouding and variable iridolenticulocorneal adhesions, plus other features. The other features may include macrocephaly or hydrocephaly with cerebral atrophy on CT scan, narrow palpebral fissures with depressed nasal bridge, smooth philtrum, thin upper lip, hearing loss, cleft lip and palate, short hands with tapering fingers, and short limbs. The condition is inherited in an autosomal recessive fashion.

        McKusick, 1995

Prenatal Diagnosis: Diagnostic criteria have not been established; however, any of the physical findings of the syndrome present in an at-risk fetus would be suggestive of the diagnosis.

Differential Diagnosis: Martsolf syndrome; Robinow syndrome (PD 168500); Walker–Warburg syndrome (PD 130750)

Ultrasound[c,d]: growth dficiency

        Jung et al., 1995

Method not stated[c]: hydramnios

        Frydman et al., 1991; Ishikiriyama et al., 1992

PD 192950 PFEIFFER SYNDROME (Acrocephalosyndactyly type V; ACS V; Noack syndrome) (McKusick No. 101600)

Ultrasound: hydrocephalus[h]

        Palumbos and Stierman, 1989

    hydramnios[c,h]

        Bader and Bixler, 1990

PD 193000 PILONIDAL SINUS (McKusick No. Unknown; see 173000)

Alpha-fetoprotein[c]: elevated in amniotic fluid

        Jandial et al., 1976

PD 193030 PITT–ROGERS–DANKS SYNDROME (Pitt syndrome) (McKusick No. 262350)

Syndrome Note: The Pitt–Rogers–Danks syndrome, an apparent autosomal recessive condition, has microcephaly, prominent eyes with telecanthus, short upper lip, wide mouth, pre- and postnatal growth deficiency, and mental retardation.

Oorthuys and Bleeker-Wagemakers, 1989; McKusick, 1996

Method not stated[c,h]: severe IUGR

Oorthuys and Bleeker-Wagemakers, 1989

PD 193100 POLYASPLENIA–CAUDAL DEFICIENCY–AGENESIS OF THE CORPUS CALLOSUM SYNDROME (Poly/asplenia–agenesis of the corpus callosum–caudal deficiency) (McKusick No. None; see 208530)

Syndrome Note: The above condition appears to be distinct from bilateral right-sidedness and left-sidedness sequences (PD 187250 and PD 187230, respectively) in that there is agenesis of the corpus callosum and deficiency of the sacrum and lumbar vertebrae. In some cases, there has been asplenia; others polysplenia. Thus, the term polyasplenia is in the title. The disorder probably is inherited in an autosomal dominant fashion.

Prenatal Diagnosis: The findings of absence of the corpus callosum, complex heart defects, and/or lumbar vertebral and/or sacral dysgenesis in an at-risk fetus would be suggestive of the diagnosis.

Differential Diagnosis: Bilateral left-sidedness sequence (PD 187230); Bilateral right-sidedness sequence (PD 187250); Corpus callosum, partial or complete agenesis (PD 119750 and PD 119700); Hydrolethalus syndrome (PD 191330)

Ultrasound[c,d]: single atrium, short femora

Rodriquez et al., 1991

Comments: The fetus reported by Rodriguez and co-authors (1991) was delivered at 37 weeks of gestation. She had low-set and malformed ears; short neck, trunk, and femora; complex congenital heart problems involving aortic atresia proximally and hypoplasia of the ascending aorta, single atrium and persistent atrioventricular canal, and a patent ductus arteriosus; polysplenia; right-sided spleens, stomach duodenum and pancreas; symmetric liver; malrotation of the bowel; agenesis of the right kidney and ureter; duplication of the uterus and vagina with ambiguous genitalia; imperforate anus; and contractures of the lower extremities. The child died at 2 days of age. On examination of the brain, there was absence of the corpus callosum, anomalies of the cerebral cortex, and heterotopias.

PD 193150 PRADER–WILLI SYNDROME (Prader–Labhart–Willi syndrome; PWS) (McKusick No. 176270)

Condition Note: In the infant with Prader–Willi syndrome, there is usually marked hypotonia, feeding difficulties, hyporeflexia, and cryptorchidism with hypoplastic penis and scrotum in males, or hypoplastic labiae in females. Later in childhood and as adults, these individuals have compulsive eating habits, obesity, small hands and feet, short stature, hypogonadotropic hypogonadism, and mental retardation.

In approximately 70% of cases, the etiology of Prader–Willi syndrome is a deletion of the 15q11,q13 segment with paternal origin of the deleted chromosome, or in about 20% of affected, maternal uniparental disomy (both number

15 chromosomes derived from the mother). If similar deleted chromosome 15 {del(15)(q11q13)} is from the mother, then the child has Angelman syndrome.
> McKusick, 1990

Prenatal Diagnosis: Deletion of 15(q11q13) with fetal structural abnormalities consistent with the Prader–Willi syndrome, or paternally derived deleted 15(q11q13), or maternal uniparental disomy in the fetus would be sufficient to make the diagnosis.

Differential Diagnosis: Angelman syndrome (McKusick No. 105830)

Alpha-fetoprotein[c]: low levels in the maternal serum
> Le Bris-Quillevere et al., 1990

Amniocentesis: karyotype of amniotic fluid cells showed microscopic del(15)(q11q13)
> Le Bris-Quillevere et al., 1990; Toth-Fejel et al., 1995

> de novo inversion of chromosome 15 with breakpoints of (pter q12::q26 q12::q26qter)
> > Toth-Fejel et al., 1995

> demonstration of maternal uniparental heterodisomy of chromosome 15 by DNA analysis of seven informative microsatellite markers using DNA from uncultured amniotic fluid cells and parental blood
> > Wang et al., 1993b; Verp et al., 1995

> > *Comment:* The study reported by Wang and associates (1993b) and Verp and co-workers (1995) was initiated by the finding of trisomy 15 mosaicism (46,XY/47,XY,+15) in two chorionic villus cultures.

> utilizing a modified polymerse chain reaction method and microsatellite analysis on uncultured amniotic fluid cells revealed maternal uniparental disomy
> > Kubota et al., 1996

> > *Comment:* In the fetus reported by Kubola and co-workers (1996), chorionic villus analysis indicated mosaic trisomy 15.

Chorionic villus sampling[c,g]: trisomy 15 mosaicism in short-term cultured chorionic villi
> Wang et al., 1993b; Verp et al, 1995

> *Comment:* See additional information under amniocentesis.

Cordocentesis (PUBS)[d]: del(15)(q11q13) chromosomal abnormality in the fetal white cells
> Le Bris-Quillevere et al., 1990

Ultrasound[c]: reduced femoral length, micrognathia[d], micropenis[d], hypoplastic scrotum[d], reduced fetal movements[d]
> Le Bris-Quillevere et al., 1990

> *Comments:* The fetus reported by Le Bris-Quillevere and associates (1990) was aborted at 29 weeks of gestation. Autopsy findings included abnormally lobulated ears, prominent metopic suture, small saddle-shaped nose, thin upper lip, micrognathia, simian crease, fifth finger clinodactyly, small penis, right unilateral cryptorchidism, and on radiograph, 13 ribs bilaterally. These features were consistent with the diagnosis of Prader–Willi syndrome.

PD 193300 PRIMARY LYMPHATIC MALFORMATION, MIXED VASCULAR TYPE (McKusick No. None)

Physical examination[c,d]: hydramnios
> Windeband et al., 1987

Comments: The child reported on by Windeband and co-workers (1987) had an unusual condition that ultimately led to the death of the child. The child was delivered at 34 weeks of gestation with extensive hydrops fetalis. The placenta also was grossly edematous. The mother was found to be blood group A, Rh-positive, and the child was blood group O, Rh-positive. The albumin level in the child was low—2.2 g/dL (normal 3.5–5.0 g/dL), and hyperbilirubinemia developed at 3 days of age. She was also found to have a normal chromosomal constitution. Later her hemoglobin concentration fell to 5.9 g/dL.

Contrast material injected into the groin of this child showed abnormal abdominal and thoracic lymphatic vessels ending by the right axilla. Labeled red blood cells indicated pooling of cells in lymphatic vessels in the lower half of the body.

After initial improvement and discharge from the hospital, the child became worse with recurrence of the edema, a drop in the plasma albumin level, and progressive renal failure. Chylous fluid was obtained from the subcutaneous tissue. She died at the age of 66 days. Autopsy was refused.

The diagnosis was thought to be a primary lymphatic malformation with abnormal vascular connection leading to abnormal loss of albumin and red blood cells into the lymphatic system.

PD 193400 PROTEUS SYNDROME (McKusick No. 176920)

Condition Note: Proteus syndrome was named after the Greek god Proteus because of this god's polymorphic nature (McKusick, 1992). The disorder is characterized by hydrocephalus; macrocephaly; cranial, facial, and limb asymmetry; retinal detachment; scleral tumors; prognathism; malocclusion; hyperostoses; lymphangioma; lipomata; large hands and feet; macrodactyly; abnormal pigmentation; varicose veins; warty, hyperplastic plantar overgrowth; and mental retardation in some individuals (Winter and Baraitser, 1990). The condition may be inherited as an autosomal dominant disorder in some families.

Prenatal Diagnosis: Not established.

Differential Diagnosis: Klippel–Trenaunay–Weber syndrome (PD 191530); Maffucci syndrome, Neurofibromatosis, tye I (PD 269250); Ollier disease

Ultrasound: hydramnios[c]

Ram and Noor, 1993

PD 193450 PSEUDOTRISOMY 13 SYNDROME

(Holoprosencephaly–polydactyly syndrome) (McKusick No. 264480)

Syndrome Note: As the name implies, pseudotrisomy 13 syndrome has a similar phenotype to that of trisomy 13 syndrome (PD 103000). The major features of pseudotrisomy 13 syndrome include holoprosencephaly with associated facial abnormalities, pre- and postaxial polydactyly, congenital heart defects, and a normal chromosomal constitution. The inheritance is probably autosomal recessive.

Norman and Donnai, 1991; Boles et al., 1992; McKusick, 1996

Ultrasound[c]: holoprosencephaly

Boles et al., 1992

cleft lip

Boles et al., 1992

cleft palate
Norman and Donnai, 1991
atrioventricular canal
Boles et al., 1992
polydactyly
Norman and Donnai, 1991
intrauterine growth retardation
Boles et al., 1992

PD 193520 RADIAL–RENAL SYNDROME (Acrorenal syndrome) (McKusick No. 179280)

Syndrome Note: Radial–renal syndrome consists of bilateral absence of the radius and thumb, external ear malformations, renal anomalies, and short stature. The exact mode of inheritance has not been determined. The disorder may be heterogeneous.
McKusick, 1986
Continuous-wave Doppler evaluation[c,d]: increased peripheral arterial resistance
Meizner et al., 1987
Ultrasound: absent thumb and radius, shortened ulna with lateral deviation of hand, both kidneys on the left side (crossed renal ectopia)
Meizner et al., 1986b

PD 193540 RAG SYNDROME (McKusick No. None)

Syndrome Note: RAG syndrome consists of *R*obin sequence, *a*niridia, and severe *g*rowth and developmental delay; it appears to be inherited in an autosomal recessive mode.
Saal et al., 1986
Ultrasound[c,d]: severe IUGR, oligohydramnios
Saal et al., 1986

PD 193550 REUSS SYNDROME (Cystic kidney disease with ventriculomegaly; Ventriculomegaly–cystic kidney syndrome) (McKusick No. 219730)

Syndrome Note: Reuss and associates (1989) described an apparently new syndrome characterized by ventriculomegaly and normal-sized cystic kidneys. On microscopic examination of the kidneys, a pattern of cystic dilatation of the renal tubules that could not be classified according to the Potter classification was seen. On prenatal ultrasonic examination, the kidneys were of normal size but very echodense, the amniotic fluid volume was normal, and the AFP was elevated. Acetylcholinesterase also was present in the amniotic fluid.

Five affected fetuses and one premature stillborn were reported by Reuss and colleagues (1989) from two sets of consanguineous parents from the same family. The inheritance of this disorder appears to be by an autosomal recessive mode.

Prenatal Diagnosis: The diagnosis appears to be established by the prenatal detection of ventriculomegaly, normal-sized but echodense kidneys, and elevated levels of AFP and acetylcholinesterase in amniotic fluid in fetuses at risk.

Differential Diagnosis: Congenital nephrosis, Finnish type (PD 176000) is associated with elevated amniotic fluid AFP and acetylcholinesterase; Meckel syndrome (PD 192140) is associated with encephalocele, polycystic kidney disease, and polydactyly. Other conditions in the differential diagnosis include Smith–Lemli–Opitz syndrome (PD 194160); Zellweger syndrome (PD 234500), and other conditions associated with hydrocephaly (see Hydrocephaly in the Index).

Alpha-fetoprotein[c,i]: elevated levels in the amniotic fluid
>Reuss et al., 1989

Acetylcholinesterase[c,i]: rapid-migrating isozyme present on polyacrylamide gel electrophoresis
>Reuss et al., 1989

Ultrasound[i]: ventriculomegaly; normal-sized, very echodense kidneys; hydramnios
>Reuss et al., 1989

PD 193555 RICHARDSON–KIRK SYNDROME (Hypoparathyroidism with short stature, mental retardation, and seizures) (McKusick No. 241410)

Syndrome Note: Richardson and Kirk (1990) have reported eight children, four girls and four boys, who had hypoparathyroidism, extreme failure to thrive, and developmental delay, and who were dysmorphic. All were offspring of consanguineous matings. Dysmorphic features included microcephaly, deep-set eyes, depressed nasal bridge with beaked nose, long philtrum, thin upper lip, micrognathia and large floppy ear lobes. In addition there were low birth weight, hypocalcemia associated with low parahormone levels, reduced numbers of T cells and medullary bone stenosis in most. Other similar cases have been reported (McKusick, 1994).

Prenatal Diagnosis: None has been established.

Differential Diagnosis: Kenny–Caffey syndrome (McKusick No. 24460); DiGeorge syndrome (PD 100995)

Maternal urine testing[c,h]: low urinary estriol levels
>Richardson and Kirk, 1990

PD 193560 RITSCHER–SCHINZEL SYNDROME (Cranio–cerebello–cardiac dysplasia; Dandy–Walker-like malformation with atrioventricular septal defect; 3C syndrome) (McKusick No. 220210)

Syndrome Note: The major characteristics of this syndrome include a distinct facial appearance with ocular colobomata, ocular hypertelorism, and apparent low-set ears; short neck; congenital heart defects; hand anomalies; and macrocephaly with posterior fossa malformations. The condition appears to be inherited in an autosomal recessive mode.
>Marles et al, 1995

Ultrasound[i]: hypertelorism, abnormalities of the posterior fossa resembling a Dandy–Walker malformation, oligohydramnios
>Marles et al., 1995

PD 193570 ROBERTS SYNDROME (Appelt–Gerken–Lenz syndrome; Pseudothalidomide syndrome; SC phocomelia) (McKusick No. 268300, 269000)

Syndrome Note: The salient features of this disorder include severe phocomelia of all limbs, and bilateral cleft lip and palate. Other features include severe growth deficiency, mental retardation in survivors, absent or malformed thumbs, and cryptorchidism. Cytogenetically there is premature separation of the centromeres. It is inherited as an autosomal recessive disorder.
>Smith, 1982; Romke et al., 1987

Prenatal Diagnosis: The presence of limb reduction deformity, cleft lip and palate, and premature separation of the centromeres in an isolated case, or any one of these features in a fetus at risk should be sufficient to establish the diagnosis.

Alpha-fetoprotein[c]: elevated in maternal serum
> Stanley et al., 1988

Amniocentesis: poorly defined centromeres with G-banding
> Willner et al., 1979

> localized repulsion of sister chromatids
>> Stanley et al., 1988

> puffed-out centromeres with both C- and G-banding
>> Willner et al., 1979; Stanley et al., 1988

>> *Comments:* The patient reported by Stanley and colleagues (1988) had birth weight, length, and head circumference below the fifth percentiles; nevus flammeus lesions over the nose and upper lip; and cystic lesions in the right kidney that were detected by postnatal ultrasound. At 11 months he was noted to have brachycephaly, a round face, anteverted nares, micrognathia, and short wide feet with mild metatarsus adductus deformities. Because this patient did not have a cleft lip/palate or reduction in limb length, the diagnosis of Roberts syndrome is suspect.

> premature centromere separation
>> Stanley et al., 1988; Stioui et al., 1992

Chorionic villus sampling[g,i]: premature centromere separation on cytogenetic analysis of chorionic villi
> Stioui et al., 1992; Otano et al., 1993

Ultrasound: hydrocephalus
> Palumbos and Stierman, 1989

> shortened and/or absent long bones of the extremities, polycystic kidneys, oligohydramnios, nonvisualization of bladder, growth deficiency, premaxillary protuberance or swelling, claw-like deformity of distal extremity, phocomelia
>> Kaffe et al., 1977b; Hobbins et al., 1979; Willner et al., 1979; Hobbins et al., 1982; Romke et al., 1987

> tetraphocomelia[i]
>> Otano et al., 1993

> humeroradial synostosis
>> Stioui et al., 1992

PD 193600 ROBIN SEQUENCE (Pierre Robin syndrome) (McKusick No. Unknown; see 261800)

Sequence Note: The primary defect in the Robin sequence appears to be hypoplasia and/or shortening of the mandible. This defect in turn causes the tongue to be uplifted and posteriorly positioned. The uplifting causes the tongue to mechanically block the fusion of the lateral palatine shelves with the nasal septum in the midline. As a result the child is born with micrognathia, glossoptosis, and a U-shaped cleft palate. Major, if not life-threatening, airway obstruction problems may result from the glossoptosis. Fortunately, many children with this condition have catch-up growth of their mandible during the first year of life, and the respiratory problem disappears. The cause of the micrognathia has not been established.

Romero et al., 1988 pp. 109–110

Prenatal Diagnosis: The diagnosis should be considered whenever micrognathia is discovered prenatally, particularly when the abnormality is associated with oligohydramnios. Because about 60% of infants with the Robin sequence have other findings, additional physical defects should be sought in the fetus discovered to have micrognathia.

Differential Diagnosis: There is a large number of syndromes which have the Robin sequence as a feature. The syndrome most frequently associated with the Robin sequence is Stickler syndrome. If shortened limbs are associated findings, Spondyloepiphyseal dysplasia congenita (PD 173500) and Diastrophic dysplasia (PD 154000) should be considered.

Ultrasound[c,d]: micrognathia
> Bundy et al., 1986b; Pilu et al., 1986

cleft in the palate
> Bundy et al., 1986b

nonvisualization of the fetal stomach
> Bundy et al., 1986b

hydramnios
> Bundy et al., 1986b

PD 193610 RUSSELL–SILVER SYNDROME (Silver syndrome; Silver–Russell dwarfism; Silver–Russell syndrome) (McKusick No. 270050)

Syndrome Note: Pre- and postnatal growth deficiency, and a small triangular face with a normal head size are the usual features of the Russell–Silver syndrome. Variable features include body asymmetry, clinodactyly and shortening of the fifth finger, and cafe-au-lait spots. The condition is usually sporadic in an otherwise phenotypically normal family. However, autosomal dominant inheritance with variable expressivity and an X-linked recessive form have been reported in some families.

Jones, 1988

Prenatal Diagnosis: None has been established.

Differential Diagnosis: Any condition that is associated with intrauterine growth deficiency should be considered in the differential (see Intrauterine growth deficiency in the Index). In addition 18p- syndrome should be considered as a diagnostic possibility.

Ultrasound[c,d]: discordant in size of monozygotic twins at 28 weeks' gestation
> Samn et al., 1989; Samn et al., 1990

PD 193620 RUTLEDGE SYNDROME (Rutledge lethal multiple congenital anomaly) (McKusick No. 268670)

Syndrome Note: Rutledge and co-authors (1984) described a lethal malformation syndrome in three children that appears to be distinct from the Smith–Lemli–Opitz syndrome (PD 194160). Major features of this condition include closed fontanels; cerebellar hypoplasia; V-shaped upper lip; microglossia with inclusion cysts of the tongue; high arched palate; micrognathia; webbed neck; congenital heart defect; pulmonary, laryngeal and gallbladder hypoplasia; polydactyly; mesomelic shortening of the limbs; and clubfeet. All three children died within the first 2 weeks after birth. The disorder is inherited as an autosomal recessive condition.

Prenatal Diagnosis: Criteria for prenatal diagnosis have not been established; however, the findings of features of the syndrome in an at-risk fetus would be suggestive of the diagnosis.

Differential Diagnosis: Diastrophic dysplasia (PD 154000); Smith–Lemli–Opitz syndrome (PD 194160)

Ultrasound[c,d]: shortened humerus, IUGR
Rutledge et al., 1984

PD 193624 SCHINZEL–GIEDION SYNDROME (Schinzel–Giedion midface-retraction syndrome) (McKusick No. 269150)

Syndrome Note: The major features of this syndrome include severe midface retraction, congenital heart defect, hydronephrosis, hypertrichosis, clubfeet, multiple telangiectases over the nose and cheeks, syndactyly, and embryonal tumors. Radiographic changes in the skull include a short and sclerotic base, multiple wormian bones, wide cranial sutures and fontanels, and increased density of the long bones. Death may occur in the neonatal period, and those that live usually develop intractable seizures and spasticity, and have severe growth and developmental retardation.

Antich et al., 1995; McKusick, 1995

Prenatal Diagnosis: None has been established. Hydronephrosis and hydramnios in the at-risk child would be presumptive evidence for the diagnosis

Ultrasound[c,d]: hydronephrosis, hydramnios
Antich et al., 1995

PD 193630 SECKEL SYNDROME (Bird-head dwarfism) (McKusick No. 210600)

Ultrasound: microcephaly, prominent nose, hypoplastic face, severe IUGR
de Elejalde and Elejalde, 1984

PD 193750 SEQUESTRATION OF LUNG (Accessory lung; Bronchopulmonary sequestration; Pulmonary extralobar sequestration) (McKusick No. None)

Condition Note: A sequestered lobe of lung is an abnormal and nonaerated mass of extra lung tissue in which the blood supply is usually derived from systemic rather than pulmonary sources. Furthermore, the dysplastic lung segment does not communicate with the rest of the bronchial tree. The sequestered lung may be either intralobar or extra lobar. Other congenital defects may be present in 15–40% of cases. When hydrops fetalis is present, the fetus usually succumbs shortly after birth from pulmonary hypoplasia.

Weiner et al., 1986; Reece et al., 1987; Romero et al., 1988, pp. 202–205

Prenatal Diagnosis: Extralobar lung sequestration should be considered whenever there is a discrete echodense or echogenic, intrathoracic, or intraabdominal mass.

Reece et al., 1987; Romero et al., 1988, pp. 203–204

Differential Diagnosis: Congenital bronchial cyst (PD 272380); Cystic adenomatoid malformation of lung (PD 272500); Hamartoma of the lung; Mesoblastic nephroma (PD 276750); Sequestration of lung (PD 193750); Teratoma, lung (PD 281750); Teratoma, mediastinal (PD 281770)

Prenatal Treatment: The experience is limited with this condition, but the method of choice when there is pleural effusion present that is causing mediastinal shift and associated with hydrops fetalis would be pleuroamniotic shunt (Weiner et al., 1986).

Treatment Modality: Transcutaneous fetal pleuroamniotic shunting
Weiner et al., 1986

Methods and Findings: Ultrasound: mass impinging on the mediastinum and heart, hypoplastic lungs
Kleinman et al., 1982; Weiner et al., 1986
hydrothorax[c,d]
Reece et al., 1987; Romero et al., 1988, p. 204; Slotnick et al., 1990
increase echogenicity of portions of the left lung
Slotnick et al., 1990
severe compression of the pulmonary structures and downward displacement of the diaphragm
Slotnick et al., 1990
echo-dense mass in the chest[c,d]
Mayden et al., 1984; Reece et al., 1987; Romero et al., 1988, p. 204
left-side homogeneous echogenic thoracic mass
Bernier et al., 1995
uniformly echogenic dense retroperitoneal mass in the right upper quadrant of the abdomen[c,d]
Mariona et al., 1986
displacement of the heart to the right hemithorax[c]
Slotnick et al., 1990; Bernier et al., 1995
pleural effusion
Weiner et al., 1986
ascites
Slotnick et al., 1990
bilateral hydrocele
Slotnick et al., 1990
hydrops fetalis[c,d]
Kleinman et al., 1982; Mayden et al., 1984; Weiner et al., 1986; Slotnick et al., 1990
hydramnios
Weiner et al., 1986; Slotnick et al., 1990

PD 193850 SHPRINTZEN–GOLDBERG SYNDROME (Marfanoid craniosynostosis syndrome; Shprintzen–Goldberg craniosynostosis syndrome) (McKusick No. 182212)

Syndrome Note: The Shprintzen–Goldberg syndrome is the combination of a marfanoid phenotype and craniosynostosis, in particular a cloverleaf skull (kleeblattschadel). Specific other features include exophthalmos, low-set ears, hypoplasia of the maxilla and mandible, hyperplasia of the soft palatal tissue, pectus carinatum, multiple abdominal hernias, arachnodactyly, and camptodactyly. Neurologically, there is hypotonia and mental retardation. One patient at the age of 18 years had a dilated aortic root that progressed to aortic dissection, rupture, and death.
McKusick, 1985; Saal et al., 1995

Prenatal Diagnosis: No definitive method exists to establish the diagnosis. Clover-leaf skull in the at-risk fetus would be presumptive evidence for the diagnosis. **Differential Diagnosis:** Amniotic band disruption sequence (PD 185000); Antley–Bixler syndrome (PD 185500); Apert syndrome (PD 148500); Congenital contractural arachnodactyly; Crouzon syndrome (PD 153200); Kleeblattschadel syndrome (PD 161000); Marfan syndrome (PD 267470); Pfeiffer syndrome (PD 192950); Short rib–polydactyly syndrome, Beemer–Langer type (PD 169220); Thanatophoric dysplasia (PD 174000)

Ultrasound[c,d]: abnormally shaped skull including bulged appearance of the frontal and temporal bones, and unusually flattened occiput; hydrocephalus; unusual convolutions of the posterior brain.

Saal et al., 1995

ocular hypertelorism

Saal et al., 1995

PD 193900 SIMPSON–GOLABI–BEHMEL SYNDROME (Golabi–Rosen syndrome; Simpson dysmorphia syndrome) (McKusick No. 312870)

Syndrome Note: The Simpson–Golabi–Behmel syndrome, an X-linked recessive condition, is characterized by pre- and postnatal overgrowth, macrocephaly, coarse facies, upslanting palpebral fissures, large mouth with a central cleft of the lower lip, cleft palate, postaxial polydactyly, hypoplastic index finger, supernumerary nipples, ventricular septal defect, and other abnormalities.

McKusick, 1994

Prenatal Diagnosis: Because features in this syndrome are variable, DNA linkage appears to be the most reliable method of diagnosis. However, detection of birth defects and excessive fetal growth in an at-risk fetus would be strong evidence in favor of the diagnosis.

Alpha-fetoprotein[c]: elevated in maternal serum

Chueh et al., 1993; Hughes-Benzie et al., 1995

Amniocentesis: linkage of gene with polymorphic Xq26 microsatellite markers

Hughes-Benzie et al., 1995

Ultrasound[i]: bilateral cleft lip

Chueh et al., 1993

cystic hygroma of the neck

Chueh et al., 1993

diaphragmatic hernia, right-sided

Chueh et al., 1993

single umbilical artery

Chueh et al., 1993

PD 193910 SIMPSON–GOLABI–BEHMEL SYNDROME, INFANTILE LETHAL VARIANT (McKusick No. None; see 312870)

Syndrome Note: The Simpson–Golabi–Behmel syndrome is an X-linked reces-sive disorder with pre- and postnatal overgrowth, facial anomalies, and various visceral, skeletal, and neurologic abnormalities. Normally the condition is not lethal, and affected individuals are mentally retarded. Listed in this entry is a more severe form characterized by hydrops fetalis, dysplastic kidney, severe neurologic impairment, and death during infancy. This variant has been separated form the milder form because of the severity of the disorder.

Terespolsky et al., 1995

Prenatal Diagnosis: Finding of kidney abnormalities and/or hydrops fetalis in the at-risk fetus is presumptive evidence for the condition.

Differential Diagnosis: Simpson–Golabi–Behmel syndrome (PD 193900)

Ultrasound[i]: renal abnormalities, hydramnios

Terespolsky et al., 1995

Comments: Post-termination, the fetus who was reported by Terespolsky and associates (1995) had a short neck, broad nose with anteverted nares, immobile shoulders and hips, mild bilateral hydronephrosis, and a dilated urinary bladder. On microscopic examination, there were dysplastic changes in the kidneys.

PD 194000 SINGLE UMBILICAL ARTERY (Two vessel umbilical cord; SUA) (McKusick No. None)

Condition Note: A study by Herrmann and associates (1988) of fetuses at higher than normal obstetrical risk were studied prospectively for the presence of a single umbilical artery (SUA). In these fetuses, six were found with SUA, as well as having IUGR. Of these fetuses, one was found to have the de Lange syndrome (PD 191200), another microcephaly, a third truncus arteriosus (PD 115250), in a fourth respiratory distress syndrome developed after birth, and two were normal after birth.

In the neonate, the association of a single umbilical artery with other congenital anomalies is well established (Tortora et al., 1984). In fact 20–28% of newborns with single umbilical arteries have significant defects (Froehlich and Fujikura, 1966; Heifetz, 1984). The systems most frequently involved include the skeletal, gastrointestinal, genitourinary, cardiovascular, and central nervous systems. Because of this high association, whenever a single umbilical artery is identified prenatally, a careful sonographic search for other fetal anomalies is clearly indicated (Tortora et al., 1984).

Prenatal Diagnosis: The presence of a single umbilical artery can be seen readily on ultrasonic transverse sections of the umbilical cord by identifying only two vessels in the cord. Typically the vein is larger than the artery. In longitudinal section of the cord, when only one artery is present, loss of the braiding pattern can be noted.

Romero et al., 1988, pp. 387–390

Ultrasound[d]: only two vessels in the umbilical cord

Jassani et al., 1980; Spirt et al., 1987

a single umbilical vein and artery present in the umbilical cord

Tortora et al., 1984; Romero et al., 1988, pp. 387–388

enlarged umbilical vein

Spirt et al., 1987

intrauterine growth retardation[c]

Jassani et al., 1980; Tortora et al., 1984

duodenal atresia[c]

Tortora et al., 1984

hydramnios[c]

Tortora et al., 1984

oligohydramnios[c]

Tortora et al., 1984

PD 194130 SIRENOMELIA (Symmelia) (McKusick No. None)

Differential Diagnosis: Diabetic embryopathy (PD 243500); Sacral agenesis (PD 169000); Sacral agenesis/spina bifida, familial (PD 169020); Spina bifida cystica (PD 129000); Spina bifida occulta (PD 130000)

Radiograph[d]: fusion of lower limbs, abnormal sacrum
>> Russell, 1969

Ultrasound[c]: hydrocephalus, fetal growth retardation, polycystic kidneys, oligohydramnios
>> Chervenak et al., 1983b; von Lennep et al., 1985; Stevenson et al., 1986

hydrocephalus
>> Harris et al., 1987

lack of visualization of lower extremities, decreased biparietal diameter
>> Stevenson et al., 1986

sacral agenesis
>> Harris et al., 1987

renal agenesis
>> Stevenson et al., 1986; Harris et al., 1987; Gembruch and Hansmann, 1988

lack of bladder filling
>> Gembruch and Hansmann, 1988

oligohydramnios
>> Harris et al., 1987; Gembruch and Hansmann, 1988

PD 194160 SMITH–LEMLI–OPITZ SYNDROME (Acrodysgenital dwarfism; Gardner–Silengo–Wachtel syndrome; Genitopalatocardiac syndrome; Lowry–Miller–Maclean syndrome; RSH syndrome; SLO syndrome; Smith–Lemli–Opitz syndrome, type I; Smith–Lemli–Opitz syndrome, type II) (McKusick No. 270400)

Syndrome Note: Smith–Lemli–Opitz syndrome is depicted by microcephaly, ptosis, cataracts, anteverted nares, cleft palate, small tongue, micrognathia, congenital heart disease, ambiguous genitalia with hypospadias, cleft scrotum, cryptorchidism, postaxial polydactyly, 2–3 toe syndactyly, varying degrees of mental retardation, and death in infancy in some cases (Curry et al., 1987). The condition is inherited in an autosomal recessive mode and diagnosed more often in males than females because ambiguous genitalia occurs more frequently in males.

The cause of Smith–Lemli–Opitz syndrome is a deficiency of 3 beta-hydroxysteriod-delta-7-reductase (7-dehydrocholesterol reductase), the enzyme that converts 7-dehydrocholesterol to cholesterol (Tint et al., 1994a). The affected child, as would be expected, has elevated serum levels of 7-dehydrocholesterol and low levels of serum cholesterol. Patients with type I and II Smith–Lemli–Opitz syndrome have elevated levels of serum 7-dehydrocholesterol and reduced levels of cholesterol, and the difference in severity in this condition is probably related to the relative deficiency of the enzyme produced by different mutations within the gene.
>> McGaughran et al., 1994

Prenatal Diagnosis: The only reliable reported method of diagnosis is the determination of elevated levels of 7-dehydrocholesterol in amniotic fluid.

Differential Diagnosis: Alstrom syndrome (retinitis pigmentosa, obesity, diabetes mellitus, and perceptive deafness); Bardet–Biedl syndrome (PD 186500); Biemond syndrome II (iris coloboma, hypogenitalism, obesity, polydactyly, and mental retardation); Hydrolethalus syndrome (PD 191300); Laurence–Moon syndrome (mental retardation, pigmentary retinopathy, hypogenitalism, and spastic paraplegia); Meckel syndrome (PD 192140); Short rib–polydactyly syndromes (PD 169250, PD 169500, PD 170000, PD 171000); Trisomy 13 syndrome (PD 103000)

> Creech et al., 1988; McKusick, 1988

Alpha-fetoprotein[c]: lowered levels in maternal serum

> Rossiter et al., 1995

Amniocentesis[i]: elevated levels of amniotic-fluid 7-dehydrocholesterol (cholesta-5,7-dien-3 beta-ol)

> Abuelo et al., 1994; Kelley et al., 1994; McGaughran et al., 1994; Rossiter et al., 1994; Tint et al., 1994b; Abuelo et al., 1995; McGaughran et al., 1995; Rossiter et al., 1995

elevated level of 7-dehydrocholesterol in amniotic fluid cells

> Kelley et al., 1994

reduced levels of amniotic fluid cholesterol

> McGaughran et al., 1994; Tint et al., 1994b; McGaughran et al., 1995

> *Comments:* Not all reported cases of Smith–Lemli–Opitz syndrome have shown reduced levels of amniotic fluid cholesterol during the second trimester, and therefore, this test is only helpful when the amniotic fluid level is low.

> Abuelo et al., 1994; Abuelo et al., 1995

increased ratio of 7-dehydrocholesterol to cholesterol is cultured amniotic fluid cells

> Abuelo et al., 1995

low levels of amniotic fluid unconjugated estriol

> Abuelo et al., 1994

increased level of 7-dehydrocholesterol in amniotic fluid

> Abuelo et al., 1995

increased level of isomeric 7-dehydrocholesterol in amniotic fluid

> McGaughran et al., 1995

increased level of delta lathosterol (cholest-7-en-3 beta-ol) in amniotic fluid

> Abuelo et al., 1994; Kelley et al., 1994; Rossiter et al., 1994; Rossiter et al., 1995

> *Comment:* Lathosterol is a precursor to 7-dehydrocholesterol (Rossiter et al., 1995).

Echocardiography[c]: congenital heart defect

> Greenberg et al., 1987; Gelman-Kohan et al., 1990

Fetoscopy[c]: female genitalia in the presence of a normal male karyotype as determined from chorionic villi and fetal blood

> Hyett et al., 1995

Maternal blood sampling[i]: low levels of serum cholesterol

> Tint et al., 1994b; Abuelo et al., 1995

low level of serum hCG

> Rossiter et al., 1995

low level of serum unconjugated estriol

> Hyett et al., 1995; Rossiter et al., 1995

Maternal urine sampling[c]: low estriols in the maternal urine

> Curry et al., 1987

Ultrasound: short noses, long upper lip, micrognathia[c]

> McGaughran et al., 1995

congenital heart defect[c]
  Greenberg et al., 1987
right cardiac ventricular enlargement[c]
  Rossiter et al., 1995
cystic mass in right renal fossa (uretero–pelvic junction obstruction)[c]
  Rossiter et al., 1995
abdominal calcifications[c]
  Rossiter et al., 1995
increased nuchal translucency with a thickness of 5 mm[g]
  Hyett et al., 1995
  Comments: The above finding was observed at 11 weeks of gestation but was not detected by ultrasound at 16 and 20 weeks. The nuchal translucency was thought by Hyett and co-workers (1995) to be normal appearing female genitalia in the presence of a normal male karyotype (46,XY) as determine from chorionic villi and fetal blood.[c]
  Hyett et al., 1995
female-appearing genitalia in a 46,XY fetus
  McGaughran et al., 1995
cystic hygroma[c]
  Greenberg et al., 1987
no detectable bladder or kidneys[i]
  Seller et al., 1995
hydronephrosis, hydroureter[c]
  Greenberg et al., 1987
intrauterine growth retardation[c]
  Belmont et al., 1987; Curry et al., 1987; Greenberg et al., 1987; Rossiter et al, 1995
lack of fetal movement[h]
  Curry et al., 1987
clubfeet[c]
  McGaughran et al., 1995; Seller et al., 1995
hydrops fetalis[c]
  Greenberg et al., 1987
oligohydramnios
  Belmont et al., 1987; Curry et al., 1987; Seller et al., 1995

PD 194180 TETRAAMELIA SYNDROME (Tetraamelia with pulmonary hypoplasia) (McKusick No. 273395)

Syndrome Note: Rosenak and associates (1991) have reported the tetraamelia syndrome in three of seven children in an Arabic family. The condition is characterized by amelia of all four limbs, agenesis or hypoplasia of the lungs with associated peripheral pulmonary vessel aplasia, and neonatal death. Other reported findings include low-set ears, micrognathia, cleft lip and hydrocephalus. The condition appears to be inherited in an autosomal recessive mode.

Prenatal Diagnosis: The diagnosis is established in a fetus at risk who has tetraamelia. The disorder should be considered in any fetus with amelia.

Differential Diagnosis: Amelia/hemimelia syndrome (PD 202500); Amniotic band disruption sequence (PD 185000); Ectromelia (PD 157000); Ohdo syndrome (PD 192780); Roberts syndrome (PD 193570); Tetraamelia, isolated (PD 173550); Tetraamelia syndrome (PD 194180)

Alpha-fetoprotein[c]: low level in the maternal serum
Rosenak et al., 1991
Ultrasound[g,i]: absence of limbs (tetraamelia)
Rosenak et al., 1991

PD 194184 TETRALOGY OF FALLOT–DUODENAL ATRESIA, FAMILIAL (McKusick No. None)

Condition Note: Lemire and associates (1996) have reported a sister and a brother, both of whom had tetralogy of Fallot and duodenal atresia. In addition, the sister had a right facial palsy, while the brother had bilateral microtia without facial palsy. The parents were clinically normal.

Alpha-fetoprotein[c]: elevated in maternal serum
Lemire et al., 1996
Ultrasound[i]: tetralogy of Fallot, duodenal atresia, hydramnios
Lemire et al., 1996

PD 194190 ALPHA-THALASSEMIA/MENTAL RETARDATION SYNDROME, X-LINKED RECESSIVE TYPE (Alpha-thalassemia/mental retardation syndrome, nondeletion type; ATR-X; X-linked alpha-thalassemia/mental retardation) (McKusick No. 301040)

Syndrome Note: This condition is characterized by a mild alpha-thalassemia, severe mental retardation, and dysmorphic features. The hemoglobin problem consists of a form of hemoglobin H disease with mild hypochromia, and the presence of HbH. The levels of HbH may be low and may require demonstration of hemoglobin H inclusions on brilliant crest blue stained peripheral smears. There is usually almost complete absence of speech. The physical findings include telecanthus, hypertelorism, flat nasal bridge, midfacial hypoplasia, carp-shaped mouth, and ambiguous genitalia. The gene for the condition is located between Xq12-q21.3.

McKusick, 1994; McPherson et al., 1995
Prenatal Diagnosis: Not established.
Ultrasound[c,h]: hydramnios
McPherson et al., 1995

PD 194200 THALIDOMIDE EMBRYOPATHY (Thalidomide syndrome) (McKusick No. None)

Condition Note: The teratogenic effects of thalidomide are well recognized and include shortening or absence of long bones (phocomelia), clubhands and clubfeet, and other defects of ears, eyes, teeth, and intestines.

Gollop et al., 1987
Ultrasound[i]: upper limbs reduced to nubbins, absence of tibiae and fibulae with feet connected directly to the femora in a fetus unintentionally exposed to thalidomide until the 35th day of pregnancy
Gollop et al., 1987

PD 194230 THYMIC APLASIA–FETAL DEMISE (Thymic aplasia with fetal death) (McKusick No. 274210)

Condition Note: Shepard and co-authors (1976) reported two fetuses with IUGR present by the second trimester, thymic aplasia, and fetal demise. In the first fetus, there also were agenesis of the right kidney and ureter, and marked hypoplasia of both lungs. In the second fetus, there were also agenesis of the left main stem bronchus, truncus arteriosus, a single atrium, and a single ventricle.

Ultrasound[i]: fetal demise, IUGR
>Shepard et al., 1976

PD 194250 TORSION OF THE TESTIS (McKusick No. 187400)

Ultrasound[c,d]: cystic swelling projecting into the amniotic fluid close to the fetal buttock and containing a small solid mass
>Hubbard et al., 1984

PD 194500 TREACHER COLLINS SYNDROME (Mandibulofacial dysostosis) (McKusick No. 154500)

Syndrome Note: Treacher Collins syndrome is an autosomal dominant disorder characterized by down-slanting palpebral fissures, lower eyelid colobomata, malar hypoplasia, hypoplastic or absent external ears, ear tags, defects of the middle and inner ears, conductive hearing loss, micrognathia, cleft palate, and variable expressivity.
>Crane and Beaver, 1986

Prenatal Diagnosis: Presence of microtia and micrognathia in a fetus at risk would be presumptive evidence of the diagnosis.

Amniocentesis[i]: DNA linkage analysis indicating that the fetus possessed the gene for the disorder
>Hansen et al., 1996

>DNA linkage analysis with Treacher Collins gene (TCOF1), and short tandem repeat polymorphism using polymerase chain reaction amplification indicated the fetus possessed the gene.
>>Edwards et al., 1996

Fetoscopy[i]: severely deformed external ears
>Tolarova and Zwinger, 1981; Nicolaides et al., 1984

>absent external auditory canal
>>Nicolaides et al., 1984

>low set ears
>>Tolarova and Zwinger, 1981

>open eyelids
>>Nicolaides et al., 1984

>down slanting palpebral fissures
>>Tolarova and Zwinger, 1981; Nicolaides et al., 1984

>abnormal facies
>>Tolarova and Zwinger, 1981

>micrognathia
>>Tolarova and Zwinger, 1981; Nicolaides et al., 1984

>cleft palate
>>Nicolaides et al., 1984

Ultrasound[i]: down slanting palpebral fissures
>Hansen et al., 1996

>virtually complete absence of the nose
>>Hansen et al., 1996

>microtia
>>Crane and Beaver, 1986

maxillary hypoplasia
> Edwards et al., 1996

micrognathia
> Crane and Beaver, 1986; Edwards et al., 1996; Hansen et al., 1996

visible stomach bubble
> Edwards et al., 1996

hydramnios
> Edwards et al., 1996

PD 194600 VAN DER WOUDE SYNDROME (Cleft lip and/or palate with mucous cysts of lower lip) (McKusick No. 119300)

Syndrome Note: Van der Woude syndrome is an autosomal dominant disorder characterized by lower lip pits, fistulas of the lip, hypodontia of the second premolars, and cleft lip with or without cleft palate.
> Tolarova and Zwinger, 1981

Prenatal Diagnosis: The only successful method of diagnosis has been direct visualization of the lip fistulas by fetoscopy.

Differential Diagnosis: Cleft lip (PD 189000) and other disorders associated with cleft lip (see Cleft lip in the Index).

Fetoscopy[i]: visualization of lower lip fistulas
> Tolarova and Zwinger, 1981

PD 194650 VATER ASSOCIATION (VACTERL association) (McKusick No. 192350)

Condition Note: In 1973, Quan and Smith delineated the VATER association as a nonrandom association of *v*ertebral, *a*nal atresia (imperforate anus), *t*racheo-esophageal fistula with *e*sophageal atresia, and *r*adial dysplasia. Subsequently, two other defects, renal and cardiac anomalies, have been added to the list of major defects in the association. Some investigators have suggested using the acronym VACTERL (*v*ertebral, *a*nal, *c*ardiac, *t*racheo*e*sophageal, *r*enal, and *l*imb) to denote the major components of this association.

Numerous other less frequently occurring defects have also been reported in patients with the VATER association. In addition, other patients have been reported with anomalies of both the VATER and the CHARGE association, suggesting an underlying etiologic relationship between the two.
> Weaver et al., 1986

Prenatal Diagnosis: The VATER association should be considered whenever one or more major defects of the VATER association are detected prenatally.

Amniography[d]: no swallowing of amniotic fluid, esophageal atresia
> Claiborne et al., 1986

> *Comment:* The diagnosis in the fetus reported by Claiborne and co-workers (1986) was suspected prenatally.

Ultrasound: multiple fluid-filled structures in the fetal abdomen (distended bowel)[c]
> Diament et al., 1983

> *Comments:* After delivery, the neonate reported by Diament and associates (1983) was found to have bilateral renal agenesis, esophageal atresia, duodenal stenosis, imperforate anus, lung hypoplasia, Potter sequence, and vertebral and radial defects.

abnormalities of thoracic vertebrae
    Claiborne et al., 1986
    Comment: In the case reported by Claiborne and collaborators (1986), the diagnosis was suspected prenatally.
a 90-degree lower thoracic scoliosis[c]
    Henry and Norton, 1987
    Comments: The fetus reported on by Henry and Norton (1987) was terminated and found to have an imperforate anus, multiple vertebral defects, and a two-vessel umbilical cord.
intrathoracic localization of the stomach detected after instillation of artificial amniotic fluid into amniotic cavity[c]
    Gembruch and Hansmann, 1988
dextroposition of the heart
    Gembruch and Hansmann, 1988
polydactyly
    Claiborne et al., 1986
radial aplasia
    Gembruch and Hansmann, 1988
cystic kidney (type IIb) on one side, renal agenesis on the contralateral side
    Gembruch and Hansmann, 1988
absence of kidneys and no bladder filling after instillation of artificial amniotic fluid into the amniotic cavity[c]
    Gembruch and Hansmann, 1988
dilated colon in the pelvis of a fetus with imperforate anus
    Harris et al., 1987
ascites
    Harris et al., 1987
hydramnios[c]
    Claiborne et al., 1986; Harris et al., 1987
oligohydramnios[c]
    Diament et al., 1983; Gembruch and Hansmann, 1988; Iafolla et al., 1991
intrauterine growth retardation
    Gembruch and Hansmann, 1988

PD 194660 VATER ASSOCIATION WITH HYDROCEPHALUS

(VACTERL association with hydrocephalus; VACTERL-H) (McKusick No. 276950, 314390)

Association Note: The VATER association is a nonrandom association of six major congenital abnormalities: vertebral anomalies, anal atresia, congenital heart defects, tracheoesophageal fistula, renal anomalies, and radial dysplasia and other limb defects. The VATER association with hydrocephalus has these same defects (minus anal atresia) plus hydrocephalus. This condition may be inherited in an autosomal recessive and/or X-linked fashion.
    Wang et al., 1993a
Prenatal Diagnosis: The diagnosis should be considered whenever congenital hydrocephalus with one or more of the major anomalies of the VATER association is found prenatally.

Ultrasound: hydrocephalus[i]
>
> Grix, 1989; Iafolla et al., 1991; Wang et al., 1993a; Froster et al., 1996b

biventicular hydrocephalus[d,i]
>
> Genuardi et al., 1993a

rapidly progressive hydrocephalus[c,d]
>
> Iafolla et al., 1989

bilateral radial agenesis[i]
>
> Froster et al., 1996b

abnormal forearms with flexed wrists
>
> Wang et al., 1993a
>
> *Comments*: After termination, the fetus reported by Wang and co-workers (1993b) had absent thumbs and radii, and 2–3 syndactyly of the right hand.

no stomach bubble
>
> Wang et al., 1993a

renal agenesis[d,i]
>
> Genuardi et al., 1993a

renal hypoplasia[d,i]
>
> Genuardi et al., 1993a

oligohydramnios[d,i]
>
> Genuardi et al., 1993a

intrauterine growth retardation[d,i]
>
> Genuardi et al., 1993a

PD 194665 VELOCARDIOFACIAL SYNDROME (Shprintzen syndrome; VCF syndrome) (McKusick No. 192430)

Condition Note: The major features of velocardiofacial syndrome include cleft palate, velopharyngeal insufficiency, congenital heart defect, and a characteristic facial appearance with a prominent tubular nose. Numerous other features also may be present including microcephaly, dysmorphic ears, slender hands and digits, inguinal hernial, learning disabilities or mental retardation, and short stature. The condition is frequently inherited in an autosomal dominant mode produced by a microdeletion of 22q11.
>
> McKusick, 1995

Chorionic villus sampling[c,g]: presence of both copies of DNA polymorphic markers in the syndrome's critical region indicating that the fetus did not have the deletion associated with the syndrome.
>
> Driscoll et al., 1993a

Amniocentesis: in amniotic fluid cells, the presence of both copies of a DNA polymorphic marker in the syndrome's critical region indicating that the fetus did not have the deletion associated with the condition[c]
>
> Driscoll et al., 1993a
>
> fluorescence in situ hybridization (FISH) done on amniotic fluid cells revealed the presence of both copies of probes in the syndrome's critical region indicating that the fetus did not have the deletion associated with the syndrome[c]
>
> Driscoll et al., 1993a

Ultrasound[c,h]: bilateral hydronephrosis and hydroureters
>
> Bars et al., 1995

Comments: In the fetus reported by Bars and colleagues (1995), the child following birth had no anatomic site of urinary obstruction. She did, however, have a neurogenic bladder of unknown etiology, microcephaly, hypoplastic nasal alae, Robin sequence, and slender fingers. Her mother also was dysmorphic; both had a 22q11 deletion.

PD 194670 WATERS–WEST SYNDROME (Hemolytic anemia, lethal congenital nonspherocytic, with genital and other abnormalities) (McKusick No. 600461)

Syndrome Note: Waters and West (1995) described two brothers with an apparently new hematologic-multiple congenital anomaly syndrome that consists of severe, non-spherocytic, nonimmune hemolytic amenia of congenital onset; flat occiput; dimpling of the earlobes; ascites with hepatosplenomegaly; micropenis; hypospadias; increased gap between the first and second toes; deep plantar furrow; and other features consistent with Potter phenotype (fetal compression secondary to oligohydramnios). These children died 8 and 25 hours after birth from respiratory insufficiency caused by pulmonary hypoplasia. At autopsy, there was exuberant hematopoiesis in the liver and kidneys. After extensive evaluation no explanation for the anemia was found.

Ultrasound: hydramnios in the late second trimester followed by oligohydramnios in the third, ascites
Waters and West, 1995

PD 194700 WEYERS SYNDROME (Deficient ulnar and fibular rays with bilateral hydronephrosis syndrome; Weyers oligodactyly syndrome) (McKusick No. None)

Ultrasound: short and deformed ulnae and fibulae; shortened humerus, radius, femur, and tibia; bell-shaped chest with short and horizontal ribs; decreased mineralization of vertebral bodies; bilateral hydronephrosis; and oligohydramnios, poorly coordinated, and decreased in frequency and range of fetal movements
Elejalde et al., 1985a

PD 194725 YUNIS–VARON SYNDROME (Cleidocranial dysplasia with micrognathia, absent thumbs, and distal aphalangia) (McKusick No. 216340)

Syndrome Note: The features of the Yunis–Varon syndrome include macrocephaly; sparse eyebrows and lashes; small nose with anteverted nostrils; abnormal pinnae with absence of the tragus, antitragus, and ear lobe; short philtrum; micrognathia; absent clavicles; absent or hypoplastic thumbs and hallaces; and variable agenesis/hypogenesis of the other digits. Radiographically, there may be absent sternal ossification, hip dislocation, and agenesis/hypogenesis of the phalanges. Death usually occurs during the first few months of life. The condition is inherited in an autosomal recessive fashion.

Gorlin et al., 1990; McKusick, 1995, Rabe et al, 1996
Ultrasound[c,d]: ventriculomegaly, intrauterine growth retardation
Rabe et al., 1996

Chapter 3

Dermatologic Disorders[a]

Review Articles: Anton-Lamprecht, 1984; Anton-Lamprecht and Arnold, 1987a; Anton-Lamprecht and Arnold, 1987b; Arnold and Anton-Lamprecht, 1987

PD 194750 ALBINISM, OCULOCUTANEOUS TYPE I (Albinism I; Oculocutaneous albinism, type I; Oculocutaneous albinism, tyrosinase-negative) (McKusick No. 203100)

Condition Note: Oculocutaneous albinism (OCA) is a heterogeneous group of disorders characterized by various degrees of reduced or absence of melanin pigmentation in skin, hair, and eyes; and ocular abnormalities including nystagmus, photophobia, and reduced visuality. The two principle types of OCA include OCA, type I, that is tyrosinase deficient, and OCA type II, that is tyrosinase "positive." Tyrosinase catalyses the first two and rate-limiting steps in melanin biosynthesis. The gene for this enzyme has been sequenced and multiple mutations have been reported. OCA type I is located at 11q14-q21. The condition is an autosomal recessive disorder.

                Falik-Borenstein et al., 1995; McKusick, 1996

Prenatal Diagnosis: When the mutations in the OCA, type I gene are identified within a family then the mutations can be sought in the at-risk fetus. If the above information is not available, then the diagnosis may be established by detection of lack of melanosomal development in the affected fetus. However, when utilizing this method, caution needs to be taken if the parents are light complected because their fetus may have later onset of melanization than do fetuses from dark-skinned parents (Anton-Lamprecht and Arnold, 1987a).

    Amniocentesis[i]: appropriate molecular genetic testing determining the presence of mutations in both OCA, type I gene

        Falik-Borenstein et al., 1995

    Fetal skin biopsy obtained during fetoscopy[i]: lack of melanosomal development beyond stage II by electron microscopy

        Eady et al., 1983; Falik-Borenstein et al., 1995

        absence of melanin pigment in both the epidermis and the fetal hair by light microscopy

        Falik-Borenstein et al., 1995

PD 194920 APLASIA CUTIS CONGENITA (McKusick No. Unknown; see 107600, 207700)

Condition Note: Congenital and localized deficiency of skin usually of full thickness, characterizes this condition. Although most lesions are small and present on the scalp, they may involve larger segments such as the entire scalp and other regions of the body. Although the condition is inherited as an autosomal dominant trait in some families and an autosomal recessive in others, it is usually sporadic. Prognosis for normal functioning in an affected child is usually excellent.

Prenatal Diagnosis: In the presence of an elevation of the maternal serum and/or amniotic fluid alpha-fetoprotein (AFP), in the presence of amniotic fluid fast-migrating acetylcholinesterase isozyme and the absence of detectable fetal or chromosomal defects, the condition should be considered.

Differential Diagnosis: Adams–Oliver syndrome, Deletion of chromosome 4p, Johanson–Blizzard syndrome, and Trisomy 13 syndrome (PD 103000) are conditions associated with similar defects to those seen in this condition. Unexplained elevation of AFP and the presence of amniotic fluid fast-migrating acetylcholinesterase can also be seen in a number of disorders (see Acetylcholinesterase isozyme, rapidly migrating amniotic fluid in the Index).

Acetylcholinesterase[c]: presence of fast-migrating amniotic fluid isozyme
> Bick et al., 1985; Bick et al., 1987; Vieira-Rush et al., 1988

Alpha-fetoprotein[c]: elevated in amniotic fluid
> Bick et al., 1985; Bick et al., 1987; Vieira-Rush et al., 1988

elevated in maternal serum
> Vieira-Rush et al., 1988

> *Comments:* In the patient reported on by Vieira-Rush and associates (1988), the infant was born at term with skin lesions present on both flanks. These lesions measured 3.5 × 1 cm and 3.0 × 1.5 cm on the right and left sides, respectively. The infant had no other problems and was progressing normally.

PD 195000 CONGENITAL BULLOUS ICHTHYOSIFORM ERYTHRODERMA (Bullous erythroderma ichthyosiformis congenita; Bullous congenital ichthyosiform erythroderma; Bullous CIE; Bullous ichthyosiform erythroderma; Epidermolytic hyperkeratosis) (McKusick No. 113800)

Prenatal Diagnosis: The diagnosis appears feasible by demonstrating one or more of the abnormal skin changes presented below in a fetus at risk. However, caution needs to be taken in the diagnosis of this condition, because there appears to be considerable interfamilial variation in the disorder.
> Anton-Lamprecht and Arnold, 1987a

Amniocentesis[i]: amniotic fluid cells studied by light microscopy revealed the presence of abnormal intracytoplasmic dense inclusions and pyknotic nuclei
> Holbrook et al., 1983; Eady et al., 1986

electron microscopic studies of amniotic fluid cells revealed cytolysis of suprabasal cells, and erosions and clumping of tonofilaments (keratin filaments)
> Holbrook et al., 1983; Eady et al., 1986

electron microscopic studies of amniotic fluid cells revealed tonofibrillar clumps and hyperkeratosis
> Anton-Lamprecht and Arnold, 1987a

Fetal skin biopsy obtained during fetoscopy[i]: light microscopy revealed intracytoplasmic dense inclusions and vacuolate cytoplasm in all cell layers between the stratum basale and periderm
> Golbus et al., 1980; Holbrook et al., 1983; Lofberg and Gustavii, 1984; Eady et al., 1986

electron microscopic studies demonstrated cytolysis and specific clumping of tonofilaments

Anton-Lamprecht and Arnold, 1987a

electron microscopic studies revealed intracellular edema and cytolysis within the epidermis, and intracellular clumping of tonofilaments in all cells except those of the basal and periderm layers; the desmosomes also were abnormal

Anton-Lamprecht, 1981; Holbrook et al., 1983; Eady et al., 1986

PD 195500 EPIDERMOLYSIS BULLOSA DYSTROPHICA, HALLOPEAU–SIEMENS TYPE (Hallopeau–Siemens type epidermolysis bullosa; Epidermolysis bullosa dystrophica, recessive; Recessive dystrophic epidermolysis bullosa) (McKusick No. 226600)

Disease Note: This type of epidermolysis bullosa is one of the more severe forms of these disorders. Complications include corneal erosion and symblepharon, scarring, formation of synechias, esophageal stenosis, and mutilations of the hands and feet. Blisters develop just below the basal lamina in the uppermost papillary dermis. The cause for the blistering is a deficiency of type VII collagen which is the major component of the anchoring fibrils. The deficiency appears to be caused by a mutation in the COL 7A1 gene. This form of epidermolysis bullosa is inherited as an autosomal recessive disorder; others (epidermolysis bullosa dystrophica, Pasini type [McKusick No. 131750]) are inherited as an autosomal dominant disorder, but still have a mutation in the COL7A1 gene.

Anton-Lamprecht and Arnold, 1987a; Anton-Lamprecht and Arnold, 1987b; McKusick, 1995

Prenatal Diagnosis: The diagnosis in the past has been made by fetal skin biopsy and the demonstration of the appropriate pathologic findings associated with this condition in fetuses at risk. Because the mode of inheritance and severity of the condition varies with the type of epidermolysis bullosa, the exact type of epidermolysis bullosa in the family needs to be determined prior to prenatal evaluation. Furthermore, because the density of the connective tissue fibrils of the fetal papillary dermis shows considerable variation and increases steadily with gestational age, the diagnosis of this condition from fetal skin needs to be made by personnel experienced with both normal fetal skin at various gestational ages and with the pathologic changes of this type of epidermolysis bullosa.

Now that a mutation in the gene (COL7A1) has been found to cause this condition, the diagnosis can be made by molecular techniques. However, before this approach can be utilized, the mutation has to be identified in a family. If the mutation cannot be determined, then the diagnosis prenatally will need to be made by fetal skin biopsy.

Dunnill et al., 1995; McKusick, 1995

Differential Diagnosis: Other forms of epidermolysis bullosa need to be considered and excluded.

Acetylcholinesterase[c]: presence of fast-migrating amniotic fluid isozyme

Bick et al., 1985; Bick et al., 1987

Alpha-fetoprotein[c]: elevated in amniotic fluid

Bick et al., 1985; Bick et al., 1987

Amniocentesis[i]: linkage analysis using polymerase chain reaction (PCR) and detection of an intragenic restriction-fragment-length polymorphism (RFLP) in the COL7A1 gene

Witt et al., 1995

identification of a specific mutation within the COL7A1 gene
Witt et al., 1995; Hovnanian et al., 1995
Comments: The fetuses tested by Hovnanian and co-workers (1995) and Witt and associates (1995) were found to be heterozygous for the condition, and were normal at birth.
Chorionic villus sampling (CVS)[g,i]: linkage analysis utilizing PCR and detection of an intragenic or extragenic RFLP in the COL7A1 gene
Dunnill et al., 1995; Hovnanian et al., 1995
Comments: In the fetus assessed by Dunnill and colleagues (1995), the fetus tested to be heterozygous for the condition, and was normal at birth.
detection of the specific mutation within the COL7A1 gene
Hovnanian et al., 1995
Fetal skin biopsy obtained during fetoscopy[i]: separation of the skin below the basal lamina, which remained attached to the fetal epithelium; focal collagenolysis below the basal lamina
Anton-Lamprecht et al., 1981; Anton-Lamprecht and Arnold, 1987a; Anton-Lamprecht and Arnold, 1987b
bulla separating epidermis and basement membrane from the dermis, absence of anchoring fibrils
Bick et al., 1987

PD 195550 EPIDERMOLYSIS BULLOSA HERPETIFORMIS, DOWLING–MEARA TYPE (Epidermolysis bullosa simplex, Dowling–Meara type) (McKusick No. 131760)

Condition Note: The condition cited under this entry is inherited as an autosomal dominant disorder and is characterized by formation of blisters of the skin from minimal trauma. The definitive diagnosis of the disorder in adults is based on the electron microscopic appearance of involved and uninvolved skin where there is a split within the basal epidermal layer and aggregation K14 and K5 keratin filaments in the basal layer and in the immediate suprabasal, spinous layer keratinocytes.
Holbrook et al., 1992
Fetal skin biopsy by ultrasonic-guided fetoscopy[i]: light microscopic evaluation revealed separation of the epidermis and the dermis
Holbrook et al., 1992
electron microscopic evaluation revealed aggregation of the keratin filaments within the basal cells of the detached epidermis, and in the attached basal cell remnants
Holbrook et al., 1992

PD 196000 EPIDERMOLYSIS BULLOSA LETALIS (EBA-G; Epidermolysis bullosa atrophicans generalizata gravis; Epidermolysis bullosa Herlitz type; Epidermolysis bullosa letalis, junctional type; Herlitz syndrome; Junctional epidermolysis bullosa of the Herlitz type; Junctional Herlitz–Pearson type epidermolysis bullosa; R-EBA-6; Recessive epidermolysis bullosa atrophicans generalisata gravis) (McKusick No. 226700)

Disease Note: Epidermolysis bullosa letalis (EBL) is the most common of the inherited epidermolyses accounting for up to 50% of newborns with these disorders. As the name implies, the disease is an early lethal one, with affected infants dying within a few weeks or months after birth. The degree of severity of the disorder is similar among siblings but may be remarkably different between children of unrelated families. Blister formation, the major hallmark of the condition, is always generalized and involves the skin, mucous membranes, and epithelium of many internal organs. Blister formation in this disease is junctional with separation occurring in the space of the lamina rara. The basal lamina and well-formed anchoring fibrils cover the blister's floor, while intact basal cells form the undersurface of the blister's roof. The basic defect involves the hemidesmosomes, which are either severely hypoplastic or missing entirely. In this specific disorder, there is always lack of a region of intense interfacing filaments of the hemidesmosomes that normally traverse the lamina rara beneath the attachment plates.

The case of EBL is a deficiency of or complete lack of laminin 5, an anchoring filament protein, that is involved in the formation of hemidesmosomes. There are three genes that encode for the constitutive polypeptides that make up laminin 5. A mutation in any one of these genes, LAMA3, LAMB3, LAMC2, leads to EBL. However, the mutations must be allelic in one of these genes; both mutations must be in the LAMA3 gene, or the LAMB3 gene, or the LAMC2 gene, and the mutations must be such that there is complete absence of the protein. All mutations found to produce this disorder, thus far, result in premature termination codons.

> Anton-Lamprecht and Arnold, 1987a; Anton-Lamprecht and Arnold, 1987b; Christiano et al., 1997

Prenatal Diagnosis: Demonstration of allelic mutations in the genes, LAMA3, LAMB3 or LAMC2, that cause this condition appears to be the method of choice for diagnosis. Otherwise demonstration of absent or hypoplastic hemidesmosomes at the dermoepidermal junction in a fetus at risk can be used for the diagnosis. To state that the diagnosis has been excluded, one needs to either show that the fetus carries only one or none of the mutations causing the disorder, or to have ultrastructural demonstration of well-formed, completely normal hemidesmosomes in the fetal skin sample (Anton-Lamprecht and Arnold, 1987a). Epidermolysis bullosa letalis can be safely excluded by demonstrating the presence of complete hemidesmosomes (Hausser et al., 1989).

Differential Diagnosis: Other forms of epidermolysis bullosa need to be considered and excluded.

Amniocentesis[i]: demonstration of mutations in the genes causing this condition by molecular genetic techniques

> Christiano et al., 1997

> no complete hemidesmosomes in amniotic fluid cells, presence of small densifications along the plasma membrane facing the basal lamina (incomplete hemidesmosome formation)

> Hausser et al., 1989

> demonstration of heterozygosity by molecular genetic techniques

> Christiano et al., 1997

Chorionic villus sampling[g,i]: demonstration of mutations in the genes causing this conditin by molecular genetic techniques

> Christiano et al., 1997

> demonstration of heterozygosity by molecular genetic techniques

> Christiano et al., 1997

Fetal amnion biopsy[i]: hypoplastic hemidesmosomes

> Hausser and Anton-Lamprecht, 1990

Fetal skin biopsy obtained during fetoscopy[i]: separation of the epidermis from the dermis at the lamina lucida, reduced number of and malformed and/or hypoplastic hemidesmosomes
> Rodeck et al., 1980; Anton-Lamprecht and Arnold, 1987a; Hausser et al., 1989

Fetal skin biopsy by ultrasound directed biopsy forceps[i]: junctional separation of the epithelium, hypoplasia of hemidesmosomes in fetuses at risk
> Elias et al., 1988

PD 196500 EPIDERMOLYSIS BULLOSA LETALIS WITH PYLORIC ATRESIA (Aplasia cutis congenita with gastrointestinal atresia; Bull–Carmi syndrome; Carmi syndrome) (McKusick No. 226730)

Syndrome Note: This condition is characterized by junctional epidermolysis bullosa, pyloric atresia present at birth, and death in infancy. Other features may include pyelonephrosis with ureterovesical-junction stenosis, protein-losing gastroenteropathy, pterygia, and contractures. The condition is an autosomal recessive disorder caused by a mutation in the integrin-beta-4 gene.
> McKusick, 1995

Fetal skin biopsy guided by ultrasound[i]: electron microscopic examination of fetal skin showed separation between the basal cell plasma membrane and lamina densa, hypoplastic hemidesmosomes, atrophic sub-basal dense plagues, and invagination of the plasma membranes within the cytoplasm of the basal keratinocytes
> Nazzaro et al., 1990

Ultrasound[i]: dilatation of the stomach, hydramnios
> Nazzaro et al., 1990

PD 197000 EPIDERMOLYSIS BULLOSA SIMPLEX (McKusick No. Unknown; see 131900, 131950, 131960)

Alpha-fetoprotein[c]: elevated in maternal serum
> Yacoub et al., 1979

PD 197500 HYPOHYDROTIC ECTODERMAL DYSPLASIA, X-LINKED FORM (Anhydrotic ectodermal dysplasia; Christ–Siemens–Touraine syndrome) (McKusick No. 305100)

Chorionic villus sampling[g,i]: linkage of the gene for the condition with various RFLPs utilizing DNA from chorionic villi
> Zonana et al., 1990

Fetal skin biopsy obtained during fetoscopy[i]: absence of sebaceous glands and other skin appendages
> Anton-Lamprecht et al., 1982; Arnold et al., 1984; Anton-Lamprecht and Arnold, 1987a

PD 197750 ICHTHYOSIS CONGENITA (Collodion fetus; Congenital ichthyosis; Congenital nonbullous ichthyosiform erythroderma; Desquamation of newborn; Lamellar exfoliation of newborn; Lamellar ichthyosis, type 1; Nonbullous congenital ichthyosiform erythroderma) (McKusick No. 242300)

Condition Note: Ichthyosis congenita is an autosomal recessive condition with marked cornification of the skin that is present at birth. The skin often is collodion-like with neonatal desquamation. The latter condition may lead to life-threatening sepsis and protein and electrolyte losses. Mutations in the gene that encode for keratinocyte transglutaminase cause this condition.

McKusick, 1997; Schorderet et al., 1997

Prenatal Diagnosis: Demonstration of mutations in keratinocytic transglutaminase genes in a homozygous state probably is the method of choice in most cases. Otherwise, the diagnosis must be established by finding the dermatologic changes on skin obtained by fetal skin biopsy.

Chorionic villus sampling[g,i]: finding mutations in the keratinocytic transglutaminase genes by molecular genetic techniques

Schorderet et al., 1997

Fetal skin biopsy obtained during fetoscopy[i]: light microscopic studies revealed a thickened interfollicular epidermis with multiple layers of flattened cells and excessive keratinization of the epidermal lining of the follicular infundibulum

Perry et al., 1987

increased amounts of horn lamellae in the orifices of hair follicles and an increase of unkeratinized flattened regressive cell layers in the interfollicular epidermis

Arnold and Anton-Lamprecht, 1987

electron microscopy evaluation of the epidermis revealed granular cells that contained larger-than-normal keratohyalin granules and multiple layers of parakeratotic cornified cells; the granules in the granular cells were increased in both number and size

Perry et al., 1987

PD 198000 ICHTHYOSIS CONGENITA, HARLEQUIN FETUS TYPE

(Congenital ichthyosis; Harlequin fetus type; Harlequin fetus; Harlequin ichthyosis; Ichthyosis fetalis) (McKusick No. 242500)

Fetal skin biopsy obtained during fetoscopy[i]: by light microscopy hyperkeratosis with formation of plugs of keratin debris around hair follicles, acanthosis

Elias et al., 1980b; Blanchet-Bardon et al., 1983; Blanchet-Bardon and Dumez, 1984

by electron microscopy, thickened stratum corneum with involvement of both follicular and interfollicular epidermis; abnormal vesicular keratinosomes with no lamellar configuration; keratohyalin granules in granular cells

Blanchet-Bardon et al., 1983; Blanchet-Bardon and Dumez, 1984; Arnold and Anton-Lamprecht, 1987

Ultrasound[c]: shortening of the long bones

Charles et al., 1989

Comments: Shortening of the long bones in the fetus reported by Charles and associates (1989) was thought to be related to restricted fetal movement (the fetal akinesis/hypokinesis sequence [PD 191232]), which was secondary to the skin condition.

PD 198250 RESTRICTIVE DERMOPATHY, LETHAL (Fetal hypokinesia

sequence due to restrictive dermopathy; Hyperkeratosis–contracture syndrome; Lowry hyperkeratosis syndrome; Tight skin contracture syndrome, lethal) (McKusick No. 275210)

Syndrome Note: This condition is depicted by intrauterine growth retardation (IUGR); congenital contractures (arthrogryposis); decreased fetal movement;

taut, shiny, and restrictive skin; narrow and pinched nose; small mouth with limited jaw mobility, ectropion; enlarged fontanels; abnormalities of the clavicles and long bones; and pulmonary hypoplasia. Neonatal death normally ensues. Histologically, the skin shows hyperkeratosis, parakeratosis, and absence of elastin fibers in a thin dermis. Electromicroscopic studies reveal keratin filaments and abnormal globular-shaped keratohyalin granules. The condition is inherited in an autosomal recessive mode. Disturbingly, a fetal skin biopsy showed normal skin at 19.5 weeks of gestation in a fetus who later was shown to have the condition (Hamel et al., 1992).

> McKusick, 1995

Maternal report[c]: decreased fetal movement

> Lowry et al., 1985; Holbrook et al., 1987a; Hamel et al., 1992
> fetal movements ceased after about 6 months of gestation
> Lowry et al., 1985; Holbrook et al., 1987a; Hamel et al., 1992

Ultrasound: decreased fetal movements[d,i]

> Lowry et al., 1985; Holbrook et al., 1987a
> intrauterine growth retardation
> Lowry et al., 1985
> hydramnios
> Lowry et al., 1985; Holbrook et al., 1987a; Hamel et al., 1992
> oligohydramnios [c,d]
> Lowry et al., 1985

PD 198450 SJOGREN SYNDROME (McKusick No. 270150)

Syndrome Note: This condition is characterized by xerostomia and xerophthalmia, and may be found in association with rheumatoid arthritis and other immunologic diseases affecting the skin.

> McKusick, 1988

Prenatal Diagnosis: No definitive method of diagnosis has been accepted. Complete heart block secondary to complete atrioventricular block has been reported in a fetus whose mother had the condition (Carpenter et al., 1986).

Differential Diagnosis: Atrioventricular node, absence of (PD 108120); Bilateral left-sidedness sequence (PD 187230); Complete heart block (PD 109000); Lupus erythematosus (PD 267450)

Prenatal Treatment: Terbutaline has been used to increase the fetal ventricular rate. Transuterine transthoracic fetal ventricular pacing has also been successful on a short-term basis (Carpenter et al., 1986).

Methods and Findings: Doppler auscultation[c]: bradycardia at 55 beats per minute

> Carpenter et al., 1986

Echocardiography[d,i]: complete atrioventricular block with an atrial rate of 128 beats per minute and a ventricular rate of 32 beats per minute, pericardial effusion, right atrial-wall hypertrophy, right ventricular enlargement

> Carpenter et al., 1986
> *Comments:* In the above fetus reported on by Carpenter and associates (1986), the mother had Sjogren syndrome. The authors thought that the fetus was similarly affected.

Ultrasound[i]: depressed right ventricular contractility,[d] right ventricular dilation,[d] bilateral pleural effusion[d]

> Carpenter et al., 1986

lack of fetal movements[d]
>Carpenter et al., 1986

hydramnios[c]
>Carpenter et al., 1986

PD 198500 SJOGREN–LARSSON SYNDROME (Fatty alcohol : NAD+ oxidoreductase deficiency; Fatty aldehyde dehydrogenase deficiency) (McKusick No. 270200)

Condition Note: The features of Sjogren–Larsson syndrome, an autosomal recessive disorder, include congenital ichthyosis, spastic quadriplegia, seizures, and mental retardation. The disorder is a result of fatty aldehyde dehydrogenase deficiency which is a component of fatty alcohol : NAD+ oxidoreductase.
>Rizzo et al., 1993; McKusick, 1995

Prenatal Diagnosis: Although the diagnosis of this condition can be and has been made by fetal skin biopsy, the more reliable and safer method appears to be the determination of fatty aldehyde dehydrogenase activity in cultured chorionic villus or cultured amniotic fluid cells.

Amniocentesis[i]: deficiency of fatty aldehyde dehydrogenase and fatty alcohol : NAD+ oxidoreductase activities in cultured amniotic fluid cells
>Rizzo et al., 1993

Chorionic villus sampling[g,i]: deficiency of fatty aldehyde dehydrogenase and fatty alcohol : NAD+ oxidoreductase activities in cultured chorionic villi
>Rizzo et al., 1993

Fetal skin biopsy obtained during fetoscopy[i]: skin showed prominent granular layer with enlarged granules, orthokeratotic and thickened keratin layer with densely packed keratin, papillomatosis, and separation of dermis from epidermis
>Kousseff et al., 1982

prominent granular layer covered by continuous thickened horny cell layers
>Arnold and Anton-Lamprecht, 1987

Chapter 4

Fetal Infections[a]

PD 198700 CANDIDA ALBICANS (McKusick No. None)

Amniocentesis: organism cultured from amniotic fluid where preterm prelabor amniorrhexis had occurred
Carroll et al., 1990
Cordocentesis (percutaneous umbilical blood sampling or PUBS): organism cultured from fetal blood where preterm prelabor amniorrhexis had occurred
Carroll et al., 1990

PD 198750 CAPNOCYTOPHAGA (McKusick No. None)

Disease Note: Infection prenatally of the various species of capnocytophaga, a fastidious gram-negative gliding bacterium normally found in oral flora, will cause amnionitis and probably preterm labor. However, the infection is not known to cause fetal defects.
McDonald and Gordon, 1988
Prenatal Diagnosis: The diagnosis is established by isolating capnocytophaga species from amniotic fluid.

Amniocentesis[d]: elevated amniotic fluid white cell count, numerous gram-negative fusiform bacilli in amniotic fluid, culture and isolation of capnocytophaga from amniotic fluid
McDonald and Gordon, 1988

PD 198760 *CHLAMYDIA TRACHOMATIS* (McKusick No. None)

Amniocentesis[h]: culture of organism from amniotic fluid
Pao et al., 1991
identification of organism in amniotic fluid by polymerase chain reaction (PCR) and specific DNA probe
Pao et al., 1991

PD 198770 CITROBACTER (McKusick No. None)

Cordocentesis (PUBS): organism cultured from fetal blood where preterm prelabor amniorrhexis had occurred
Caroll et al., 1990

PD 198775 CRYSEOMONAS (McKusick No. None)

Amniocentesis: organism cultured from amniotic fluid where preterm prelabor amniorrhexis had occurred
Carroll et al., 1990

PD 198800 COXSACKIE (Coxsackievirus) (McKusick No. None)

Ultrasound[c]: increased echogenicity of fetal bowel
       Strasberg et al., 1995
   cerebral calcifications
       Strasberg et al., 1995
   oligohydramnios
       Strasberg et al., 1995

PD 199000 CYTOMEGALOVIRUS (CMV) (McKusick No. None)

Disease Note: Prenatal infection of the mother by CMV has been associated with abnormalities in the fetus and infant. Fetal infections may occur either with primary infections or with reinfection of the mother. As such, results of maternal serology are of little assistance in determining if the fetus has or has not been infected, except when the results are negative.

   Abnormalities of the fetus associated with this infection include microcephaly, hydrocephaly, hydranencephaly, intracranial calcification, bradycardia, hydrops fetalis, and intrauterine growth retardation (IUGR). Developmental delay and mental retardation may also be present in those children who suffered prenatal infections.
       Romero et al., 1988, p. 420; Hogge et al., 1989b
Prenatal Diagnosis: Diagnosis of CMV infection in the fetus can be reliably accomplished by culturing the virus from amniotic fluid or fetal blood. Levels of CMV-specific IgM antibody in fetal serum have been shown to be unreliable for establishing the diagnosis.
       Hogge et al., 1993
Differential Diagnosis: Other fetal infections such as Coxsackievirus (PD 198800); Parvovirus (PD 200750); Syphilis (PD 202000) and Toxoplasmosis (PD 202250) have been associated with hydrops fetalis noted either prenatally or postnatally. Thus, fetal infections should be considered whenever hydrops fetalis is discovered. The presence of Hydrocephalus (PD 125000), Hydranencephaly (PD 124000), Microcephaly, unspecified type (PD 128300), or intracranial calcifications can also be caused by other fetal infections.

   Alpha-fetoprotein (AFP)[c]: elevated in maternal serum
       Katz et al., 1986b
   Amniocentesis: recovery of CMV from amniotic fluid[i]
       Davis et al., 1971; Hogge et al., 1989b; Hogge et al., 1993
    dark brown amniotic fluid[c]
       Katz et al., 1986b
   Cordocentesis (PUBS): elevated CMV-specific IgM antibody level in fetal serum
       Hogge et al., 1989b; Hohlfeld et al., 1991
    low hemoglobin levels in fetal blood[i]
       Hohlfeld et al., 1991

low hematocrit in fetal blood[i]
>Hohlfeld et al., 1991

elevated white count in fetal blood[i]
>Hohlfeld et al., 1991

elevated percentage of moncytes in fetal blood[i]
>Hohlfeld et al., 1991

reduced platelet count in fetal blood[i]
>Hohlfeld et al., 1991

Electrocardiogram[c,d]: fetal bradycardia
>Lewis et al., 1980

Radiograph[c,d]: brain calcification
>Marquis and Lee, 1976

Ultrasound[c]: hydranencephaly
>Rutledge et al., 1986; Hogge et al., 1993

microcephaly with intracranial calcification
>Hogge et al., 1989b

hydrocephalus
>Hogge et al., 1989b; Palumbos and Stierman, 1989

fetal scalp edema
>Gollop and Eigier, 1986b

fetal bradycardia[d]
>Lewis et al., 1980

ascites
>Gollop and Eigier, 1986b; Hohlfeld et al., 1991; Strasberg et al., 1992; Hogge et al., 1993

increased echogenicity of fetal bowel
>Strasberg et al., 1992

hydrops fetalis
>Gollop and Eigier, 1986b; Nicolaides et al., 1986a; Hohlfeld et al., 1991

intrauterine growth retardation
>Katz et al., 1986b; Hogge et al., 1989b

thickened placenta
>Gollop and Eigier, 1986b

Method not stated[i]: abnormal fetal heart rate pattern
>Hohlfeld et al., 1991

PD 199250 ENTEROBACTOR (McKusick No. None)

Amniocentesis: organism cultured from amniotic fluid where preterm prelabor amniorrhexis had occurred
>Carroll et al., 1990

Cordocentesis (PUBS): organism cultured from fetal blood where preterm prelabor amniorrhexis had occurred
>Carroll et al., 1990

PD 199500 ENTEROVIRUS (McKusick No. None)

Ultrasound[c,d]: hydrocephalus with enlargement of the lateral and third ventricles, increased biparietal diameter
>Dommergues et al., 1994

fetal tachycardia, myocardial wall and interventicular septal hyperplasia, pericardial effusion
Dommergues et al., 1994
Cordocentesis (PUBS)[c,d]: elevated level of serum alpha interferon
Dommergues et al., 1994

PD 199600 FUSOBACTERIUM (McKusick No. None)

Cordocentesis (PUBS): organism cultured from fetal blood where preterm prelabor amniorrhexis had occurred
Carroll et al., 1990

PD 199700 *GARDNERELLA VAGINALIS* (McKusick No. None

Amniocentesis: organism cultured from amniotic fluid where preterm prelabor amniorrhexis had occurred
Carroll et al., 1990

PD 199800 *HEMOPHILUS INFLUENZAE* (McKusick No. None)

Amniocentesis: organism cultured from amniotic fluid where preterm prelabor amniorrhexis had occurred
Carroll et al., 1990
Cordocentesis (PUBS): organism cultured from fetal blood where preterm prelabor amniorrhexis had occurred
Carroll et al., 1990

PD 200000 HERPES TYPE I (Necrosis of fetal liver) (McKusick No. None)

Alpha-fetoprotein[c]: elevated in maternal serum
Seppala, 1976

PD 200250 HUMAN IMMUNODEFICIENCY VIRUS (Acquired immunodeficiency syndrome; AIDS; HIV) (McKusick No. None)

Amniocentesis[d]: human immunodeficiency virus (HIV) cultured from both amniotic fluid and amniotic fluid cells from fetuses whose mothers had antibodies to HIV
Sprecher et al., 1986; Mundy et al., 1987
Comment: HIV antibody may be present in amniotic fluid because of specific IgG antibody of maternal origin (Lifson and Rogers, 1986).

PD 200450 LACTOBACILLUS (McKusick No. None)

Cordocentesis (PUBS): organism cultured from fetal blood where preterm prelabor amniorrhexis had occurred
Carroll et al., 1990

PD 200500 LISTERIOSIS (McKusick No. None)

Alpha-fetoprotein[c,d]: elevated in amniotic fluid
Yarberry-Allen et al., 1983
Amniocentesis[c,d]: elevated levels of IgA and IgG in amniotic fluid by hydroxyethylcellulose–agarose gel electroimmunodiffusion
Yarberry-Allen et al., 1983
Ultrasound[c]: pleural effusion,[d] ascites,[d] hydrops fetalis[d]
Gembruch et al., 1987

fetal demise
> Ramsden et al., 1989

hydramnios[d]
> Gembruch et al., 1987

PD 200620 MYCOPLASMA (*Acholeplasma oculi*) (McKusick No. None)

Disease Note: Only *Acholeplasma laidlawii* and *oculi* have been found in man. *A. oculi* has been isolated from amniotic fluid but has not been associated with fetal disease (Waites et al., 1987).

Prenatal Diagnosis: Isolation of organism from amniotic fluid is considered diagnostic at present.

> Amniocentesis[c]: isolation of *A. oculi* in pure culture from human amniotic fluid at 19 weeks of gestation, demonstration of organism directly in amniotic fluid
> Waites et al., 1989

PD 200640 *MYCOPLASMA HOMINIS* (McKusick No. None)

> Amniocentesis: organism cultured from amniotic fluid where preterm prelabor amniorrhexis had occurred
> Carroll et al., 1990

PD 200750 PARVOVIRUS (Erythema infectiosum; Fifth disease; Human parvovirus) (McKusick No. None)

Disease Note: Human parvovirus B19 is thought to produce disease that is usually a benign infection in otherwise healthy children. However, in individuals with hemolytic anemias such as sickle cell disease or thalassemias, it may cause aplastic crises. In infected fetuses, the virus may cause the same crises, leading to severe anemia, hydrops fetalis, and in some cases, death. Infection in the fetus may also produce viral myocarditis and damage to the myocardium (Elliott et al., 1994). The anemia resulting from this intrauterine infection has been successfully treated by in utero transfusion (see Preferred Treatment and Treatment Modalities below).

In one report of 42 pregnancies, where the mothers became seropositive for parvovirus B19 during their pregnancies (Schwarz et al., 1988), erythema infectiosum or an atypical form of the condition developed in 27 (64%), and 15 (36%) were clinically symptom-free. Three (7%) of the pregnancies were terminated. No complications were seen in 29 (74%) and hydrops fetalis occurred in 10 (26%). In 7 of the 10 fetuses with hydrops fetalis, death occurred; the other three received in utero transfusions and two survived to term. These latter two were healthy. The other one had not yet delivered.

Because elevation of maternal serum AFP levels prior to the onset of hydrops has been associated with fetal infections of this virus, Roberts (1988) recommends weekly maternal serum AFP determinations, and fetal ultrasound assessments for hydrops for the first 8 weeks following maternal infection, then biweekly until delivery. Unexplained AFP elevation and/or hydrops fetalis warrants further fetal evaluation, including fetal blood drawing, to determine the presence of the virus and anemia.

> Roberts, 1988; Naides and Weiner, 1989

Prenatal Diagnosis: Presumptive diagnosis can be made if there is an unexplained elevation of maternal AFP and onset of hydrops fetalis in the fetus of a pregnant woman shown immunologically to have had a recent parvovirus infection

(Schwarz et al., 1988). Alternatively, the definitive diagnosis can be made by identifying the virus by immunoelectron microscopy (Naides and Weiner, 1989; Sahakian et al., 1991) or by DNA techniques (Peters and Nicolaides, 1990)

Differential Diagnosis: Amegakaryocytic thrombocytopenia (PD 202500); Maternal chronic immune thrombocytopenia (PD 207700); Maternal idiopathic thrombocytopenia (PD 207750); Neonatal alloimmune thrombocytopenia (PD 207850); Thrombocytopenia–absent radius syndrome (PD 175000)

Prenatal Treatment: The treatment of choice at the present time is fetal blood transfusion or exchange transfusion by cordocentesis. Complete reversal of the congestive heart failure and hydrops fetalis, requiring in some cases repeat transfusions, have been reported in a number of cases (Schwarz et al., 1988; Peters and Nicolaides, 1990; Soothill, 1990; Sahakian et al., 1991). Healthy nonanemic children have been born subsequently.

Treatment Modality: Intravascular fetal transfusion via ultrasound-guided cordocentesis

        Schwarz et al., 1988; Peters and Nicolaides, 1990; Soothill, 1990; Sahakian et al., 1991

Methods and Findings: AFP[c]: elevated in maternal serum

        Brown et al., 1984

  Cordocentsis (PUBS)[i]

        Naides and Weiner, 1989; Peters and Nicolaides, 1990; Soothill, 1990

    reticulocytopenia

        Peters and Nicolaides, 1990

    thrombocytopenia

        Naides and Weiner, 1989; Peter and Nicolaides, 1990

    neutropenia

        Naides and Weiner, 1989

    erythroblastemia

        Peters and Nicolaides, 1990

    identification of B19 parvoviral DNA by dot hybridization

        Peters and Nicolaides, 1990

    umbilical venous pressure elevated (consistent with congenital heart failure)[c]

        Sahakian et al., 1991

    identification of B19 parvoviral DNA from fetal serum by using polymerase chain reaction, B19-specific probe, and Southern analysis

        Sahakian et al., 1991

    elevated serum lactate dehydrogenase activity[c]

        Sahakian et al., 1991

    reduced serum aspartate aminotransferase activity

        Sahakian et al., 1991

    parvovirus B19 particles detected by electron microscopy in fetal blood

        Soothill, 1990

Maternal blood sampling[c]: elevated anti-B19 IgG and IgM antibody levels

        Naides and Weiner, 1989

Paracentesis, fetal abdominal[i]: identification in ascitic fluid of nonenveloped icosahedral-appearing viral particles approximately 23 nm in diameter using transmission electron microscopy

        Naides and Weiner, 1989; Sahakian et al., 1991

identification in ascitic fluid of the B19 parvovirus by specific monoclonal antibody and a second-stage colloidal gold conjugated antibody
label using immune electron microscopy

>Naides and Weiner, 1989; Sahakian et al., 1991

Pulsed-wave Doppler analysis[d,i]: increased time-averaged, mean intensity-
weight blood velocity in the fetal descending thoracic aorta

>Peters and Nicolaides, 1990

Ultrasound[i]: hydrops fetalis

>Brown et al., 1984; Schwarz et al., 1987; Rosengren et al., 1988;
>Schwarz et al., 1988; Naides and Weiner, 1989; Chiba et al., 1990;
>Peters and Nicolaides, 1990; Sahakian et al., 1991

anencephaly

>Rosengren et al., 1988

ventriculomegaly

>Sahakian et al., 1991

scalp edema

>Peters and Nicolaides, 1990

cardiomegaly

>Naides and Weiner, 1989; Peters and Nicolaides, 1990; Sahakian
>et al., 1991

bulging of the right atrium during systole

>Naides and Weiner, 1989

pericardial effusion

>Peters and Nicolaides, 1990; Sahakian et al., 1991

ascites

>Naides and Weiner, 1989; Peters and Nicolaides, 1990; Soothill,
>1990; Sahakian et al., 1991

fetal demise

>Rosengren et al., 1988; Naides and Weiner, 1989

placental hydrops

>Naides and Weiner, 1989

oligohydramnios

>Sahakian et al., 1991

hydramnios

>Soothill, 1990

PD 201000 RUBELLA (McKusick No. None)

Amniocentesis: recovery of rubella virus from amniotic fluid

>Cederqvist et al., 1977b; Morgan-Capner et al., 1984; Morgan-
>Capner et al., 1986

transmission electron microscope (TEM) studies of amniotic fluid cells
revealed lack of nuclear heterochromatin, almost complete disappearance of electron-dense cytoplasmic layer, increased number of mitochondria, decreased number and size of microvilli, distortion of microvilli, amorphous appearing nuclei, microfilaments in the vicinity of the
nuclear membrane, myelin figures, and cytoplasmic virus-like inclusions[i].

>Straussberg et al., 1995

scanning electron microscope studies of amniotic fluid cells showed
smaller and rounded cells, decreased number of membranal microvilli,

rudimentary and clubbed microvilli, and irregular membrane between microvilli[i]

Straussberg et al., 1995

Fetoscopy with fetal blood sampling: elevated rubella-specific IgM antibodies

Daffos et al., 1984b; Morgan-Capner et al., 1984; Morgan-Capner
et al., 1985; Enders and Jonatha, 1987

Comment: False negative results may occur if sampling is done before 22
weeks by this method (Morgan-Capner et al., 1985; Enders and Jonatha, 1987).

Ultrasound[c,d]: hydrops fetalis

Spahr et al., 1980

PD 201600 *STAPHYLOCOCCUS EPIDERMIDIS* (McKusick No. None)

Amniocentesis: organism cultured from amniotic fluid where preterm prelabor amniorrhexis had occurred

Carroll et al., 1990

Cordocentesis (PUBS): organism cultured from fetal blood where preterm
prelabor amniorrhexis had occurred

Carroll et al., 1990

PD 201700 *STREPTOCOCCUS AGALACTIAE* (McKusick No. None)

Amniocentesis: organism cultured from amniotic fluid where preterm prelabor amniorrhexis had occurred

Carroll et al., 1996

Cordocentesis (PUBS): organism cultured from fetal blood where pretem
prelabor amniorrhexis had occurred

Carroll et al., 1996

PD 201750 *STREPTOCOCCUS MILLERI* (McKusick No. None)

Amniocentesis: organism cultured from amniotic fluid where preterm prelabor amniorrhexis had occurred

Carroll et al., 1990

Cordocentesis (PUBS): organism cultured from fetal blood where preterm
prelabor amniorrhexis had occurred

Carroll et al., 1996

PD 201800 STREPTOCOCCUS VIRIDANS TYPE (McKusick No. None)

Cordocentesis (PUBS): organism cultured from fetal blood where preterm
prelabor amniorrhexis had occurred

Carroll et al., 1990

PD 202000 SYPHILIS (McKusick No. None)

Amniocentesis[i]: identification of *Treponema pallidum* organism by rabbit
infectivity testing or PCR followed by identification of organism with appropriate DNA probe

Nathan et al., 1997

Maternal blood sampling: positive maternal VDRL[d]

Cremin and Shaff, 1975

Radiograph[d]: symmetrical periosteal cloaking of tibiae and humeri, hydramnios

Cremin and Shaff, 1975

PD 202250 TOXOPLASMOSIS (McKusick No. None)

General Reference: Lynfield and Eaton, 1995

Disease Note: In a study reported by Blaakaer (1986), *Toxoplasma gondii* infection of the mother during early pregnancy will lead to fetal infection in approximately 40–50% of cases with about 10–20% of these fetuses presenting with some symptoms after birth. In contrast to the above report, Hohlfeld and co-workers (1994) studied 2632 women who became infected during their pregnancies, and found that only 7.4% of the fetuses developed the infection. In this latter study, the incidence of congenital toxoplasmosis increased with gestational age with the highest rates being after 23 weeks. Between 23 and 26 weeks of gestation, the percent incidence of infection was 26; this figure raised to 67% between 31 and 34 weeks. But the total at-risk number of fetuses was only six at the latter time. The total number of infected fetuses in the study was 194. In some cases of fetal infections, there may be major brain damage with significant microcephaly and associated mental retardation in the surviving children. The incidence of congenital infection in the United States is estimated to be from 1:1000 to 1:8000 live births (McCabe and Remington, 1988). The maternal infections are contracted in part by handling feces of infected animals, primarily domesticated cats, and by eating meat that has been insufficiently cooked.

The diagnosis of acute toxoplasma infection in the mother can be made by detecting a seroconversion, or a significant rise in toxoplasma-specific IgA and IgG titers, or by demonstrating toxoplasma-specific IgM by capture enzyme-linked immunosorbent assey (ELISA) (Lynfield and Eaton, 1995). Detection of the organism in the fetus now can be made by PCR and appropriate DNA probes. Hohlfeld and associates (1994) amplified and detected the B1 gene of *T. gondii.* Using this technique, they found the overall sensitivity of the test to be 97.4%, the specificity to be 100%, and the negative predictive valve to be 99.7%. Similar results were found by Cazenave and associates (1992).

Prenatal Diagnosis: Detection of the *Toxoplasma gondii* organism in amniotic fluid sediment and/or fetal blood in suspected or at-risk pregnancies by PCR techniques now appears to be the most reliable method.

Prenatal Treatment: The most important form of treatment is prevention of infection in the first place. This may be accomplished by avoiding animal feces and undercooked meat during pregnancy. If an infection does occur and is recognized during pregnancy, it is possible to treat the pregnant woman and her fetus. Doing so may avoid or decrease some of the fetal damage. However, once it has been established that the mother has been infected, she should be treated with a course of leucomycin, 50 mg/kg/day, for 3 weeks (Blaakaer, 1986,) or longer (Daffos et al., 1988a), and if the fetus is recognized also to be infected, pyrimethamine and either sulfadoxine or sulfadiazine should be added to the treatment regimen (Daffos et al., 1988a). More recently the use of pyrimethamine (50 mg/d), sulfadiazine (3000 mg/d) and spiramycine (3000 mg/d), all for 1 to 4 months have been found to be efficacious (Couvreur et al., 1993).

Hohlfeld and associates (1994) used a slightly different approach. They started all patients on 3 g/d of spiramycin as soon as the maternal infection was confirmed or strongly suspected, and before doing prenatal diagnosis.

Treatment Modalities: Maternal medications
> leucomycin (used singly when fetus not recognized to be infected)
>> Blaakaer, 1986; Daffos et al., 1988a
> pyrimethamine plus either sulfadoxine or sulfadiazine (if the fetus is recognized to be infected)
>> Daffos et al., 1988a; Couvreur et al., 1993
> pyrimethamine, sulfadiazine, and spiramycine in combination when the fetus is infected
>> Couvreur et al., 1993

Methods and Findings: Amniocentesis: identification of the *Toxoplasma gondii* in amniotic fluid by PCR and appropriate genetic testing
> Cazenave et al., 1992; Hohlfeld et al., 1994;
>> isolation of organism from amniotic fluid sediment by inoculating sediment into mice
>> Desmonts et al., 1985; Daffos et al., 1988a; Hohlfeld et al., 1994
>> isolation of the organism after inoculation of amniotic fluid
>> Cazenave et al., 1992; Hohlfeld et al., 1994

Cordocentesis (PUBS): identification of the *T. gondii* in fetal blood by PCR and appropriate molecular genetic testing
> Hohlfeld et al., 1994
>> isolation of *T. gondii* by inoculation of fetal blood into mice
>> Desmonts et al., 1985; Daffos et al., 1988a; Couvreur et al., 1993
>> elevated specific IgM antibodies
>> Desmonts et al., 1985; Daffos et al., 1988a; Couvreur et al., 1993; Hohlfeld et al., 1994
>> increased leukocytic and eosinophilic counts in fetal blood[c]
>> Hohlfeld et al., 1994
>> thrombocytopenia[c]
>> Hohlfeld et al., 1994
>> increased serum gamma-glutamyl transferase activity
>> Hohlfeld et al., 1994

Ultrasound[c]: enlarged cerebral ventricles as indicated by an increase in the ventricle/hemisphere ratio
> Desmonts et al., 1985; Daffos et al., 1988a
>> intracranial calcification[h]
>> Daffos et al., 1988a
>> intracranial densities[c,d]
>> Hohlfeld et al., 1996
>> intrahepatic calcification[h]
>> Daffos et al., 1988a
>> hydrops fetalis
>> Spahr et al., 1980
>> ascites[c,d]
>> Blaakaer, 1986; Daffos et al., 1988a

PD 202400 VARICELLA (Chickenpox; Congenital varicella syndrome; Fetal varicella syndrome; Varicella embryopathy; Varicella-zoster viral infection) (McKusick No. None)

Disease Note: Varicella infection during pregnancy may result in a serious, if not life-threatening, disease to both the mother and the fetus. Although the fetus may remain unaffected, varicella infection in early pregnancy has been associated with multiple congenital defects involving multiple organs, and has been denoted as the varicella embryopathy (Alkalay et al., 1987b; Cuthbertson et al., 1987). Higa and associates (1987) have analyzed data from 52 infants whose mothers had contracted varicella during pregnancy. In this group of infants, 27 had congenital defects while 25 developed herpes zoster in the early postnatal period. Most of the mothers whose infants had congenital defects contracted their infections within the first 20 weeks of gestation, whereas the mothers of the infants in whom herpes zoster developed postnatally had their infections after 20 weeks. These authors postulate that the congenital abnormalities found in the affected infants were the result of the fetuses developing in utero varicella-herpes zoster infections and/or central nervous system (CNS) infections secondary to varicella-herpes zoster infections.

Prenatal Diagnosis: The demonstration of elevated varicella (varicella-zoster) virus-specific immunoglobulin M in fetal serum is one specific mode of diagnosis (Cuthbertson et al., 1987); the culture of the virus from the amniotic fluid is another (Pons et al., 1992). In one reported case the culture of amniotic fluid was positive for virus although there was no elevation in IgM varicella virus-specific antibody (Pons et al., 1992).

Isada and associates (1991) have performed PCR on chorionic villi from two women who contracted varicella infections during the first trimester. The chorionic villi on both tested positive for the virus. However, assessment of one fetus who was terminated at 23 weeks of gestation and the newborn who was delivered at term revealed no evidence of fetal infection. Kustermann and co-workers (1996) found four of five fetuses who tested positive by DNA methodology prenatally were DNA positive for the virus from paraffin-embedded tissue sections posttermination. Infection in these five fetuses occurred between 10 and 24 weeks' gestation for a 36% rate of placental/fetal infection in the 14 fetuses at risk for contracting the infection.

Differential Diagnosis: The specific maternal infection acquired during pregnancy needs to be determined, particularly other exanthems and venereal diseases.

    Alpha-fetoprotein[c]: elevated levels in maternal serum
            Meschino et al., 1993

      Comments: In the case cited by Meschino and associates (1993), the mother contracted chickenpox at 13 weeks of gestation. She was found to have elevated levels of maternal serum AFP at 15 and 17 weeks. Following amniocentesis, the amniotic fluid AFP level was normal, with no acetylcholinesterase activity present. Subsequently, progressive IUGR developed. At birth the neonate had multiple, punctate skin and died at 22 days of age from progressive respiratory distress and hepatic failure.

    Amniocentesis[i]: identification of varicella virus by viral culture from amniotic fluid sample, and by visualizing virus particles by electron microscope and immunofluorescence using monoclonal anti-varicella primers specific for varicella glycoprotein II DNA
            Pons et al., 1992
        identifying the virus by DNA testing in amniotic fluid
            Kustermann et al., 1996

Chorionic villus sampling (CVS)[g,i]:
    identifying the virus by DNA testing
        Kustermann et al., 1996
Cordocentesis (PUBS)[d,i]: elevated fetal serum varicella-specific IgM titer, fetal IgM antibody present to all three major varicella glycoproteins (gpI, gpII, and gpIII)
        Cuthbertson et al., 1987
Nonstress test[c,d]: flat base line with occasional variable
    decelerations
        Cuthbertson et al., 1987
    identifying the virus by DNA testing
        Kustermann et al., 1996
Ultrasound: ventriculomegaly,[d,i] hydramnios[d,i]
        Cuthbertson et al., 1987
    hydrocephalus[i]
        Kustermann et al., 1996
    intrauterine growth retardation[c]
        Meschino et al., 1993

PD 202450 UREAPLASMA UREALYTICUM (McKusick No. None)

Amniocentesis: organism cultured from amniotic fluid where preterm prelabor amniorrhexis had occurred
        Carroll et al., 1990

Chapter 5

Hematologic Disorders and Hemoglobinopathies[a]

General Review Articles: Alter, 1980; Alter, 1987

HEMATOLOGIC DISORDERS

PD 202500 AMEGAKARYOCYTIC THROMBOCYTOPENIA (McKusick No. Unknown; see 187950, 188000)

Fetal blood obtained at fetoscopy[i]: low platelet count (8×10^9/L)
Mibashan and Millar, 1983

PD 202600 ANTI-TJa ALLOIMMUNIZATION (Anti-P1PK alloimmunization) (McKusick No. None; see 111400)

Condition Note: The blood group P system has a number of serologic phenotypes including TJa (also known as P1PK). Because most individuals carry the TJa (or P1PK) antigen (99.0995%), alloimmunization secondary to transfusions (whole blood or as a result of pregnancy) or immunization is rare. When alloimmunization occurs in a woman who does not carry the TJa antigen, hydrops fetalis and fetal death may occur as a result of severe fetal anemia. When fetal death and the resulting miscarriage does occur, these events usually occur before the 20th week of pregnancy.
Haentjens-Verbeke et al., 1996
Cordocentesis (percutaneous umbilical blood sampling, or PUBS)[d,i]: fetal anemia
Haentjens-Verbeke et al., 1996
Ultrasound[c,d]: intrauterine growth retardation (IUGR)
Haentjens-Verbeke et al., 1996

PD 202740 BLACKFAN–DIAMOND SYNDROME, AUTOSOMAL DOMINANT TYPE (Congenital hypoplastic anemia of Blackfan–Diamond) (McKusick No. 105650)

Syndrome Note: The disorder is characterized by congenital hypoplastic anemia that is inherited in an autosomal dominant fashion. The condition is caused by defective erythroid stem cells.
McLennan et al., 1996

Prenatal Diagnosis: In the at-risk fetus, demonstration of anemia by cordocentesis should be diagnostic.

Prenatal Treatment: In the fetus who is in significant heart failure, intrauterine transfusion by cordocentesis currently is the treatment of choice.

Treatment Modality: Transfusion by cordocentesis
McLennan et al., 1996

Methods and Findings: Cordocentesis (PUBS)[d,i]: severe fetal anemia
McLennan et al., 1996

Ultrasound[i]: cardiomegaly, pericardial effusion, ascites,[d] short long bones, oligohydramnios
McLennan et al., 1996

PD 202750 BLACKFAN–DIAMOND SYNDROME, AUTOSOMAL RECESSIVE TYPE (Chronic congenital aregenerative anemia; Congenital hypoplastic anemia of Blackfan–Diamond; DBS; Diamond–Blackfan anemia; Erythrogenesis imperfecta; Pure red cell anemia) (McKusick No. 205900)

Syndrome Note: Blackfan–Diamond syndrome is a congenital deficiency of erythroid precursors leading to a hypoplastic macrocytic anemia that may be present prenatally and, if severe, may lead to heart failure and death in the neonatal period. Normally, the anemia is detected during infancy, and treatment is successfully accomplished by blood transfusions and use of steroids. The condition is inherited in an autosomal recessive fashion. The gene for this condition seems to be linked to the 19q13 chromosome region.
Visser et al., 1988, McKusick, 1997

Prenatal Diagnosis: In a fetus at risk, the detection of anemia or increased cardiac output in the absence of Rh or irregular antibodies, or fetomaternal transfusion most likely is diagnostic of the condition.

Differential Diagnosis: Blackfan–Diamond syndrome, autosomal dominant type (PD 202740); Erythroblastosis fetalis (PD 204000); Fetomaternal transfusion; Twin transfusion syndrome (PD 115500)

Doppler echocardiography[d]: increased cardiac output, increased mean temporal right and left ventricular blood velocities, large single-peak right ventricular flow velocity wave form
Visser et al., 1988

PD 202950 CHRONIC GRANULOMATOSIS DISEASE, AUTOSOMAL CYTOCHROME-b-POSITIVE, FORM II (Deficiency of neutrophil cytosol factor 2; Deficiency of p67-phox) (McKusick No. 233710)

Disease Note: The characteristics of this entry include the same as those found in the X-linked form of the disease (Chronic granulomatous disease, X-linked form, [PD 203000]). There are two genes that produce the chronic granulomatosis disease, autosomal cytochrome-b-positive types: one causes a deficiency of a 47-KD neutrophil cytosol factor, NCF-1, and a second results in a deficiency of 65-KD factor, NCF-2. The NCF-2 gene product is referred to as p67-phox (phox standing for phagocyte oxidase), and is deficient in the condition listed under this entry.

Amniocentesis[g,i]: gene linkage with an intragenic polymorphic marker after amplification by PCR
Kenney et al., 1993

Comment: The fetus reported by Kenney and co-workers (1993) was found to be heterozygous for the condition.

PD 203000 CHRONIC GRANULOMATOUS DISEASE, X-LINKED FORM
(McKusick No. 306400; see also 233650, 233690, 233700, 233710)

Disease Note: Chronic granulomatous disease is a group of disorders character-ized by an increased susceptibility to certain bacterial and fungal infections. These infections are due to a congenital deficiency of intracellular microorganism killing resulting from impaired production of microbicidal oxygen metabolites. It is usually an X-linked recessive disorder, but in 10% of cases the condition is inherited in an autosomal recessive fashion.

Huu et al., 1987

Prenatal Diagnosis: The diagnosis of the disorder has been accomplished by detecting decreased oxidative metabolic function in fetal neutrophils obtained by fetal blood drawing. Huu and associates (1987) recommend using all three tests listed below to increase the confidence level of diagnosis. These tests have been adapted to the small blood volumes normally obtained by fetal blood sampling. More recently a molecular genetic method has been reported for the diagnosis of this condition. This approach may be more reliable.

Chorionic villus sampling (CVS)[g,i]: the mutant gene was detected in chorionic villi after DNA extraction, polymerase chain reaction (PCR), and specific molecular testing

De Boer et al., 1992

Cordocentesis (PUBS)[i]: decreased ability of fetal phagocytes to generate superoxide free radicals

Newburger et al., 1979; Borregaard et al., 1982; Huu et al., 1987

decreased ability of neutrophils to reduce nitroblue tetrazolium (NBT)

Newburger et al., 1979; Borregaard et al., 1982; Huu et al., 1987

lack of formazan black deposits in the cytoplasm of neutrophils after incubation of the neutrophils with phorbol myristate acetate and NBT

Johansen, 1983; Levinsky et al., 1986

reduced production of chemiluminescence of whole blood in the pres-ence of luminol and serum-treated zymosan or phorbol myristate ac-etate

Huu et al., 1987

PD 203200 COMPLEMENT C4 PARTIAL DEFICIENCY (McKusick No. 120790, 120820)

Condition Note: The fourth component of the human complement, C4, is con-trolled by two genes that are very closely linked and located near the HLA-B region. The two C4 genes are C4F (Rodgers) and C4S (Chido). Deficiency alleles are relatively common at both C4 loci, and individuals homozygous for deficiency at either locus have less-than-normal levels of C4 complement activity. Complete deficiency (i.e., homozygous recessive at both loci), is rare and is associated with a lupus-like syndrome in the affected individual.

Pollack et al., 1980a; McKusick, 1996

Amniocentesis: linkage of C4 with HLA haplotype

Pollack et al., 1980a

Comment: The fetus reported by Pollack and associates (1980a) was found to be heterozygous for complete deficiency of complement C4.

PD 204000 ERYTHROBLASTOSIS FETALIS (Hemolytic disease of the newborn; Kell isoimmunization; Rh isoimmunization) (McKusick No. None)

Condition Note: Erythroblastosis fetalis is the destruction of fetal erythrocytes by maternal antibodies that have been produced in response to a fetomaternal bleed or other sensitization mechanisms. The normal situation for maternal sensitization is a fetus who is Rh positive and a mother who is Rh negative, although other isoimmune situations may occur. If the hemolysis of fetal red cells is severe enough, hydrops fetalis, congestive heart failure, and death may occur in the fetus.

The severity of the fetal hemolysis can be judged by measuring the indirectly reacting bilirubin in the amniotic fluid. This is accomplished by measuring the optical density of amniotic fluid at 450 nm. Three zones of density have been established by Liley (1961), and include the following: zone I incudes unaffected or mildly affected fetuses; zone II represents moderately to severely affected fetuses; and zone III includes severely affected fetuses (Grannum et al., 1986). This method, however, no longer is considered to be a reliable indicator of the degree of fetal anemia in the second trimester of pregnancy (Nicolaides et al., 1986c). Rather, ultrasonographic evidence or direct analysis of fetal blood is preferred (Nicolaides et al., 1986c).

Prenatal Diagnosis: The finding of increased amniotic fluid optic density at a wavelength of 450 nm in a fetus at risk is reasonable evidence for the diagnosis. Direct hematocrit measurement is possible for detection of fetal anemia by obtaining fetal blood via cordocentesis (PUBS). Hydrops fetalis and associated findings in a fetus at risk are also presumptive evidence of erythroblastosis fetalis.

Differential Diagnosis: Cobalamin E disease (PD 240700), Parvovirus (PD 200750), Alpha-thalassemia (PD 210000), and other conditions that give rise to hydrops fetalis need to be considered. For these latter conditions, see Hydrops fetalis in the Index.

Prenatal Treatment: Initial treatment of this condition was by injection of erythrocytes into the fetal abdomen. When this procedure was done blindly, little success was achieved. Greater success was achieved with the aid of fluoroscopic guidance of the needle into the fetal abdomen (Frigoletto et al., 1981). With the development of ultrasound, however, intraabdominal transfusion was successfully achieved with relative ease. The mortality rate was reduced to between 29 and 50% (Berkowitz and Hobbins, 1981; Barss et al., 1986). The problem with this method, however, is that the absorption of red cells from the peritoneum is erratic. A more successful method is direct umbilical vein transfusion either following fetoscopy or by cordocentesis. Because cordocentesis is safer than fetoscopy, fetoscopy for fetal blood transfusion now is not used often. Benacerraf and Frigoletto (1985) have suggested that treatment may be delayed until signs of decompensation in the fetus are seen. They observed edema of the bowel wall before treatment with glucocorticoids and early delivery. Hydrops fetalis when present often is reversed by intravascular transfusion (Rodeck et al., 1984; Grannum et al., 1988). The success rate in completely reversing the hydrops fetalis in the hands of Grannum and associates was 13 of 16 fetuses, or 81%.

Linch et al., 1986; Grannum et al., 1986; Keckstein et al., 1990; Utter et al., 1990

Treatment Modalities: Early delivery (third trimester)
Benacerraf and Frigoletto, 1985

Fetal direct transfusion using various veins isolated after hysterotomy
        Queenan, 1969
Fetal exchange transfusion using a fetal vein or artery after laparotomy
and hysterotomy
        Freda and Adamsons, 1964; Asensio et al., 1966
        Comments: Freda and Adamsons (1964) reported direct in utero exchange
        transfusion of a fetus with severe erythroblastosis fetalis whose hematocrit
        at the time of the initial exchange was 14%. The exchange transfusion was
        accomplished by making an incision through the uterus over a foot, bring-
        ing the foot and leg to the outside, and then cannulating the femoral
        artery. Although the exchange transfusion was a success, the fetus was
        precipitately delivered vaginally on the second day following the procedure
        and died of prematurity. A similar procedure was reported by Asensio
        and associates (1966) with the exchange occurring at 31 weeks' gestation
        with the delivery at 34 weeks' gestation. The child survived.
Fetal exchange transfusion using a placental vein after laparotomy and hyster-
otomy
        Seelen et al., 1966
        Comments: Seelen and co-workers (1966) accomplished an exchange trans-
        fusion in a severely affected fetus by cannulating a placental vein after
        laparotomy and hysterotomy. The procedure was successful and the fetus
        was delivered in a healthy state 18 hours post–exchange-transfusion at a
        gestational age of 34 weeks.
Feticide induced by intraamniotic instillation of dinoprost trometamel
(Amoglandin)
        Bang et al., 1982
Intraarterial injection of furosemide (2–4 mg) in hydropic fetuses
        Rodeck et al., 1984
Intravenous injection of furosemide (2–5 mg) directly into the umbilical vein
        Rodeck et al., 1981
Intrahepatic vein fetal transfusion of Rh-negative blood
        Nicolini et al., 1989a
Intraperitoneal fetal transfusion of group O, rhesus-negative erythrocytes or
maternal blood using radiographic or fluoroscopic guidance with or without
first injecting air, agitated saline, or Renografin to determine that the needle
was in the peritoneal cavity
        Liley, 1963; Queenan and Douglas, 1965; Fairweather et al., 1967;
        Queenan, 1969; Whitefield, 1970; Bock, 1976; Brown and Robert-
        son, 1973; Robertson et al., 1976; Palmer and Gordon, 1976;
        Hamilton, 1977; Frigoletto et al., 1981; Bowman and Manning,
        1983; Harman et al., 1989
        Comments: Treatment has been started as early as 20.5 weeks gestational
        age in severe cases (Bowman and Manning, 1983). Salvage rate was greater
        if done after 25 weeks' gestation (Queenan, 1969).
Intraperitoneal fetal transfusion of group O, rhesus-negative erythrocytes
after use of intraamniotic and intraabdominal contrast material, and radiographic and fluoroscopic guidance
        Kwi and Hing, 1974
Intraperitoneal fetal transfusion of compatible packed red blood cells using

a small-gauge needle under ultrasound guidance with or without the use of an indwelling catheter

     Cooperberg and Carpenter, 1977; Frigoletto et al., 1978; Callen et al., 1979; Platt et al., 1979a; Berkowitz and Hobbins, 1981; Frigoletto et al., 1981; Rodeck et al., 1981; Rodeck et al., 1984; Barss et al., 1986; Berkowitz et al., 1986a; Nicolini et al., 1989b

Comments: Barss and associates (1986) state that this approach to treatment of severely affected fetuses with erythroblastosis fetalis is a good therapeutic option to direct fetal transfusion. Nicolini and co-workers (1989a) have used both intraperitoneal and intravascular transfusions in the same fetus, and were able to lengthen the time between transfusions.

Intraperitoneal fetal transfusion done under ultrasound guidance after introducing intraabdominal air

     Lee et al., 1981

Intravascular fetal transfusion of group O, rhesus-negative blood via fetoscopy

     Rodeck et al., 1981; Rodeck et al., 1984; Nicolaides et al., 1985; Nicolaides et al., 1986d

Intravascular fetal transfusion of Group O, rhesus-negative erythrocytes via ultrasound-guided cordocentesis using an umbilical vein or artery

     Bang et al., 1982; Berkowitz et al., 1986a; Berkowitz et al., 1986b; Nicolaides et al., 1986d; Grannum et al., 1988; Harman et al., 1988; Nicolini et al., 1989a; Millard et al., 1990

Comments: Washed, packed, and irradiated O rhesus-negative or Kell-negative blood was used for transfusions (Grannum et al., 1988). The blood was obtained from anonymous donors, and transfusions given by puncturing an umbilical vein at the placental insertion site (Grannum et al., 1988).

Intravascular fetal transfusion of group O, rhesus-negative blood into the umbilical vein at its deepest most fixed point within the liver with or without intramuscular curare injection of the fetus for immobilization

     de Crespigny et al., 1985; Berkowitz et al., 1986a

Maternal treatment: cortisone given to the mother by mouth

     Hunter and Washington, 1955

hydrocortisone succinate intravenous injection of the mother every 8 hours for 4 doses[d]

     Anderson and Cordero, 1980

Comments: Anderson and Cordero (1980) observed a significant drop in the optical density (OD_{450}) in pregnancies where fetuses had severe erythroblastosis fetalis, and the mothers were treated with hydrocortisone to advance lung maturation of the fetuses. All five women were between 32 and 34 weeks of gestation. Only one of the five fetuses appeared to have progression of his disease (development of hydrops fetalis) and all five survived.

promethazine hydrochloride (Phenergan) starting with 150 mg/d and increasing 25 mg/d until 300 mg/d is reached

     Charles and Blumenthal, 1982

Comments: Promethazine appears to produce its effect on leukocyte's ability to phagocytize opsonized red blood cells. The medication is given by mouth to the mother starting as early as 8 weeks of gestation.

     Charles and Blumenthal, 1982

Methods and Findings: Alpha-fetoprotein[c]: elevated in amniotic fluid
        Adinolfi et al., 1975
Amniocentesis[i]: elevated bilirubin levels in amniotic fluid
        Fairweather et al., 1976; Berkowitz and Hobbins, 1981; Frigoletto
        et al., 1981; Bang et al., 1982; Grannum et al., 1986
    increased optical density values of the amniotic fluid[i]
        Liley, 1963; Freda and Adamsons, 1964; Queenan and Douglas,
        1965; Asensio et al., 1966; Seelen et al., 1966; Fairweather et al.,
        1967; Powell, 1968; Queenan, 1969; Clark et al., 1970; Whitefield,
        1970; Brown and Robertson, 1973; Kwi and Hing, 1974: Bock,
        1976; Fairweather et al., 1976; Palmer and Gordon, 1976; Robert-
        son et al., 1976; Hamilton, 1977; Frigoletto et al., 1978; Callen
        et al., 1979; Anderson and Cordero, 1980; Rodeck et al., 1981;
        Frigoletto et al., 1981; Bang et al., 1982; Bowman and Manning,
        1983; Rodeck et al., 1984; de Crespigny et al., 1985; Nicolaides
        et al., 1985; Berkowitz et al., 1986a; Berkowitz et al., 1986b;
        Nicolaides et al., 1986; Grannum et al., 1988; Keckstein et al., 1990
    increased insulin levels in amniotic fluid[c]
        Weiss et al., 1984
    increased activity of amniotic fluid disaccharidases prior to 21 weeks'
    gestation[c]
        Morin et al., 1980
Amniography[d,i]: fetal scalp edema
        Shaub and Wilson, 1976
Cardiotocogram[i]: flat curve
        Harman et al., 1988
Chorionic villus sampling[g]: identification of Rh positive D red blood cells;
cells were isolated from chorionic villi
        Kanhai et al., 1984
Cordocentesis (PUBS)[i]: anemia with hematocrits varying from 5–28% and
hemoglobin levels down to as low as 2 g/dL
        Rodeck et al., 1984; Berkowitz et al., 1986a; Grannum et al.,
        1986; Nicolaides et al., 1986; Grannum et al., 1988; Nicolini et
        al., 1989a; Millard et al., 1990; Utter et al., 1990; Murotsuki et
        al., 1992
    reddish screen
        Bang et al., 1982
    strongly positive reaction to a direct Coombs' test
        Bang et al., 1982
    elevated bilirubin in fetal serum (hyperbilirubinemia)
        Berkowitz et al., 1986a; Berkowitz et al., 1986b
    total serum protein of less than 3 g/dL and total serum albumin of less
    than 2 g/dL
        Grannum et al., 1988
      Comment: When the above findings were present, affected fetuses
      also had hydrops fetalis (Grannum et al., 1988).
    direct Coombs' test positive
        Berkowitz et al., 1986a; Rightmire et al., 1986
    reticulocytosis
        Nicolaides et al., 1985

erythroblastosis
Nicolaides et al., 1985
leukocytosis
Nicolaides et al., 1985
leukopenia
Nicolaides et al., 1985
Doppler velocity determinations[d,i]: increased left and right cardiac output
Rizzo et al., 1990
increased mean aortic blood velocities
Rightmire et al., 1986
increased mean inferior vena cava blood velocities
Rightmire et al., 1986
Echocardiography[c]: pericardial effusion
DeVore et al., 1982b
Fetal blood drawn from a placental vein isolated following hysterotomy[d,i]: severe anemia
Seelen et al., 1966
elevated fetal serum bilirubin
Seelen et al., 1966
Coombs' test positive
Seelen et al., 1966
Fetal blood drawn directly form the fetal leg following uterine surgery[d,i]: severe anemia
Freda and Adamsons, 1964; Asensio et al., 1966
Coombs' test positive
Freda and Adamsons, 1964; Asensio et al., 1966
elevated fetal serum bilirubin
Freda and Adamsons, 1964; Asensio et al., 1966
Fetal blood drawing by fetoscopy[i]: severe anemia in the fetus
Rodeck et al., 1981; Nicolaides et al., 1985; Linch et al., 1986; Nicolaides et al., 1986c
Maternal blood sampling: elevate Rh antibody levels
Liley 1963; Queenan and Douglas, 1965; Powell, 1968; Fraser et al., 1976; Rodeck et al., 1981; de Crespigny et al., 1985; Nicolaides et al., 1985; Berkowitz et al., 1986a; Berkowitz et al., 1986b
Physical examination of the mother[c]: hydramnios
Queenan and Gadow, 1970
Ultrasound: thickened placenta, distended fetal abdomen, fetal ascites, hydrops fetalis, pericardial effusion, visualization of both sides of the bowel wall
Shaub and Wilson, 1976; DeVore et al., 1982b; Benacerraf and Frigoletto, 1985
scalp edema
Berkowitz et al., 1986a
right atrial dilatation[c]
Grannum et al., 1986
cardiomegaly[c]
de Crespigny et al., 1985
poor myocardial contractility
Grannum et al., 1986

multiple prolonged fetal heart rate decelerations[c]
> Grannum et al., 1986

pleural effusion[i]
> Rodeck et al., 1981; Nicolaides et al., 1986d; Harman et al., 1988

pericardial effusion[i]
> Rodeck et al., 1984; Berkowitz et al., 1986a; Grannum et al., 1986; Nicolaides et al., 1986d; Harman et al., 1988

ascites[i]
> Callen et al., 1979; Frigoletto et al., 1981; Lee et al., 1981; Rodeck et al., 1981; Bang et al.; 1982; de Crespigny et al., 1985; Berkowitz et al., 1986a; Grannum et al., 1986; Nicolaides et al., 1986d; Harman et al., 1988

decreased head circumference-to-abdominal circumference ratio
> Rodeck et al., 1981

hepatomegaly
> Berkowitz et al., 1986a

hydrops fetalis[i]
> Frigoletto et al., 1978; Callen et al., 1979; Anderson and Cordero, 1980; Berkowitz and Hobbins, 1981; Frigoletto et al., 1981; Rodeck et al., 1984; de Crespigny et al., 1985; Nicolaides et al., 1985; Barss et al., 1986; Berkowitz et al., 1986a; Grannum et al., 1986; Nicolaides et al., 1986d; Rightmire et al., 1986; Harman et al., 1988; Millard et al., 1990

fetal skin edema
> Rodeck et al., 1984; Nicolaides et al., 1986d

reduced or absent movement, or poor response to stimulation[c]
> Ianniruberto and Tajani, 1981; Harman et al., 1988

absence of fetal respiratory movements
> Grannum et al., 1986; Harman et al., 1988

intrauterine growth retardation
> Rodeck et al., 1981

no fetal limb movements
> Grannum et al., 1986

increase in the umbilical vein diameter as it courses through the liver
> Holzgreve et al., 1985c

fetal death
> Rodeck et al., 1981; Grannum et al., 1986

oligohydramnios[c]
> de Crespigny et al., 1985; Berkowitz et al., 1986a

enlarged or thickened placenta[i]
> Spirt et al., 1987; Rodeck et al, 1981; de Crespigny et al., 1985; Harman et al., 1988

PD 204250 ERYTHROBLASTOSIS FETALIS INDUCED THROMBOCYTOPENIA (McKusick No. None)

Condition Note: In some severe cases of erythroblastosis fetalis, unexplained thrombocytopenia has been found. In some of these cases, the thrombocytopenia has been severe enough to result in fetal bleeding following intravascular transfusions by cordocentesis.
> Harman et al., 1988

Prenatal Treatment: Intravascular transfusion of both group A rhesus-negative erythrocytes and platelets have been effective in treating both the anemia and the thrombocytopenia in one reported case.
> Harman et al., 1988

Treatment Modalities: Intravascular fetal transfusion of both group A rhesus-negative erythrocytes and platelets.
> Harman et al., 1988

Methods and Findings: Cordocentesis (PUBS)[i]: prolonged umbilical vein bleeding following blood transfusion
> Harman et al., 1988
>> thrombocytopenia
>>> Rodeck et al., 1984; Harman et al., 1988

PD 204500 FACTOR FIVE DEFICIENCY (McKusick No. 227400; see also 134400, 227300, 227310)

> Ultrasound[c,d]: biparietal diameter greater than the 90th percentile, dilatation of the right ventricle
>> Whitelaw et al., 1984

> *Comment:* The above problems were later shown to be from intraventricular hemorrhage.

PD 205000 FANCONI ANEMIA (Fanconi pancytopenia) (McKusick No. 227650, 227660)

Condition Note: Fanconi anemia is an autosomal recessive disorder characterized by progressive pancytopenia, and in many cases death from hemorrhage, infection, or leukemia. Physical findings include abnormal skin pigmentation, short stature, and defects of the skeleton, kidneys, and heart. In addition, there is increased chromosomal breakage in cells from affected individuals. The latter finding has been used to confirm the diagnosis.
> Auerbach et al., 1986

Prenatal Diagnosis: Demonstration of an increased per cell mean chromosomal breakage utilizing amniotic fluid cells, chorionic villus cells, or fetal white blood cells is sufficient to establish the prenatal diagnosis of this condition in fetuses at risk. Detection of the mutant gene is also possible now.

> Amniocentesis[i]: increased chromosomal breakage and sister chromatid exchange in cultured amniotic cells both before and after exposure to diepoxybutane
>> Auerbach et al., 1980; Auerbach et al., 1981; Auerbach, 1984; Trunca et al., 1984; Auerbach et al., 1985
> poor growth of cultured amniotic fluid cells
>> Shipley et al., 1984

> Chorionic villus sampling[g,i]: increased chromosomal breakage in cultured chorionic villus cells after exposure to diepoxybutane
>> Auerbach et al., 1986; Murer-Orlando et al., 1993
>> identification of two mutations in the Fanconi anemia gene using molecular techniques
>>> Murer-Orlando et al., 1993

> Fetal blood drawing by fetoscopy[i]: increased chromosomal breakage both with and without the use of mitomycin C
>> Shipley et al., 1984

PD 205500 FETAL BLEEDING (Fetal hemorrhage) (McKusick No. None)

Condition Note: Fetal bleeding usually has occurred as the result of procedures done to the fetus or the fetal circulatory system. Minor bleeding may occur following cordocentesis (backbleeding) and normally is self-limiting. More serious bleeding has occurred when there has been fetal thrombocytopenia and cordocentesis or transfusions have been done, or where the umbilical cord inadvertently has been punched by a needle (Romero et al., 1982a; Sutro et al., 1984; Romero et al., 1988, pp 396–397; Keckstein et al., 1990).

Prenatal Treatment: Only cases of fetal bleeding associated with thrombocytopenia have been treated successfully by intravascular transfusion of blood enriched with platelets.

> Harman et al., 1988

Treatment Modality: Intravascular fetal transfusion of platelets

> Harman et al., 1988

Methods and Findings: Cordocentesis (PUBS)[i]: prolonged umbilical vein bleeding following blood transfusion

> Harman et al., 1988

PD 206000 GLUCOSE PHOSPHATE ISOMERASE DEFICIENCY
(McKusick No. 172400)

> Amniocentesis[d,i]: decreased glucose phosphate isomerase activity in cultured amniotic fluid cells
>
> > Whitelaw et al., 1979

PD 207000 HEMOPHILIA A (Classic hemophilia; Factor VIII deficiency)
(McKusick No. 306700)

> Amniocentesis[i]: linkage of gene with various polymorphic markers
>
> > Antonarakis et al., 1985; Phillips et al., 1985; Baty et al., 1986; Malcolm et al., 1986; Schwartz et al., 1986; Brocker-Vriends et al., 1988
>
> *Comments:* Four of 14 families evaluated by Phillips and associates (1985) were not informative for carrier status and/or prenatal diagnosis using the DNA polymorphic sites available at that time. Brocker-Vriends and coworkers (1988), based on the frequency of the RFLPs associated with the hemophilia H gene, estimate that 97% of women will be heterozygous for at least one of the linked RFLP sites; 3% will be homozygous for all markers. Of all women, 37% will be heterozygous only at an extragenic site.
>
> Chorionic villus sampling (CVS)[g,i]: sex determination by chromosomal analysis of chorionic villi followed by DNA analysis demonstrating linkage of various RFLP sites both within and outside of the hemophilia gene
>
> > Vidaud et al., 1986; Kaplan et al., 1988b; Ko et al., 1990; Wehnert et al., 1990; Lebo et al., 1993a
>
> Cordocentesis by fetoscopy[i]: deficiency of factor VIIIC
>
> > Rodeck et al., 1982b
>
> Cordocentesis by ultrasound guidance (PUBS)[i]: deficient procoagulant factor VIII (VIIIC) and procoagulant factor VIII antigen (VIIICAg) in fetal blood
>
> > Firshein et al., 1979; Mibashan et al., 1979; Mibashan et al., 1980; Ljung et al., 1982; Forestier et al., 1983; Mibashan and Millar,

1983; Antonarakis et al., 1985; Hoyer et al., 1985; Forestier et al., 1986; Miller and Hoyer, 1986; Miller et al., 1987
deficiency of factor VIII in fetal blood
Ko et al., 1990
Ultrasound[c,d]: bilateral hydronephrosis and hydroureter
Diament et al., 1983

PD 207500 HEMOPHILIA B (Christmas disease; Factor IX deficiency) (McKusick No. 306900)

Amniocentesis[i]: using molecular genetic techniques, the mutation in the hemophilia beta gene that was present in the mother of the fetus was found in the fetus
Vielhaber et al., 1994
Chorionic villus sampling (CVS)[g,i]: DNA analysis demonstrating linkage of various restriction-fragment-length polymorphism (RFLP) sites both within and outside of the hemophilia gene.
Vidaud et al., 1986; Kaplan et al., 1988b
male sex determined by Y-specific DNA probe and the fetus shown to have the hemophiliac gene by *Xmn*I restriction mapping of the fetal DNA
Zeng et al., 1987
direct detection of deletion in the gene
Vidaud et al., 1986
Cordocentesis (PUBS)[i]: deficient factor IX antigen (IXAg) and plasma IXC as determined by immunoradiometric assay
Holmberg et al., 1980; Ljung et al., 1982; Mibashan and Millar, 1983; Forestier et al., 1986; Miller et al., 1987

PD 207650 HEREDITARY ELLIPTOCYTOSIS, TYPE I (Defective self-association of spectrin dimer type of hereditary elliptocytosis; type 1 HE) (McKusick No. 130600)

Disease Note: Heterozygous hereditary elliptocytosis is a relatively common and mild congenital hemolytic disease inherited in an autosomal dominant fashion. In contrast, the homozygous state, homozygous elliptocytosis, results in a severe transfusion-dependent hemolytic anemia. Both conditions are produced by abnormalities of one of several red cell membrane proteins. In hereditary elliptocytosis type I there is a defect in spectrin, which is one of the self-association dimeric proteins.
Dhermy et al., 1987
Prenatal Diagnosis: Diagnosis is accomplished by demonstrating the findings noted below.
Cordocentesis (PUBS)[i]: decreased erythrocyte deformability, defective spectrin self-association protein with an excess of dimeric species in the red cell membrane, abnormal tryptic digest pattern of spectrin with a decrease in the 80,000-dalton peptide and an increase in the 74,000-dalton peptide
Dhermy et al., 1987

PD 207700 MATERNAL CHRONIC IMMUNE THROMBOCYTOPENIA (McKusick No. Unknown; see 188030)

Condition Note: Maternal chronic immune thrombocytopenia is thrombocytopenia in the mother that is normally associated with maternal platelet antibodies.

In some fetuses of these mothers, the platelet count is also low and the fetus is at a higher risk for development of intracranial hemorrhage.

> Kaplan et al., 1990

Prenatal Diagnosis: The diagnosis is established by demonstrating thrombocytopenia in fetal blood obtained by cordocentesis.

Differential Diagnosis: Amegakaryocytic thrombocytopenia (PD 202500); Maternal idiopathic thrombocytopenia (PD 207750); Thrombocytopenia, neonatal alloimmune (PD 207850); Parvovirus (PD 200750); Thrombocytopenia–absent radius syndrome (PD 175000)

> Cordocentesis (PUBS)[i]: thrombocytopenia in fetal blood
>> Kaplan et al., 1990
> anemia (low hematocrit)[c]
>> Murotsuki et al., 1992

PD 207750 MATERNAL IDIOPATHIC THROMBOCYTOPENIA (Idiopathic thrombocytopenia purpura) (McKusick No. None)

Condition Note: The etiology of the thrombocytopenia in the mother in this condition is unknown. In some of the fetuses of these mothers, there is also thrombocytopenia. In these fetuses, the risk of intracranial hemorrhage is increased.

> Kaplan et al., 1990

Prenatal Diagnosis: The diagnosis is established by demonstrating fetal thrombocytopenia in blood obtained by cordocentesis.

Differential Diagnosis: Amegakaryocytic thrombocytopenia (PD 202500); Maternal chronic immune thrombocytopenia (PD 207700); Neonatal alloimmune thrombocytopenia (PD 207850); Parvovirus (PD 200750); Thrombocytopenia–absent radius syndrome (PD 175000)

> Cordocentesis (PUBS)[i]: thrombocytopenia in fetal blood
>> Kaplan et al., 1990

PD 207775 MAY–HEGGLIN ANOMALY (Dohle leukocyte inclusions with giant platelets) (McKusick No. 155100)

Condition Note: The May–Hegglin anomaly is a rare, autosomal dominant hematologic disorder characterized by thrombocytopenia, giant platelets, and basophilic inclusion bodies within the cytoplasm of the granulocytes (Dohle bodies). Most affected individuals are asymptomatic but on occasion they may experience bleeding episodes as a result of their thrombocytopenia.

> Takashima et al., 1992

Prenatal Diagnosis: Demonstration of Dohle bodies and giant platelets in fetal blood from at-risk fetuses appears to be adequate for making the diagnosis.

> Cordocentesis (PUBS)[c,i]: granulocytes with Dohle bodies and giant platelets on fetal blood smear
>> Takashima et al., 1992

PD 207800 METHEMOGLOBINEMIA, TYPE II (Congenital enzymopenic methemoglobinemia, type II) (McKusick No. 250800)

Condition Note: Type I methemoglobinemia or recessive congenital methemoglobinemia is usually due to a deficiency of erythrocytic NADH-diaphorase or NADH-cytochrome b_5 reductase. The condition cited here, type II methemoglobinemia, involves a deficiency of the same enzyme, but the enzyme is deficient in a number of cell types, including erythrocytes, leukocytes, myocytes, fibroblasts, and brain cells. Clinical features include methemoglobinemia, severe psychomotor retardation, microcephaly hypotonia, and growth failure.

Kaftory et al., 1986

Prenatal Diagnosis: The demonstration of NADH-diaphorase deficiency in cultured amniotic fluid cells in fetuses at risk establishes the diagnosis.

Differential Diagnosis: Methemoglobinemia, type I, and other forms of methemoglobinemia

Amniocentesis[i]: deficient NADH-diaphorase (NADH-methemoglobin reductase, NADH-cytochrome b_5 reductase) in cultured amniotic fluid cells

Junien et al., 1981; Kaftory et al., 1986

PD 207825 OROTICACIDURIA I (Hereditary orotic aciduria) (McKusick No. 258900)

Disease Note: Oroticaciduria is characterized by megaloblastic anemia that is unresponsive to vitamin B_{12} and folic acid treatment; hypochronic, microcytic erthrocytes; growth retardation; and excessive excretion of orotic acid in the urine. Two enzymes, orotate phosphoribosyl transferase and orotidylate decarboxylase, are deficient in activity in this condition. These enzymes are involved in pyrimidine nucleotide synthesis. Treatment of affected individuals with uridine usually leads to reduced urinary excretion of orotic acid, improvement of the anemia, and catch-up growth.

Ohba et al., 1993; McKusick, 1994

Prenatal Diagnosis: Not established; only carriers detected prenatally so far.

Amniocentesis[i]: 56% reduction in orotidylate decarboxylase activity in amniotic fluid cells

Ohba et al., 1993

Comment: Both cases reported by Ohba and associates (1993) were heterozygous for the condition.

two to three times normal levels of orotic acid in amniotic fluid

Ohba et al., 1993

Comment: Both cases reported by Ohba and associates (1993) were heterozygous for the condition.

Chorionic villus sampling[g,i]: 15% orotidylate decarboxylase activity of control values

Ohba et al., 1993

Comment: Both cases reported by Ohba and associates (1993) were heterozygous for the condition.

PD 207830 PROTEIN C DEFICIENCY, HETEROZYGOUS FORM
(Congenital thrombotic disease due to protein C deficiency; Hereditary protein C deficiency; Hereditary thrombophilia) (McKusick No. 176860)

Condition Note: Protein C is a naturally occurring vitamin K-dependent serine protease zymogen. In its activated form, protein C selectively destroys factors Va and VIII:C in human plasma, and as such plays an important anticoagulant role. Deficiency of protein C results in a hypercoagulant state, and the affected individual may experience thromboses, recurrent thrombophlebitis, pulmonary emboli, premature myocardial infarctions, cerebrovascular accidents, and bilateral adrenal hemorrhage that may result in hypotension and hyponatremia. The condition is treated with oral anticoagulants. The homozygous state is associated with overwhelming venous thrombosis or purpura fulminans in the neonatal period, and a high mortality rate. The gene for the condition is located at 2q13-q14, and has been sequenced.

> Mibashan et al., 1985; McKusick, 1995

Fetal-blood sampling by fetoscopy[i]: protein C antigen plasma level between 4.7% and 5.2% of normal (heterozygous range) with normal factors II, VII, IX, and X levels

> Mibashan et al., 1985

PD 207840 THROMBASTHENIA, GLANZMANN TYPE (Deficiency of platelet fibrinogen receptor; Glanzmann thrombasthenia, type A) (McKusick No. 273800)

Disease Note: Thrombasthenia, Glanzmann type, is an autosomal recessive bleeding disorder characterized by severe and lifelong bleeding tendency secondary to impaired platelet function. The platelet function abnormality is related to a deficiency of platelet membrane glycoproteins IIb/IIIa which act as receptors for fibrinogen. Other findings in the condition include purpura despite normal bleeding time, platelet count and coagulation time; deficient clot retraction; reduced platelet adhesiveness; isolated platelets on a blood smear; and correction of the bleed problems by platelet transfusion.

> Seligsohn et al., 1985; McKusick, 1995

Prenatal Diagnosis: The diagnosis of affecteds and heterozygotes can be made by determining the binding of radioactive glycoproteins IIb/IIIa monoclonal antibody on fetal platelets.

> Cordocentesis by fetoscope[i]: heterozygous stage diagnosed by determining intermediate binding of ^{125}I-labelled glycoprotein IIb/IIIa antibody to fetal platelet

> Seligsohn et al., 1985

> *Comment:* The fetus reported by Seligsohn and colleagues (1985) was also found to have ventricular enlargement and a trisomy 18 karyotype.

PD 207850 THROMBOCYTOPENIA, NEONATAL ALLOIMMUNE (Alloimmune thrombocytopenia; NAIT; Neonatal isoimmune thrombocytopenia) (McKusick No. None; see 173470, 122974)

Condition Note: Neonatal alloimmune thrombocytopenia is a recognized cause of prenatal and neonatal hemorrhage. The hemorrhage can be intracranial and lead to the formation of porencephalic cysts.

The disorder is analogous to erythroblastosis fetalis in that maternal antibodies form against fetal platelets, cross the placenta, and destroy the fetal platelets. Unlike erythroblastosis fetalis, platelets may cross the placenta during the first pregnancy and the first born may be affected. The majority of the maternal–fetal platelet incompatibilities involve the platelet PLA-1 (P1[A1]) antigen and about 2% of the population is negative for this antigen. The incidence of this condition is estimated to be about 1 per 5000 births.

In affected fetuses and neonates, extensive hemorrhage is possible. Mortality rate is up to 14%, with the majority being due to intracranial hemorrhage.

> Lester and Sty, 1987; Lynch et al., 1988

Prenatal Diagnosis: Diagnosis may be made by demonstrating maternal antibodies to fetal platelets and a low platelet count in fetal blood, or assumed to be present by detecting hydrocephalus, porencephalic cysts, or intracranial hemorrhage in a fetus at risk.

Differential Diagnosis: Other conditions that have been associated with thrombocytopenia in the fetus include Amegakaryocytic thrombocytopenia (PD 202500); Maternal chronic immune thrombocytopenia (PD 207700); Maternal idiopathic thrombocytopenia (PD 207750); Parvovirus (PD 200750); and Thrombocytopenia–absent radius syndrome (PD 175000). Conditions associated with hydrocephaly, porencephalic cysts, and intracranial hemorrhage also should be considered. (See these items in the Index.)

Prenatal Treatment: As with Erythroblastosis fetalis (PD 204000) effective and life-saving intrauterine transfusions have been accomplished. In particular the condition has been treated by the transfusion of antigen-1-negative concentrated platelets via cordocentesis. Transfusions normally have to be repeated weekly. Delivery by cesarean section to reduce the risk of intracranial hemorrhage should be considered (Daffos et al., 1984a).

Treatment Modalities: Intravascular transfusion of platelets via ultrasonic-guided cordocentesis

> Daffos et al., 1984; Kaplan et al., 1988a; Nicolini et al., 1990; Rodeck and Roberts, 1994
>
> *Comments:* Daffos and associates (1984) performed their intrauterine platelet transfusion 6 hours before the mother was delivered by cesarean section. This procedure was done to reduce the risk of intracranial hemorrhage during delivery. This approach does not avoid the risk of hemorrhage prior to delivery, however.

Maternal intravenous gamma-globulin infusion

> Bussel et al., 1988; Nicolini et al., 1990
>
> *Comments:* Although improved, the platelet counts in four of six fetuses reported by Bussel and co-authors (1988) were less than 100×10^9/L (normal = $150–400 \times 10^9$/L. Treatment with this modality alone may make affected fetuses at increased risk for intrauterine or perinatal hemorrhage.

Maternal medication

> dexamethasone by mouth (3–5 mg/d)
>
> Bussel et al., 1988

Methods and Findings: Cordocentesis (PUBS)[i]: low platelet count

> Daffos et al., 1984a; Bussel et al., 1988; Kaplan et al., 1988a; Lynch et al., 1988; Nicolini et al., 1990

Maternal blood sampling[d,i]: anti-PLA-1 antibody present in maternal serum

> Daffos et al., 1984a; Bussel et al., 1988; Kaplan et al., 1988a; Lynch et al., 1988; Nicolini et al., 1990

> low maternal platelet counts
>
> Kaplan et al., 1988a

Ultrasound[c,d]: hydrocephalus, multiple cystic lesions in the brain, oligohydramnios

> Lester and Sty, 1987
>
> *Comment:* After the birth of the patient reported by Lester and Sty (1987), the multiple cystic lesions turned out to be porencephalic cysts.

PD 207900 VON WILLEBRAND DISEASE (McKusick No. 193400; see also 277480, 314560)

> Chorionic villus sampling[g,i]: detection of von Willebrand gene by PCR and other molecular techniques not specified
>
> Ash et al., 1988

detection of same number of von Willebrand disease variable number of tanden repeats (ATCT-vWF.VNTR) in homozygous pattern in the fetus corresponding to the same pattern in the affected sister
> Peake et al., 1990

Cordocentesis (PUBS)[i]: low levels of procoagulant factor VIII (VIIIC), von Willebrand factor antigen (VIIIWF), and von Willebrand ristocetin cofactor (VIIIRAg)
> Mibashan and Miller, 1983; Ash et al., 1988; Peake et al., 1990

HEMOGLOBINOPATHIES[a]

General Review Articles: Alter and Nathan, 1978; Leonard and Kazazian, 1978; Nathan et al., 1979; Anderson, 1984; Weatherall et al., 1985

PD 208000 HEMOGLOBIN H DISEASE (McKusick No. 142309)

Amniocentesis[i]: determination of the number of alpha-genes present by molecular hybridization of DNA from cultured amniotic fluid cells with alpha-globin gene probes
> Koenig et al., 1978; Rubin and Kan, 1985

Chorionic villus sampling[g,i]: determination of the number of alpha-genes present by using restriction endonucleases, and alpha and zeta globin gene probes on DNA obtained from chorionic villi
> Liming et al., 1986

PD 208250 HEMOGLOBIN LEPORE–BOSTON DISEASE (McKusick No. 142000.0020)

Disease Note: Hemoglobin Lepore–Boston is an abnormal hemoglobin that is the fusion product of the delta and beta globin genes.
> Camaschella et al., 1990

Chorionic villus sampling[g,i]: detection of hemoglobin Lepore–Boston gene by specific DNA probes for this type of hemoglobin
> Camaschella et al., 1990

Maternal blood sampling[g,i]: detection of hemoglobin Lepore–Boston gene, in DNA obtained from maternal peripheral-blood buffy coat after amplification by PCR, and the use of specific DNA probes
> Camaschella et al., 1990

PD 208500 HEMOGLOBIN SC DISEASE (Heterozygous S/C disease; Sickle-C disease) (McKusick Nos. 141900.0038 and 141900.0243)

Chorionic villus sampling[g,i]: DNA analysis of chorionic villus tissue using RFLPs, and appropriate DNA probes
> Vidaud et al., 1986

Cordocentesis (PUBS): absence of HbA peak, presence of both an HbS and HbC peak on chromatography analyzed by optical density, and H-3 radioactivity
> Rouyer-Fessard et al., 1989

Method not stated: direct detection of the gene by hybridization to an allele-

specific oligonucleotide probe following PCR technique to amplify DNA sequence containing the gene[i]
> Boehm et al., 1987

PD 208750 HEMOGLOBIN SE DISEASE (McKusick No. 141900.0071 and 141900.0243)

Direct detection of gene by hybridization to an allele-specific oligonucleotide probe following PCR technique to amplify DNA sequence containing the gene[i]; source of the tissue was not stated
> Boehm et al., 1987

PD 208950 SICKLE-BETA-THALASSEMIA (McKusick No. 141900.0243)

Amniocentesis[i]: direct detection of HbS gene using the restriction endonuclease, *Mst*II, in conjunction with a 1.8-kb *Bam*HI DNA probe, followed by RFLP analysis for the beta-thalassemia
> Driscoll et al., 1987

PD 209000 SICKLE CELL ANEMIA (Sickle cell disease) (McKusick No. 141900.0243)

Amniocentesis[i]: DNA analysis of amniotic fluid cells using RFLPs and appropriate DNA probes
> Kan and Dozy, 1978; Panny et al., 1979; Jones et al., 1982; Old et al., 1986; Chang et al., 1982; Chang and Kan, 1982; Orkin et al., 1982; Boehm et al., 1983; Hoar et al., 1984; Driscoll et al., 1987
Chorionic villus sampling[g,i]: DNA analysis of chorionic villus tissue using RFLPs and appropriate DNA probes
> Goossens et al., 1983; Old et al., 1986; Vidaud et al., 1986
> DNA analysis of cultured chorionic villi
> Horwell et al., 1985
> direct DNA analysis of chorionic villi obtained transabdominally from the placenta using an ultrasound-guided needle at 14 weeks of gestation
> Nicolaides et al., 1986b
Cordocentesis (PUBS)[i]: determination of beta[s]-globin chain synthesis by chromatography or isoelectric focusing
> Alter et al., 1976; Dubart et al., 1980
> absence of HbA
> Blouquit et al., 1982; Rouyer-Fessard et al., 1989
> *Comment:* Hemoglobins were separated by chromatography and analyzed by optical density and/or radioactivity (Blouquit et al., 1982; Rouyer-Fessard et al., 1989).
Direct detection of the gene by hybridization to an allele-specific oligonucleotide probe following PCR technique to amplify DNA sequences containing the gene;[i] source of tissue was not stated
> Boehm et al., 1987; Chehab et al., 1987; Impraim and Teplitz, 1987

PD 209600 SICKLE CELL TRAIT/MATERNAL THIAMINE DEFICIENCY (McKusick No. None)

Condition Note: Thiamine is an essential cofactor for transketolase, an enzyme important in the production of NADPH in the pentose phosphate pathway. NADPH is a coenzyme for glutathione reductase and methemoglobin reductase which are of prime importance in maintaining heme in an inactive form (Fe^{2+}).

In individuals with sickle cell anemia and sickle cell trait, a deficiency of thiamine may lead to hypoxemia and sickling.

> Multon et al., 1994

Ultrasound[c,d]: fetal demise

> Multon et al., 1994

Comments: In the case presented by Multon and associates (1994), a pregnant woman, who was a sickle cell trait individual, developed thiamine deficiency because of recurrent vomiting and inanition. Her fetus died suddenly at 34 weeks' gestation. At autopsy the placenta had multiple infarctions with accumulation of maternal red blood sickle cells and fibrin within the intervillous spaces enclosing the chorionic villi. The authors postulated that the sickling occurred secondary to the thiamine deficiency. The placental infarctions then lead to the death of the fetus.

PD 210000 ALPHA-THALASSEMIA (Homozygous alpha-thalassemia; Hydrops fetalis) (McKusick Nos. 141800 and 141850)

Disease Note: Homozygous alpha-thalassemia is a disease produced by the deficiency of alpha-globin chains, and results from the individual having no normal alpha-globin genes. It is the most common cause of hydrops fetalis in southeast Asia (Ghosh et al., 1987), and leads to either fetal demise or death soon after birth. The hydrops fetalis probably results from the severe anemia that develops with this condition and the associated heart failure. Pregnancies with fetal alpha-thalassemia are often complicated by preeclampsia and hemorrhage resulting in significant maternal mortality and morbidity (Ghosh et al., 1987).

Prenatal Diagnosis: Diagnosis is accomplished by demonstrating complete deficiency of alpha-globin genes in the DNA of amniotic fluid cells or chorionic villi, or the presence of hydrops fetalis in fetuses at risk.

Alpha-fetoprotein (AFP)[c]: elevated in maternal serum

> Thomas et al., 1993

Amniocentesis[i]: determination of the number of alpha-globin genes present using molecular hybridization of DNA from cultured or uncultured amniotic fluid cells with alpha-globin cDNA using either Southern blot or rapid micro-DNA hybridization techniques

> Kan et al., 1976; Dozy et al., 1979; Alter et al., 1980; Rubin and Kan, 1985; Zeng and Huang, 1985; Old et al., 1986

Chorionic villus sampling[g,i]: determination of the number of alpha-globin genes present by using restriction endonucleases, and appropriate DNA probes on DNA obtained from chorionic villi

> Liming et al., 1986; Old et al., 1986; Vidaud et al., 1986

Cordocentesis[i]: fetal blood indicated alpha-thalassemia

> Thomas et al., 1993

Radiograph[d]: hydropic fetus

> Wong et al., 1978

Ultrasound: hydropic fetus with scalp edema,[d] increased pericardial, pleural, and peritoneal fluids,[d] enlarged liver and placenta[d]

> Wong et al., 1978; Kurtz et al., 1981; Nicolaides et al., 1986a; Ghosh et al., 1987

> progressive fetal ascites that may appear as early as 20 weeks' or as late as 36 weeks' gestation

> > Holzgreve et al., 1985c; Chehab et al., 1987

abnormal estimated fetal weight–placental volume ratio, and fetal growth retardation by 28 weeks' gestation; increased transverse cardiac diameter; enlarged liver presenting as a uniformly echogenic area occupying most of the abdomen; splenic enlargement with absence of the stomach shadow

    Ghosh et al., 1987

thickened right ventricular wall[c]

    Thomas et al., 1993

umbilical vein visualized as free-floating structure in the ascites before it enters the liver

    Holzgreve et al., 1985c

free-floating intestines in ascitic fluid

    Holzgreve et al., 1985c

intrauterine growth retardation[c]

    Thomas et al., 1993

oligohydramnios[c]

    Thomas et al., 1993

Absence of a 300-base pair alpha-globin-gene-amplified product, amplified by the PCR technique using a and b primers; source of tissue was not stated

    Chehab et al., 1987

PD 211000 beta⁰-THALASSEMIA, HOMOZYGOUS (beta⁰-Thalassemia major) (McKusick No. 141900)

Amniocentesis[i]: elevated sigma-aminolevulinic acid in amniotic fluid[c]

    Phadke et al., 1979

DNA analysis in amniotic fluid cells: recognition of RFLPs and appropriate DNA probes

    Boehm et al., 1983; Old et al., 1986

determination of beta⁰39 mutant by synthetic oligonucleotide method from cultured and uncultured cells

    Rosatelli et al., 1985; Monni et al., 1986

detection of beta⁰39 and beta⁰6 mutations in uncultured amniotic fluid cells using PCR, RFLP, and ethidium-bromide–stained polyacrylamide gels after electrophoresis

    Pirastu et al., 1989

Chorionic villus sampling[g,i]: RFLP analysis of DNA isolated from chorionic villi using appropriate DNA probes

    Old et al., 1982; Old et al., 1986

homozygous beta-thalassemia determining oligonucleotide analysis from DNA extracted from chorionic villi

    Monni et al., 1988; Aulehla-Scholz et al., 1989a

beta-thalassemia beta⁰-39 and beta⁺ 110 heterozygous fetuses diagnosed by appropriate beta⁰-39 and beta⁺ 110 DNA probes testing

    Rosatelli et al., 1985; Loi et al., 1986; Monni et al., 1986; Rosatelli et al., 1988

beta⁰39/frame-shift 44 mutation thalassemia diagnosed by utilizing PCR, dot blot hybridization, and DNA analysis

    Aulehla-Scholz et al., 1989b

Cordocentesis (PUBS)[i]: quantification of beta-globin chain synthesis

    Kan et al., 1975; Kan et al., 1977; Jensen et al., 1979; Alter et al.,

1980; Dubart et al., 1980; Boccacci et al., 1981; Antsakilis et al., 1984; Dash et al., 1984; Walters et al., 1984; Cao et al., 1986; Rouyer-Fessard et al., 1987

Comments: In the above analysis, separation of globin chains was accomplished by isoelectric focusing, chromatography, or electrophoresis.

little or no HbA in fetal blood sample

Blouquit et al., 1982; Rouyer-Fessard et al., 1989

Comments: Hemoglobins separated by chromatography and analysed by optical density and/or radioactivity (Blouquit et al., 1982; Rouyer-Fessard et al., 1989).

beta/gamma ratio less than 0.025

Alter et al., 1980

Fetal blood sampling by placental aspiration[i]: no beta-chain synthesis detected by means of ^{3}H-leucine incorporation and separation of the chains on carboxymethyl-cellulose columns

Cao et al., 1982

PD 211250 BETA$^+$-THALASSEMIA, HOMOZYGOUS (beta$^+$/beta^o-Thalassemia genetic compound) (McKusick No. 141908)

Cordocentesis (PUBS)[i]: beta-globin–psi ratio of less than 0.02 in fetal blood

Cao et al., 1986

PD 211370 THALASSEMIA INTERMEDIA (McKusick No. 273500)

Chorionic villus sampling[g,i]: determination of beta$^+$IVS-lnt6 and $^+$IVS-nt 110 genes using appropriate oligonucleotides

Rosatelli et al., 1988

Cordocentesis (PUBS)[i]: microerythrocytosis (microcytes), and globin-chain synthesis ratio (beta/gamma = 0.010 and alpha/nonalpha = 0.75) alteration in fetal blood

Ferrari et al., 1982

PD 211500 BETA-THALASSEMIA MAJOR-BETA-THALASSEMIA/ LEPORE GENOTYPE (McKusick Nos. 141900 and 142000)

Cordocentesis (PUBS)[i]: no beta-globin chain synthesis in fetal blood

Furbetta et al., 1981; Cao et al., 1986

Comments: In the case reported by Furbetta and associates (1981), the father of the fetus was a Lepore (Hb Lepore Boston-Washington [delta 87 Gln, beta 116 His]) heterozygote and the mother was a high HbA$_2$ beta-thalassemia carrier.

Chapter 6

Inborn Errors of Metabolism[a]

Ira K. Brandt, M.D., and David D. Weaver, M.D.

DISORDERS OF AMINO ACID METABOLISM

PD 211900 ARGININEMIA (Arginase deficiency; Hyperargininemia)
(McKusick No. 207800)

Disease Note: Argininemia is an autosomal recessive disorder that is characterized by progressive spastic tetraplegia, hyperactivity, seizures, psychomotor retardation, and growth failure.

Prenatal Diagnosis: Fetal blood sampling for erythrocytic arginase activity and
restriction-fragment-length polymorphisms (RFLPs) are considered to be diagnostic (Brusilow and Horwich, 1989).

    Cordocentesis (percutaneous umbilical blood sampling, or PUBS)[i]: erythro-
cytic arginase deficiency

        Caruso et al., 1994; Kamoun et al., 1995

        elevated plasma arginine concentration

            Caruso et al., 1994

PD 212000 ARGININOSUCCINIC ACIDURIA (McKusick No. 207900)

Disease Note: An autosomal recessive disorder of urea synthesis typically characterized by early—even neonatal—onset of trichorrhexis nodosa, maculopapular
rashes, hepatomegaly, and occasional episodes of hyperammonemia. Argininosuccinate lyase deficiency results in a marked decrease in urea synthesis; nitrogen
excretion is accomplished by markedly increased argininosuccinic acid excretion
with a resulting depletion of arginine.

Prenatal Diagnosis: Methods that have been used include measurement of argininosuccinic acid (ASA) concentration in amniotic fluid (none present in normal
pregnancies),[14]C-citrulline incorporation into amniotic fluid cells or chorionic
villi, and argininosuccinate lyase assays (either direct or indirect, using ^{14}C-ASA
accumulation during the ^{14}C-citrulline incorporation test). Direct metabolite
measurement in amniotic fluid or the incorporation tests on chorionic villi and
cultured chorionic villus cells were more reliable than the use of cultured amniocytes (Kamoun et al., 1995).

Amniocentesis[i]: accumulation of argininosuccinic acid-^{14}C in cultured amniotic fluid cells

Goodman et al., 1973; Kamoun et al., 1983

Comment: Enzyme assay of amniotic fluid may give erroneous results when testing for this condition (Mandell et al., 1996).

increased levels of argininosuccinic acid in amniotic fluid and maternal urine

Goodman et al., 1973; Chadefaux et al., 1989b; Mandell et al., 1996

Comments: The above determination should be done along with enzyme activities (Kamoun and Chadefaux, 1991).

Chorionic villus sampling (CVS)[g,i]: deficiency of ^{14}C-citrulline incorporation into protein in villus fragments

Kleijer, 1986; Pijpers et al., 1990; Chadefaux et al., 1989b; Kamoun and Chadefaux, 1991

Comment: The above cited, indirect methodology may give erroneous results.

Chadefaux et al., 1988b

PD 212150 BIOTINIDASE DEFICIENCY (Multiple carboxylase deficiency, late onset) (McKusick No. 253260)

Disease Note: Patients with this autosomal recessive disorder present in infancy or early childhood with skin rashes, alopecia, respiratory disorders, hypotonia, seizures, myoclonus, ataxia, and optic nerve atrophy. Treatment with pharmacologic doses of biotin will prevent and ameliorate many manifestations, but some neurologic damage may be permanent.

Chorionic villus sampling[g,i]: a heterozygous fetus was identified by demonstrating decreased levels of biotinidase activities

Chalmers et al., 1994

PD 212250 CARBAMOYLPHOSPHATE SYNTHETASE DEFICIENCY (CPS 1; Hyperammonemia II) (McKusick No. 237300)

Disease Note: Carbamoylphosphate synthetase catalyzes the first step of the urea cycle. A deficiency of this enzyme leads to hyperammonemia and neonatal death in the severe form, or less significant problems with delayed onset in a second form. The disorder is inherited as an autosomal recessive condition.

McKusick, 1988

Prenatal Diagnosis: Since a reliable enzyme assay of tissues other than liver has not been developed for carbamoylphosphate synthetase activity, the only reported method of prenatal diagnosis of this condition is by the direct liver assay of this enzyme.

Differential Diagnosis: Other disorders of the urea cycle should be considered.

Fetal liver biopsy[i]: complete deficiency of carbamoylphosphate synthetase in fetal liver

Piceni Sereni et al., 1988

PD 212375 CARNITINE TRANSPORTER DEFICIENCY (McKusick No. 212140)

Disease Note: Carnitine transporter deficiency is an autosomal recessive disorder of carnitine transport across cell membranes resulting in early childhood onset of hypoketotic hypoglycemia, cardiomyopathy, or skeletal myopathy. Successful

treatment with large doses of carnitine has been reported; treatment must be maintained indefinitely, however.
> Christodoulou et al., 1996.

Amniocentesis[i]: cultured amniocytes demonstrated marked diminished carnitine transport across cell membranes
> Christodoulou et al., 1996.

PD 212500 CITRULLINEMIA (Argininosuccinate synthetase deficiency; Citrullinuria) (McKusick No. 215700)

Disease Note: Citrullinemia is an autosomal recessive disorder of the urea cycle, and is caused by a deficiency of argininosuccinate synthetase activity. Clinical features include episodes of severe vomiting, beginning in infancy, and mental deficiency. Elevated levels of citrulline are found in most body fluids including serum, spinal fluid, and urine.
> McKusick, 1988

Prenatal Diagnosis: Methods that have been used for making the diagnosis prenatally include direct enzyme assay of cultured amniotic fluid cells and chorionic villi, measurement of citrulline levels in amniotic fluid, and incorporation of ^{14}C-citrulline into protein of cultured cells. Each method, however, is problematic because of low enzyme levels in available tissues, false-negative levels of citrulline in amniotic fluid, and the limited number of laboratories offering testing of these three methods. Although Northrup and associate's (1988) method of incorporation of ^{14}C-citrulline is the best available enzymatic method, linkage analysis of RFLPs within the gene, when informative, is preferable when the risk is 25% (Northrup et al., 1990). Northrup and associates believe that if the risk is less than 25%, prenatal diagnosis is of "questionable value." Discrepancies have been noted between the non-molecular methods, but these, although very few, make it advisable to use more than one testing method (Kamoun et al., 1995; Mandell et al., 1996).

Amniocentesis[i]: deficient argininosuccinic acid synthetase activity in cultured amniotic fluid cells
> Fleisher et al., 1983

increased concentration of citrulline in amniotic fluid
> Fleisher et al., 1983; Kleijer et al., 1984a

deficient ^{14}C-citrulline incorporation into cultured amniotic fluid cells
> Kleijer et al., 1984a
> *Comment:* The above method may give false results (Mandell et al., 1996).

Chorionic villus sampling[g,i]: decreased incorporation of ^{14}C-citrulline into cultured villus cells or uncultured villus fragments
> Kleijer et al., 1984b; Kleijer, 1986; Kamoun and Chadefaux, 1991
> linkage analysis using Southern blot technique accurately predicted unaffected children
> Northrup et al., 1990

PD 213000 CYSTINOSIS (Cystinosis, early-onset or infantile nephropathic; Nephropathic cystinosis) (McKusick No. 219800)

Disease Note: An autosomal recessive disorder characterized by Fanconi syndrome leading to renal failure, retinal degeneration, corneal crystals, photophobia, growth failure, and other findings consistent with a lysosomal disorder.

This condition results from a defective transport of cystine across lysosomal membranes by facilitated diffusion; presumably a defective carrier molecule is present. Lysosomal cysteine, generated from the breakdown of proteins, is converted to cystine which remains trapped in the lysosomes in these patients. Accumulation of cystine results in reduction in cell function, particularly in those organs manifesting signs of the disorder.

Amniocentesis[i]: accumulation of ^{35}S-cystine in cultured amniotic fluid cells

> Schneider et al., 1974; Boman and Schneider, 1981

> prolonged retention of ^{35}S-L-cystine within cultured amniotic fluid cells

> States et al., 1975

Chorionic villus sampling[g,i]: elevated level of cystine in homogenized chorionic villi from a fetus at risk

> Smith et al., 1987

> increased percentage of ^{35}S-cystine in cultured chorionic villi after incubation with ^{35}S-cystine

> Smith et al., 1987; Patrick et al., 1987

> increased uptake and retention of ^{35}S-cystine in intact biopsy samples of chorionic villi

> Patrick et al., 1987

PD 214000 CYSTINURIA (McKusick No. 220100)

Disease Note: Cystinuria is an autosomal recessive disorder characterized by stone-formation in any region of the urinary tract, recurring urinary tract infections, and renal failure in untreated patients. The condition is due to defective renal tubular transport of the dibasic amino acids lysine, arginine, ornithine, and cystine; insolubility of the latter leads to stone formation.

Prenatal Diagnosis: Detection of elevated cystine in the amniotic fluid in at-risk fetuses appears to be diagnostic.

Amniocentesis[d,i]: elevated cystine in amniotic fluid

> Komrower, 1974

PD 214500 FUMARASE DEFICIENCY (McKusick No. 136850)

Disease Note: The disorder is an autosomal recessive condition characterized by congenital hydrocephalus, progressive brain atrophy, infantile spasms, fumaric aciduria, and virtual absence of fumarase in the cytosolic or both cytosolic and mitrochondrial fractions of lymphocytes and fibroblasts.

Prenatal Diagnosis: The diagnosis probably could be accomplished by enzyme assay in the first trimester, but doing so has not been reported.

Ultrasound[c]: hydrocephalus,[d] hydramnios[d]

> Remes et al., 1992

PD 215000 GLUTARICACIDEMIA, TYPE I (McKusick No. 231670)

Disease Note: This disorder is an autosomal recessive condition classically characterized by the relatively sudden onset in early childhood of hypotonia, generalized movement disorders, dystonia, and seizures. These signs may partially remit but recur during episodes of ketoacidosis precipitated by episodes of infections. There is progressive neurologic deterioration until death in mid-childhood during one of the exacerbations. Glutaricacidemia results from glutaryl-CoA dehydrogenase deficiency, and the consequent accumulation of its hydrolyzed substrate.

Treatment by dietary restriction of substrate precursors and supplementation with vitamin cofactor is of no avail.

Amniocentesis[i]: presence of glutaric acid in amniotic fluid
        Goodman et al., 1979
        deficient glutaryl-CoA dehydrogenase activity in cultured amniotic fluid cells
        Goodman et al., 1979
Chorionic villus sampling[g,i]: glutaryl-CoA dehydrogenase activity of uncultured and cultured cells reduced
        Christensen, 1994

PD 215500 GLUTARICACIDURIA, TYPE IIA (Glutaricaciduria, neonatal-lethal type; Multiple acyl-CoA dehydrogenase deficiencies) (McKusick No. 305950)

Disease Note: Glutaricaciduria, type IIA, is an autosomal recessive disorder of mitochondrial electron transport characterized by neonatal onset of severe hypoglycemia and acidosis resulting in death in the first days of life. Renal cysts are present in all cases, and cerebral dysplasia, facial anomalies (high forehead, flat nasal bridge, low-set ears), and the odor of sweaty feet may also be present. Electron transfer flavoprotein:ubiquinone oxidoreductase is the deficient enzyme.

Alpha-fetoprotein (AFP)[c]: elevated in maternal serum
        Boue et al., 1984
Amniocentesis[i]: elevated levels of amniotic fluid glutaric acid and 2-hydroxy-glutaric acid
        Mitchell et al., 1983; Boue et al., 1984; Jakobs et al., 1984b; Chalmers et al., 1985; Yamaguchi et al., 1991
        increased concentration of glutaric acid in amniotic fluid
        Jakobs, 1989
        elevated levels of other dicarboxylic acids (adipic acid, suberic acid, and sebacic acid) in amniotic fluid
        Jakobs et al., 1984b
        reduced fatty acid (palmitate and octanoate) oxidation in cultured amniotic fluid cells
        Mitchell et al., 1983; Bennett et al., 1984
        reduced oxidation of 1-^{14}C-butyrate in amniotic fluid cells
        Boue et al., 1984; Chalmers et al., 1985
        cultured amniocytes: immunoblot analysis of electron transferring flavoprotein (ETF) demonstrated beta-subunit deficiency
        Yamaguchi et al., 1991
Chorionic villus sampling[i]: cultured trophoblastic cells oxidized palmitate at a rate enabling correct prediction of an unaffected fetus
        Medlock et al., 1991
Maternal urine[i]: fast atom bombardment mass spectrometry reveals elevated tigly1-, isovalery1-, and glutaryl-carnitine levels
        Sakuma et al., 1991
Ultrasound[c]: cystic kidneys
        Boue et al., 1984; Hockey et al., 1993

PD 215550 GLUTATHIONE SYNTHASE DEFICIENCY (5-Oxoprolinuria; Pyroglutamic aciduria) (McKusick No. 266130)

Disease Note: This condition is a rare autosomal recessive disorder presenting in its severest form with fatal, untreatable, neonatal acidosis and hemolysis. Milder forms exist in the form of chronic acidosis with neurologic deficits of vary severity.

Amniocentesis[i]: 40-fold increase in the amniotic fluid 5-oxoproline concentration

Manning et al., 1994

Comment: The diagnosis in the fetus reportedly by Manning and colleagues (1994) was confirmed by reduced glutathione synthase activity in cultured fibroblasts obtained from the fetus after termination of the pregnancy.

PD 216000 HOMOCYSTINURIA (McKusick No. 236200)

Disease Note: This disorder represents a group of autosomal recessive disorders of sulfur-amino-acid metabolism characterized by marfanoid appearance, subluxated lenses, scoliosis, hernias, and vascular thromboses resulting in strokes, heart attacks, and mental retardation in patients who are not treated appropriately.

Amniocentesis[i]: deficient cystathionine synthase activity in cultured amniotic fluid cells

Fowler et al., 1982

reduced conversion of ^{35}S-homocystine to cysteine and methionine in amniotic fluid cell monolayer culture

Fowler et al., 1982

PD 216050 HOMOCYSTINURIA: 5,10-METHYLENE TETRAHYDROFOLATE REDUCTASE DEFICIENCY TYPE (McKusick No. 236250)

Disease Note: The clinical picture of this condition is variable, but in general is similar to that of patients with cystathione synthase deficiency (PD 216000); however, homocystine excretion is less and methionine concentration is reduced.

Amniocentesis[i]: cultured amniotic fluid cells had very low enzyme activity.

Wendel et al., 1983; Christensen et al., 1985

Comment: In the case reported by Christenson and associates (1985), the family decided to continue the pregnancy which resulted in a homocystinuric infant with reduced leukocyte-enzyme activity.

5, 10-methylene tetrahydrofolate reductase activity studies that indicated reduced but not very low activity enabled diagnosis of heterozygosity

Marquet et al., 1994

Chorionic villus sampling[g,i]: enzyme studies indicate reduced but not very low activity using uncultured and cultured material enabled a diagnosis of heterozygosity

Marquet et al., 1994

PD 216300 4-HYDROXYBUTYRIC ACIDURIA (Succinic semialdehyde dehydrogenase deficiency) (McKusick No. 271980)

Disease Note: Hypotonia, ataxia, seizures, delayed speech and language development, and mental retardation characterize this autosomal recessive disorder.

Prenatal Diagnosis: Elevated amniotic fluid 4-hydroxybutyric acid levels and virtually undetected cultured amniocytic enzyme activity have been used to make the diagnosis.

Amniocentesis[i]: elevated amniotic fluid 4-hydroxybutyric acid levels
        Jakobs et al., 1993; Gibson et al., 1994
    deficiency of succinic semialdehyde dehydrogenase activity in cultured amniotic fluid cells
        Jakobs et al., 1993
Chorionic villus sampling[i]: deficiency of succinic semialdehyde dehydrogenase in uncultured chorionic villi
        Gibson et al., 1994

PD 216500 3-HYDROXY-3-METHYLGLUTARYL COENZYME A LYASE DEFICIENCY (HMG-CoA lyase deficiency; Hydroxymethylglutaricaciduria) (McKusick No. 246450)

Disease Note: This condition is an autosomal recessive disorder characterized by severe episodes of encephalopathy, metabolic acidosis, and non-ketotic hypoglycemia, and may be lethal.

Prenatal Diagnosis: Elevated amniotic fluid levels of 3-hydroxy-3-methylglutaric and other acids, virtually undetectable enzyme activity in chorionic villus tissue, and DNA studies checking for mutations in the gene all are reliable for establishing the diagnosis.

Amniocentesis[i]: increased amniotic fluid levels of 3-hydroxy-3-methylglutaric, 3-methylglutaconic, 3-methylglutaric, and 3-hydroxyisovaleric acids as determined by gas chromatography/mass spectrometry
        Chalmers et al., 1989b; Mitchell et al., 1995
    homozygosity for a frameshift mutation [N46fs(+1)] was found by single-strand conformation polymorphism migration-profile analysis of DNA obtained from uncultured amniotic fluid cells
        Mitchell et al., 1995
    reduced HMG-CoA lyase activity in cultured amniotic fluid cells
        Chalmers et al., 1989b; Mitchell et al., 1995
Chorionic villus sampling[i]: HMG-CoA lyase activity essentially absent
        Chalmers et al., 1989a; Chalmers et al., 1989b
Maternal urine testing: elevated levels of 3-hydroxy-3-methylglutaric, 3-methylglutaconic, 3-methylglutaric, and 3-hydroxyisovaleric acids in maternal urine[i]
        Duran et al., 1979

PD 216550 HYPERORNITHINEMIA, HYPERAMMONEMIA, AND HOMOCITRULLINURIA SYNDROME (HHH syndrome) (McKusick No. 238970)

Disease Note: The above cited condition is a rare autosomal recessive disorder that probably is due to a defect in ornithine uptake by the mitochondria. This defect results in ornithine accumulation and reduced ability to detoxify ammonia. Some cases are severe enough to result in neonatal death.

Amniocentesis[i]: cultured amniocytes demonstrated reduced incorporation of ^{14}C ornithine
        Shih et al., 1992; Kamoun et al., 1995

PD 216600 HYPEROXALURIA, TYPE I (Glycolicaciduria; Hepatic AGT deficiency; Oxalosis I; Peroxisomal alanine:glyoxylate aminotransferase deficiency) (McKusick No. 259900)

Disease Note: The autosomal recessive disease, hyperoxaluria, type I, is caused by the deficiency of peroxisomal alanine : glyoxylate aminotransferase, an enzyme found only in the liver. Clinical manifestations include high urinary oxalate excretion leading to progressive, bilateral oxalate urolithiasis, and nephrocalcinosis. Deposit of oxalate occurs elsewhere later in life. Progressive renal failure develops with time, and death ensues during childhood or as a young adult. For additional details, see Peroxisomal disorders (PD 231625).

Danpure et al., 1989a; McKusick, 1990

Prenatal Diagnosis: The diagnosis is made prenatally by demonstrating deficiency or absence of peroxisomal alanine:glyoxylate aminotransferase in fetal liver obtained by percutaneous liver biopsy. Because some affected fetuses have only partial deficiencies of the latter enzyme activity, or deficient enzyme protein, or both, enzyme assay, immunochemistry, and immunoblotting should all be employed to establish the diagnosis (Danpure et al., 1989b).

Differential Diagnosis: Hyperoxaluria, type II, and other conditions that produce urolithiasis should be considered.

Percutaneous fetal liver biopsy[i]: reduced levels of peroxisomal alanine:glyoxylate aminotransferase activity

Danpure et al., 1989a; Danpure et al., 1989b

no immunoreactive alanine:glyoxylate aminotransferase protein following protein A-gold immunocytochemical localization on electron microscopic sections

Danpure et al., 1989a; Danpure et al., 1989b

no residual alanine:glyoxylate aminotransferase activity or immunoreactivity on immunoblotting

Danpure et al., 1989a; Danpure et al., 1989b

PD 216800 ISOVALERIC ACIDEMIA (Isovaleric acid CoA dehydrogenase deficiency; Isovaleryl-CoA dehydrogenase deficiency; Sweaty feet syndrome) (McKusick No. 243500)

Amniocentesis[i]: elevated concentrations of isovalerylglycine (IVG) in amniotic fluid

Hine et al., 1986; Dumoulin et al., 1991; Kleijer et al., 1995

amniotic fluid collected at 12 weeks' gestation was positive for increased IVG in an affected fetus

Kleijer et al., 1995

reduced incorporation of ^{14}C-isovaleric acid into cultured amniotic fluid cells

Dumoulin et al., 1991; Kleijer et al., 1995

Maternal urine sampling[i]: elevated levels of IVG in maternal urine

Hine et al., 1986

Chorionic villus sampling[g,i]: uncultured and cultured material assayed by ^{14}C isovaleric acid incorporation showed decreased incorporation.

Kleijer et al., 1995

Comment: Kleijer and associates (1995) considered the use of uncultured villi the best strategy for establishing the diagnosis.

PD 216900 LONG-CHAIN 3-HYDROXYACYL-CoA-DEHYDROGENASE DEFICIENCY (Long-chain 3-hydroxy dicarboxylic aciduria) (McKusick No. 143450)

Disease Note: This disorder, an autosomal-recessive, mitochondrial disease is characterized by episodic non-ketotic hypoglycemia, hepatomegaly, cardiomyopathy, rhabdomyolysis, hepatopathy, coma, dicarboxylic acid urine (both hydroxylated and non-hydroxylated forms), and a high mortality rate. Episodes vary in severity, and are precipitated by fasting or infection. Urinary ketones and carnitine levels are low, and long-chain dicarboxylic acid levels are elevated during episodes.

Prenatal Diagnosis: Chorionic villus biopsy material is deficient in the enzyme, long-chain 3-hydroxy-acyl-CoA-dehydrogenase in this disorder, and appears to be diagnostic.

  Chorionic villus sampling[g,i]: long-chain 3-hydroxyacyl-CoA-dehydrogenase deficiency in cultured and uncultured (at 10 weeks) chorionic villi

    Perez-Cerda et al., 1993; von Dobeln et al., 1994

PD 217000 MAPLE SYRUP URINE DISEASE (McKusick No. 248600)

  Amniocentesis[i]: deficient branched-chain ketoacid decarboxylase activity in cultured amniotic fluid cells

    Cox et al., 1978; Wendel and Claussen, 1979; Carmi et al., 1986

  Chorionic villus sampling[g,i]: deficiency of decarboxylation of branched-chain ketoacids in uncultured chorionic villi

    Kleijer et al., 1985a; Kleijer, 1986

PD 217750 3-METHYLGLUTACONIC ACIDURIA (3-Methylglutaconyl-CoA hydratase deficiency; 3-MG-CoA-hydratase deficiency) (McKusick No. 250950)

Disease Note: This disease represents a small, heterogeneous group of disorders in which four types have been characterized. Type 1 is autosomal recessive, and associated with impaired speech development. Type 2 is X-linked, with short stature, mitochondrial cardiomyopathy, skeletal myopathy and recurrent infections, and normal cognitive development. Type 3 is found in Iraqi Jews with optic atrophy, spastic paraplegia, and movement disorder. Type 4 has severe psychomotor retardation, cerebellar dysgenesis, normal enzyme activity, and autosomal recessive inheritance (Chitayat et al., 1992).

Prenatal Diagnosis: Presumably, increased 3-methylglutaconic and 3-methylglutaric acids in amniotic fluid is diagnostic.

  Amniocentesis[i]: normal 3-methylglutaconic and 3-methylglutaric acid concentrations in amniotic fluid correctly predicted a normal fetal sibling of a type 4 patient

    Chitayat et al., 1992

PD 218000 METHYLMALONIC ACIDURIA (5′-Deoxyadenosylcobalamin deficiency and Methylmalonyl CoA mutase deficiency) (McKusick Nos. 251000, 251100, 251110)

Disease Note: Methylmalonic aciduria is a group of disorders resulting from a failure of the cell to convert L-methylmalonyl CoA to succinyl CoA. As a result, methylmalonate accumulates in the body and subsequently is excreted in large amounts in the urine. Clinically, the disorder is noted by recurrent vomiting, dehydration, failure to thrive, developmental delay, hepatomegaly, muscular hypotonia, coma, and in some cases, death. Laboratory findings in affected patients include metabolic acidosis, anemia, neutropenia, thrombocytopenia, hyperglycinemia, hyperammonemia, ketonemia/ketonuria, and hypoglycemia. These disorders are inherited in an autosomal recessive fashion.

Wajner et al., 1986

Prenatal Diagnosis: Diagnosis of this condition has been made by demonstrating a deficiency of methylmalonyl CoA mutase in amniotic fluid cells and chorionic villus tissue in fetuses at risk. It also has been detected by demonstrating elevated levels of methylmalonate and methylcitrate in amniotic fluid of affected fetuses and elevated levels of methylmalonate in maternal urine of affected fetuses.

Differential Diagnosis: Other inborn errors of metabolism that produce metabolic acidosis and hyperammonemia need to be considered.

Prenatal Treatment: Treatment of affected fetuses has been accomplished by giving the mother daily cyanocobalamin (vitamin B_{12}) orally or intravenously beginning as early as the 21st and as late as the 39th week of gestation. At birth high, levels of circulating vitamin B_{12} have been noted, and the neonates have been clinically normal. The advantage of treating this disorder prenatally as opposed to immediate postnatal treatment is not clear at this time (Ampola et al., 1975; Zass et al., 1995; Soda et al., 1995). From an historical point, the report by Ampola and co-workers (1975) was the first report where prenatal treatment of a vitamin-responsive inborn error of metabolism was undertaken (Harrison et al., 1984, p 185).

Methods and Findings: Amniocentesis[i]: deficient methylmalonyl CoA mutase activity in cultured and uncultured amniotic fluid cells

Ampola et al., 1975; Mahoney et al., 1975; Morrow et al., 1977; Trefz et al., 1981

elevated levels of methylmalonate in amniotic fluid and maternal urine

Mahoney et al., 1975; Nakamura et al., 1976; Trefz et al., 1981; Zinn et al., 1982; Sweetman, 1984; Sweetman, 1985

elevated levels of methylmalonate and methylcitrate in amniotic fluid

Sweetman et al., 1982; Holm et al., 1989; Jakob, 1989

elevated levels of methylcitrate in amniotic fluid

Buchanan et al., 1980; Naylor et al., 1980; Sweetman et al., 1982; Sweetman, 1984; Fensom et al., 1984; Sweetman, 1985; Holm et al., 1989

elevated levels of propionylcarnitine in amniotic fluid

Penn et al., 1987; Sugiyama et al., 1990

Chorionic villus sampling[g,i]: deficiency of methylmalonyl CoA mutase activity in uncultured chorionic villi

Fowler et al., 1988

Maternal urine sampling[d,i]: elevated levels of methylmalonate in the maternal urine

Wajner et al., 1986

PD 218100 MEVALONIC ACIDURIA (McKusick No. Unknown)

Disease Note: An autosomal recessive disorder, mevalonic aciduria is characterized by psychomotor retardation, severe failure to thrive, diarrhea, hepatosplenomegaly, cataracts, and other dysmorphic features. There are pronounced mevalonic aciduria and marked reduction in mevalonate kinase activity in lymphocytes and fibroblasts; heterozygotes are readily detected. Intermediate and mild forms of the disorder exist, and are consistent within families.

Prenatal Diagnosis: The diagnosis of this condition can be accomplished by several methods: measurement of maternal urinary mevalonic acid and amniotic fluid mevalonic acid, and mevalonate–kinase activity in cultured amniocytes or chorionic villi.

> Amniocentesis[i]: elevated level of mevalonic acid in amniotic fluid
> > Sweetman, 1985
> Maternal urine[i]: increased levels of mevalonic acid
> > Mancini et al., 1993

PD 218150 MULTIPLE CARBOXYLASE DEFICIENCY, BIOTIN-RESPONSIVE (Holocarboxylase synthetase deficiency; Multiple carboxylase deficiency, neonatal or early onset form) (McKusick No. 253270)

Disease Note: This disorder is produced by a deficiency in holocarboxylase synthetase which is the enzyme that attaches biotin to inactive apocarboxylases to make the active forms of these enzymes, holocarboxylases. Clinical manifestations include hypotonia, vomiting, developmental delay or regression, skin rash, and alopecia. Biochemical characteristics include severe metabolic acidosis, ketosis, lactic acidosis, hyperammonemia, and organic aciduria. If untreated the condition may lead to coma and death. Biotin, 10 mg/d orally, is the usual treatment.

> Sweetman, 1990

Prenatal Diagnosis: Diagnosis of this condition can be made prenatally by finding elevated 3-hydroxyisovaleric acid in the amniotic fluid and biotin-responsive deficiencies of carboxylases in cultured cells.

> Packman et al., 1982; Sweetman, 1990

Differential Diagnosis: Biotinidase deficiency; Biotin-unresponsive 3-beta-methylcrotonylglycinuria; Multiple carboxylase deficiency, late-onset form

Prenatal Treatment: Treatment as early as 23 weeks of gestation has been accomplished by giving the mother 10 mg/d of biotin by mouth. The goal of treatment has been to prevent possible prenatal neurologic damage and severe ketoacidosis in the perinatal period. With treatment, affected fetuses have had uncomplicated postnatal courses (Packman et al., 1982; Roth et al., 1982).

Methods and Findings: Amniocentesis[i]: elevated level of 3-hydroxyisovaleric acid in amniotic fluid

> Jakobs et al., 1984a
> elevated level of methylcitrate in amniotic fluid
> > Packman et al., 1982
> low levels of activity of propionyl CoA carboxylase, pyruvate carboxylase, and 3-methyl-crotonyl CoA carboxylase in amniotic fluid cells grown in media not supplemented with biotin
> > Packman et al., 1982

PD 218200 NONKETOTIC HYPERGLYCINEMIA, TYPICAL (D-glycericacidemia; Glycine encephalopathy) (McKusick No. 220120)

Disease Note: The condition is an autosomal recessive one produced by a defect in the glycine cleavage pathway and results in markedly elevated levels of glycine in body fluids. There are two types of nonketotic hyperglycinemia, typical (neonatal) and atypical (late onset). The former is characterized by rapid development of postnatal neurologic symptoms, and weeks to months of respiratory and deglutition failure which results in death during infancy if not treated properly. Neurologic symptoms usually include lethargy, hypotonia, apnea, and seizures; survivors have severe psychomotor retardation. Brain abnormalities have been reported (Johnston and Weinstein, 1989). The atypical cases have had less dramatic clinical courses and milder residual developmental disabilities.

Hayasaka et al., 1987

Prenatal Diagnosis: Diagnosis is established by demonstrating reduced to absent glycine-cleavage enzyme in chorionic villus samples. Less reliable methods are the detection of elevated glycine concentrations in the amniotic fluids of fetuses at risk, and demonstrating a mutational change in DNA and enzyme.

Differential Diagnosis: Acyl-CoA dehydrogenase, long-chain, deficiency of; Non-ketotic hyperglycinemia, atypical type; Propionicacidemia (PD 219000)

Amniocentesis[i]: elevated levels of glycine, increased glycine/serine ratio, and reduced levels of serine in amniotic fluid of affected fetuses

Garcia-Castro et al., 1982a; Garcia-Castro et al., 1982b; Wendt et al., 1983; Applegarth et al., 1986; Toone and Applegarth, 1989

Comments: Wendt and associates (1983) have shown that there is an overlap of values in the glycine/serine ratio between the amniotic fluid of normal and affected fetuses at 38 to 40 weeks' gestation. Thus, the use of the above ratio may not be reliable for prenatal diagnosis in later gestational ages. Normal amniotic fluid levels of glycine and a normal glycine/serine ratio in an affected fetus at 16 weeks of gestation have also been reported by Garcia-Munoz and co-workers (1989). False-positive results have been reported by Parvy and colleagues (1990); this group believes that "this unreliable method should not be used." Toone and associates (1992) believe that amniotic fluid glycine concentration should be determined as an adjunct to CVS enzyme assay.

elevated glycerine/serine ratio in amniotic fluid at 12 weeks' gestation[g]

Hayasaka et al., 1987

Chorionic villus sampling[g,i]: deficient glycine-cleavage enzyme activity

Hayasaka et al., 1990; Tada et al., 1992; Toone et al., 1992; Rolland et al., 1993b; Toone et al., 1994

detection of G1556A mutation in DNA resulting in a S564I change in enzyme structure; allele-specific oligonucleotide hybridization technique was employed

Tada et al., 1992

Ultrasound[c,d]: ventriculomegaly

Johnston and Weinstein, 1989

PD 218500 ORNITHINE TRANSCARBAMYLASE DEFICIENCY (Ornithine carbamyl transferase deficiency) (McKusick No. 311250)

Disease Note: Ornithine transcarbamylase is a hepatic urea cycle enzyme. A deficiency of this enzyme results in lethal neonatal ammonia intoxication in hemizygous affected males. The condition is inherited in an X-linked recessive mode.

Fox et al., 1985

Prenatal Diagnosis: The diagnosis may be accomplished by demonstration of enzyme deficiency in fetal liver, by Southern analysis, by RFLP linkage in informative families (Kamoun et al., 1995), or by direct mutation detection of the defective gene.

Amniocentesis[g,i]: amniocyte DNA RFLP used to rule out the disorder
Pembrey et al., 1985; Nussbaum et al., 1986; Hoshide et al., 1996

Chorionic villus sampling[g,i]: linkage of the defective gene to RFLPs
Fox et al., 1985; Pembrey et al., 1985; Fox et al., 1986; Spence et al., 1989; Liechti-Gallati et al., 1991; Hoshide et al., 1996

Fetal liver biopsy[i]: undetectable ornithine transcarbamylase activity in fetal liver obtained by biopsy
Rodeck et al., 1982a; Holzgreve and Golbus, 1984; Fox et al., 1986
direct mutation detection
Liechti-Gallati et al., 1991

PD 218750 PHENYLKETONURIA (Phenylalanine hydroxylase deficiency; PKUI) (McKusick No. 261600)

Amniocentesis[g,i]: linkage of human cDNA for phenylalanine hydroxylase to RFLPs
Lidsky et al., 1985; Speer et al., 1986
linkage of various RFLPs to the gene for phenylketonuria using DNA from amniotic fluid cells[i]
Huang et al., 1990

Chorionic villus sampling[g,i]: linkage of cDNA for phenylalanine hydroxylase to informative RFLPs
Lidsky et al., 1985; Speer et al., 1986; Wulff et al., 1989
Comment: In the NICHD collaborative study one of three cases gave inconclusive results by this method; the infant was affected.
Desnick et al., 1992
minisatellite analysis of short tandem repeats in intron 3, and variable number of tandem repeats in area flanked by two Hind III sites downstream of exon 13
Romano et al., 1994
Comments: Polymerase chain reaction (PCR) amplification of three polymorphisms (short tandem repeats, variable number of tandem repeats, and Xmnl restriction-fragment-length polymorphisims) provides material for greater informativity for analysis; no prenatal diagnosis was reported, however.
Eisensmith et al., 1994

PD 219000 PROPIONICACIDEMIA (Propionic acidemia) (McKusick No. Unknown; see 232000, 232050)

Disease Note: Propionicacidemia is an autosomal recessive disorder produced by a deficiency in propionyl CoA carboxylase. As a result, proprionyl CoA accumulates. This latter compound is an intermediate in the distal and common pathway of the metabolism of isoleucine, valine, methionine, threonine, cholesterol, and odd-chain fatty acids. The classical presentation of the disorder include severe acidosis and hyperammonenia by 2 days of age. Followed by anorexia, lethargy, hyperventilation, seizures, coma, and death in untreated cases.

Prenatal Diagnosis: The diagnosis can be made by detecting deficiency of propionyl CoA carboxylase activity in cultured amniotic fluid cells of fetuses at risk.

Amniocentesis[i]: deficient propionyl CoA carboxylase activity in cultured amniotic fluid cells

> Gompertz et al., 1973; Gompertz et al., 1975; Sweetman et al., 1979

elevated concentrations of methylcitrate in amniotic fluid[g]

> Sweetman et al., 1979; Buchanan et al., 1980; Naylor et al., 1980; Sweetman et al., 1982; Sweetman, 1984; Sweetman, 1985; Chadefaux et al., 1988a; Chadefaux et al., 1989a; Holm et al., 1989; Jakobs, 1989

> *Comments:* Elevated concentrations of methylcitrate in amniotic fluid are not reliable for establishing the diagnosis, and the diagnosis should be confirmed by enzyme studies.

> Fensom et al., 1984

elevated level of 3-hydroxypropionate in amniotic fluid[g]

> Chadefaux et al., 1989a

elevated acylcarnitines in amniotic fluid

> Van Hove et al., 1993

Chorionic villus sampling[g,i]: deficient propionyl CoA carboxylase activity in direct assay of chorionic villi

> Chadefaux et al., 1988a; Perez-Cerda et al., 1989

Comments: Caution is necessary with the use of chorionic villi for the diagnosis of this condition. Chadefaux and co-workers (1988a) reported a study of a fetus who was at risk and who had 50% of normal propionyl CoA carboxylase activity in chorionic villi. Amniotic fluid levels of methylcitrate and 3-hydroxypropionate at 11 and 15 weeks of gestation were elevated. The pregnancy was terminated and liver assay of fetal liver showed only 3% of normal activity of propionyl CoA carboxylase.

> Chadefaux et al., 1989a; Kamoun and Chadefaux, 1991

Maternal urine[d]: elevation of methylcitrate

> Aramaki et al., 1989

Ultrasound[c]: increased echogenicity of fetal bowel

> Pallante et al., 1995

PD 219500 TETRAHYDROBIOPTERIN DEFICIENCY, DIHYDROPTERIDINE REDUCTASE DEFICIENCY TYPE (BH_4 deficiency; Phenylketonuria variant; Phenylketonuria II; PKU, atypical) (McKusick No. 261630)

Disease Note: In this condition, a deficiency of tetrahydrobiopterin, a coenzyme for phenylalanine, tyrosine and tryptophan hydroxylases, exists, leading to a reduction in the conversion of phenylalanine to tyrosine and an accumulation of the former. Tetrahydrobiopterin is regenerated by a cyclic pathway in which three metabolic blocks are known, each of which may lead to phenylketonuria. Mental retardation is not prevented by dietary restriction of phenylalanine in this condition because of the involvement of tyrosine and tryptophan hydroxylases.

> McKusick, 1986; Niederwieser et al., 1986

Amniocentesis[i]: deficiency of dihydropteridine reductase activity in cultured amniocytes

> Firgaira et al., 1983; Blau et al., 1989

linkage analysis with the dihydropteridine reductase gene in informative families

> Dahl et al., 1988

Chorionic villus sample[h,i]: DNA isolated, PCR performed, and gel electrophoretic analyses of products detected mutation in the dihydropteridine reductase gene
> Smooker et al., 1993

PD 219600 TETRAHYDROBIOPTERIN DEFICIENCY, 6-PYRUVOYL TETRAHYDROBIOPTERIN SYNTHASE DEFICIENCY TYPE
(Phenylketonuria III; PKU variant; Phosphate-eliminating enzyme [PEE] deficiency) (McKusick No. 261640)

Amniocentesis[i]: high concentration of total neopterin and extremely low total levels of biopterin in amniotic fluid
> Niederwieser et al., 1986; Blau et al., 1989; Shintaku et al., 1994

Cordocentesis (PUBS)[i]: very low PEE activity in erythrocytes
> Niederwieser et al., 1986; Blau et al., 1989

DISORDERS OF CARBOHYDRATE METABOLISM[a]

PD 219650 ACETOACETYL-COENZYME A THIOLASE DEFICIENCY
(McKusick No. 203750)

Disease Note: This condition is an autosomal recessive disorder of mitochondrial acetoacetyl-CoA thiolase characterized by recurrent episode of ketoacidosis and increased urinary excretion of 2-methylacetoacetate, 2-methyl-3-hydroxybuyrate, and tiglyglycine. The severity of the episodes varies from being asymptomatic to life-threatening; there is no correlation between the clinical picture, and the particular mutation within families (Fukao et al., 1995).

Amniocentesis[i]: cultured amniocytes' DNA was employed for PCR amplification and several genomic regions, including exon 8 and exon 9 fragments, were analyzed for the presence of the heteroduplex of mutations IVS (+1) and A301P. These were present in the affected proband. Only IVS (+1) was found, thus, correctly diagnosing the fetus as a carrier. Fragments around exon 9 were analyzed for polymorphism in intron 9, which was associated with the A310P mutation; the fetus showed the same Taq I fragment pattern as the proband, but by Msp I fragment analysis, but this was found to be due to a recombination between exons 1 and 9 in the father. This latter finding suggests that more than one polymorphism needs to be used in prenatal diagnosis.
> Fukoa et al., 1995

> cultured amniocytes were used for immunoblotting studies. The fetus had appreciable enzyme protein; the latter was virtually absent in fibroblasts form the proband. Thus the fetus was considered a carrier.
> Fukao et al., 1995

PD 219750 FRUCTOSE-1:6-DIPHOSPHATASE DEFICIENCY (McKusick No. 229700)

Ultrasound[g]: reduced crown-to-rump length
> Tchobroutsky et al., 1985

PD 220000 GALACTOSEMIA, CLASSIC FORM (Galactose-1-phosphate uridyl transferase deficiency) (McKusick No. 230400)

> Amniocentesis[i]: deficient galactose-1-phosphate uridyl transferase activity in cultured amniotic fluid cells
>> Nadler, 1968; Fensom and Benson, 1975; Ng et al., 1977a; Ng et al., 1977b; Shin et al., 1983; Jakobs et al., 1988; Holton et al., 1989
>> increased levels of galactitol in amniotic fluid[i]
>>> Jakobs et al., 1984c; Jakobs et al., 1988; Holton et al., 1989; Jakobs, 1989
> Chorionic villus sampling[g,i]: deficient galactose-1-phosphate uridyl transferase activity in uncultured chorionic villi
>> Kleijer, 1986; Kleijer et al., 1986b

PD 220475 GLYCOGEN STORAGE DISEASE, TYPE IA (Glucose-6-phosphatase deficiency; von Gierke disease) (McKusick No. 232200)

Disease Note: Glycogen storage disease, type IA, is an autosomal recessive disorder resulting from a deficiency in glucose-6-phosphatase in the tissues in which the enzyme is normally present: liver, kidney, and intestine. Growth retardation, hepatomegaly, renomegaly, hypoglycemia, hyperlipidemia, lactic acidosis, and hyperuricemia are characteristic.

> Amniocentesis[i]: amniotic fluid cells, uncultured and cultured, provided DNA for PCR amplification of specific exons and allele-specific oligonucleotides used for dot-blot hybridization analysis to detect mutation in the gene
>> Wong, 1996
>> *Comment:* The fetus reported by Wong (1996) was correctly diagnosed by the above procedure as being a carrier of the disorder.
> Fetal liver biopsy[i]: deficiency of glucose-6-phosphatase activity
>> Golbus et al., 1988

PD 220500 GLYCOGEN STORAGE DISEASE, TYPE III (Cori disease; Forbes disease; Amylo-1,6-glucosidase deficiency) (McKusick No. 232400)

> Amniocentesis[i]: deficiency of amylo-1,6-glucosidase activity in cultured amniotic fluid cells by either qualitative assay or immunoblot analysis
>> Brown, 1984; Yang et al., 1990
> Chorionic villus sampling: uncultured and cultured chorionic villi were found deficient in debranching-enzyme activity[i]
>> Maire et al., 1989
>> deficiency of amylo-1,6-glucosidase in uncultured chorionic villi[i,g]
>>> Shin et al., 1989

PD 220520 GLYCOGEN STORAGE DISEASE, TYPE IV (Amylopectinosis; Amylo-1,4→1,6 transglucosylase deficiency; Andersen disease) (McKusick No. 232500)

Disease Note: Deficiency of glycogen-branching enzyme results in the presence of normal amounts of an abnormal glycogen (reduced percentage of branch points) which irritates the liver. Symptoms and signs of cirrhosis appear in infancy, and death from liver failure during early childhood is the usual outcome of this autosomal recessive disorder.

Prenatal Diagnosis: The diagnosis has been accomplished by enzyme assay of cultured amniocytes and probably could be done using cultured chorionic villi;

uncultured normal chorionic villi give inconsistent results (Brown and Brown, 1989). The assay is an indirect one that measures the enzyme's ability to stimulate phosphorylase and glycogen synthase activities.

Differential Diagnosis: Other causes of cirrhosis should be considered.

Amniocentesis[i]: deficient branching-enzyme activity in cultured amniocytes
> Brown and Brown, 1989

PD 220650 LEIGH SYNDROME (Subacute necrotizing encephalomyelopathy) (McKusick No. see below)

Disease Note: This syndrome may be caused by any one of a number of genetically determined biochemical disorders that have in common necrosis, gliosis, cavitation and capillary proliferation in the brain (tegmental gray matter), brainstem (basal ganglia and thalamus), and the posterior column of the spinal cord. The pathologic findings may be ascertained by imaging procedures which may be indicated in patients who usually present in early infancy with varying degrees of chronic lactic acidosis, developmental delay, hypotonia, feeding and swallowing difficulties, vomiting, lethargy, failure to thrive, ataxia, tremors, nystagmus, respiratory irregularities, optic atrophy, and external ophthalmoplegia. Delayed forms of the syndrome may be seen in adults (Kalimo et al,. 1979). Abnormalities noted to cause the syndrome are: pyruvate dehydrogenase, E1 component (pyruvate decarboxylase) deficiency (PD 221550); pyruvate dehydrogenase, E2 (dihydrolipoyl transacetylase) deficiency; pyruvate dehydrogenase, E3 (dihydrolipoyl dehydrogenase) deficiency; pyruvate dehydrogenase phosphatase deficiency; pyruvate carboxylase deficiency (PD 221500); cytochrome C oxidase (Complex IV) deficiency (PD 243250); NADH-CoQ oxidoreductase (complex I) deficiency; and thiamine triphosphate synthesis inhibitor.

PD 220750 ALPHA-MANNOSIDOSIS (McKusick No. 248500)

Amniocentesis[i]: deficient acid alpha-mannosidase activity in cultured and uncultured amniotic fluid cells, decreased ratio between the activities of acid alpha-mannosidase and alpha-fucosidase, increased thermal lability of deficient acid alpha-mannosidase
> Poenaru et al., 1979

Chorionic villus sampling[g]: deficient alpha-mannosidase activity
> Petushkova, 1991

PD 220800 MITOCHONDRIAL DISORDERS

Disorder Note: Ruitenbeek and co-authors (1996) reviewed mitochondrial disorders, dividing them into groups according to their genetic implications for prenatal diagnosis. In their publication, they also pointed out a number of caveats. A summary follows along with pertinent PD numbers.

Mitochondrial DNA (mtDNA) is characterized by variation in numbers of chromosomes per mitochondrium and of mitochondria (Mt) per cell (both in proportion to energy requirement of the tissue involved), by high mutation rate, by heteroplasmy, by changing ratio of mutated to wild-type Mt during life, by a threshold ratio for abnormal phenotype, by maternal inheritance, and by unpredictability of the ratio of mutated to wild-type mtDNA in a given oocyte.

Heteroplasmic point mutations thus are not amenable to reliable prenatal diagnosis using mtDNA analysis; only one case has been recorded, Mitochondrial DNA^{T8993G} disease (PD 248500). Others may be diagnosed by other techniques.

Listing of mitochondrial disorders:

- Leigh syndrome (PD 220650)
- Mitochondrial encephalomyopathy with lactic acidosis and stroke-like episodes (MELAS)
- Mitochondrial DNA^{T8993G} disease (PD 248500)
- Myoclonic epilepsy and ragged-red fibers (MERRF)
- Neuropathy, ataxia and retinitis pigmentosa (NARP)

    Comment: Homoplasmic point mutations are more amenable to mtDNA analysis.

- Leber hereditary optic neuropathy

    Comments: Large deletions or duplications of mtDNA cannot be detected in somatic cells of first-degree relatives, and recurrence risk is not increased; prenatal diagnosis is not appropriate. Occurrence is sporadic except that in progressive external ophthalmoplegia some families have multiple small deletions and inheritance is autosomal dominant.

- Progressive external ophthalmoplegia (PEO)
- Kearns–Sayre syndrome (KSS)
- Pearson syndrome

    Comment: Depletion of mtDNA due to deficiency of synthetic factors results in varying reductions in mtDNA in various tissues, thus preventing reliable prenatal diagnosis.

- Infantile mitochondrial myopathy–Barth syndrome (cardioskeletal myopathy with neutropenia and abnormal Mt) is X-linked recessive and linkage studies may enable prenatal diagnosis.
- Pyruvate dehydrogenase complex deficiencies are listed under Leigh syndrome (PD 220650)
- Citric acid cycle enzyme deficiencies are autosomal recessive disorders.

    aconitase

    2-oxoglutarate dehydrogenase complex

    fumarase

- Succinyl-coenzyme A:3 ketoacid coenzyme A transferase deficiency (PD 221580)
- Medium-chain acylcoenzyme A dehydrogenase deficiency (PD 227500)
- Long-chain 3-hydroxyacyl CoA dehydrogenase deficiency (PD 216900)
- Very-long-chain acylcoenzyme A dehydrogenase deficiency (PD 233750)
- Acetoacetyl coenzyme A thiolase deficiency (PD 219650)
- Respiratory-chain enzyme deficiency without mtDNA mutation

    succinic dehydrogenase, flavoprotein subunit

    cytochrome C oxidase deficiency (PD 243250) (see Leigh syndromes [PD 220650])

    NADH-CoQ oxidoreductase deficiency (see Leigh syndrome [PD 220650])

PD 221000 POMPE DISEASE (Glycogen storage disease, type IIa; Glycogenosis, type IIa) (McKusick No. 232300)

Disease Note: Pompe disease is an autosomal recessive disorder characterized by the lysosomal accumulation of glycogen. The accumulation of glycogen results from an impaired breakdown of glycogen, a result of a deficiency in alpha-1,4-

glucosidase. The age at onset of the usual form of the disease is during early infancy, with nearly all tissues being affected, resulting in hepatosplenomegaly, muscular weakness, and cardiac failure. The latter problem is caused by glycogen accumulation in the heart and usually results in death of the individual by the end of the first year of life.

Besancon et al., 1985

Prenatal Diagnosis: The condition is diagnosed by demonstrating deficiency of alpha-1,4-glucosidase in cultured amniotic fluid cells or chorionic villus tissue, or uncultured chorionic villus tissue in a fetus at risk.

Differential Diagnosis: Other forms of Pompe disease and other glycogen storage diseases should be considered.

Amniocentesis[i]: deficient alpha-1,4-glucosidase (acid maltase) activity in cultured amniotic fluid cells

Niermeijer et al., 1975; Fensom et al., 1976; Brown, 1984; Ezaki et al., 1987; Lin et al., 1987

glycogen-filled lysosomes on electron microscopic examination of uncultured amniotic fluid cells

Hug et al., 1970; Hug et al., 1984b

Chorionic villus sampling[g,i]: reduced level of alpha-1,4-glucosidase activity in cultured and uncultured chorionic villi

Besancon et al., 1985; Ezaki et al., 1987; Shin et al., 1989

electron microscopy of uncultured and cultured chorionic villi showed multiple vacuoles packed with glycogen particles and vacuoles that are almost empty

Hug et al., 1991

enzyme assay using maltose as substrate showed reduced activity of alpha-1,4-glucosidase

Park et al., 1992

PD 221500 PYRUVATE CARBOXYLASE DEFICIENCY (Leigh encephalomyelopathy; Leigh encephalopathy; Leigh syndrome) (McKusick No. 266150)

Disease Note: See Leigh Syndrome (PD 220650)

Amniocentesis[i]: deficiency of pyruvate carboxylase activity in cultured amniotic fluid cells

Marsac et al., 1981; Marsac et al., 1982; Robinson et al., 1985

deficiency of pyruvate carboxylase subunit on polyacrylamide-gel electrophoresis of cultured amniotic fluid cell extracts

Robinson et al., 1985

PD 221550 PYRUVATE DEHYDROGENASE, E1 COMPONENT DEFICIENCY (Intermittent ataxia with pyruvate dehydrogenase deficiency; Leigh syndrome: subacute necrotizing encephalomyelopathy; Pyruvate decarboxylase deficiency; SNE) (McKusick No. Unknown; see 208800, 312170)

Disease Note: Pyruvate dehydrogenase is a complex of multiple copies of three enzymes: pyruvate decarboxylase (E1), dihydrolipoyl transacetylase (E2), and dihydrolipoyl dehydrogenase (E3). The complex is composed of 60 E2 subunits, which form the core of the complex, with the other components attached to the surface. The E1 component is formed from two alpha and two beta subunits, while E2 and E3 are each single polypeptide chains. The E1-alpha subunit gene is located on the X chromosome at Xp22.1. Despite the location of the E1-alpha subunit on the X chromosome, equal numbers of males and females are affected. Different mutations have been found in the alpha and beta subunits of the E1 enzyme, and these different mutations account for the variation in severity seen in this disorder. Clinical manifestations vary from mild ataxia with carbohydrate intolerance to severe infantile lactic acidosis, which is lethal. Physical abnormalities of the brain have been reported, and a large number of these patients have Leigh syndrome or partial manifestations of Leigh syndrome. See also Leigh syndrome (PD 220650).

> Johnston and Weinstein, 1989; McKusick, 1990; Brown and Brown., 1994; Brown et al., 1994

Chorionic villus sampling[g,i]: cultured cells show reduced pyruvate dehydrogenase, E1 component, activity

> Brown and Brown, 1994

> *Comments*: Heterozygous females may not show a clear-cut reduction in pyruvate dehydrogenase, E1, activity. X-inactivation pattern may be helpful, but because of variable patterns of methylation, direct DNA analysis may be necessary to obtain a reliable diagnosis.

> Brown and Brown, 1994

Ultrasound[c,d]: cerebral ventriculomegaly

> Johnston and Weinstein, 1989

> *Comments*: In the case reported by Johnston and Weinstein (1989), persistent and severe lactic acidosis developed in the neonate shortly after birth. The infant died on the third day. An autopsy revealed massive ventriculomegaly, microencephaly, hypoplasia of the white matter with microcysts, abnormal gyral formation, heterotopias, and absent pyramids and corpus callosum. E1 component of pyruvate dehydrogenase complex was deficient in the liver and fibroblasts.

PD 221580 SUCCINYL-COENZYME A:3 KETOACID COENZYME A TRANSFERASE DEFICIENCY (McKusick No. 245050)

Disease Note: This enzyme deficiency is characterized by severe recurrent ketoacidic attacks, acetoacetate and 3-hydroxybutyrate accumulation in blood and urine, and absence of the mitochondrial enzyme in tissues. Inheritance is autosomal recessive.

Amniocentesis[i]: amniotic fluid 3-hydroxybutyrate concentrations were not informative

> Fukao et al., 1996

> cultured amniocytes had no succinyl-coenzyme A:3 ketoacid coenzyme A transferase activity

> Fukao et al., 1996

> *Comment*: The diagnosis of this condition in the fetus reported by Fukao and associates (1996) was confirmed after birth.

Chorionic villus sampling[g,i]: direct assay of succinyl-coenzyme A:3 ketoacid coenzyme A transferase revealed no activity to be present

> Fukao et al., 1996

> *Comments*: The control material in the case reported by Fukao and colleagues (1996) had almost no enzyme activity. Therefore the results on the fetus by this approach were not significantly informative.

PD 221585 TRIOSE PHOSPHATE ISOMERASE DEFICIENY (McKusick No. 190450)

Disease Note: This condition is an autosomal recessive disorder characterized by accumulation of dihydroxyacetone phosphate (DHAP), early onset of non-spherocytic hemolytic anemia, central nervous system (CNS) degeneration, cardiomyopathy, increased susceptibility to infections, and death in childhood. The gene appears to be located on chromosome 12.

Prenatal Diagnosis: In cells with nuclei (amniocytes, chorionic villus cells), DHAP concentration may not be a reliable marker because another enzyme (glyerol-3-phosphate dehydrogenase) might metabolize the DHAP (Bellingham et al., 1990).

Cordocentesis (PUBS)[i]: erythrocytes demonstrated half the normal triose phosphate isomerase activity, and were otherwise normal including dihydroxyacetone phosphate concentration. The heterozygous state was confirmed at 4 months of age.

Bellingham et al., 1989

normal erythrocyte enzyme activity and heat stability, whole blood dihydroxyacetone phosphate concentration, and DNA sequence (index case mutation in exon 3, G312C) indicated a normal fetus

Pekrun et al., 1995

PD 221600 TYROSINEMIA, TYPE I (Fumarylacetoacetate hydrolase deficiency; Hereditary tyrosinemia, type I) (McKusick No. 276700)

Disease Note: Tyrosinemia, type I, is an autosomal recessive disorder characterized by progressive liver disease, renal tubular dysfunction, and rickets. The condition is produced by a deficiency of fumarylacetoacetase activity, which results in the excretion of succinylacetone in the urine of affected individuals.

Kvittingen et al., 1986

Prenatal Diagnosis: The diagnosis is established in fetuses at risk by demonstrating deficiency of fumarylacetoacetase activity in direct chorionic villus preparations or cultured amniotic fluid cells, or elevation of succinylacetone in the amniotic fluid.

Differential Diagnosis: Other types of tyrosinemia need to be considered.

Amniocentesis[i]: elevated levels of succinylacetone in amniotic fluid

Gagne et al., 1982a; Gagne et al., 1982b; Jakobs et al., 1985; Pettit et al., 1985; Kvittingen et al., 1986; Jakobs, 1989

no activity of fumarylacetoacetate hydrolase in cultured amniotic fluid cells

Steinmann et al., 1984; Jakobs et al., 1985

high level of succinylacetone as determined by its inhibitory effects on delta-aminolevulinate dehydratase

Gagne, 1984; Gagne et al., 1984

analysis of RFLPs in DNA from cultured aminocytes of both carrier and affected

Demers et al., 1994

elevated levels of succinylacetone in amniotic fluid[g]

Jakobs et al., 1990

Chorionic villus sampling[g,i]: deficiency of fumarylacetoacetate hydrolase activity in chorionic villi

Kvittingen et al., 1986

DISORDERS OF LIPID METABOLISM[a]

PD 221700 ADRENOLEUKODYSTROPHY, NEONATAL (McKusick No. 202370)

Disease Note: See Peroxisomal disorders (PD 231625)

Amniocentesis[i]: elevated amniotic fluid very-long-chain fatty acids (C26:0/C22:0; C26:1/C22:0) and certain bile acids (trihydroxycoprostanic acid/cholic acid; dihydroxycoprostanic acid/chenodeoxycholic acid)

Verhoeven et al., 1995

Comments: Neither pipecolic- nor phytanic-acid concentrations were informative in the case published by Verhoeven and co-workers (1995). Furthermore, the index cases were not clearly defined in this article.

elevated hexacosanoic acid (C26) and C26:C22 fatty acid ratio in cultured amniotic fluid cells from a male fetus who was at risk

Moser et al., 1982; Wanders et al., 1991

Chorionic villus sampling[g,i]: elevated hexacosanoic acid (C26) in cultured chorionic villi

Boue et al., 1985

RFLP linkage to the Xq28 region using restriction endonuclease *MspI* and probe ST14-9

Boue et al., 1985

PD 221705 ADRENOLEUDODYSTROPHY, X-LINKED (McKusick No. 300100)

Amniocentesis[i]: cultured amniocytes had increased concentration of C26:0 very-long chain fatty acid

Moser and Moser, 1989

Comments: According to data presented by Moser and Moser (1989), amniotic fluid levels of very-long-chain fatty acids are not reliable for diagnosis of this condition.

cultured amniocytes used for preparation of cDNA fragments: patterns revealed heterozygosity for the affected gene; the fetus was confirmed to be female. A carrier female was predicted and verifed postnatally.

Imamura et al., 1996

lignoceric acid oxidation was slightly lower than the normal range in a carrier female

Imamura et al., 1996

Chorionic villus sampling[g,i]: DNA digests from cultured cells revealed heterozygosity and thus a carrier female fetus

Imamura et al., 1996

Comments: Very-long-chain fatty acid profile may be normal in material from affected fetus especially in first subculture. Further subculturing may reveal diagnostic pattern.

Carey et al., 1994; Gray et al., 1995b

PD 221850 CHOLESTEROL ESTER STORAGE DISEASE (Cholesteryl ester storage disease; Lysosomal acid lipase deficiency) (McKusick No. 215000)

Amniocentesis[i]: deficiency of lysosomal lipase A activity in cultured amniotic fluid cells

Desai et al., 1987

PD 222000 FABRY DISEASE (Diffuse angiokeratoma) (McKusick No. 301500)

Amniocentesis[i]: deficient alpha-galactosidase activity in cultured and uncultured amniotic fluid cells and amniotic fluid
        Brady et al., 1971; Kleijer et al., 1987
    cytoplasmic lipid storage bodies on electron microscopic examination of cultured amniotic fluid cells
        Wyatt and Cox, 1977
Chorionic villus sampling[g,i]: deficiency of alpha-galactosidase activity by direct analysis of chorionic villi with and without the use of N-acetylgalactosamine to inhibit alpha-N-acetylgalactosaminidase
        Kleijer et al., 1987

PD 223000 FARBER DISEASE (Lipogranulomatosis, familial) (McKusick No. 228000)

Disease Note: Farber disease is an autosomal recessive disorder characterized by deficient lysosomal ceramidase resulting in lysosomal ceramide accumulation, subcutaneous nodules, cherry-red macula, aphasia, painful swelling of joints, and death in early childhood.
    Amniocentesis[i]: deficient ceramidase activity in cultured amniotic-fluid cells
        Fensom et al., 1979; Carey et al., 1984
    Chorionic villus sampling[g,i]: normal ceramidase activity enabled the correct prediction of an unaffected child; repeat CVS in the second trimester confirmed the results, as did postnatal studies
        Akhunov et al., 1995

PD 223500 FUCOSIDOSIS (alpha-L-Fucosidase deficiency) (McKusick No. 230000)

Disease Note: Fucosidosis in characterized by autosomal recessive inheritance, coarse facies, skeletal deformities, growth retardation, high sweat chloride concentration, and psychomotor retardation appearing by 1 year of age in the severe, fatal form (type I), or by 2 years of age in a milder form (type II) with survival to adult years. Angiokeratoma and normal sweat chloride concentrations are found in type II.
Prenatal Diagnosis: The diagnosis prenatally is established by finding decreased fucosidase activity in cultured amniocytes.
    Amniocentesis[i]: cultured amniocytes revealed decreased fucosidase activity in affected fetuses
        Poenaru et al., 1976; Durand et al., 1979

PD 224000 GANGLIOSIDOSIS, GM$_1$-TYPE 1, INFANTILE (McKusick No. 230500)

Amniocentesis[i]: absent beta-galactosidase activity in cultured amniotic fluid cells and in amniotic fluid
        Lowden et al., 1973
    cytoplasmic vacuoles on phase-contrast microscopic examination of cultured amniotic fluid cells
        Kudoh et al., 1978
    elevated levels of galactosyl-oligosaccharides in amniotic fluid as determined by high-performance liquid chromatography
        Warner et al., 1983

Chorionic villus sampling[g,i]: deficiency of beta-galactosidase activity in chorionic villi
>> Gatti et al., 1985

PD 225000 GANGLIOSIDOSIS, GM₁-TYPE 2, JUVENILE (McKusick No. 230600)

Amniocentesis[i]: absent beta-galactosidase activity in cultured amniotic fluid cells
>> Booth et al., 1973

PD 226000 GAUCHER DISEASE, INFANTILE CEREBRAL, JUVENILE, AND NORRBOTTNIAN FORMS (McKusick No. 230900, 231000)

Amniocentesis[i]: deficient glucocerebrosidase (beta-glucosidase) activity in cultured amniotic fluid cells using labeled glycosylceramide, the natural substrate
>> Schneider et al., 1972; Svennerholm et al., 1981; Heilbronner et al., 1981; Suchlandt et al., 1982

>> mutational analysis enabled prenatal diagnosis of specific type of Gaucher disease
>> Zimran et al., 1995

Chorionic villus sampling[g,i]: deficient glucocerebrosidase (beta-glucosidase) activity in fresh chorionic villi
>> Besley et al., 1988

PD 227000 KRABBE DISEASE (Globoid-cell leukodystrophy) (McKusick No. 245200)

Disease Note: Krabbe disease is an autosomal recessive disorder of sphingolipid metabolism characterized by onset usually within the first few weeks of life. The disorder produces hypersensitivity to external stimuli, irritability, hypertonicity, increased tendon reflexes, opisthotonos, seizures, and fever. There is rapid motor and mental deterioration. Death usually occurs by the third year of life. A deficiency of the lysosomal enzyme, cerebroside beta-galactosidase, results in this disorder.
>> Giles et al., 1987

Prenatal Diagnosis: A demonstration of a deficiency in cerebroside beta-galactosidase in amniotic fluid cells or chorionic villi is diagnostic for this condition.

Amniocentesis[i]: deficient cerebroside beta-galactosidase (galactosylceramide beta-galactosidase) activity in cultured amniotic fluid cells
>> Suzuki et al., 1971; Ellis et al., 1973; Harzer, 1977; Besley, 1978; Farrell et al., 1978; Tsutsumi et al., 1982; Suchlandt et al., 1982; Giles et al., 1987

Chorionic villus sampling[g,i]: deficient cerebroside beta-galactosidase activity in chorionic villi
>> Kleijer et al., 1984d; Kleijer, 1986; Giles et al., 1987; Harzer et al., 1987

Comments: Uncultured chorionic villi are inadequate for diagnostic purposes in this condition (Harzer et al., 1989). In a further report, the NICHD collaborative study found that 1 of 11 cases gave inconclusive results because of a pseudo-deficiency allele. Even loading studies with cultured amniocytes were inconclusive; the pregnancy resulted in an affected child (Desnick et al., 1992).

PD 227500 MEDIUM-CHAIN ACYL-COENZYME A DEHYDROGENASE DEFICIENCY (MCAD deficiency) (McKusick No. 201450)

Disease Notes: The disease is produced by an inborn error in the mitochondrial beta-oxidation pathway of straight-chain monocarboxylic fatty acids resulting from a deficiency in medium-chain acyl-coenzyme A dehydrogenase (MCAD). The clinical manifestation is usually fasting hypo- to nonketotic hypoglycemia that may lead to the death of the child. The disorder may present as sudden death. Onset may be any time during the first 2 years. Laboratory findings include hypoglycemia, and a marked C6-C10 dicarboxylic aciduria with an inappropriately low ketosis during an acute attack. Definitive diagnosis depends on demonstration of reduced activity of MCAD.

Bennett et al., 1987

Amniocentesis[i]: reduced rate of oxidation of 1-^{14}C-octanoic acid in cultured amniotic fluid cells

Comments: Although the predominant cell type (epithelial, large epithelial, fibroblast) does not appear to matter, enzyme activity significantly decreases after the 5th cell passage, so that control samples should be of similar passage numbers.

Bennett et al., 1987

cultured amniocytes incubated with stable-isotope-labelled palmitate and L-carnitine resulted in increased octanoyl- and decanoylcarnitine, indicating an affected fetus

Nada et al., 1996

Chorionic villus sampling[g,i]: reduced rate of [14]CO_2 release from 1-^{14}C octaoate by cultured cells

Comments: Although the clinical picture (a fatal Reye-like illness following a respiratory infection), and the defective release of CO_2 from octanoate in the patient reported by Pollitt and colleagues (1994) suggested this disorder, normal amounts of hexanoylglycine suggested that the patient had another, as yet uncharacterized disorder of medium-chain fatty acid oxidation.

polymerase chain reaction assay for the A985G (K304E) mutation led to a correct diagnosis of an affected fetus

Gregersen et al., 1995

PD 228000 METACHROMATIC LEUKODYSTROPHY (McKusick No. 250100; see also 249900; 250100)

Prenatal Diagnosis: Prenatal diagnosis of this disorder is complicated by the finding that some healthy individuals have a mutation in the gene that results in low arylsulfatase A activity when assayed with natural and artificial substrates using standard techniques, but have normal metabolism (hydrolysis of ^{14}C-sulfatide) by intact cells, including cultured amniocytes and cultured chorionic villus cells.

Baldinger et al., 1987

Amniocentesis[i]: deficient arylsulfatase A activity in cultured amniotic fluid cells and amniotic fluid

Nadler and Gerbie, 1970; Borresen and van der Hagen, 1973;

van der Hagen et al., 1973; Wiesmann et al., 1975; Rattazzi and
Davidson, 1977; Suchlandt et al., 1982
deficient arylsulfatase A in amniotic fluid
Eto et al., 1982
deficient cerebroside sulfatase in cultured amniotic fluid cells
Baier and Harzer, 1983
cytoplasmic inclusions on electron microscopic examination of cultured
amniotic fluid cells
Wyatt and Cox, 1977
deficiency of arylsulfatase A activity in cultured amniotic fluid cells
Sanguinetti et al., 1986
Chorionic villus sampling[g,i]: deficient arylsulfatase A activity in direct villus
assay and in cultured chorionic villi
Fensom et al., 1988
Comments: The NICHD collaborative study reported inconclusive results
in three cases, including one with a pseudo-deficiency allele.
Desnick et al., 1992
immunoprecipitation followed by electrophoresis and then enzyme ac-
tivity visualization using 4-methylumbelliferyl sulfate enabled demon-
stration of arylsulfatase A activity deficiency.
Poenaru et al., 1988

PD 229000 MUCOLIPIDOSIS, TYPE II (Leroy disease, I-cell disease) (McKusick No. 252500)

Disease Note: Mucolipidosis, type II, results from a deficiency of UDP-*N*-
acetylglucosamine produced by a deficiency of *N*-acetylglucosamine 1-
phosphotransferase (GlcNAc-PO$_4$ transferase). The latter is an enzyme that
specifically phosphorylates mannose residues of lysosomal glycoproteins which
then allows these enzymes to enter into the lysosomes. As a result of GlcNAc-
PO$_4$ transferase deficiency, the enzymes are secreted from the cell rather than
into the lysosomes (Ben-Yoseph et al., 1988).

The clinical features of this condition include slow development in infancy
(reaching a plateau at about 18 months), low nasal bridge with anteverted nostril,
progressive hypertrophy of the alveolar ridges, joint limitation in flexion particularly the hips, broadening of the wrists and fingers, periosteal new bone formation
of long tubular bones, and minimal hepatomegaly. The urinary mucopolysaccharides are usually normal to mildly increased. Death usually occurs by 5 years of
age from congestive heart failure. The disorder is inherited as an autosomal
recessive condition.
Jones, 1988

Prenatal Diagnosis: Diagnosis in the second trimester has been based on the
intracellular deficiency of several lysosomal enzyme activities of cultured amniotic fluid cells, cytoplasmic inclusion bodies in cultured amniotic fluid cells,
and elevated levels of total hexosaminidase in maternal serum. First trimester
diagnosis has been made by demonstrating deficiency of beta-galactosidase activity in chorionic villi.

Differential Diagnosis: Mucolipidosis type III (Pseudo-Hurler polydystrophy)
(PD 229050) also has a defect in lysosomal enzyme packaging, and needs to be
differentiated from Mucolipidosis II (PD 229000). Mucopolysaccharidoses and
lipidoses also must be considered.

Amniocentesis[i]: decreased activity of several lysosomal enzymes (hexosamini-dase, beta-galactosidase, and alpha-fucosidase) in cultured amniotic fluid cells, increased lysosomal enzyme activities in amniotic fluid

> Aula et al., 1975; Hug et al., 1984a; Besley et al., 1990

cytoplasmic inclusions on electron microscopic examination of cultured amniotic fluid cells

> Aula et al., 1984

elevated levels of beta-glucuronidase, alpha-fucosidase, alpha-mannosi-dase, beta-glucosaminidase, and beta-galactosidase in amniotic fluid[g,i]

> Poenaru et al., 1990

Chorionic villus sampling[g,i]: deficiency of beta-galactosidase activity by direct biochemical assay of chorionic villi

> Poenaru et al., 1984

Maternal blood sampling: elevated levels of hexosaminidase (total A and B) activity in maternal serum

> Hug et al., 1984a

PD 230000 MUCOLIPIDOSIS, TYPE IV (Berman disease) (McKusick No. 252650)

Disease Note: Mucolipidosis IV is an autosomal recessive lysosomal storage disease. The onset of the disease occurs during infancy, and is characterized by cloudy cornea, retinal degeneration, athetosis, and psychomotor retardation. The condition has been reported to be a deficiency of ganglioside neuraminidase, but the deficiency has not been used for prenatal diagnostic purposes.

> Kohn et al., 1982; Ornoy et al., 1987

Prenatal Diagnosis: The demonstration of increased numbers of inclusion, stor-age, or lamellar bodies in cultured amniotic fluid and chorionic villus cells appears to be adequate for the prenatal diagnosis of this condition.

Amniocentesis[i]: cultured amniotic fluid cells: multiple abnormal cytoplasmic storage (inclusion) bodies on electron microscopy

> Kohn et al., 1977; Kohn et al., 1982; Ornoy et al., 1986; Ornoy et al., 1987

accumulation of phospholipids and gangliosides in cultured amniotic fluid cells

> Zeigler et al., 1992

Chorionic villus sampling[g,i]: increased frequency of cells with abnormal inclu-sion (lamellar) bodies on electron microscopic examination of cultured chori-onic villi

> Ornoy et al., 1986; Ornoy et al., 1987

Comment: The above findings were not found in uncultured chorionic villus trophoblastic cells (Ornoy et al., 1987).

PD 230250 MULTIPLE SULFATASE DEFICIENCY (Juvenile sulfatidosis, Austin type; MSD; Mucosulfatidosis; Sulfatidosis, juvenile, Austin type) (McKusick No. 272200)

Disease Note: This disorder, which clinically is a combination of metachromatic leukodystrophy and a mucopolysaccharidosis, results from deficiencies of two or more sulfatases (e.g., arylsulfatases A, B, and C) and heparin sulfamidase. Increased amounts of acid mucopolysaccharides are present in several tissues and in the urine of patients with the disease. Excessive levels of sulfatide are also found in the urine. Although the facial features are only mildly coarse, the neurologic deterioration in affected individuals is rapid. The disorder is inherited as an autosomal recessive one.

McKusick, 1988; Patrick et al., 1988

Prenatal Diagnosis: The demonstration of two or more sulfatase deficiencies in chorionic villi in fetuses at risk is necessary for the diagnosis.

Differential Diagnosis: See various listings under Mucopolysaccharidoses in the Index; and Metachromatic leukodystrophy (PD 228000)

Chorionic villus sampling[g,i]: undetectable levels of arylsulfatase activity in cultured and uncultured chorionic villi

Patrick et al., 1988

reduced levels of heparin sulfamidase activity in cultured and uncultured chorionic villi

Patrick et al., 1988

PD 230750 NEURONAL CEROID LIPOFUSCINOSIS, INFANTILE
FINNISH TYPE (Infantile Finnish type of neuronal ceroid lipofuscinosis; Infantile neuronal ceroid lipofuscinosis; Santavuori disease) (McKusick No. 256730)

Condition Note: This form of neuronal ceroid lipofuscinosis is characterized by ataxia, minor motor seizures with myoclonic jerks, microcephaly, loss of speech, mental retardation, regression of motor and psychologic development, and onset during infancy. Total derangement of cortical cytoarchitecture, severe degeneration of white matter and deposits of granular material are seen on histologic examination of the brain. The disease is mainly found in Finns, with an incidence in Finland of $1:13,000$. The condition is inherited as an autosomal recessive trait.

McKusick, 1988; Rapola et al., 1988

Prenatal Diagnosis: Pathologic inclusion bodies in chorionic villi in a fetus at risk are sufficient to establish the diagnosis.

Differential Diagnosis: One should consider other forms of neuronal ceroid lipofuscinoses and in particular, Late amaurotic idiocy with multilamellar cytosomes, Neuronal ceroid lipofuscinosis, late infantile type (PD 230800), and Neuronal ceroid lipofuscinosis, juvenile type (PD 230765).

Chorionic villus sampling[g,i]: presence of pathologic inclusion bodies, consisting of unit-membrane-bound, electron-dense amorphic material in the endothelial cells of the capillaries of the chorionic villi and, on occasion, the mesenchymal cells of the villous stroma

Rapola et al., 1988; Rapola et al., 1990; Rapola et al., 1993

DNA-based linkage analysis in informative families

Vesa et al., 1993

PD 230765 NEURONAL CEROID LIPOFUSCINOSIS, JUVENILE TYPE
(Amaurotic family idiocy, juvenile type; Batten disease; Ceroid lipofuscinosis, neuronal 3, juvenile; Spielmeyer–Sjogren–Vogt disease; Spielmeyer–Vogt disease; Vogt–Spielmeyer disease) (McKusick No. 204200)

Disease Note: This type of fuscinosis is one of the most common causes of hereditary, progressive encephalopathy in children. The onset of symptoms begins normally at 5–10 years of age, and includes rapid deterioration of vision with pigmentary degeneration in the fundus, progressive deterioration of intellectual function, seizures, psychotic behavior, and kyphoscoliosis. The diagnosis is made by finding vacuolation in lymphocytes, fingerprint and curvilinear structures in electron micrographs of skin, and lipid-laden nerve cells obtained by rectal or brain biopsy. Mutations in the ceroid lipofuscinosis neuronal 3 (CLN3) gene that is located at 16p11.2 to p12.1 causes this condition.

Conradi et al., 1989; McKusick, 1990

Prenatal Diagnosis: There is no biochemical test that can be used for the prenatal diagnosis of this condition. The diagnosis may be established by demonstrating the characteristic electron micrographic structures in syncytiotrophoblastic cells in fetuses at increased risk (Conradi et al., 1989).

Differential Diagnosis: Neuronal ceroid lipofuscinosis, infantile Finnish type (PD 230750); Neuronal ceroid lipofuscinosis, late infantile type (PD 230800); and other lipidoses

Chorionic villus sampling[g,i]: fingerprint inclusions, and membrane-bound vacuoles that were sometimes found in combination with granular material in electron micrographic sections

Conradi et al., 1989

restriction-fragment-length polymorphism analysis and linkage to mutant gene

Jarvela et al., 1991

PD 230800 NEURONAL CEROID LIPOFUSCINOSIS, LATE INFANTILE TYPE (Amaurotic idiocy, late infantile type; Batten disease; Batten–Vogt syndrome; Ceroid lipofuscinosis, neuronal 2, late infantile type; Jansky–Bielschowsky disease) (McKusick No. 204500)

Amniocentesis[i]: trilamellar curvilinear deposit in lysosomes, demonstrated by electron microscopic examination of amniotic fluid cells

MacLeod et al., 1984a; MacLeod et al., 1984b; MacLeod et al., 1985; MacLeod et al., 1988; Chow et al., 1993

PD 231000 NIEMANN–PICK DISEASE, TYPE A (McKusick No. 257200)

Amniocentesis[i]: deficient sphingomyelinase activity in cultured amniotic fluid cells

Epstein et al., 1971; Patrick et al., 1977; Wenger et al., 1978; Donnai et al., 1981; Schoenfeld et al., 1982

PD 231500 NIEMANN–PICK DISEASE, TYPE B (McKusick No. 257200)

Amniocentesis[i]: deficient sphingomyelinase activity in cultured amniotic fluid cells

Wenger et al., 1981

Chorionic villus sampling[g,i]: deficient sphingomyelinase activity in cultured and uncultured chorionic villi

Vanier et al., 1985

PD 231600 NIEMANN–PICK DISEASE, TYPE C (McKusick No. 257220)

Disease Note: Nieman–Pick disease, type C, is a neurovisceral lysosomal lipid-storage disorder that is inherited in an autosomal recessive mode. Although a deficiency in lysosomal sphingomyelinase has been reported, a primary enzyme deficiency has yet to be found, and the detection of a deficiency in sphingomyelinase is not reliable for prenatal diagnosis of the disorder (Vanier et al., 1989)

Prenatal Diagnosis: The diagnosis in a fetus at risk can be made by demonstrating low levels of lipoprotein-stimulated cholesteryl ester formation and accumulation of perinuclear storage of unesterified cholesterol in chorionic villus cells.

Differential Diagnosis: Other forms of Nieman–Pick disease (PD 231000 and PD 231500) and other lysosomal storage diseases need to be considered.

Amniocentesis[i]: deficient sphingomyelinase activity in cultured amniotic fluid cells

Suchlandt et al., 1982

Chorionic villus sampling[g,i]: low levels of lipoprotein-stimulated cholesteryl ester formation in cultured chorionic villi

Vanier et al., 1989; Vanier et al., 1992

massive perinuclear storage of unesterified cholesterol demonstrated by fluorescence of filipin stained unesterified cholesterol in chorionic villus cells

Vanier et al., 1989; Vanier et al., 1992

PD 231625 PEROXISOMAL DISORDERS

Disease Note: As a group of at least 12 conditions, peroxisomal disorders are conventionally divided into three groups according to anatomic and biochemical characteristics.

Wanders and co-workers (1996) have also presented a clinical classification which is of additional help in the differential diagnosis of these disorders. A list follows of peroxisomal disorders with individual enzyme defects and PD numbers.

1. Absence of peroxisomes and deficiency of all peroxisomal enzymes:
   Zellweger syndrome (cerebrohepatorenal syndrome) (PD 234500)
   Neonatal adrenoleukodystrophy (PD 221700)
   Infantile Refsum disease (PD 231850)
   Pipecolic acidemia (probably not a distinct clinical entity (no PD number)
2. Peroxisomes present but lack two or more enzymes:
   Rhizomelic chondrodysplasia punctata: lacks dihydrohydroxy acetone phosphate-acyltransferase, dihydroxyacetone phosphate synthase, and phytanic acid oxidase (PD 150500)
   Zellweger-like syndrome: lacks dihydroxyacetone phosphate-acyltransferase and peroxisomal beta-oxidation enzyme proteins (no PD number)
3. Peroxisomes present but lack one enzyme:
   Adrenoleukodystrophy, X-linked: lack peroxisomal very-long-chain fatty acid-CoA synthase (PD 221705)
   Pseudo-neonatal adrenoleukodystrophy: lack acetyl CoA oxidase (no PD number)
   Bifunctional enzyme protein deficiency (no PD number)
   Pseudo-Zellweger syndrome: lack peroxisomal 3-oxyacyl CoA thiolase (no PD number)
   Hyperoxaluria, type I: lacks alanine:glyoxylate aminotransferase (PD 216600)
   Acatalasemia (no PD number)
   Adult Refsum disease: lacks phytanic acid oxidase; it is uncertain that this is a peroxisomal defect (no PD number)
   Dihydroxyacetone phosphate acyltransferase deficiency (no PD number)
   Alkyl dihydroxyacetone phosphate synthase deficiency (no PD number)
   Glutaryl-CoA oxidase deficiency (no PD number)

Di- and trihydroxycholestanoic acidemia (no PD number)
Mevalonate kinase deficiency (PD 218100)
Schutgens et al., 1989; Wanders et al., 1990; Theil et al., 1990;
Aikawa et al., 1994; Suzuki et al., 1994; Verhoeven et al., 1995;
Wanders et al., 1996

PD 231630 PEROXISOMAL DISORDERS: UNCLASSIFIED (McKusick No. None)

Disease Note: A new disorder has been reported that is characterized by unusual facies, hypotonia, hepatomegaly, retinal degeneration, and mental and physical retardation. The livers of patients with this disorder have absence of peroxisomes (Aikawa et al., 1994).

Amniocentesis[i]: increased amniotic fluid and cultured amniocyte levels of very-long-chain fatty acids (C26:0/C22:0, C26:0/C22:0)
Aikawa et al., 1994
subcellular fractionation of cultured amniocytes showed absence of mature peroxisomes on equilibrium density centrifugation
Aikawa et al., 1994

PD 231700 PSEUDOARYLSULFATASE A DEFICIENCY (McKusick No. 250100)

Amniocentesis[i]: deficient arylsulfatase A activity in cultured amniotic fluid cells in the presence of normal cerebroside sulfate hydrolyzation (cerebroside sulfate loading test using ^{35}S-labeled sulfatide)
Kihara et al., 1983

PD 231850 REFSUM DISEASE, INFANTILE TYPE (Infantile Refsum disease) (McKusick No. 266500)

Disease Note: Refsum disease of the infantile type is an autosomal recessive disorder involving the metabolism of phytanic acids, very-long-chain fatty acids, pipecolic acid, bile acids, and impaired biosynthesis of plasmalogens. It is a disorder of peroxisomes and, on ultrastructural analysis of affected livers, there is absence of peroxisomes. The condition presents in the first year of life with transient jaundice, hepatomegaly, sensorineural deafness, retinitis pigmentosa, osteopenia, failure to thrive, and psychomotor delay. The disorder is produced by a deficiency of phytanic acid oxidase activity. See also peroxisomal diseases (PD 231625).
Poll-The et al., 1985; Poll-The et al., 1987

Prenatal Diagnosis: The diagnosis can be established in at-risk fetuses by demonstrating low levels of activity for phytanic acid oxidase or acyl-CoA dihydroxyacetone phosphate acyltransferase in either chorionic villus or amniotic fluid cells.

Amniocentesis[i]: low phytanic acid oxidase activity in cultured amniotic fluid cells
Poll-The et al., 1985; Poulos et al., 1986
elevated C_{26}/C_{22} fatty acid ratio in cultured amniotic fluid cells
Poll-The et al., 1985; Poulos et al., 1986
reduced level of acyl-CoA dihydroxyacetone phosphate acyltransferase activity in cultured amniotic fluid cells
Poulos et al., 1986

Chorionic villus sampling[g,i]: elevated C_{26}/C_{22} fatty acid ratio
>Poll-The et al., 1987

reduction in acyl-CoA dihydroxyacetone phosphate acyltransferase activity
>Poll-The et al., 1987

impairment of de novo biosynthesis of ether lipids demonstrated by a significant reduction in incorporation of the radioactive precursor ^{14}C-hexadecanol into plasmalogens
>Poll-The et al., 1987

abnormal subcellular catalase activity localization
>Poll-The et al., 1987

PD 232000 SANDHOFF DISEASE (Gangliosidosis, Gm_2-type 2; Gm_2 gangliosidosis variant O) (McKusick No. 268800)

Disease Note: Sandhoff disease is an autosomal recessive storage disease resulting from a deficiency of lysosomal beta-N-acetyl-hexosaminidase A and B activities. As a result of these deficiencies, there is an accumulation of a variety of glycoconjugates and gangliosides in various tissues, including the central nervous system. Infantile (the most common and severe type), juvenile, and adult variants have been described.
>Giles et al., 1988

Prenatal Diagnosis: Diagnosis prenatally is established by demonstration of deficient beta-*N*-acetyl-hexosaminidase A and B total activities in amniotic fluid cells and/or chorionic villi in a fetus at risk.

Differential Diagnosis: The main conditions that should be considered in the differential are other lipidoses and mucolipidoses, primarily Gangliosidosis, Gm_1-type 1 (PD 224000), Gangliosidosis, Gm_1-type 2 (PD 225000), and Tay–Sachs disease (PD 233000).

Amniocentesis[i]: deficient beta-N-acetyl-hexosaminidase A and B activity in cultured and uncultured amniotic fluid cells
>Desnick et al., 1973; Suchlandt et al., 1982; Warner et al., 1986; Giles et al., 1988

presence of types 5, 6, and 7 N-acetylglucosaminyl-oligosaccharide in amniotic fluid
>Warner et al., 1986

Chorionic villus sampling[g,i]: deficient beta-N-acetyl-hexosaminidase activity in uncultured chorionic villi
>Giles et al., 1988

abnormal isozyme, beta-hexosaminidase S (Hex S), in uncultured chorionic villi as demonstrated by column chromatography
>Giles et al., 1988

PD 233000 TAY–SACHS DISEASE (Gangliosidosis, Gm_2-type 1) (McKusick No. 272800)

Amniocentesis[i]: deficient beta-N-acetyl-hexosaminidase A activity in cultured amniotic fluid cells and amniotic fluid
>O'Brien et al., 1971; Navon and Padeh, 1971; Saifer et al., 1973; Kustermann-Kuhn and Harzer, 1983; Redwine and Petres, 1984; Inui et al., 1986

Comments: Several families have been reported with heat-labile beta-hexosaminidase. An incorrect diagnosis of Tay–Sachs disease in the fetus may be made if the heat-inactivation method is used in this situation (Momoi et al., 1983).

absence of beta-N-acetyl-hexosaminidase A isozyme after electrophoretic separation of amniotic fluid cell extracts

Kustermann-Kuhn and Harzer, 1983

membranous cytoplasmic bodies on electron microscopic examination of cultured amniotic fluid cells

Wyatt and Cox, 1977

Chorionic villus sampling[g,i]: deficient hexosaminidase A activity in chorionic villi

Grebner et al., 1983; Grebner et al., 1984; Grabowski et al., 1984; Grebner and Jackson, 1985; Inui et al., 1986; Callahan et al., 1990

failure to break down a specific hexosaminidase A substrate, 4-methylumbelliferyl-6-sulfo-2-acetamido-2-deoxy-beta-D-glucopyranoside; reaction product was detected by fluorescence, using short-wave ultraviolet radiation

Grebner and Wenger., 1986; Grebner and Wenger, 1987

in a qualitative test, lack of ultraviolet light (254 nm) fluorescent "halo" around whole chorionic villi when using 4-methylumbelliferyl-6-sulfo-2-acetamido-2-deoxy-beta-D-glucopyranoside as a substrate

Grebner and Wenger, 1987

absence of hexosaminidase A isozyme on polyacrylamide gel and Cello-gel electrophoresis

Grebner and Jackson, 1985

DNA analysis using a 169-bp fragment containing a 4-bp insertion mutation in exon 11 (found in both parents) permitted exclusion of Tay–Sachs disease

Triggs-Raine et al., 1990

PD 233500 TAY–SACHS DISEASE, ATYPICAL TYPE (Adult-onset Gm_2 gangliosidosis) (McKusick No. 272800)

Amniocentesis[i]: deficiency but not total absence of hexosaminidase A activity in cultured amniotic fluid cells

Besancon et al., 1984; Navon et al., 1986

total deficiency of hexosaminidase A activity when using the heat inactivation method

Navon et al., 1986

Chorionic villus sampling[g,i]: deficiency but not total absence of hexosaminidase A in cultured chorionic villi

Besancon et al., 1984

PD 233600 TAY–SACHS DISEASE, B1 VARIANT (Gangliosidosis Gm_2-type B1; Tay–Sachs disease, late-infantile and juvenile forms) (McKusick No. 272800.0006ff)

Amniocentesis[i]: cultured amniocytes had virtually no hexosaminidase A activity when assayed with 4-methylumbelliferyl-N-acetylglucosanine-6-sulphate

Lemos et al., 1995

PD 233750 VERY-LONG-CHAIN ACYL-COENZYME A
DEHYDROGENASE DEFICIENCY (McKusick No. 201475)

Amniocentesis [i]: amniocytes were cultured in medium containing deuterium-labelled palmitic acid and L-carnitine; abnormal accumulation C_{16} acylcarnitine led to the diagnosis

Nada et al., 1996

Comments: The diagnosis of this condition was confirmed after birth in the patient reported by Nada and colleagues (1996). The index case, a sibling, had died during a severe metabolic acidosis not specifically diagnosed; mitochondrial membrane-enzyme activity was markedly reduced.

cell-free amniotic fluid did not show diagnostic acylcarnitine levels

Nada et al., 1996

deficiency of very-long-chain acyl-coenzyme A dehydrogenase in amniotic fluid cells

Nada et al., 1996

PD 234000 WOLMAN DISEASE (McKusick No. 278000)

Disease Note: Wolman disease is an autosomal recessive disorder produced by a deficiency of acid lipase (acid esterase). The enzyme deficiency produces a characteristic clinical picture with onset of the disease occurring early in infancy with recurrent vomiting and persistent diarrhea. Hepatosplenomegaly, abdominal distention, calcification of enlarged adrenal glands, and severe wasting develops, with death occurring before 6 months of age. Foamy cells are present in the viscera and contain excessive amounts of triglycerides and cholesteryl esters that are confined to the lysosomes.

Patrick et al., 1976

Prenatal Diagnosis: The diagnosis is established by demonstrating deficiency of acid lipase (acid esterase) in cultured or uncultured chorionic villi or cultured amniotic fluid cells.

Differential Diagnosis: Analphalipoproteinemia; Biliary duct atresia, complete (PD 131380); Cholesteryl ester storage disease (PD 221850); Farber disease (PD 223000); Niemann–Pick disease, types A, B, and C (PD 231000, PD 231500, and PD 231600, respectively)

Amniocentesis[i]: deficient acid lipase (acid esterase) activity in cultured amniotic fluid cells

Patrick et al., 1976; Coates et al., 1978; Christomanou and Cap, 1981

Comment: Some discrepancies between results of enzyme assay employing fluorescent substrate versus radiolabelled substrate suggest that the latter should be employed.

Iavarone et al., 1989

Chorionic villus sampling[g,i]: reduced levels of acid lipase (acid esterase) activity in both cultured and uncultured chorionic villi, using both 4-methylumbelliferyl-palmitate and radiolabeled cholesterol oleate as substrate

van Diggelen et al., 1988

Comment: Some discrepancies between results of enzyme assay employing fluorescent substrate versus radiolabelled substrat suggest that the latter should be employed.

Iavarone et al., 1989.

PD 234500 ZELLWEGER SYNDROME (Cerebrohepatorenal syndrome)
(McKusick No. 214100)

Syndrome Note: Zellweger syndrome is an autosomal recessive disease clinically characterized by severe hypotonia, distinctive facies, hepatomegaly, failure to thrive, and psychomotor retardation. Death usually occurs during the first year of life.

Peroxisomes are absent and the resulting lack of peroxisomal enzymes results in medium- and long-chain dicarboxylic aciduria, decreased synthesis of tissue plasmalogens, an accumulation of very-long-chain fatty acids and trihydroxycoprostanic acid in the plasma, and increased levels of pipecolic acid in the blood and urine. See also Peroxisomal disorders (PD 231625).

> Wanders et al., 1986a; Rocchiccioli et al., 1987

Amniocentesis[i]: elevated levels of very-long-chain fatty acids (C26:0/C22:0; C26:1/C22:0) and certain bile acids (trihydroxycoprostanic acid/cholic acid; dihydroxycopostanic acid/chenodeoxycholic acid) in amniotic fluid

> Verhoeven et al., 1995

> *Comments:* In the fetus reported by Verhoeven and associates (1995) neither phytanic- nor pipecolic-acid concentrations were informative; also the index cases were not clearly defined.

cultured and uncultured amniotic fluid cells showed presence of peroxisomes (cells do not showed punctate immunofluorescense after staining with anticatalase); normal fetus diagnosed

> Suzuki et al., 1994

deficiency of acyl-CoA-dihydroxyacetone phosphate acyltransferase (ACDHPA) activity in cultured amniotic fluid cells

> Schutgens et al., 1985; Kleijer, 1986; Poulos et al., 1986; Wanders et al., 1986a; Wanders et al., 1986b; Wanders et al., 1995

impaired de novo plasmalogen biosynthesis in cultured amniotic fluid cells

> Schutgens et al., 1985

elevated levels of the very-long-chain fatty acid, hexacosanoic (C26:0) acid, in cultured amniotic-fluid cells

> Moser et al., 1984; Solish et al., 1985; Wanders et al., 1991

decreased peroxisomal bound catalase activity ($<5\%$) in cultured amniotic fluid cells by means of digitonin titrations; most catalase activity was found in the soluble cytoplasm

> Wanders et al., 1986a; Wanders et al., 1986b

increased C_{26}/C_{22} fatty acid ratio in cultured amniotic fluid cells

> Poulos et al., 1986; Wanders et al., 1991

decreased beta oxidation of C26:0 fatty acid in cultured amniotic fluid cells

> Wanders et al., 1991

decreased lignoceric acid (C24:0) oxidation in cultured amniocytes

> Suzuki et al., 1994

> *Comment:* In spite of the above finding in the fetus reported by Suzuki and colleagues (1994), the fetus was unaffected.

two of six clones of cultured amniocytes had point mutations (C to T) in the peroxisomal assembly factor-1 (PAF-1) gene on PCR sequencing studies; peroxisomes were present and enzymes activities were normal; diagnosis of carrier state

> Shimozawa et al., 1993

increased requirement of digitonin to release latency of catalase
>Wanders et al., 1986b

Chorionic villus sampling[g,i]: elevated level of the very-long-chain fatty acid, hexacosanoic (C26:0) acid in chorionic villi
>Hajra et al., 1985

decreased beta-oxidation of C26:0 fatty acid by cultured chorionic villus cells
>Wanders et al., 1991

increased C_{26}/C_{22} fatty acid ratio in cultured chorionic villus cells
>Poulos et al., 1986; Wanders et al., 1991

elevation of very-long-chain fatty acids C24:0 and C26:0 by direct assay of chorionic villi using a gas chromatographic mass spectrometric method
>Rocchiccioli et al., 1987

deficiency of acyl-CoA:dihydroxyacetone phosphate acyltransferase activity
>Hajra et al., 1985; Schutgens et al., 1985; Carey et al., 1986; Poulos et al., 1986; Wanders et al., 1995

decreased phytanic acid oxidase activity in cultured chorionic villus cells
>Poulos et al., 1986

impaired de novo plasmalogen biosynthesis in cultured chorionic villi
>Schutgens et al., 1985

no acyl-CoA oxidase and peroxisomal 3-ketoacyl-CoA thiolase detected in cultured chorionic villi by immunoblot analysis
>Shimozawa et al., 1988

absence of punctate fluorescence in chorionic villus fibroblasts by immunofluorescency microscopy using an anti-catalase antiserum
>Wanders et al., 1989

DISORDERS OF MUCOPOLYSACCHARIDE METABOLISM[a]

Recent advances in the prenatal diagnosis of the mucopolysaccharidoses have been reviewed by Fenson and Bensom (1994).

PD 235000 HUNTER SYNDROME (Mucopolysaccharidosis, type II) (McKusick No. 309900)

Amniocentesis[i]: deficient iduronate sulfatase activity in amniotic fluid
>Liebaers et al., 1977; Archer et al., 1984; Lissens et al., 1988

abnormal intracellular accumulation of ^{35}S-mucopolysaccharides in cultured amniotic-fluid cells
>Liebaers et al., 1977

abnormal two-dimensional electrophoretic pattern of amniotic fluid glycosaminoglycans (dermatan and heparan sulfates)
>Mossman and Patrick, 1982; Archer et al., 1984; Lissens et al., 1988

Chorionic villus sampling[g,i]: deficient iduronate sulfatase activity in chorionic villi (direct enzyme assay) in male fetuses
>Kleijer et al., 1984c; Kleijer, 1986; Pannone et al., 1986; Cooper et al., 1991; Besley et al., 1992

increased incorporation of ^{35}S-sulfate in cultured chorionic villus cells
> Kleijer et al., 1984c

Cordocentesis (PUBS)[i]: less than 1% normal plasma iduronate sulfatase (idur-onate 2-sulfate sulfatase) activity in a male fetus
> Lissens et al., 1988

Maternal blood sampling: no increase in maternal serum iduronate sulfatase activity during pregnancy when an affected fetus was present[i]
> Bach and Zlotogora, 1984; Bach and Zlotogora, 1985; Zlotogora and Bach, 1986

Method not stated[i]: direct detection of the mutation
> Bunge et al., 1994

> *Comments:* Prenatal diagnosis of two affected fetuses and one heterozygous XXY male was reported by Burge and associates (1994). Diagnosis was accomplished by direct detection of the gene mutation; source of the tissue for each affected fetuses was not stated.

PD 236000 HURLER SYNDROME (Mucopolysaccharidosis, type HI) (McKusick No. 252800)

Amniocentesis[i]: decreased alpha-L-iduronidase activity in cultured amniotic fluid cells
> Aberg et al., 1978; Stirling et al., 1979; Ikeno et al., 1981; Kleijer et al., 1983; Simoni et al., 1984

> presence of glycosaminoglycans (dermatan and heparan sulfates) in amniotic fluid
>> Henderson and Nelson, 1977; Ikeno et al., 1981; Mossman et al., 1981

> analysis of mucopolysaccharide metabolism in cultured amniotic fluid cells: abnormal accumulation of ^{35}S-sulfate intracellular mucopolysac-charides
>> Henderson and Nelson, 1977; Aberg et al., 1978; Kleijer et al., 1983

> abnormal two-dimensional electrophoretic patterns of amniotic fluid glycosaminoglycans
>> Mossman and Patrick, 1982

Chorionic villus sampling[g,i]: deficiency of alpha-L-iduronidase activity
> Desnick et al., 1992

> *Comments:* Fresh and cultured material gave inconclusive results using enzyme assay in three of nine cases in the NICHD collaborative study; the authors of this study recommend that only cultured villi or amniocytes be used for the diagnosis of this condition.
> Desnick et al., 1992

PD 237000 MAROTEAUX–LAMY SYNDROME (Mucopolysaccharidosis, type VI) (McKusick No. 253200)

Amniocentesis[i]: deficient arylsulfatase B activity in cultured amniotic fluid cells
> Kleijer et al., 1976; Van Dyke et al., 1981; Carey et al., 1984

> accumulation of ^{35}S-sulfate intracellular mucopolysaccharides in cul-tured amniotic fluid cells
>> Kleijer et al., 1976

abnormal two-dimensional electrophoretic patterns of amniotic fluid glycosaminoglycans
>Mossman and Patrick, 1982

PD 237500 MORQUIO SYNDROME, TYPE A (Mucopolysaccharidosis, type IVA; Galactose-6-sulfatase deficiency) (McKusick No. 253000)

Amniocentesis[i]: deficient N-acetylgalactosamine-6-sulfate sulfatase activity in cultured amniotic fluid cells
>von Figura et al., 1982; Yong et al., 1987; Zhao et al., 1990; Beck et al., 1992
>abnormal glycosaminoglycan pattern on one-dimensional electrophoresis of amniotic fluid
>Zhao et al., 1990; Beck et al., 1992
>deficient galactose-6-sulfate sulfatase activity in cultured amniotic fluid cells using 4-methylumbelliferyl-6-sulfogalactoside as a substrate
>Zhao et al., 1990

Ultrasound[i]: bilateral pleural effusions, ascites, hydrops fetalis
>Yong et al., 1987; Beck et al., 1992

PD 238000 SANFILIPPO DISEASE, TYPE A (Mucopolysaccharidosis, type IIIA) (McKusick No. 252900)

Amniocentesis[i]: deficient heparan sulfatase (heparan sulfamidase) activity in cultured amniotic fluid cells
>Harper et al., 1974; Kleijer et al., 1996

Comments: Using 4-methylumbelliferone-alpha-D-N-sulfoglucosaminide as a substrate, Kleijer and associates (1996) were able to establish the diagnosis in an affected fetus. The advantage of this substrate is the ease of testing and apparent reliability.

>increased levels of heparan sulfate in amniotic fluid
>Harper et al., 1974
>abnormal two-dimensional electrophoretic patterns of amniotic fluid glycosaminoglycans
>Mossman and Patrick, 1982

Chorionic villus sampling[g,i]: deficiency of heparan sulfatase activity in direct assay of villi
>Kleijer et al., 1986a; Kleijer et al., 1996

Comments: Using 4-methylumbelliferone-alpha-D-N-sulfoglucosaminide as a substrate, Kleijer and associates (1996) were able to establish the diagnosis in an affected fetus. The advantage of this substrate is the ease of testing and apparent reliability.

PD 238500 SANFILIPPO DISEASE, TYPE B (Mucopolysaccharidosis, type IIIB) (McKusick No. 252920)

Amniocentesis[i]: increased amounts of heparan sulfate in amniotic fluid
>Mossman et al., 1983; Kleijer et al., 1984e; Maire et al., 1995
>undetectable levels of N-acetyl-alpha-D-glucosaminidase activity in cultured amniotic fluid cells
>Mossman et al., 1983; Beratis et al., 1984; Kleijer et al., 1984e; Maire et al., 1993

Chorionic villus sampling[g,i]: reduced level of N-acetyl-alpha-D-glucosaminidase activity in homogenates of cultured and uncultured chorionic villi

Minelli et al., 1988

PD 238750 SANFILIPPO DISEASE, TYPE C (Mucopolysaccharidosis, type IIIC) (McKusick No. 252930)

Disease Note: This condition is a mucopolysaccharide storage disease with progressive mental retardation and death that usually occurs in the teenage years. The deficient enzyme that normally catalyzes the N-acetylation of alpha-glycoaminide linked glucosamine residues at the nonreducing terminal of heparan sulfate, using acetyl-CoA as a cosubstrate, is acetyl-CoA:alpha-glucosaminide N-acetyltransferase.

Di Natale et al., 1987

Prenatal Diagnosis: Detection of acetyl-CoA: alpha-glucosaminide N-acetyltransferase deficiency in a fetus at risk is considered diagnostic.

Amniocentesis[i]: increased heparan sulfate in amniotic fluid supernatant

Maire et al., 1993

absence of acetyl-CoA: alpha-glucosaminide N-acetyltransferase activity in cultured amniotic fluid cells

Maire et al., 1993; He et al., 1994

Comments: According to a study published by He and associates (1994), 4-methylumbelliferyl-beta-D-glucosamide is a reliable substrate for enzyme assay in amniotic fluid cells.

a 14:21 Robertsonian translocation was noted in the karyotypes of a mother and her two affected children (one unaffected child had a normal karyotype), the second having been diagnosed fetally by excessive heparan sulfate in amniotic fluid

Zaremba et al., 1992

Chorionic villus sampling[g,i]: deficiency of acetyl-CoA:alpha-glucosaminide N-acetyltransferase activity by direct assay of chorionic villi

Di Natale et al., 1987

Comments: According to a study published by He and associates (1994), 4-methylumbelliferyl-beta-D-glucosaminide is a reliable substrate for enzyme assay of either uncultured or cultured chorionic villus cells.

PD 238800 SLY SYNDROME (Beta-Glucuronidase deficiency; Mucopolysaccharidosis VII) (McKusick No. 253220)

Disease Note: Sly disease is an autosomal recessive disorder characterized by a Hurleroid phenotype, and moderate mental retardation, usually manifested in early childhood. Severe cases may present at birth with hydropic fetalis, and mild cases, presenting after 4 years of age, may have few, if any, symptoms and signs of the disorder.

Prenatal Diagnosis: Cultured amniocytes enable diagnostic enzyme studies and demonstration of beta-glucuronidase deficiency.

Neufeld and Muenzer, 1989

Amniocentesis[i]: enzyme assay and glycosaminoglycan electrophoresis of amniotic fluid demonstrated deficiency of beta-glucuronidase

Kagie et al., 1992

Comment: The diagnosis of Sly syndrome was confirmed in fibroblasts of a fetus reported by Kagie and associates (1992) after the pregnancy was terminated.

Ultrasound: hydrops fetalis[i]

Lissens et al., 1991; Stangenberg et al., 1992

OTHER METABOLIC DISORDERS[a]

PD 239000 ACUTE INTERMITTENT PORPHYRIA (McKusick No. 176000)

Amniocentesis[i]: decreased activity of uroporphyrinogen I synthetase in cultured amniotic fluid cells

Sassa et al., 1975

PD 240000 ADENOSINE DEAMINASE DEFICIENCY (Combined immunodeficiency disease) (McKusick No. 102700)

Amniocentesis[i]: deficient adenosine deaminase activity in cultured amniotic fluid cells

Hirschhorn et al., 1975; Chen et al., 1980; Ziegler et al., 1981; Dooley et al., 1987

Chorionic villus sampling[g,i]: deficient adenosine deaminase activity by direct assay of chorionic villi

Dooley et al., 1987

Cordocentesis (PUBS)[i]: profound lymphopenia and complete absence of T and B cells in fetal blood

Durandy et al., 1982a; Durandy et al., 1982b

deficient adenosine deaminase activity in fetal blood

Simmonds et al., 1983; Dooley et al., 1987

elevated levels of erythrocytic deoxyadenosine triphosphate in fetal blood

Simmonds et al., 1983

PD 240250 ADRENOCORTICOTROPIN DEFICIENCY, FAMILIAL ISOLATED (ACTH deficiency) (McKusick No. 201400)

Condition Note: Familial isolated adrenocorticotropin deficiency is a relatively rare condition characterized by adrenal hypoplasia and corticosteroid deficiency due to a lack of production of adrenocorticotropic hormone (ACTH). The condition may present in the newborn period and may lead to death at that time if not recognized and treated, or the onset may occur during infancy or later. Levels of other tropic hormones are normal. The disorder under this entry varies from the X-linked type of congenital adrenal hypoplasia (PD 241500) because this condition is inherited as an autosomal recessive trait, and has normal adrenal architecture. Replacement hormone therapy is the treatment of choice.

Malpuech et al., 1988

Prenatal Diagnosis: Diagnosis prior to birth has been accomplished by detecting low levels of maternal plasma estriol during the third trimester, a reflection of the underactivity of the fetal adrenal gland.

Differential Diagnosis: Congenital adrenal hypoplasia, X-linked type (PD 241500)

Maternal blood sampling[d,i]: low levels of estriol in maternal plasma
Malpuech et al., 1988

PD 240500 ALPHA-1-ANTITRYPSIN DEFICIENCY (McKusick No. 107400)

Disease Note: The plasma protease inhibitor, alpha-1-antitrypsin, is deficient in about 1 in 7000 North American Caucasians and some 1 in 2000 to 3000 northern Europeans. Although there are a number of different alleles, the Z allele in the homozygous state produces the most severe clinical disorder. Homozygous ZZ newborns have approximately a 17% chance of having liver disease that may progress to cirrhosis. In about one third of these cases, the cirrhosis will be fatal. In adults, the homozygous ZZ individual will usually develop obstructive lung disease in early adult life if they smoke or if they are in a smoke-filled environment for any appreciable amount of time. Many parents request prenatal diagnosis because of the risk of the fatal liver disease during infancy in their affected offspring. Subsequent children with Pi type ZZ, whose sibling had progressive liver disease in early childhood from alpha-1-antitrypsin deficiency, have a risk of 40% or more of having severe liver disease themselves (Cox and Billingsley, 1986).
Cox and Mansfield, 1987

Prenatal Diagnosis: Pi typing, either from fetal blood or by DNA methods (linkage analysis or direct detection of the mutant gene), or a combination of these methods, appears to be the appropriate approach to the diagnosis of this condition. Using RFLP or oligonucleotide probes appears to be equally reliable. However, the RFLP method is easier to use (Hejtmancik et al., 1986b)

Amniocentesis[c,i]: heterozygous state, MZ, demonstrated by the use of synthetic M and Z oligonucleotides and appropriate restriction endonucleases
Kidd et al., 1984

Chorionic villus sampling[g,i]: determination of Pi ZZ type by RFLPs using various restriction endonucleases
Kidd et al., 1984; Cox et al., 1985; Hejtmancik et al., 1986b; Cox and Mansfield, 1987

use of M and Z allelic oligonucleotide probes
Hejtmancik et al., 1986b

demonstration of the Pi ZZ genotype by PCR technique and appropriate molecular genetic techniques
Abbott et al., 1988; Abbott et al., 1992

detection of the gene mutation by use of denaturing gradient gel electrophoresis after PCR amplification
Dubel et al., 1991

determination of the heterozygous state by PCR and molecular genetics techniques
Forrest et al., 1992

Cordocentesis (PUBS)[i]: decreased concentration of serum alpha-1-antitrypsin in fetal blood
Jeppsson et al., 1981

Pi ZZ typing of fetal blood as determined by electrofocusing and immunofixation
Jeppsson et al., 1981; Corney et al., 1987

PD 240600 ANDROGEN INSENSITIVITY, PARTIAL (Reifenstein syndrome) (McKusick No. 312300)

Disease Note: Partial androgen insensitivity represents a group of X-linked disorders resulting from defects in the intracellular androgen receptor. The phenotypes vary from testicular feminization (PD 249800) to male pseudoher-maphroditism to normal but infertile males.

Chorionic villus sampling[i]: RFLPs and DNA androgen-binding linkage
Lobaccaro et al., 1994

PD 240680 ASPARTYLGLUCOSAMINURIA (Aspartylglycosaminuria) (McKusick No. 208400)

Disease Note: Aspartylglucosaminuria is an autosomal recessive disorder pro-duced by a deficient activity of the lysosomal enzyme, aspartylglucosaminidase. Features of this disorder include severe mental retardation, sagging cheeks, broad nose and face, asymmetry of the skull, scoliosis, hyperactivity, and vacuolated lymphocytes. Affected individuals excrete abnormal amounts of 2-acetamido-1-(bet-L-aspartamido)-1,2-dideoxyglucose in their urine. The carrier frequency in the Finnish population is 1 in 40, but the gene is much rarer in other populations.
Aula et al., 1989; McKusick, 1990

Prenatal Diagnosis: The diagnosis of this condition prenatally is made by detect-ing low levels of aspartylglucosaminidase activity in uncultured chorionic villi or cultured amniotic fluid cells.

Differential Diagnosis: Congenital sialidosis (PD 243000); Mannosidosis (PD 220750); Mucolipidosis, type II (PD 229000); Mucolipidosis, type III; Various types of Mucopolysaccharidoses (see Mucopolysaccharidosis in the Index); Salla disease (PD 249250)

Amniocentesis[i]: deficiency of N-aspartylglucosaminidase activity in cultured amniotic fluid cells
Aula et al., 1984; Aula et al., 1989

Chorionic villus sampling[g,i]: deficiency of N-aspartylglucosaminidase activity in uncultured chorionic villi
Aula et al., 1989

PD 240690 BARTTER SYNDROME (McKusick No. 241200)

Syndrome Note: The characteristic findings of Bartter syndrome include hypoka-lemia, hyperkaliuria, antidiuretic-hormone-resistant polyuria, hyperaldosteron-ism, hyperreninemia, overproduction of renal prostaglandins, and hypertrophy of the renal juxtaglomerular apparatus. The condition is inherited as an autosomal recessive syndrome. The primary defect in the disorder is not known.

Clinically, Bartter syndrome can be divided into an early-neonatal onset type and a late-onset type. Neonatal-onset Bartter has intrauterine onset of polyuria leading to hydramnios as early as the 22nd week of gestation. If the hydramnios is not treated by repeat amniocentesis, preterm labor and delivery may ensue.
Proesmans et al., 1987

Prenatal Diagnosis: The presumptive diagnosis can be made if hydramnios devel-oped at the end of the second or during the third trimester in a fetus at risk. If hydramnios does develop in the above situation, the fetus should be carefully evaluated by ultrasound for fetal abnormalities, and if none is found, then the chloride concentration of the amniotic fluid should be determined. If elevated, the diagnosis is most likely Bartter syndrome.

On the other hand, when there is unexplained hydramnios with no history of maternal diabetes or Bartter syndrome, and an ultrasonic evaluation has not revealed any fetal abnormalities, an amniotic fluid chloride concentration should be done. The diagnosis of Bartter syndrome is important to establish because the affected newborns may experience life-threatening water and electrolyte disturbances if the condition is not treated.

> Proesmans et al., 1987

Differential Diagnosis: Congenital chloride diarrhea (PD 131750) also gives hydramnios and elevated concentrations of chloride in the amniotic fluid; other causes of hydramnios should be ruled out (see Hydramnios in the Index).

Amniocentesis[d,i]: elevated levels of potassium and chloride in amniotic fluid

> Proesmans et al., 1987

Ultrasound[d]: hydramnios

> Pereira and Hasaart, 1982; Sieck and Ohlsson, 1984

PD 240695 CANAVAN DISEASE (Aspartoacylase deficiency; Spongy degeneration of the central nervous system) (McKusick No. 271900)

Disease Note: This disorder is characterized by onset in early infancy of hypotonia, macrocephaly and developmental regression that progresses over a period of several years to optic atrophy, spasticity, posturing, seizures, and death. Inheritance is autosomal recessive, and the condition occurs predominantly in Ashkenazi Jews.

Prenatal Diagnosis: The diagnosis may be established by amniocentesis that reveals increased N-acetylaspartate (NAA) concentration in the fluid (Matalon et al., 1992; Jakobs et al., 1992); and reduced aspartoacylase activity in cultured amniocytes. Enzyme assay of cultured chorionic villi is not reliable, however (Matalon et al., 1992). Fresh chorionic villi have shown aspartoacylase deficiency during the first trimester when the amniotic fluid N-acetylaspartate concentration is unreliable (Rolland et al., 1993a).

Bennett and associates (1993) have shown that amniotic fluid N-acetylaspartic acid levels determined by stable isotope dilution have been a reliable predictor of pregnancy outcome, whereas amniocyte aspartoacylase activity was not adequate. Kelley (1993) was not so sanguine, finding NAA levels to vary with gestational age. DNA analysis for mutations in the gene appears to be reliable as well (Matalon et al., 1995).

Amniocentesis[i]: increased N-acetylaspartate concentration in amniotic fluid by isotope dilution

> Matalon et al., 1992; Bennett et al., 1993; Elpeleg et al., 1994

reduced aspartoacylase activity in cultured amniotic fluid cells

> Matalon et al., 1992

polymerase chain reaction amplification of DNA for mutation analysis by RFLP

> Elpeleg et al., 1994; Matalon et al., 1995

analysis by single-strand conformation polymorphism and nucleotide sequencing demonstrated mutation in the gene.

> Matalon et al., 1995

Chorionic villus sampling[g,i]: aspartoacylase deficiency in fresh chorionic villi

> Rolland et al., 1993a

Comment: Reduced aspartoacylase activity in cultured chorionic villus samples is not entirely reliable according Matalon and associates (1992).

Maternal urine sampling[i]: N-acetylaspartic acid increased after 4 months' gestation

> Ozand et al., 1991

PD 240698 CARBOHYDRATE-DEFICIENT-GLYCOPROTEIN
SYNDROME, TYPE I (Jaeken syndrome; Neonatal olivopontocerebellar atrophy) (McKusick No. 212065)

Disease Note: This condition is an autosomal recessive disorder characterized by mental retardation, ataxia and other neuromotor disabilities, retinal degeneration, and skeletal deformities. In the neonatal period, patients may have peculiar skin ("peau d'orange" and uneven consistency), restricted movement of large limb joints, and general truncal floppiness. Although a number of glycoproteins are affected in this condition, the carbohydrate deficit is most conveniently estimated on transferrin in blood samples even using blood from filter-paper blood spots (Hagberg et al., 1993). The syndrome cannot be diagnosed prenatally by analysis of transferrin and AFP on samples obtained at 11 weeks (chorionic villus samples) and at 17 weeks (amniotic fluid) (Stibler et al., 1994), however.

    Fetal electrocardiography[d,i]: hypertrophic non-obstructive cardiomyopathy and pericardial effusion
               Garcia Silva et al., 1996

PD 240700 COBALAMIN E DISEASE (Methylcobalamin deficiency)
(McKusick No. 236270)

Disease Note: Cobalamin E disease is an autosomal recessive disorder characterized by early neurologic deterioration, hypotonia, developmental delay, seizures, dislocation of lenses, and usually death during childhood.

Prenatal Diagnosis: The diagnosis may be made by demonstrating reduced sulfate and increased S-sulfocysteine in amniotic fluid; and reduced sulfite oxidase activity in cultured amniotic fluid cells. Chorionic villus tissue can be used to determine sulfite-oxidase activity, but has not been used for the diagnosis of this condition (Bamforth et al., 1990)

    Amniocentesis[i]: deficiency of methylcobalamin in cultured amniotic fluid cells
               Rosenblatt et al., 1985
        decreased incorporation of ^{14}C from labeled 5-methyltetrahydrofolate into methionine in cultured amniotic fluid cells
               Rosenblatt et al., 1985
        normal sulfite oxidase activity in cultured amniocytes correctly indicated an unaffected fetus
               Bamforth et al., 1990
        normal sulfate concentration in amniotic fluid correctly indicated an unaffected fetus
               Bamforth et al., 1990

PD 240750 COMBINED XANTHINE OXIDASE–SULFITE OXIDASE
DEFICIENCIES (McKusick No. 252150)

    Amniocentesis[i]: increased levels of S-sulfocysteine in amniotic fluid
               Ogier et al., 1983
        undetectable sulfite oxidase activity in cultured amniotic fluid cells
               Ogier et al., 1983

PD 240950 CONGENITAL ADRENAL HYPERPLASIA, 11-BETA-
HYDROXYLASE DEFICIENCY TYPE (Adrenal hyperplasia IV; Adrenogenital syndrome; 11-beta-hydroxylase deficiency; P450 steroid 11-beta-hydroxylase deficiency) (McKusick No. 202010)

Prenatal Diagnosis: The definitive diagnosis is established by demonstrating elevated levels of deoxycortisol in the amniotic fluid of a fetus at risk during

the second trimester. This finding should be correlated with the ultrasound findings of the external genitalia, the fetal karyotype, and HLA linkage studies.
        Wong and Lessick, 1988
    Amniocentesis: elevated levels of deoxycortisol in amniotic fluid[i]
        Rosler et al., 1979; Wong and Lessick, 1988
    Maternal urine sampling[g,i]: increased excretion of tetrahydro-11-deoxy cortisol
        Rosler et al., 1979
    Ultrasound[c]: demonstration of male-appearing external genitalia in a chromosomally normal female (46, XX)
        Wong and Lessick, 1988

PD 241000 CONGENITAL ADRENAL HYPERPLASIA, 21-HYDROXYLASE DEFICIENCY TYPE (Adrenal hyperplasia III; Adrenogenital syndrome; CAH1; 21-Hydroxylase deficiency) (McKusick No. 201910)

Disease Note: Congenital adrenal hyperplasia (CAH) is one of the more common inborn errors of metabolism, occurring with a frequency of between $1:5000$ and $1:10,000$ births, and is inherited as an autosomal recessive condition. Nearly 95% of all cases of CAH are due to a deficiency of 21-hydroxylase (21-HO) activity. The deficiency of this enzyme leads to a failure of the conversion of 17-hydroxyprogesterone (17-HOP) to 11-deoxycortisol. As a result there is a deficient production of cortisol and an increase in ACTH level. The latter causes overproduction and accumulation of 11-deoxycortisol precursors, particularly 17-HOP, which is metabolized to androgens. In turn, the excessive androgens cause virilization of the external genitalia in females prenatally, and rapid growth, penile or clitoral enlargement, precocious sexual development, and premature closures of the epiphyses postnatally if the child is not treated. About one half of all individuals with 21-HO deficiency also have a defect in aldosterone synthesis. If this deficiency is untreated, shock and death may develop in the neonatal period from failure to conserve urinary sodium. Clinically there are four forms of 21-HO deficiency, including salt-losing, simple virilizing, late-onset, and cryptic forms.
    The gene for 21-hydroxylase (CYP21B) has been identified and sequenced (New, 1992; Strachan, 1993). It is closely linked to component C4 of serum complement. Mutations at different locations in CYP21B gene account for the various clinical manifestations of this disorder (New, 1992). A pseudogene to CYP21B, denoted as CYP21A, is located 30 kb from the former gene, and is nonfunctional (Strachan, 1993). Because of sequence homology between the two genes, CAH may be produced by unequal crossing over, and deletion of the CYP21B gene (Strachan, 1993).
        McKusick, 1988; Forest et al., 1989
Prenatal Diagnosis: It appears that the detection of elevated levels of 17-HOP in the amniotic fluid is only reliable in diagnosing the salt-losing variant of 21-hydroxylase deficiency (Hughes et al., 1987). Otherwise, the diagnosis is accomplished by linkage with HLA typing, RFLPs to the HLA region, or direct detection of the mutation. The advantage of the latter two methods is that they can be done on chorionic villi in the first trimester. Elevated levels of 17-HOP have been reported in the first trimester and can be used for the diagnosis of

this condition during this period (Mornet et al., 1986; Raux-Demay et al., 1989). Grosse-Wilde and associates (1988) have compared the reliability of using both the HLA and 17-HOP methods and found 88% concordance. The two cases not diagnosed were missed by the HLA method, because one antigen was "missed" and there was serologically cross-reactive HLA antigen in the second (Grosse-Wilde et al., 1988). DNA from chorionic villus tissue has been used in gene-probe analysis, a method that should be able to detect all the reported mutations of the CYP21B gene (Honour et al., 1993).

Prenatal Treatment: Prevention of the external virilization of affected female embryos has been accomplished by treating the mothers of embryos at risk with dexamethasone (20 μg/kg/d) beginning not later than in the eighth gestational week of pregnancy (Forest et al., 1989; Loeuille et al., 1990; Pang et al., 1990; Speiser et al., 1990), but starting at 5–6 weeks gestation is preferable (Migeon, 1990). The treatment of the mother (and the fetus) is continued until term if subsequent prenatal diagnosis indicates an affected female fetus. The treatment is stopped if the fetus is male or an unaffected female. Prevention of virilization in the affected female fetus has not been consistent, however (Pang et al., 1990), unless treatment is started before 8 weeks' gestation and given in 2 or 3 divided doses daily (Forest and Dorr, 1993; Speiser, 1993).

Forest and Dorr (1993) have reported data on 70 fetuses diagnosed with CAH who were treated prenatally. Treatment was stopped in 32 cases because the fetuses were male or the pregnancies were terminated (2 males, 4 females). Of the 38 female fetuses where treatment was continued until term, 27 were born with normal or slightly virilized genitalia, none of whom required surgery. Eleven cases had significantly abnormal genitalia attributed to late initiation of therapy or the use of only a single daily dose of dexamethasone.

Treatment Modality: Maternal ingestion of dexamethasone

> Forest et al., 1989; Loeuille et al., 1990; Migeon, 1990; Pang et al., 1990; Speiser et al., 1990; Karaviti et al., 1992; Forest and Dorr, 1993; Pang et al., 1993

Methods and Findings: Amniocentesis[i]: elevated 17-HOP,[g] delta[4]-androstenedione, 17-hydroxypregnenolone, testosterone (female fetuses only), and/or pregnanetriol levels in amniotic fluid

> Jeffcoate et al., 1965; Nichols and Gibson, 1969; Hughes and Laurence, 1979; Marcus et al., 1979; Warsos et al., 1980; Forest et al., 1981; Carson et al., 1982; Hughes and Laurence, 1982; Mornet et al., 1986; Pang et al., 1986; Hughes et al., 1987; Grosse-Wilde et al., 1988; Reindollar et al., 1988; Raux-Demay et al., 1989; Karaviti et al., 1992

HLA-A and B antigen typing on cultured amniotic-fluid cells and genetic linkage to the gene for 21-hydroxylase deficiency

> Pollack et al., 1979; Couillin et al., 1981; Forest et al., 1981; Pang et al, 1985; Grosse-Wilde et al., 1988

HLA-C, DQ, and/or DR typing of cultured amniotic fluid cells and genetic linkage to the gene for 21-hydroxlase deficiency

> Grosse-Wilde et al., 1988; Keller et al., 1991

use of complementary DNA (cDNA) probe to show lack of the TagI 3.7 kb cytochrome P-450$_{C-210H}$ fragment

> Reindollar et al., 1988

Chorionic villus sampling[g,i]: RFLP linkage of HLA class I and II probes to gene for 21-hydroxylase deficiency

> Mornet et al., 1985; Mornet et al., 1986; Raux-Demay et al., 1989; Keller et al., 1991; Karaviti et al., 1992; New, 1992

gene-probe analysis of DNA obtained after PCR revealed mutation in affected fetuses

> Honour et al., 1993

polymerase chain reaction/single-strand-conformation-polymorphism-profile analysis suggested a carrier female fetus; this finding was confirmed by direct nucleotide sequencing and allele-specific oligonucleotide hybridization

> Hayashi iet al., 1997

Maternal blood sampling: increased concentration of 17-HOP in maternal serum after 34 weeks of gestation

> Nagamani et al., 1978

PD 241500 CONGENITAL ADRENAL HYPOPLASIA, X-LINKED TYPE
(Adrenal hypoplasia; X-linked adrenal hypoplasia congenita) (McKusick No. 300200)

Condition Note: This X-linked recessive condition is characterized by cytomegalic adrenal cortical hypoplasia and hypogonadism. As a result, affected males have glucocorticoid, mineralocorticoid, and testosterone deficiency. If untreated, these males may develop vomiting, dehydration, listlessness, and electrolyte imbalance, and die during the neonatal or early infancy period. Appropriate steroid treatment normally successfully treats the condition, and allows for normal growth and development (Guo et al., 1995).

The gene for this condition is located at Xp21, and is distal to the glycerol kinase gene. The gene is also near the dosage-sensitive sex (DSS) reversal locus, and has been termed the DAXI (for DSS-AHC critical region on X, gene 1), AHC meaning adrenal hypoplasia congenita, which is one of the alternate names for this condition. Mutations found in various families vary from a single base pair deletion causing a premature transcription termination, to deletion of the entire gene or larger segmental deletions involving regions beyond the gene. These larger deletions have been detected by fluorescene in situ hybridization (FISH) using a cosmid probe (Guo et al., 1995).

Prenatal Diagnosis: Although the definitive diagnosis of congenital adrenal hypoplasia, X-linked type, using FISH has not been reported, this method appears to be the technique of choice where deletion of the gene is a sizable one. Otherwise, detection of the specific mutation in the involved gene will be necessary.

Alternatively, the diagnosis can be made by finding low levels of maternal serum or urine estriol with normal or low maternal urine levels of dehydroepiandrosterone sulfate (DHEAS), 16 alpha-hydroxy dehydroepiandrosterone sulfate (16OH-DHEAS), and androstenetriol (5-AT), and by decreased levels of cortisol, DHEAS, and 17 alpha-hydroxy pregnenolone in amniotic fluid.

> Bradly et al., 1994

Differential Diagnosis: Placental steroid sulfatase deficiency (PD 249000)

Amniocentesis[i]: low levels of amniotic fluid cortisol, dehydroepiandrosterone,

dehydroepiandrosterone sulfate, 17-alpha-hydroxypregnenolone, and 17-alpha-hydroxypregnenolone sulfate[d]
> Hensleigh et al., 1978

Maternal urine analysis: low levels of maternal urine estriol and conjugated serum estriol (E_3)[d]
> Hensleigh et al., 1978

PD 242000 CONGENITAL ERYTHROPOIETIC PORPHYRIA (Gunter disease, Uroporphyrin III synthetase deficiency) (McKusick No. 263700)

Amniocentesis: reddish brown amniotic fluid containing massive amounts of porphyrin
> Kaiser, 1980

uroporphyrin I dramatically elevated in amniotic fluid
> Ged et al., 1996

restriction analysis of the relevant PCR-amplified DNA fragment and direct sequencing for the C73R mutation enabled diagnosis using cultured amniocytes
> Ged et al., 1996

PD 243000 CONGENITAL SIALIDOSIS (Mucolipidosis, type I; Neuramidase deficiency) (McKusick No. 256550)

Disease Note: Congenital sialidosis is an autosomal recessive disorder manifested by hydrops fetalis, viceromegaly, severe psychomotor retardation, and death during infancy, all resulting from sialidase deficiency.

Amniocentesis[i]: deficient sialidase activity, increased bound neuraminic acid, and ultrastructural abnormalities in amniotic fluid cells
> Kleijer et al., 1979; Johnson et al., 1980b

increased sialo-oligosaccharides in amniotic fluid
> Johnson et al., 1980b

cultured amniotic fluid cells had deficiency of sialidase activity
> Sasagasako et al., 1993

PD 243250 CYTOCHROME C OXIDASE DEFICIENCY (Leigh encephalomyelopathy; Leigh syndrome; Necrotizing encephalopathy, infantile subacute type) (McKusick No. 220110)

Disease Note: See Mitochondrial disorders (PD 220800)

Amniocentesis[i]: deficiency of cytochrome C oxidase activity in cultured amniotic fluid cells
> Ruitenbeek et al., 1988

Chorionic villus sampling[g,i]: deficiency of cytochrome C oxidase activity in uncultured chorionic villus cells
> Ruitenbeek et al., 1988

PD 243500 DIABETIC EMBRYOPATHY (Diabetic macrosomia; Fetal macrosomia secondary to maternal diabetes mellitus; Infant of diabetic mother) (McKusick No. None)

Differential Diagnosis: Sacral dysgenesis (PD 169040); Sacral agenesis/spina bifida, familial (PD 169020); Sirenomelia (PD 194130); Spina bifida cystica (PD 129000); Spina bifida occulta (PD 130000)

Amniocentesis[i]: increased insulin levels in amniotic fluid[d]
>> Ogata et al., 1980

Radiograph[d]: abnormal lower thoracic and upper lumbar vertebrae, absent femora and lower spine, relatively large head
>> Griscom, 1974

Ultrasound: hydrocephalus
>> Palumbos and Steirman, 1989; Kousseff, 1990

abdominal circumference greater than 2 standard deviations (SD) above the mean after 32 weeks' gestation[d]
>> Ogata et al., 1980; Langer et al., 1991

abdominal circumference greater than 2 SD below the mean
>> Langer et al., 1991

moderately shortened limbs
>> Weldner et al., 1985

short femora
>> Meaders et al., 1995

macrosomia index (chest diameter in centimeters minus biparietal diameter in centimeters) of greater than 1.4[d]
>> Elliott et al., 1982

increased thickness of subcutaneous fat[d]
>> Jeanty et al., 1985

reduced crown–rump length [g]
>> Tchobroutsky et al., 1985

single umbilical artery[c,d]
>> Herrmann and Sidiropoulos, 1988

hydramnios[c]
>> Kouseff, 1990

oligohydramnios
>> Hill et al., 1983b

intrauterine growth retardation[c,d]
>> Herrmann and Sidiropoulos, 1988; Langer et al., 1991

large-for-gestational age
>> Leonard, 1989; Langer et al., 1991

PD 243750 FETAL HYPERTHYROIDISM (McKusick No. Unknown; see 145680)

Amniocentesis[d,i]: low level of thyroxine in amniotic fluid
>> Pekonen et al., 1984

elevated level of reverse triiodothyroxine in amniotic fluid
>> Pekonen et al., 1984

Cordocentesis (PUBS[d,i]: elevated reverse T_3, total T_4, and thyroid-stimulating immunoglobulin (Ig); low level of thyroid stimulating hormone (TSH) in fetal blood
>> Wenstrom et al., 1990

polycythemia, thrombocytopenia, and leukocytosis in fetal blood

Fetal electrocardiogram: tachycardia in fetuses whose mothers have long-acting thyroid stimulator (LATS) and previously have had thyrotoxicosis[d,i]
>> Maxwell et al., 1980; Cove and Johnston, 1985; Bruinse et al., 1988; Wenstrom et al., 1990

Ultrasound[d]: cyst-like formation in thyroid region, tachycardia
>Pekonen et al., 1984

PD 243860 GALACTOSIALIDOSIS (Goldberg syndrome; GSL;
Neuraminidase/beta-galactosidase deficiency) (McKusick No. 256540)

Syndrome Note: Galactosialidosis is produced by the combined deficiency of
beta-galactosidase and alpha-neuraminidase, both of which are lysosomal
enzymes. Their simultaneous deficiency is due to various deficiencies of the
32-kD protective protein, or its 52-kD precursor the latter of which is responsible
for the stabilization of the alpha-neuraminidase/beta-galactosidase complex.
Clinically there are three forms. The early infantile form has severe symptoms
and early death. In this form, there is marked deficiency of both the 32- and
the 52-kD proteins. Patients with the late infantile form, the second type, are
dysmorphic, have visceromegaly, and survive longer. Here there is a deficiency
of the 32-kD protein and an accumulation of the 52-kD precursor. The third
form, the juvenile-adult type, has some 52-kD precursor, but no 32-kD protein
and is characterized by a skeletal dysplasia, corneal opacities, cherry-red spot
of the retina, neurologic deficiencies, and mental retardation. All three forms
are inherited in an autosomal recessive mode.
>McKusick, 1988; Sewell and Pontz, 1988

Prenatal Diagnosis: Diagnosis is made by detection of deficiencies of both beta-
galactosidase and alpha-neuraminidase in cultured amniotic fluid cells in a fetus
at risk

Differential Diagnosis: Congenital sialidosis (PD 213000) and other forms of
neuraminidase deficiencies

Amniocentesis[i]: deficiencies of both beta-galactosidase and neuraminidase
(sialidase) activities in cultured amniotic fluid cells
>Kleijer et al., 1979; Sewell and Pontz, 1988
elevated sialic acid in cultured amniotic fluid cells
>Kleijer et al., 1979
abnormal oligosaccharides in amniotic fluid demonstrated by thin-layer
chromatography
>Sewell and Pontz, 1988

**PD 244000 HYPERCHOLESTEROLEMIA, FAMILIAL HOMOZYGOUS
FORM** (McKusick No. 143890)

Amniocentesis[i]: absence of low-density lipoprotein (LDL) cell-surface receptors on cultured amniotic fluid cells by measurement of the binding, uptake,
and degradation of ^{125}I-LDL
>Brown et al., 1978; Rose et al., 1982; de Gennes et al., 1985
Fetal blood sampling[i]: increased total cholesterol, LDL cholesterol, and apoli-
poprotein B
>de Gennes et al., 1985
Comment: The above method enables quicker diagnosis than by the cultured amniotic fluid cells approach (de Gennes et al., 1985).

PD 244500 HYPERGLYCEROLEMIA (GK1 deficiency; Glycerol kinase
deficiency) (McKusick No. 307030)

Disease Note: Isolated glycerol kinase deficiency may give rise to episodes of
vomiting, hypoglycemia, and somnolence in young children, but also may be
asymptomatic. The condition is inherited as an X-linked recessive trait.
>Borresen et al., 1987

Prenatal Diagnosis: The diagnosis is determined as noted below in fetuses at risk. Amniocentesis[i]: elevated amounts of glycerol in amniotic fluid, low levels of glycerol kinase activity in cultured amniotic fluid cells

Borresen et al., 1987

PD 244750 HYPOPHOSPHATASIA, ADULT FORM (Autosomal dominant hypophosphatasia) (McKusick No. 146300)

Condition Note: The adult form of hypophosphatasia is inherited in an autosomal dominant mode, and is characterized by low serum alkaline phosphatase, elevated urinary phosphoethanolamine, early loss of teeth, bowed legs, short stature, and variable expressivity.

McKusick, 1988

Prenatal Diagnosis: The presence of shortened and bowed leg bones in a fetus at risk should normally be sufficient for the diagnosis. In sporadic cases, the diagnosis should be considered whenever there is a fetus with mild shortening and bowing of the long bones of the legs.

Differential Diagnosis: Achondroplasia, heterozygous type (PD 146000); Campomelic dysplasia, short limb type (PD 150000); Congenital bowed long bones, isolated (PD 151750); Osteogenesis imperfecta, type I (PD 163500); Osteogenesis imperfecta, type II (PD 164000); and Proximal focal femoral deficiency (PD 168000) are the major conditions to be considered in the differential. In Osteogenesis imperfecta, type II, and Hypophosphatasia, infantile form, (PD 245000), there may be failure of or poor visualization of the fetal head and skeleton; these findings have not been reported in Hypophosphatasia, adult form (PD 244750).

Ultrasound[i]: symmetrical tibial and femoral shortening with marked midshaft bowing, intrauterine growth retardation (IUGR), normal-appearing cranial vault ossification

Curry et al., 1988

PD 245000 HYPOPHOSPHATASIA, PERINATAL LETHAL AND INFANTILE FORMS (Congenital hypophosphatasia; Congenital lethal form of hypophosphatasia; Infantile hypophosphatasia; Phosphoethanolaminuria; Spurlimbed dwarfism) (McKusick No. 241500)

Amniocentesis[i]: deficient bone/liver alkaline phosphatase isozyme activity in cultured amniotic fluid cells and amniotic fluid

Mulivor et al., 1978; Warren et al., 1985

deficiency of total alkaline phosphatase activity in cultured amniotic fluid cells

Rattenbury et al., 1976; Blau et al., 1978; Spranger, 1988

Comments: Vanneuville and colleagues (1982) found normal enzyme activity in cultured amniocytes, and at delivery characteristic radiologic findings, enzyme deficiency, and neonatal death were reported.

low to undetectable levels of alkaline phosphatase in amniotic fluid

Benzie et al., 1976; Shohat et al., 1991

amniocyte DNA and allele-specific oligonucleotide probes for missense mutations present in the index case (a compound heterozygote), hybridization studies revealed only one of the mutations, enabling the diagnosis of a heterozygous fetus, which was later confirmed

Henthorn and Whyte, 1995

Chorionic villus sampling[g,i]: low level of bone/liver alkaline phosphatase isozyme in chorionic villi assayed by monoclonal antibodies

Warren et al., 1985; Brock and Barron, 1991

restriction-fragment-length polymorphic studies and linkage to alkaline phosphatase gene correctly predicted an unaffected heterozygous infant

Greenberg et al., 1990

polymerase chain reaction–restriction-fragment-length polymorphism and PCR–allele-specific oligonucleotide analysis correctly identified a compound-heterozygous fetus; PCR–single strand conformation polymorphism methodology confirmed the diagnosis

Orimo et al., 1996

very low levels of bone/liver alkaline phosphatase isozyme assayed by determining residual alkaline phosphatase activity in the presence of various inhibitors

Muller et al., 1991

Fetoscopy with fetal skin biopsy[i]: reduced levels of alkaline phosphatase in cultured skin cells

Benzie et al., 1976

Maternal examination[c,d]: hydramnios

Benzie et al., 1976

Radiograph: undermineralization or no mineralization of the fetal skeleton

Benzie et al., 1976; McGuire et al., 1987

unusual bony spurs[c]

Goldstein et al., 1987

Ultrasound: failure to visualize or poor visualization of fetal head and ribs due to deficient bone mineralization[i]

Benzie et al., 1976; Rudd et al., 1976; Mulivor et al., 1978; Kurtz and Wapner, 1983; Wladimiroff et al., 1985b; Bader and Lewis, 1988; Spranger, 1988

Comment: In this condition, the skull may appear as a very thin, faint, circular outlined structure within which a falx is more readily visualized.

relatively increased echogenicity of the falx as compared with the calvarium[c]

Laughlin and Lee, 1982; Spirt et al., 1987

unusual globular shape of the head with indentation in it by the placenta

Kurtz and Wapner, 1983

reduced fetal bone echogenicity (hypomineralization) and fractures of fetal spine and long bones

Kurtz and Wapner, 1983; Warren et al., 1985; Wladimiroff et al., 1985b; Donnenfeld and Mennuti, 1987; McGuire et al., 1987

bowing of extremities and long bones, abnormal position of the radius-ulna to the humerus and the tibia-fibula to the femur

Wladimiroff et al., 1985b

short, bowed, and thin femorae, tibiae, and fibulae; absence of ischial ossification centers

Spirt et al., 1987

shortened and angulated femora and humeri
>Bader and Lewis, 1988

dumbbell-shaped appearance to the long bones with marked irregularly flared metaphyses
>McGuire et al., 1987

shortened limbs[i]
>Wladimiroff et al., 1985b; Goldstein et al., 1987; Goldstein, 1988; Spranger, 1988; Shohat et al., 1991

oligohydramnios[c]
>Wladimiroff et al., 1985b

hydramnios[c]
>McGuire et al., 1987; Shohat et al., 1991

PD 245250 HYPOTHALAMIC CORTICOTROPIN DEFICIENCY (McKusick No. none)

Disease Note: This autosomal recessive, potentially fatal disorder is characterized by encephalopathy, hypoglycemia, hepatitis, and facial dysmorphism. During hypoglycemia episodes, cortisol and ACTH levels are nil both before and after ACTH and corticotropin-releasing hormone injection. Hypothalmic under-responsiveness is considered responsible for the disorder.

Maternal urine sampling[i]: low maternal urinary estriol in an at-risk pregnancy
>Mandel et al., 1990

>Comment: The advantage of making the diagnosis prenatally is that it allows immediate institution of cortisol therapy after birth (Mandel et al., 1990).

PD 245500 HYPOTHYROIDISM (Congenital hypothyroidism; Cretinism; Goiter; Thyroid agenesis) (McKusick No. None)

Condition Note: There are numerous causes for fetal hypothyroidism including absence of the fetal thyroid gland, defects in the metabolic pathway producing thyroxine (T_4), and deficient production of TSH. The fetus is protected to some extent from these deficiency states by transplacental transfer of maternal T_4 with fetal levels being 25–50% of normal levels in fetuses with no T_4 production (Vulsma et al., 1989). Maternal treatment of fetal hypothroidism has not been undertaken, however.

Prenatal Treatment: Experience is limited, but repeated intraamniotic cavity injection of thyroxine appears to be safe and effective. The thyroxine following injection is then swallowed and absorbed by the fetus.

Treatment Modalities: Intraamniotic caviety injection of 500 μg of Na-L-thyroxine that is repeated periodically.
>Hirsch et al., 1990

>Comments: Initial treatment in the case of Hirsch and co-workers (1990) began at 22 weeks' gestation and was repeated approximately every 2 weeks through the 36th week. Following the initiation of treatment, the fetal serum T_4 and TSH levels reached normal levels. The neonate was euthyroid and healthy after birth. Testing revealed he had an enzymatic organification defect in the thyroidine synthesis pathway as did his parents; the exact defect was not stated.

Intramuscular injection of Na-L-thyroxine (Synthroid)[j]
>Van Herle et al., 1975

>*Comments*: The fetus treated by Van Herle and associates (1975) had absence of the thyroid gland as a result of his mother having received ^{131}I therapy at 13 weeks of gestation for papillary carcinoma of the thyroid. Thyroxine (120 μg) was injected into the fetal buttock beginning at 32 weeks' and repeated every 2 weeks for a total of 4 injections. At parturition, cord blood of serum T_3 and T_4 levels were undetectable while serum TSH level was very high. The child was of normal size (4 kg), and other than for the absence of the thyroid gland and tracheal narrowing at the level of C7, was normal.

Methods and Findings: Amniocentesis[i]: low levels of T_4 and elevated levels of TSH in amniotic fluid
>Kourides et al., 1984; Hirsch et al., 1990

Cordocentesis (PUBS)[d]: low levels of T_4 and free throxine, and elevated levels of TSH in fetal blood
>Johnson et al., 1989b

Ultrasound[c]: fetal bradycardia, disproportionately large chest diameter, oligohydramnios, ascites
>Weiner et al., 1980a; Weiner et al., 1980b

>bilobed anterior neck mass
>>Johnson et al., 1989b

>hyperextended neck
>>Johnson et al., 1989b

>decrease volume of gastric fluid
>>Johnson et al., 1989b

>hydramnios
>>Johnson et al., 1989b

>>*Comments*: Landau and co-authors (1980) found no correlation between amniotic fluid levels of 3,3,5-triiodothyroxine and the presence of hypothyroidism in the fetus.

>bilobed symmetrical mass, mainly solid with some small cystic areas in the anterior neck region
>>Kourides et al., 1984

PD 245600 HYPOTHYROIDISM, PROPYLTHIOURACIL INDUCED
(McKusick No. None)

Condition Note: It has been estimated that 0.2% of pregnant women have hyperthyroidism due to Graves' disease. When the condition is diagnosed, these women are usually treated with propylthiouracil rather than methimazole, which more readily passes through the placenta, or radioactive iodine, which may destroy the fetal thyroid gland. Graves disease and/or the medications used to treat this condition may produce either hyperthyroidism or hypothroidism in the fetus. Furthermore, fetal hypothyroidism may result from transplacental passage of maternal TSH-inhibitory immunoglobins or propylthiouracil. Fetal goiter may also be produced by maternal propylthiouracil consumption.
>Davidson et al., 1991

Prenatal Diagnosis: Determination of fetal thyroid function from fetal blood obtained by cordocentesis is now the method of choice for diagnosing hypothyroidism prenatally.

> Davidson et al., 1991

Differential Diagnosis: Disorders of thyroid function such as Fetal hyperthyroidism (PD 243750), Goiter (PD 274500), and Hypothroidism (PD 245500) should be considered. Tumors of the thyroid or neck should also be included in the differential including Teratoma, neck (PD 283000); Teratoma, pharyngeal (PD 283500); and Tumor, thyroid (PD 287000).

Prenatal Treatment: In fetuses shown to have hypothyroidism, weekly intraamniotic injection of thyroxine (200–250 μg per injection) appears to be the treatment of choice (Davidson et al., 1991). In the fetus treated by Davidson and associates (1991), the treatment produced significant reduction in the size of the goiter and resulted in a euthyroid child at birth.

Treatment Modality: Intraamniotic injections of thyroxine[d]

> Weiner et al., 1980b; Davidson et al., 1991

Methods and Findings: Amniocentesis[d,i]: reduced levels of amniotic fluid thyroxine, triiodothyronine, and reverse triiodothyronine concentrations

> Davidson et al., 1991

Cordocentesis (PUBS)[d,i]: low levels of fetal serum thyroxine and thyroid-stimulating hormone–binding inhibitory immunoglobulins, and elevated levels of fetal serum TSH and thyroid-stimulating immunoglobulin bioactivity

> Davidson et al., 1991

> low levels of fetal serum T_4 and triiodothyroxine (T_3)

> > Davidson et al., 1991; Noia et al., 1992

> elevated levels of fetal serum TSH

> > Davidson et al., 1991; Noia et al., 1992

> elevated level of thyroglobulin in fetal serum

> > Noia et al., 1992

Ultrasound[d,i]: goiter that enlarged with time

> Davidson et al., 1991

> cystic-solid neck mass 4 × 6 cm in the anterior fetal neck that contained large pulsatile vessels

> > Weiner et al., 1980

> bilateral echogenic mass in the fetal neck

> > Noia et al., 1992

> fetal neck partially distended

> > Weiner et al., 1980

PD 246000 LESCH–NYHAN SYNDROME (Hypoxanthine–guanine phosphoribosyl transferase deficiency) (McKusick No. 308000)

> Amniocentesis[i]: deficient hypoxanthine–guanine phosphoribosyl transferase activity determined by measuring the incorporation of radioactive hypoxanthine into cultured amniotic fluid cells

> > Bakay et al., 1977; Hosli et al., 1977; Alford et al., 1995

> > deficient hypoxanthine–guanine phosphoribosyl transferase activity measured by incorporation of ^{14}C-hypoxanthine into ^{14}C-inosinic acid

> > > Tisenfield et al., 1979; Graham et al., 1996

> > detection of mutation in cultured amniocytes by PCR amplification and DNA sequencing, and dosage and linkage analysis

> > > Alford et al., 1995

Chorionic villus sampling[g,i]: deficient hypoxanthine–guanine phosphoribosyl transferase (HGPRT) activity using a radiochemical assay in cultured and uncultured material

> Gibbs et al., 1984; Stout et al., 1985; Marcus et al., 1992; Alford et al., 1995; Graham et al., 1996

> *Comments:* In a male fetus reported by Gruber and associates (1989), the HGPRT activity was about half normal, and the HGPRT/APRT (adenosine-phosphoribosyl transferase) ratio was normal. Postnatally, the child turned out to have no HGPRT activity and to be affected with the condition. No explanation for missing the diagnosis could be given by the authors.

> mutant gene present as demonstrated by link analysis

> > Gibbs et al., 1986; Alford et al., 1995

> mutant gene present as demonstrated by allele-specific oligonucleotide hybridization to amplified cDNA

> > Edwards et al., 1989b

> hypoxanthine-guanine phosphoribosyl transferase allele typing by PCR amplification of an STR in intron 3; and dosage analysis of HGPRT gene sequences

> > Alford et al., 1995

PD 246500 LYMPHOPROLIFERATIVE DISEASE, X-LINKED RECESSIVE TYPE (Duncan disease; Familial fatal Epstein–Barr infection; Immunodeficiency-5; X-linked lymphoprolifertive disease; X-linked progressive combined variable immunodeficiency) (McKusick No. 308240)

Disease Note: this X-linked lymphoproliferative disease is characterized by a selective immunodeficiency to the Epstein–Barr virus, severe or fatal infectious mononucleosis, acquired hypogammaglobulinemia, hyperimmunoglobulinemia M, aplastic anemia, and malignant lymphoma. The prognosis in affected males with this disease is poor with a lethality rate of approximately 77% by 10 years of age. No patients have been documented to live into their fifth decade. The gene for this condition maps to the distal long arm of the X chromosome at Xq25-q26.

> McKusick, 1995; Schuster et al., 1995

Differential Diagnosis: Adenosine deaminase deficiency (PD 240000); Purine nucleoside phosphorylase deficiency (PD 249200)

> Chorionic villus sampling[g,i]: utilizing multiplex PCR and various polymorphic markers, linkage to Xq24q25 region in a male fetus

> > Schuster et al., 1995

PD 247000 LYSOSOMAL ACID PHOSPHATASE DEFICIENCY (McKusick No. 200950)

> Amniocentesis[i]: deficient acid phosphatase activity in the lysosomal fraction of cultured amniotic fluid cells

> > Nadler and Egan, 1970

PD 248000 MENKES DISEASE (Menkes kinky hair disease) (McKusick No. 309400)

> Amniocentesis[i]: increased incorporation of ^{64}Cu into cultured amniotic fluid cells

> > Horn, 1976; Horn, 1981; Horn, 1983; Tonnesen and Horn, 1989; Tonnesen et al., 1989

Comments: There is an increased risk of false-negative results when analyzing the incorporation of labeled copper by cultured amniotic fluid cells after 18 weeks of gestation (Horn, 1983; Tonnesen et al., 1987a).

increased retention of ^{64}Cu in cultured amniotic fluid cells
    Hirschhorn and LaBadie, 1985; Tonnesen and Horn, 1989
Chorionic villus sampling[g,i]: elevated levels of copper in direct measurements of chorionic villi
    Tonnesen et al., 1985; Tonnesen et al., 1987a; Tonnesen et al., 1987b; Tonnesen and Horn, 1989; Tonnesen et al., 1989
Comments: ^{64}Cu-uptake studies cannot be used for the diagnosis of Menkes disease using chorionic villi because some control samples have taken up as much labeled copper as have samples from affected fetuses (Tonnesen et al., 1987a). Maternal decidua may contain elevated copper values and contamination of the chorionic villus samples by decidua may lead to false positive diagnoses (Tonnesen et al., 1989).

mutation analysis by allele-specific oligonucleotide hybridization and nucleotide sequencing
    Tumer et al, 1994; Das et al., 1995

PD 248500 MITOCHONDRIAL DNA^{T88993G} DISEASE (Complex V, ATP synthase, subunit ATPase 6; Leigh syndrome; Neurogenic muscle weakness, ataxia and retinitis pigmentosa) (McKusick No. 516060.01)

Disease Note: Major characteristics of this condition, which is caused by a mutation in the mitochondrial DNA, include neurogenic muscle weakness, ataxia, and retinitis pigmentosa. Mental retardation, dementia, seizures, and sensory neuropathy are additional features. The severity is roughly proportional to the percentage of mitochondria possessing the mutant DNA, which is generally uniform in various tissues.

Chorionic villus sampling[g,i]: detection of mutation in the mitochondrial DNA from chorionic villi
    Harding et al., 1992
Comments: Two affected fetuses from the same family were reported by Harding and co-workers (1992). The mutation was found in 100% of the mitochondrial DNA in chorionic villi from both fetuses, and from 68–98% in various other tissues obtained posttermination of these fetuses.

PD 249000 PLACENTAL STEROID SULFATASE DEFICIENCY (X-linked ichthyosis) (McKusick No. 308100)

Disease Note: A deficiency of placental steroid sulfatase during pregnancy is manifested by low maternal serum and urine estriol levels, increased rate of stillbirth, relative refractoriness of oxytoxic agents and delay in the onset of labor. In infants with the above enzyme deficiency, there is ichthyosis of the scalp, ears, neck, back, and the front of the legs to dorsum of the foot.
    Schleifer et al., 1993; Bradley et al., 1994; McKusick, 1995
Prenatal Diagnosis: Placental steroid sulfatase deficiency is diagnosed or suspected by finding the following: low maternal serum or urine estriol levels, elevated levels of the precursors dehydroepiandrosterone sulfate (DHEAS), 16-alpha-hydroxy dehydroepiandrosterone sulfate (16OH-DHEAS), and androstenetriol (5-AT) in maternal urine and amniotic fluid, deficiency of placental

steroid sulfatase in cultured amniotic fluid cells, or by molecular genetic demonstration of a deletion in the steroid sulfatase gene.

> Bradley et al., 1994

Differential Diagnosis: Congenital adrenal hypoplasia, X-linked type (PD 241500)

> Amniocentesis[i]: increased dehydroepiandrosterone sulfate concentration in amniotic fluid
>
> > Braunstein et al., 1976; Hahnel et al., 1982; Bick et al., 1989
>
> steroid sulfatase deficiency in cultured amniotic fluid cells
>
> > Hahnel et al., 1982; Bick et al., 1989
> >
> > *Comments*: The male fetus reported by Bick and associates (1989 and 1992) had a deletion of the distal end of the p arm of the X chromosome. The fetus also had chondrodysplasia punctata, X-linked recessive form, and Kallmann syndrome.

Maternal blood sampling[i]: increased dehydroepiandrosterone sulfate in maternal plasma

> Hahnel et al., 1982

> deficient or undetectable levels of unconjugated estriol (uE$_3$) in maternal serum

> > Hahnel et al., 1982; Schleifer et al., 1993; McGowan et al., 1995

Maternal urine sampling[i]: increased 16-alpha-hydroxydehydroepiandrosterone in maternal urine

> Hahnel et al., 1982

> deficient estriol in maternal urine

> > Hahnel et al., 1982

PD 249120 PSEUDOCHOLINESTERASE DEFICIENCY (Cholinesterase deficiency; PChE deficiency) (McKusick No. 177400)

Condition Note: Pseudocholinesterase (cholinesterase) is a normal component of both plasma and amniotic fluid, and is not to be confused with acetylcholinesterase which normally is found in low concentrations in the plasma and is absent in amniotic fluid. Pseudocholinesterase is a nonspecific esterase; acetylcholinesterase converts acetylcholine to choline at nerve endings. There are a number of genetic variants of pseudocholinesterase that result in nearly total deficiency of enzyme activity (silent allele) or reduced activity as detected by inhibition by dibucaine and fluorides.

A deficiency of pseudocholinesterase has no apparent adverse effect on the affected individual under normal circumstances but leads to prolonged apnea when succinylcholine (suxamethonium, a muscle relaxant) is administered to the affected individual (homozygous dominant). The pseudocholinesterase in amniotic fluid is apparently maternally derived because the enzyme has been found to be diminished or absent in gel electrophoresis when the mother but not the fetus has the abnormal form of pseudocholinesterase.

> Super et al., 1987; Haddow et al., 1989

Prenatal Diagnosis: The condition is suggested when there is a very faint or absent amniotic fluid pseudocholinesterase band following gel electrophoresis. The diagnosis is confirmed by appropriate pseudocholinesterase testing of the maternal serum.

Differential Diagnosis: No other condition is known to produce a deficiency of pseudocholinesterase isozyme on gel electrophoresis. Although the dibucaine variant is the only one so far reported prenatally to be associated with the deficiency of the pseudocholinesterase isozyme, the other variants, which are less frequent than the dibucaine type, most likely will be reported to produce deficiency of the pseudocholinesterase isozyme with time.

   Amniocentesis: decreased or absence of amniotic fluid pseudocholinesterase band on gel electrophoresis

   Super et al., 1987; Haddow et al., 1989

   Comments: Of the three cases reported with this condition, all had deficiency of total enzyme activity in their plasma and two had reduced dibucaine numbers (percentage inhibition by dibucaine of pseudocholinesterase) (Super et al., 1987; Haddow et al., 1989).

PD 249200 PURINE NUCLEOSIDE PHOSPHORYLASE DEFICIENCY
(PNP deficiency; Immunodeficiency, nucleoside-phosphorylase deficiency; NP deficiency; Nucleoside phosphorylase deficiency; Purine nucleoside orthophosphate ribosyltransferase deficiency) (McKusick No. 164050)

Condition Note: Deficiency of purine nucleoside phosphorylase (PNP) results in a deficiency of T cells and T-cell immunity. The affected individual may have recurrent infections, severe hemolytic anemia, and fatal varicella infection. Because PNP catalyzes the phosphorolytic cleavage of inosine to hypoxanthine, a deficiency of this enzyme leads to excessive excretion of purine nucleosides in the urine and amniotic fluid.

   Kleijer et al., 1989; McKusick, 1990

Prenatal Diagnosis: The diagnosis is established by demonstrating deficiency of purine nucleoside phosphorylase in cultured amniotic fluid cells in fetuses at risk.

Differential Diagnosis: Adenosine deaminase deficiency (PD 240000); other immunodeficiency states

   Amniocentesis[i]: no purine nucleoside phosphorylase activity in cultured amniotic fluid cells

   Kleijer et al., 1989

   elevated levels of the purine nucleosides inosine, guanosine, deoxyinosine, and deoxyguanosine in the amniotic fluid

   Kleijer et al., 1989

PD 249225 RICKETS, VITAMIN D-DEPENDENT, TYPE IIA (Vitamin D-dependent rickets–alopecia syndrome) (McKusick No. 277440)

Disease Note: This autosomal recessive disorder is characterized by hypocalcemia, severe rickets and alopecia. The condition is caused by end-organ unresponsiveness to 1,25-dihydroxy vitamin D; the serum concentration of the latter is usually high, and a number of mutations have been noted in the gene in various families.

   Weisman et al., 1990

   Amniocentesis[i]: cultured cells' 24-hydroxylase activity was not stimulated by treatment with 1,25-dihydroxy vitamin D_3 nor did their extracts bind to ^3H1,25-hydroxy vitamin D

   Weisman et al., 1990

PD 249250 SALLA DISEASE (Sialuria, Finnish type) (McKusick No. 268740)

Disease Note: Salla disease, an autosomal recessive lysosomal storage disease, is characterized by psychomotor retardation, clumsiness, and ataxia with the onset in the second year of life. Biochemically, the disease is noted by increased concentrations of free N-acetylneuraminic acid (sialic acid) both in the urine and in intracellular spaces. Histologically, there are enlarged storage lysosomes. Life expectancy can be normal. Most affected individuals have been of Finnish ancestry.

McKusick, 1986; Renlund and Aula, 1987

Prenatal Diagnosis: The diagnosis is established by prenatal identification of elevated levels of free sialic acids and increased ratio of free/total sialic acid in cultured amniotic fluid cells in fetuses at risk.

Amniocentesis[i]: elevated level of free sialic acid in cultured amniotic-fluid cells, and increased ratio of free to total sialic acid in cultured amniotic fluid cells

Renlund and Aula, 1987

PD 249500 SEVERE COMBINED IMMUNODEFICIENCY, HLA CLASS II NEGATIVE TYPE (Bare lymphocyte syndrome; HLA class II negative SCID; HLA class II negative severe combined immunodeficiency) (McKusick No. 209920)

Fetal blood drawing by fetoscopy[i]: diminished expression of HLA class I antigens and beta 2-microglobulin; poor expression of HLA class II molecules on peripheral blood mononuclear cells, and on activated T blast cells

Durandy et al., 1987

PD 249600 SEVERE COMBINED IMMUNODEFICIENCY DISEASE, X-LINKED (Agammaglobulinemia, Swiss type; IMD4; Immunodeficiency-4; SCIDX; Thymic epithelial hypoplasia; XSCID) (McKusick Nos. 300400, 308380)

Disease Note: This form of severe combined immunodeficiency disease is an X-linked recessive disorder, and is produced by a mutation in the interleukin-2 receptor, gamma chain gene. The disease is characterized by lymphocytopenia; early death; susceptibility to viral, fungal, and bacterial infections; lack of delayed hypersensitivity; thymic atrophy; and no benefit from administration of gamma globulin.

McKusick, 1995

Method for obtaining fetal tissue not stated[h]: The fetuses of known carrier females for mutants in the interleukin-2 receptor, gamma chain gene had mutations in the gene detected by various molecular genetic techniques

Pepper et al., 1995

PD 249750 SIALIC ACID STORAGE DISEASE, INFANTILE TYPE (McKusick No. 269920)

Amniocentesis[i]: marked elevation of free sialic acid in cell-free amniotic fluid and cultured amniotic fluid cells from a fetus at risk

Vamos et al., 1986; Poulain et al., 1995

elevated sialic acid in amniotic-fluid cells

Clements et al., 1988

Comments: Clements and co-workers (1988) found the amniotic fluid cells could be used for the diagnosis of this condition, but amniotic fluid could not.

increased number of vacuoles in amniotic fluid cells

Clements et al., 1988
increased accumulation of tritium-labeled sialic acid in cultured amniotic fluid cells from a fetus at risk
Vamos et al., 1986
Chorionic villus sampling[g,i]: marked vacuolization of syncytiotrophoblastic cells, fibroblasts and macrophages; excessive numbers of macrophages with cystoplasmic vacuolization; increased sialic acid content in chorionic villi
Lake et al., 1989
Comments: Lake and associates (1989) reported twins fetuses at risk for sialic acid storage disease; a previous sibling had been affected with this disorder. Both twins were tested by sampling each of their placentas. One twin was found affected. Selected fetocide was performed; the unaffected co-twin was allowed to continue to term, and was healthy at birth.
Ultrasound[c,d]: hepatomegaly, ascites, bilateral talipes, IUGR, oligohydramnios
Poulain et al., 1995
Comments: The diagnosis of the case presented by Poulain and colleagues (1995) was made by demonstration elevated sialic acid in the amniotic fluid. The diagnosis was considered after consulting the POSSUM Database (Murdock Institution for Research into Birth Defects, Melbourne, Australia).

PD 249775 TAY SYNDROME (IBIDS syndrome; Ichthyosiform erythroderma with hair abnormality and mental retardation; PIBIDS; Trichothiodystrophy, type 2; Trichothiodystrophy with congenital ichthyosis) (McKusick No. 242170)

Syndrome Note: Tay syndrome consists in part of microcephaly associated with mental retardation and ataxia, nonbullous ichthyosiform erythroderma, lack of subcutaneous fatty tissue, trichorrhexis nodosa, photosensitivity, and growth deficiency. Trichothiodystrophy is also present, and indicates sulfur-deficient hair that is brittle. PIBIDS is an acronym standing for *p*hotosensitivity *i*chthyosis, *b*rittle hair, *i*ntellectual impairment, *d*ecreased fertility, and *s*hort stature. The condition is a DNA repair deficiency, and inherited in an autosomal recessive mode.

Savary et al., 1991; McKusick, 1996
Amniocentesis[i]: deficient DNA excision repair in cultured amniotic fluid cells after exposure of cell to UV
Savary etal., 1991

PD 249800 TESTICULAR FEMINIZATION (Complete androgen insensitivity) (McKusick No. 313700)

Amniocentesis[i]: elevated amniotic fluid testosterone level, elevated above normal male fetal levels
Stephens, 1984
Ultrasound[i]: female genitalia when karyotype of amniotic fluid cells indicated 46,XY male chromosomal constitution
Stephens, 1984

PD 249880 WILLIAMS SYNDROME (Idiopathic infantile hypercalcemia; Williams–Beuren syndrome; Williams elfin face syndrome) (McKusick No. 194050)

Condition Note: The full-blown phenotype of the Williams syndrome includes mild to moderate mental retardation; a friendly and loquacious personality;

hoarse voice; characteristic facial appearance, that includes a stellate pattern of the iris, anteverted nares, long philtrum, prominent lips with open mouth, and coarse facial features in the older child and adult; supravalvular aortic stenosis; peripheral pulmonary artery stenosis; and infantile hypercalcemia. In most cases, the condition is sporadic, but may be inherited in an autosomal dominant mode, with great variability of phenotype. In inherited situations, it is not uncommon for affected family members to express only the supravalvular aortic stenosis. The condition, idiopathic infantile hypercalcemia, is most likely the same condition as Williams syndrome.

Williams syndrome, in most cases, has been found to be caused by a microdeletion at chromosome 7q11.23 location and appears to be a contiguous gene deletion syndrome. Two genes, elastin and LIM kinase 1, have been documented to be missing in many patients, and deletion of these two genes may account for a number but probably not all of the features seen in the disorder. The diagnosis of William syndrome can be confirmed normally by FISH.

Jones, 1988; McKusick, 1988; Westgren et al., 1988

Prenatal Diagnosis: The diagnosis if considered prenatally, can be made by demonstrating a deletion in chromosome 7 at 7q11.223 by appropriate FISH testing of chorionic villus or amniotic fluid cells.

Differential Diagnosis: Aortic valvular stenosis (PD 106350); Endocardial fibroelastosis (PD 109700); Pulmonary stenosis (PD 112250); Pulmonary valve atresia (PD 112380)

Cordocentesis (PUBS)[c,d]: elevated serum calcium and phosphate levels, reduced serum total protein and albumin levels

Westgren et al., 1988

Ultrasound[c,d]: cardiomegaly with enlarged left ventricle, hydrops fetalis, ascites, placentomegaly, hydramnios

Westgren et al., 1988

Comments: The fetus reported by Westgren and co-workers (1988) died 2 days after fetal blood sampling. At autopsy, the fetus had the findings noted prenatally plus aortic stenosis located 3 cm above the aortic valve, and diffuse calcification of the aorta that were seen on gross examination. Focal and subintimal microscopic calcifications were present in all major and medium-sized arteries. The parents of the fetus had previously given birth to a stillborn infant with nonimmune hydrops fetalis. The parents were first cousins. The diagnosis of Williams syndrome in the above fetus is tentative because there were no children or adults in the family with the fully expressed phenotype in the family.

PD 249900 WILSON DISEASE (Hepatolenticular degeneration) (McKusick No. 277900)

Chorionic villi sampling[g,i]: RFLP analysis revealed a heterozygous fetus at a probability level of 0.910. Proximal (Rb) and distal (D13S26) markers were used for linkage.

Cossu et al., 1992

PD 251000 XERODERMA PIGMENTOSUM III (XP, group C) (McKusick No. 278720)

Amniocentesis[i]: absent DNA excision repair synthesis by autoradiography in cultured amniotic fluid cells

Halley et al., 1979

Chorionic villus sampling[g,i]: DNA extracted from the villi and subjected to PCR amplification of intron 3 to analyze the family mutation at the alw NI site by demonstrating an RFLP linkage; the fetus was found to be a heterozygous carrier

Matsumoto et al., 1995

Chapter 7

Other Prenatal Conditions[a]

PD 251950 ABORTION, FAILED EARLY INDUCED (McKusick No. None)

Condition Note: Although failed early induced abortion is uncommon, the frequency of such happenings is inversely related to the gestational age at the time of the attempted termination. The outcome of nine early induced abortions that were completed unsuccessfully have been summarized by Arnon and Ornoy (1995). Four pregnancies ended near term or at term in normal infants, one in a near-term infant with multiple congenital abnormalities, three in missed or spontaneous abortions, and one induced abortion at 24 weeks who had severe intrauterine growth retardation (IUGR). The authors speculated that vascular disruption or insufficiency may have produced the IUGR in the latter case.

Prenatal Diagnosis: None established.

Differential Diagnosis: Other causes for birth defects or IUGR should be considered.

Ultrasound: severe IUGR
　　　　Arnon and Ornoy, 1995
　　　　Comments: In one case reported by Arnon and Ornoy (1995), the failed induction occurred at 9 weeks of gestation. At 22 and 24 weeks, severe IUGR in this pregnancy was observed. The pregnancy was then terminated, and an asymmetric IUGR fetus of 19 week size without physical birth defects or skeletal abnormalities was found.

PD 252000 ABRUPTIO PLACENTAE (Ablatio placentae; Premature separation of the placenta) (McKusick No. None)

Alpha-fetoprotein (AFP)[c]: elevated in maternal serum
　　　　Milunsky et al., 1988
Ultrasound: irregularly shaped sonolucent areas within the placenta
　　　　Gottesfeld, 1978
　　　　intrauterine growth retardation[c]
　　　　　　Gembruch and Hansmann, 1988
　　　　non-functioning kidney[c]
　　　　　　Gembruch and Hansmann, 1988
　　　　intraventricular bleeding with hydrocephalus[c]
　　　　　　Gembruch and Hansmann, 1988

PD 252125 AGAMMAGLOBULINEMIA, X-LINKED TYPE (Bruton agammaglobulinemia tyrosine kinase deficeincy; Bruton type agammaglobulinemia) (McKusick No. 300300)

Condition Note: This form of agammaglobulinemia is an X-linked recessive disorder characterized by a selective defect in the humoral immune responds. Males who are affected have very low concentrations of serum immunoglobulins in association with absent or low numbers of B lymphocytes. The deficiency of immunoglobulins leads to recurrent bacterial or viral infections beginning between 6 and 18 months of age. The condition is the result of a mutation in the Bruton agammaglobulinemia tyrosine kinase gene which is located at 1q22, and disturbs growth and differentiation of B lymphocytes precursor in the bone marrow.

Allen et al., 1994; McKusick, 1995

Method not stated[h,i]: close linkage of the gene to various polymorphic markers in a male fetus

Allen et al., 1994

PD 252175 ALPHA-FETOPROTEIN, BENIGN ELEVATION (McKusick No. None; see 104150)

Condition Note: Numerous disorders are associated with elevation of either the maternal serum AFP, or amniotic fluid AFP, or commonly both. Conditions reported with increased levels of AFP are listed in the Index under Alpha fetoprotein (AFP), elevated in amniotic fluid and Alpha-fetoprotein (AFP), elevated in maternal serum. Benign elevation of unknown etiology occasionally is found. Usually this is the situation when the chromosomal and ultrasonic analyses of the fetus are normal, and there is no detectable acetylcholinesterase activity in the amniotic fluid (Berry and Lamm, 1995).

Of a total of 13,239 amniotic fluid samples assayed for AFP, Berry and Lamm (1995) reported 230 (1.7%) with elevation of AFP. The elevation was accounted for in 80% by neural tube or ventral wall defects. Another 15% had diverse causes, while the remaining 5% had normal amniotic fluid/acetylcholinesterase and chromosomal analysis. In each of these pregnancies, a healthy, full-term infant of average birth weight was born.

Alpha-fetoprotein[c]: elevated in amniotic fluid with normal fetal chromosomes and ultrasound evaluations, and no acetylcholinesterase activity in the amniotic fluid

Berry and Lamm, 1995

PD 252180 ALPHA-FETOPROTEIN, FAMILIAL ELEVATION (McKusick No. None; see 104150)

Condition Note: Elevation of AFP both in the maternal serum and amniotic fluid has been seen in a large number of disorders (see Index under Alphafetoprotein, elevated in amniotic fluid and Alpha-fetoprotein, elevated in maternal serum.

Benign elevation of AFP in both maternal serum and amniotic fluid with no amniotic fluid acetylcholinesterase activity present, and normal chromosomal and ultrasonic evaluations of the fetus has been reported in siblings by Berry and Lamm (1995). The parents were first cousins. Both fetuses were born healthy and without congenital defects. Although the maternal AFP levels between pregnancies were not reported, the condition here as reported by Berry and Lamm (1995) does not appear to be autosomal dominant hereditary persistence of AFP because in the latter condition, amniotic fluid levels of AFP were normal (McKusick, 1994).

Alpha-fetoprotein[c]: elevation in both maternal serum and amniotic fluid in opposite sexed siblings
Berry and Lamm, 1995

PD 252250 AMNIOCHORIONIC SHEET (Amniotic sheet; Chorioamniotic sheet) (McKusick No. None)

Condition Note: An amniochorionic sheet appears to be a fetal membrane that is wrapped around an intrauterine adhesion band or synechia. The sheet usually has a characteristic appearance with a thickened free edge representing the amniochorionic sheet as it wraps around the synechia. The edge may be observed to undulate with a sheet of membranous tissue the thickness of a diamniotic dichorionic membrane trailing off from the edge. The sheet typically extends into the amniotic cavity but does not entrap the fetus, allows free fetal movement, and usually disappears by the third trimester. The synechiae are thought to result from intrauterine instrumentation. The fetus and resulting child normally have no abnormalities.
Randel et al., 1988

Prenatal Diagnosis: The ultrasound findings noted below in the presence of an intact amniotic membrane are diagnostic for this condition.

Differential Diagnosis: Amniotic band disruption sequence (PD 185000); Blighted twin (PD 253000); Circumvallate placenta; Extrachorionic hemorrhage; Nonfusion of amniotic and chorionic membranes; Septate uterus

Ultrasound: aberrant sheet of tissue that extends into the amniotic cavity and has a thickened and undulating free edge, free communication of amniotic fluid within the amniotic cavity; sheet not attached to the fetus
Randel et al., 1988

PD 252350 AMYLOID NEUROPATHY, FAMILIAL PORTUGUESE TYPE (Familial amyloidotic polyneuropathy, Portuguese type; Hereditary amyloidosis, Portuguese type) (McKusick No. 176300)

Disease Note: Familial amyloid neuropathy, Portuguese type, is an autosomal dominant disorder associated with severe neuropathy which results form amyloid deposition in tissues in general, but in particular in peripheral nerves. The onset of the disease typically occurs between 25 and 40 years of age, and leads to the death of the individual in about 10 years. The disorder is produced by a mutation in the human plasma transthyretin (thyroxine-binding prealbumin) gene. Specifically, there is a single amino acid substitution, valine to methionine at position 30 of the mature protein. The mutation in the gene occurs in the second exon, and results in a new restriction site.
Almeida et al., 1990; Morris et al., 1991

Prenatal Diagnosis: The diagnosis can be established by detecting the mutation using in the DNA from chorionic villi or amniotic fluid cells using various molecular genetic techniques.

Amniocentesis[i]: detection of the mutation causing this disease by utilizing polymerase chain reaction (PCR), and oligonucleotide probes
Almeida et al., 1990

Chorionic villus sampling (CVS)[g,i]: detection of the mutation causing this disorder by PCR, a restriction endonuclease, and restriction-fragment-length polymorphism (RFLP)

>Morris et al., 1991

PD 252500 ATAXIA TELANGIECTASIA (Louis–Bar syndrome) (McKusick No. 208900)

Condition Note: Ataxia telangiectasia is an autosomal recessive disorder of late infancy/early childhood onset. Neurologic problems include delayed walking in some, truncal ataxia, dysarthria, dystonia, athetosis, little or no facial expression, jerky eye movements, and mental retardation in some. The neurologic problems are slowly progressive. Skin findings include telangiectasias of the conjunctivae, ears, face, and neck. Other features may include short stature, increased lower respiratory infections, increased chromosomal breakage with X-ray radiation, reduced synthesis of IgA, IgG, and IgM, lymphocytopenia, and increased risk of lymphoma and leukemias. The gene for the condition has been linked to chromosome 11 at the 11q22.3 region. Death from pulmonary infection or cancer usually occurs in the second decade of life.

Prenatal Diagnosis: Either genetic linkage in informative families and/or chromosomal breakage studies in amniotic fluid cells are the currently available methods of diagnosis. The reliability of each method has not been established, however.

Differential Diagnosis: Other conditions involving the posterior fossa or foramen magnum, or a number of the degenerative or metabolic disorders should be considered including Friedreich ataxia (PD 265300); Hepatolenticular degeneration; Pelizaeus–Merzbacher disease; Hallevorden–Spatz disease; and Nijmegen breakage syndorme (PD 269350).

>Gorlin et al., 1990, pp. 469-472

Amniocentesis[i]: increased rate of spontaneous chromosome breakage in cultured amniotic fluid cells

>Shaham et al., 1982; Chessa et al., 1993

>increased chromosome breakage induced by culturing normal donor lymphocytes in cell-free amniotic fluid from a fetus at risk

>>Shaham et al., 1982

>increase chromosomal breakage induced by X-rays

>>Chessa et al., 1993

Method not stated[h]: linkage with various genetic markers

>Gatti et al., 1993

PD 252800 BECKER MUSCULAR DYSTROPHY (Muscular dystrophy, pseudohypertrophic progressive, Duchenne and Becker types) (McKusick No. 310200)

Chorionic villus sampling[g,i]: linkage between the Duchenne/Becker muscular dystrophy gene, and various DNA polymorphic markers

>Bakker et al, 1989a

PD 253000 BLIGHTED OVUM (McKusick No. None)

Condition Note: Bernard and Cooperberg (1985) have made a distinction between blighted ovum and early embryonic demise by the absence of a yolk sac in the former, and its presence in the latter. Both conditions have an absence of the embryo. Viable pregnancies where no embryo was seen have an average diameter of 1.3 cm, while both blighted ovum and early embryonic demise have a diameter on the average of 1.8 cm. However, in no sac greater than 2.0 cm, where no fetal parts were visualized, was the pregnancy viable. Other differentiating points between the three classes of pregnancies were also described by Bernard and Cooperberg (1985).

Alpha-fetoprotein[c]: undetectable levels (< 15 ng/mL) in maternal serum
>> Haddow et al., 1987

Ultrasound[g]: anembryonic gestational sac
>> Kurjak and Latin, 1979; Bernard and Cooperberg, 1985
> absence of a yolk sac
>> Bernard and Cooperberg, 1985
> poor trophoblastic reaction
>> Bernard and Cooperberg, 1985
> noncontinuous trophoblastic reaction around the gestational sac
>> Bernard and Cooperberg, 1985
> decrease growth rate of gestational sac (average rate, 0.025 cm/d; average viable pregnancy, 0.12 cm/d)
>> Bernard and Cooperberg, 1985

PD 253250 BREUS MOLE (Hematomole) (McKusick No. None)

Condition Note: A Breus mole is a massive thrombohematoma that separates the villous chorion from the membraneous chorionic plate. There generally are no associated fetal abnormalities. However, the hematoma may continue to enlarge, and be associated with IUGR, abruption of the placenta, and stillbirth. On the other hand, the hematoma may involute and cause no problems. The cause of the Breus mole is unknown.
> Evans et al., 1996

Alpha-fetoprotein[c,h]: elevated in maternal serum
> Evans et al., 1996

Cordocentesis (percutaneous umbilical blood sampling, or PUBS)[c,d]: fetal blood gases indicated fetal compromise
> Evans et al., 1996

Ultrasound: placental clots with a bilaminar appearance, subchorionic clot, enlarged placental, involution of clot, enlargement of clot with time, progressive oligohydramnios, IUGR, placental abruption, fetal demise
> Evans et al., 1996

PD 253500 CALCIFIED LIVER PLAQUES (McKusick No. None)

Ultrasound[c]: echogenic ring found in fetal abdomen, which at autopsy was found to be calcified intrahepatic subcapsular plaques
> Corson et al., 1983

PD 254000 CALCIFIED UMBILICAL CORD (McKusick No. None)

Radiograph[c,d]
> Schiff et al., 1976

PD 254250 CARBON MONOXIDE POISONING, ACUTE (McKusick No. None)

Condition Note: Carbon monoxide has a greater affinity for hemoglobin than does oxygen. Thus, sufficiently high concentrations of carbon monoxide in the blood will significantly decrease the oxygen-carrying capacity of the blood. Short- or long-term maternal exposure to carbon monoxide in high concentrations may lead to hypoxia in the fetus. The fetal hypoxia may produce organ damage, particularly in the brain, or death of the fetus.

Van Hoesen et al., 1989

Prenatal Diagnosis: The diagnosis is implied if there is fetal distress in a woman who has had significant oxygen desaturation and elevated blood levels of carboxy-hemoglobin from either short- or long-term exposure to carbon monoxide.

Differential Diagnosis: Other conditions that may produce hypoxemia in the fetus should be considered.

External electrophysiological fetal monitoring[c,d]: tachycardia, decreased beat-to-beat variability

Van Hoesen et al., 1989

PD 254325 CHARCOT–MARIE–TOOTH DISEASE, TYPE 1A (CMT1A; Hereditary motor and sensory neuropathy, type 1A) (McKusick No. 118220)

Disease Note: The various types of Charcot–Marie–Tooth (CMT) diseases constitute collectively the most common genetic neuropathies. Three inheritance patterns have been encountered including autosomal dominant and recessive, and X-linked recessive with the incidence of each being 1/2600, 1/26,000 and 1/72,000, respectively. The CMT diseases have been classified into type I, a demyelinating neuropathy with slower than normal nerve conduction velocities, and hypertrophic or onion-bulb changes in the peripheral nerves; type II is a non-demyelinating neuronal disorder with normal or near normal motor nerve conduction velocities without hypertrophic changes in the nerves. Both types are associated with pes cavus, distal muscle weakness and atrophy, absent or diminished deep tendon reflexes, and mild sensory loss.

Type 1 CMT disease maps to band 17p11.2 and is a duplication of this region which spans the peripheral myelin protein gene. This gene is considered to cause CMT type 1A disease.

Lebo et al., 1993b; McKusick, 1996

Chorionic villus sampling[g,i]: demonstration of the duplication of 17p11.2 region by multicolor fluorescence in situ hybridization (FISH) in an at-risk fetus

Lebo et al., 1993b

demonstration of the duplication of 17p11.2 region by various molecular genetic techniques in an at-risk fetus

Lebo et al., 1993b; Navon et al., 1995

DNA polymorphic markers linked CMT disease gene

Navon et al., 1995

Amniocentesis[i]: demonstration of the duplication of 17p11.2 region by multi-color FISH in at-risk fetuses

Lebo et al., 1993b

demonstration of the duplication of 17p11.2 region by various molecular genetic techniques in an at-risk fetus

Lebo et al., 1993b

PD 254400 CHEDIAK–HIGASHI SYNDROME (McKusick No. 214500)

Syndrome Note: The major features of this syndrome include partial albinism with decreased pigmentation of hair and eyes, and immunodeficiency. Other related characteristics include photophobia; nystagmus; large eosinophilic, peroxidase-positive inclusion bodies in myeloblasts and promyelocyts of the bone marrow; neutropenia; recurrent infections; and malignant lymphoma. The condition is inherited as an autosomal recessive disorder. Death often occurs before the age of 7 years.

> Durandy et al., 1993; McKusick, 1994

Prenatal Diagnosis: The diagnosis has been established by light and electron microscopic studies of neutrophils, and light microscopic studies of hair shaft. Diagnosis necessitates fetal skin biopsy and/or fetal blood drawing.

Differential Diagnosis: Albanism, oculocutaneous type (PD 194750); Griscelli syndrome (PD 265400); Hermansky–Pudlak syndrome

Cordocentesis (fetal blood drawing by fetoscopy)[i]: giant inclusions with complex structures that contained myelin figures, membranous structures, and dense material in neutrophils found by electron microscopic examination

> Durandy et al., 1993

giant and small granules that are peroxidase-positive present on electron microscopic studies of neutrophils

> Durandy et al., 1993

peroxidase-positive, large inclusions resulting from the fusion of eosinophilic granules present in electron microscopic examination of eosinophils

> Durandy et al., 1993

Fetal skin biopsy by fetoscopy[i]: direct light microscopy of the hair shaft showed clear giant and irregular melanin granules

> Durandy et al., 1993

PD 254450 COCAINE EXPOSURE (McKusick No. None)

Condition Note: No cocaine syndrome or embryopathy has been recognized. However, Hume and co-workers (1994) have found a three-fold increase in the rate of birth defects in embryos/fetuses exposed to cocaine as compared to nonexposed controls. The defects involved a wide variety of organ systems.

Ultrasound: simple and complex choroid plexus cysts

> Hume et al., 1994

omphalocele

> Hume et al., 1994

gastroschisis

> Hume et al., 1994

meconium peritonitis

> Hume et al., 1994

urethral atresia[d]

> Hume et al., 1994

anal atresia[d]

> Hume et al., 1994

PD 254500 COCKAYNE SYNDROME (McKusick No. 216400, 216410, 216411)

Amniocentesis[i]: decreased colony-forming ability of amniocytes after UV irradiation

> Sugita et al., 1982

reduced rate of RNA synthesis in amniotic fluid cells after cells were exposed to UV irradiation

> Lehmann et al., 1985

PD 254600 CONGENITAL DEFICIENCY OF ALPHA-FETOPROTEIN
(McKusick No. 104150)

Condition Note: Congenital deficiency of AFP has been reported by Faucett and colleagues (1989), and appears to be a benign disorder. In this condition, there is complete absence of AFP in the amniotic fluid and in the fetal and maternal serum during pregnancy. The two fetuses reported with this condition were born healthy (Faucett et al., 1989). The condition may be analogous to analbuminemia, also a benign condition.

Prenatal Diagnosis: The diagnosis is established whenever there are undetectable levels of AFPs in the pregnant maternal serum, amniotic fluid, and fetal or newborn serum.

Differential Diagnosis: Long-standing fetal demise for any reason will result in low levels of AFP. See listing of conditions resulting in fetal death under Fetal demise in the Index.

    Alpha-fetoprotein: undetectable levels (< 0.5 ng/mL in maternal serum)
        Faucett et al., 1989
        undetectable levels of AFP in amniotic fluid
        Faucett et al., 1989

PD 254750 CONGENITAL MYASTHENIA GRAVIS (Congenital myasthenia; Infantile myasthenia gravis; Myasthenia gravis) (McKusick No. Unknown; see 254200 and 254210)

Condition Note: Myasthenia gravis in the neonate may be produced by passive transfer of anti-AChR (acetylcholine receptor) antibodies to the fetus from a mother with myasthenia gravis or by a nonautoimmune disorder characterized by autosomal recessive inheritance and absence of myasthenia in the mother. In the former form of the disease, the child has respiratory and feeding difficulties in the neonatal and infancy periods, but typically recovers. In the latter form, the infant may also have respiratory and feeding problems, but weakness may persist into adulthood.

        McKusick, 1988

Prenatal Diagnosis: The diagnosis can be assumed to be present when there is decreased fetal movement in a fetus who has one or more affected siblings or an affected mother.

Differential Diagnosis: See Fetal movements, decreased restricted, or absent in the Index.

    Ultrasound[d]: decreased fetal movements, hydrops fetalis, small chest, hydramnios
        Chitayat et al., 1989b
    Comments: Myasthenia gravis developed in the 20-year-old mother of the above fetus when she was 7 years old. The father and she were second cousins. During this pregnancy, she took pyridostigmine bromide, 180 mg 3 times a day. Sometime after 28 weeks' gestation, she delivered a stillborn with severe arthrogryposis, generalized edema, rib abnormalities, and right-sided ureteropelvic junction obstruction which resulted in hydronephrosis. There were no cardiac defects detected (Chitayat et al., 1989b).

PD 255000 CONJOINED TWINS (Siamese twins) (McKusick No. None)

Condition Note: Conjoined literally means brought together so as to touch. Conjoined twins, then, are twins that are attached at some point, with the most common sites of attachment being thorax and abdomen. The sites of attachment are used for naming purposes (the anatomical part(s) plus "pagus"). Thus, *cephalopagus* means attachment at the heads only, *thoracopagus* at the thorax only, and *thoracoabdominopagus* refers to joining at both the thorax and the abdomen. The cause of conjoined twinning has not been determined.

There are two basic types of conjoined twins—symmetrical twins, in whom the twins are of about the same size and possess a symmetry with regard to their attachment and relative location to one another, and asymmetrical twins, in whom one twin is much smaller than the other, with no symmetry to the two twins (attachment may be anywhere, such as the smaller twin protruding from the mouth of the large twin). The latter type is also known as *parasitic* twin or *heteropagus*.

SYMMETRICAL CONJOINED TWINS

Cephalopagus (Craniopagus)

> *Comments*: Cephalopagus twins are twins in whom only part of their heads are fused together; the rest of the bodies are separate. The locations of the attachments vary from one conjoined set to another, but are normally attached at the same location on the two heads.

Computerized tomography[d]: heads joined together, encephalocele in one
> Abrams et al., 1985b

Ultrasound[d]: anencephaly in one twin, encephalocele in the other twin, heads remain in fixed relationship to each other, hydramnios, enlarged umbilical cords
> Abrams et al., 1985b

Cephalothoracopagus (Cephalothoracopagus syncephalus; Craniothoracopagus; Janiceps)

> *Comments*: These conjoined twins have fusion of the cranial and thoracic regions such that there is a face looking forward and one looking backward. It is similar to thoracopagus in that the fusion of the thoraces and abdomens is similar, but in this condition the faces are also fused.

Alpha-fetoprotein[c]: elevated in maternal serum
> Chatterjee et al., 1983

Radiograph[c]: hydramnios
> Carlson et al., 1975

Ultrasound: abnormal symmetrical cranial structure with no midline echoes, thick wedge-shaped fetal trunk
> Morgan et al., 1978; Chatterjee et al., 1983

> fusion of the skulls, thoraces, and upper abdomens, separate vertebral columns, hydramnios
> > Delprado and Baird, 1984; Fitzgerald et al., 1985

> separate vertebral columns leading to a single head, separate hearts
> > Koontz et al., 1985

> single fetus, bilobed head region, reduced crown-to-rump length, fetal demise as determined by absence of heart beat
> > Sperber and Machin, 1987

Dicephalus

> *Comments*: Dicephalus refers to twins with one body, but two separate heads and necks. There are usually two spinal cords and vertebral columns that are parallel and located next to each other.

Amniofetography[d]: two fetal heads with a single trunk but two spines
> Hubinont et al., 1984

Maternal blood sampling: low level of maternal serum human placental lactogen
> Hubinont et al., 1984

Ultrasound[d]: one fetal heart, two heads
> Hubinont et al., 1984

Diprosopus

> *Comments*: Diprosopus is partial or complete duplication of the face and head with a single neck and body. The duplication of the craniofacial structures represents a spectrum with the mildest form being isolated duplication of the nose and the more severe form complete duplication of the face. In the latter situation, there may be four eyes, with the medial two either separate or fused. If fused, the orbs may share a central orbit (Okazaki et al., 1987).

Ultrasound: increased biparietal diameter,[d] two mouths,[d] two noses,[d] four eyes,[d] single median orbit containing the two median eyes,[d] two pairs of lateral brain ventricles,[d] dilated ventricles of the brain,[d] cyst-like structure involving the posterior fossa,[d] dextrocardia,[d] fetal demise,[d] hydramnios
> Okazaki et al., 1987

anencephaly with severely malformed spine
> Moerman et al., 1983

hydramnios
> Moerman et al., 1983; Okazaki et al., 1987

Omphalopagus

> *Comments*: In omphalopagus, the twins are joined at their abdomens. There may be duplication and/or sharing of the abdominal organs.

Magnetic resonance imaging (MRI): connection of twins at their upper abdomens by a bridge of tissue, shared hepatic tissue
> Turner et al., 1986

Ultrasound: breech positioning of twins[c,d], smaller abdomen in one twin,[c,d] single placenta,[c,d] incompletely visualized divided membrane[c,d]
> Weston et al., 1990

> *Comment*: The twins reported by Weston and co-workers (1990) were monochorionic, diamniotic conjoined twins jointed by bilateral omphaloceles.

Thoracopagus

> *Comments*: In thoracopagus, the most common form of conjoined twinning, the twins are joined anteriorly at their chests, usually share a common heart, and are normally facing each other. Congenital heart defects are usually present, and separation of the twins postnatally is frequently impossible because of the shared heart.

Amniograph: common intestines
> Spirt et al., 1987

Ultrasound: twins who appeared to maintain the same positional relationship, share a common heart and liver in some cases, have two spines parallel to each other, and lie in the same amniotic sac; some have appeared to be joined at the thorax with heads that were closer together than normal
> Apuzzio et al., 1984; Maggio et al., 1985, Fitzgerald et al., 1985; Spirt et al., 1987

shared, malformed heart
Sanders et al., 1985

Thoracoabdominopagus (thoracoomphalopagus)

Comments: Here, the joining of the twins involves both the thoracic and abdominal regions. However, there is a wide spectrum of fusion with partial involvement of the thorax or abdomen to extensive fusion of both.

Radiograph[c]: hydramnios
Chan, 1976

Ultrasound: monoamniotic twin pregnancy whose fetuses maintained fixed positions to each other, had fused chest and abdominal walls, and shared a common heart and liver; separate heads, hydramnios

Schmidt and Kubli, 1982; Fitzgerald et al., 1985; Turner et al., 1986

fetal heads facing each other in close proximity, hyperextension of one head, conjoined omphaloceles
Alkalay et al., 1987a

hydrocephalus, scalp edema, pericardial effusion, ascites, intrauterine death of both twins
Turner et al., 1986

common atrium, common or single atrioventricular (AV) valve, subaortic outflow chamber, pulmonary atresia or stenosis, single ventricles, ventricular septal defect, atrial septal defect, small atrium with outlet atresia, small mitral valve, common systemic vena atrium, single six-vessel umbilical cord
Sanders et al., 1985

Comments: Thoracoabdominopagus twins have also been reported with separate hearts; one twin had a normal single heart while the other had situs inversus, a right aortic arch, single left ventricle and atrioventricular valve, and pulmonary atresia.

ASYMMETRICAL CONJOINED TWINS (Heteropagus, Parasitic twin)

Cephalic attachment

Ultrasound: Ovoid bony outlined mass attached to the head of the otherwise normal appearing cotwin, cerebral tissue present in mass, 10-mm opening between mass and fetal head at the left parietal bone
Lituania et al., 1988

Comments: After termination of the twins reported by Lituania and associates (1988), an isolated head attached to the left parietal area of the normal twin was found. The parietal bone of the normal twin was interrupted by an ovoid foramen that measured 10×8 mm. No connection of the brains existed. The brain of the parasitic head was hypoplastic and abnormally folded, with dilated ventricles and a thin cortex. In addition to brain in the parasitic head that was covered by skin, there were fairly well formed or partly formed eyes, eyelids, scapula, humerus, and clavicle, and a dentinogenic cyst. The autopsy findings in the other twin were not mentioned.

Fetus in fetu

Comments: This form of conjoined twinning is usually a benign condition in which a partly formed, small twin is located inside the host twin. The usual location for the fetus in fetu is a retroperitoneal site and either prenatally or postnatally may present as an intraabdominal mass (Farrell and Geddie, 1989).

Ultrasound[c]: abdominal wall defect, oligohydramnios
>Farrell and Geddie, 1989

Comments: In the situation reported by Farrell and Geddie (1989), the pregnancy of the abnormal fetus was terminated. At autopsy, a mass that protruded from the host's genitalia was found to contain a fetus in fetu. The latter fetus was covered by skin and the whole mass was enclosed by amnion. Within the mass was an axial skeleton with bone, cartilage, testes, and well-developed lungs and trachea. The rest of the fetus was disorganized tissue. The host twin had the following defects: facial compression from the oligohydramnios, thoracolumbar kyphoscoliosis, omphalocele, absence of external genitalia, imperforate anus, small and hypoplastic kidneys, and hypoplastic ureters.

PD 255500 CORONAL CLEFT VERTEBRA (McKusick No. None)

Radiograph[d]: anterior cleft of one or more thoracic or lumbar vertebrae
>Rowley, 1955

PD 256000 CYSTIC FIBROSIS (Mucoviscidosis) (McKusick No. 219700)

Prenatal Diagnosis: Considerable effort has been put forth to develop a prenatal diagnostic test for cystic fibrosis. With the localization of the cystic fibrosis gene to chromosome 7 at q22/31, and its close linkage to a number of RFLPs (Super et al.,1987) and to specific point mutations within the gene, especially delta F508, it is now possible to diagnose this condition with a high degree of certainty by direct gene testing or by linkage in an informative family. An informative family is one in which the DNA polymorphisms linked to the gene for cystic fibrosis are in the right phase to tell when the fetus is homozygous recessive for the gene. Using the KM-19 polymorphic locus, PstI restriction endonuclease and PCR, Feldman and associates (1988a, 1988b) found that, in 84 couples at a 1 in 4 risk for having offspring with cystic fibrosis, 48% were fully informative, 41% were informative for one parent, and 11% were uninformative. Curtis and associates (1989b) claim that given a living affected sibling and the battery of closely linked RFLPs available, that virtually all families are informative, and prenatal diagnosis is possible. By using PCR, DNA may be obtained on deceased affected individuals by utilizing the Guthrie blood spot (Curtis et al., 1989b).

The DNA approach appears to be the method of choice at present for the prenatal diagnosis of cystic fibrosis. If the specific mutations are known, then direct detections of these mutations can be done showing "homozygosity" for mutations of the cystic fibrosis gene even though the two mutations may be at different sites within the gene. If this is not possible, linkage of the cystic fibrosis gene to various DNA polymorphisms in informative families would be the next approach. If the family has only one informative parent, DNA linkage analysis may not be helpful. Where direct DNA analysis is not possible, where there is an uninformative family, and where no affected individual is available for study, assessing the activity of intestinal alkaline phosphatase in amniotic fluid may be the only alternative.

Amniocentesis: detection of delta F508 mutation by molecular techniques
>Baranov et al., 1992; Van Allen, et al., 1992; Dowman et al., 1993; Ferec et al., 1993

detection of other mutations in the cystic fibrosis gene
>Baranov et al., 1992; Dowman et al., 1993; Ferec et al., 1993; Chitayat et al., 1995b

linkage between the cystic fibrosis gene and various RFLPs in cultured or uncultured amniotic fluid cells [i]

> Spence et al., 1986; Curtis et al., 1988; Fontaine et al., 1988; Feldman et al., 1989; Lissens et al., 1989; Van Allen et al., 1989; Baranov et al., 1992

reduced methylumbelliferylguanidinobenzoate reactive proteases activity in amniotic fluid

> Nadler and Walsh, 1980; Nadler et al., 1981a
>
> *Comments:* False-negative results utilizing this method have been reported (Nadler et al., 1981b; Schwarts and Brandt, 1981; Green et al., 1982; Seale and Rennert, 1982; Brock and Hayward, 1983; Carbarns et al., 1983).

deficiency of phenylalanine-inhibitable alkaline phosphatase activity in amniotic fluid prior to 22 weeks' gestation

> Brock, 1983; Brock, 1984a; Brock, 1984b; Brock et al., 1984c; Morin et al., 1984a; Muller et al., 1984a; Muller et al., 1984b; Aitken et al., 1985; Brock, 1985; Mulivor et al., 1985; Muller et al., 1985a; Muller et al., 1985b; Carey and Pollard, 1986; Claass et al., 1986; Morin et al., 1987; Bozon et al., 1989

deficiency of homoarginine-inhibitable alkaline phosphatase activity in amniotic fluid prior to 22 weeks' gestation

> Brock, 1983; Muller et al., 1984a; Muller et al., 1984b; Aitken et al., 1985; Brock, 1985; Mulivor et al., 1985; Muller et al., 1985a; Muller et al., 1985b; Claass et al., 1986; Morin et al., 1987; Bozon et al., 1989

less than 50% residual alkaline phosphatase activity in cell-free amniotic fluid expressed as a percentage of the total activity to residual activity after l-homoarginine inhibition

> Carey and Pollard, 1986

reduced level of intestinal isozyme of alkaline phosphatase activity in amniotic fluid as determined by monoclonal antibodies

> Brock et al., 1984c; Brock et al., 1985b; Mulivor et al., 1985

greater than 50% residual alkaline phosphatase activity in cell-free amniotic fluid expressed as a percentage of the total activity to residual activity after l-phenylalanine inhibition

> Carey and Pollard, 1986

reduced levels of intestinal alkaline phosphatase activity in amniotic fluid

> Connor et al., 1988; Van Allen et al., 1989

missing amniotic fluid protease and alcohol dehydrogenase bands on polyacrylamide gels after isoelectric focusing

> Brock, 1983

altered amniotic fluid protease pattern after gel filtration [c]

> Brock, 1983

reduced activities of gamma-glutamyltranspeptidase and/or aminopeptidase M in amniotic fluid [c]

> Baker and Dann, 1983; Brock et al., 1983b; Carbarns et al., 1983; Gosden et al., 1983; Brock et al., 1984a; Brock et al., 1984b; Aitken et al., 1985; Brock, 1985; Muller et al., 1985a; Muller et al., 1985b; Bozon et al., 1989

reduced gamma-glutamyltranspeptidase activity in amniotic fluid[c]

Carey and Pollard, 1986; Morin et al., 1987; Connor et al., 1988; Van Allen et al., 1989

reduced activities of 5-nucleotide phosphodiesterase in amniotic fluid[c]

Brock et al., 1983b

reduced levels of activity of the intestinal disaccharidases sucrase, lactase, maltase, and/or trehalase[c]

Brock et al., 1983b; Morin et al., 1983; Van Diggelen et al., 1983; Brock et al., 1984; Szabo et al., 1984; Kleijer et al., 1985b; Papp et al., 1986; Schwartz and Brandt, 1985; Szabo et al., 1985b

reduced activity of aminopeptidase M in amniotic fluid prior to 22 weeks' gestation[c]

Brock et al., 1984c

reduced level of leucine aminopeptidase activity in amniotic fluid[c]

Van Allen et al., 1989

reduced levels of maltase activity in amniotic fluid[c]

Claass et al., 1986; Connor et al., 1988

unusually viscous and greenish-colored amniotic fluid[c]

Papp et al., 1986

reduced levels of microvillus bound gamma-glutamyltranspeptidase, maltase, and intestinal alkaline phosphatase activity

Connor et al., 1988

Chorionic villus sampling[g,i]: direct detection of the various mutations within the cystic fibrosis gene by molecular genetic techniques

Novelli et al., 1990; Baranov et al., 1992

linkage between the cystic fibrosis gene and various RFLPs utilizing different DNA probes in cultured or uncultured chorionic villi

Farrall et al., 1986; Spence et al., 1986; Super et al., 1987; Schwartz et al., 1988; Feldman et al., 1989; Gasparini et al., 1989; Lissens et al., 1989; Baranov et al., 1992

Preconception genetic analysis[i]: analysis of the first polar body for the presence or absense of the delta F508 mutation in an ovum at risk for possessing the gene

Strom et al., 1990

Preimplantation embryo biopsy[i]: DNA blastomeric analysis for homozygosity of the delta F508 mutation

Strom et al., 1990; Liu et al., 1994

heterozygous embryo detected by PCR and detection of the delta F508 deletion

Handyside, 1993; Liu et al., 1994

Ultrasound: dilated loops of fetal bowel distal to stomach caused by meconium ileus with perforation of the distal ileum[d]

Jassani et al., 1982

dilated and thickened loops of intestines[d]

Chemke et al., 1987

enlarged loops of bowel later shown to represent meconium ileus[i]

Caspi et al., 1988

intestinal calcification or mass

Dowman et al., 1993

meconium ileus presenting as a highly echogenic intraabdominal mass[d]

Muller et al., 1984a; Gilbert et al., 1985; Muller et al., 1985c; Papp et al., 1985
meconium peritonitis[c]
Chitayat et al., 1995b
increased echogenicity of fetal bowel[c]
Dowman et al., 1993; Pallante et al., 1995; Strasberg et al., 1995
highly echogenic meconium[c]
Van Allen et al., 1992
ascites[c,d]
Papp et al., 1985
hydramnios[c,d]
Papp et al., 1985

PD 257000 DUCHENNE MUSCULAR DYSTROPHY (McKusick No. 310200)

Condition Note: Duchenne muscular dystrophy (DMD) is a progressive muscle disease that leads to progressive muscular weakness and death in affected males with death occurring usually by the age of 20. The gene which, when mutated, causes DMD is located on the short arm of the X chromosome in band Xp21 and codes for a protein called dystrophin. The DMD gene is one of the largest known human genes (> 2000 kb). A total or near total deficiency of dystrophin is associated with DMD, whereas a 1–2% level or an abnormal form of the protein is associated with Becker muscular dystrophy. Sixty percent of the mutations in the DMD gene that produce DMD are deletions.

Ward et al., 1989; McKusick, 1996

Amniocentesis: detection of deletion in the DMD gene by molecular genetic techniques

Sugino et al., 1989

linkage of various polymorphic DNA markers and the DMD gene

Katayama et al., 1988; Sugino et al., 1989; Ward et al., 1989; Soong et al., 1991

elevated levels of myoglobin in amniotic fluid[c]

Torok et al., 1982

Chorionic villus sampling[g,i]: linkage between the DMD gene and various RFLPs utilizing different DNA probes

Bakker et al., 1985; Hejtmancik et al., 1986a; Darras et al., 1987; Ward et al., 1987; Cole et al., 1988; Burt et al., 1989; Katayama et al., 1988; Bakker et al., 1989a; Bakker et al., 1989b; Sugino et al., 1989; Ward et al., 1989

Comments: Caution must be exercised with doing linkage analysis testing for DMD because not all families are informative, and crossing over, even within the gene, can lead to false negative results (Darras et al., 1987; Fischbeck and Ritter, 1987).

In the fetus reported on by Burt and colleagues (1989), Western blot studies using dystrophin antibodies on fetal muscle obtained after termination of the pregnancy showed no detectable dystrophin.

detection of the DMD gene by PCR–RFLP analysis, multiplex PCR, and dinucleotide repeat polymorphic analysis

Katayama et al., 1994

Comment: By the techniques of Katayama and associates (1994), both affected male and carrier female fetuses were diagnosed.

detection of the deletion in the DMD gene
Sugino et al., 1989

Cordocentesis (PUBS)[c]: elevated creatine kinase activity in fetal blood
Mahoney et al., 1977; Golbus et al., 1979

Comments: This method is unreliable for the diagnosis of this disorder because false-negative and occasionally false-positive results have been reported (Ionasescu et al., 1978; Emery et al., 1979; Golbus et al., 1979; Edwards et al., 1984).

Maternal blood sampling: elevated levels of myoglobin in maternal serum[c]
Torok et al., 1982

Muscle biopsy[i]: no dystrophin present in the fetal muscle
Evans et al., 1993; Evans et al., 1995b

PD 257500 ECTOPIC PREGNANCY, ABDOMINAL LOCATION
(Abdominal pregnancy) (McKusick No. None)

Condition Note: This condition occurs when the implantation site is outside of the uterine cavity and the fallopian tube, but located intraabdominally. The placenta may be attached to any abdominal structure, and as such, is at a much greater risk of premature placental separation prior to term. Such detachment may lead to massive maternal hemorrhage with the death of both the mother and fetus.
Cohen et al., 1985

Prenatal Diagnosis: Ultrasound and MRI appear to be the most reliable modes for diagnosis of this condition, but even extensive ultrasound and MRI evaluations may fail to diagnosis the condition. The diagnosis should be considered whenever there is an abnormal relationship among the fetus, placenta, amniotic fluid, and uterus.
Spanta et al., 1987

Differential Diagnosis: Ectopic pregnancy, fallopian tube location (PD 258000)
Alpha-fetoprotein[c]: elevated levels in maternal serum
Hage et al., 1988; Bombard et al., 1993

Magnetic resonance imaging: fetus in transverse lie in the abdominal cavity[d]
Cohen et al., 1985
placenta attached to the uterus in the lower abdomen[d]
Cohen et al., 1985
enlarged uterus with a central linear area of increased signal intensity and separated from the placenta by a thin line of low signal intensity[d]
Cohen et al., 1985
abnormal relationship between the fetus, placenta, and uterus
Spanta et al., 1987; Hage et al., 1988
oligohydramnios[c]
Cohen et al., 1985

Maternal blood sampling[c]: elevated levels of maternal serum human chorionic gonadotropin (MShCG)
Bombard et al., 1993
lowered levels of matrnal serum unconjugated estriol (MSuE$_3$)
Bombard et al., 1993

Ultrasound[d]: fetus in transverse lie[c]
Cohen et al., 1985
placenta previa[c]

Cohen et al., 1985

large cervical mass, the corpus uteri, located in the cul-de-sac, and in continuity with the uterine cervix[c]

Cohen et al., 1985

a mass in the lower abdomen (the uterus) that was separate from the gestational sac

Spanta et al., 1987

arrest in fetal growth[d]

Spanta et al., 1987

oligohydramnios[c]

Tromans et al., 1984; Cohen et al., 1985

Failed prostaglandin and oxytocin induction of labor and delivery

Tromans et al., 1984

Comments: The ectopic pregnancy in the case reported by Tromans and co-workers (1984) was not detected by two abdominal ultrasound scans. The ectopic pregnancy was only discovered after failed induction. For further details of the case, see Hamartoma–vertical mouth–hypoplastic kidney (PD 330000).

PD 258000 ECTOPIC PREGNANCY, FALLOPIAN TUBE LOCATION
(Extrauterine pregnancy; tubal pregnancy) (McKusick No. None)

Ultrasound[g]: absence of normal intrauterine pregnancy or pregnancy found in fallopian tube

Cadkin and Sabbagha, 1977; Smith et al., 1981a

PD 258100 ECTOPIC PREGNANCY, INTERSTITIAL TYPE (McKusick No. None)

Condition Note: An interstitial pregnancy is an ectopic pregnancy with the gestation in that portion of the fallopian tube that lies within the wall of the uterus.

Ultrasound, transvaginal[g]: pregnancy located in an interstitial position, myometrial bridge separating interstitial gestational sac and cotwin intrauterine gestational sac

Leach et al., 1992

PD 258250 EARLY EMBRYONIC DEMISE (McKusick No. None)

Condition Note: Bernard and Cooperberg (1985) have made a distinction between blighted ovum and early embryonic demise by the absence of a yolk sac in the former, and its presence in the latter. Both conditions have an absence of an embryo. Viable pregnancies, where no embryo was seen, have an average diameter of 1.3 cm, whereas both blighted ovum and early embryonic demise have a diameter on the average of 1.8 cm. However, in no sac greater than 2.0 cm where no fetal parts were visualized was the pregnancy viable. Other differentiating points between the three classes of pregnancies were described by Bernard and Cooperberg (1985).

Ultrasound[g]: anembryonic gestational sac

Bernard and Cooperberg, 1985

presence of a yolk sac in the absence of other embryonic parts

Bernard and Cooperberg, 1985

noncontinuous trophoblastic reaction around the gestational sac

Bernard and Cooperberg, 1985

PD 258420 FAMILIAL DYSAUTONOMIA (Hereditary sensory and autonomic neuropathy III; Riley–Day syndrome) (McKusick No. 223900)

Disease Note: Familial dysautonomia is an autosomal recessive sensory neuropathy that primarily affects individuals of Ashkenazi Jewish descent. The disorder is characterized by abnormal sensory and autonomic functions manifested by episodes of protracted vomiting, decreased discrimination to pain and temperature, and cardiovascular instability. Specific problems may include lack of tearing, cold hands and feet, paroxysmal hypertension, and emotional liability. The diagnosis clinically is based on the absence of fungiform papillae on the tongue, decreased or absent deep tendon reflexes, and the absence of both overflow tears and the flare response to intradermal histamine administration. The gene for the disease has been localized to chromosome 9 at region q31-q33.

> Eng et al., 1995; McKusick, 1995

Prenatal Diagnosis: Linkage analysis at the present time is the only means of prenatal diagnosis.

> Amniocentesis[i]: linkage analysis between the gene and polymorphic markers located in the region 9q31-q33 utilizing amniotic fluid cells
> > Eng et al., 1995
> > *Comment:* By the linkage-analysis method affected, carrier, and non-affected fetuses have been detected (Eng et al., 1995).
> Chorionic villus sampling[i]: linkage analysis between the gene and polymorphic markers located in the region 9q31-q33 utilizing both cultured and uncultured chorionic villi
> > Eng et al., 1995

PD 258500 FETAL ALCOHOL SYNDROME (FAS) (McKusick No. None)

> Alpha-fetoprotein[c]: reduced level in maternal serum
> > Lazzarini et al., 1987
> > elevated level in maternal serum
> > Herrmann and Sidiropoulos, 1988
> Ultrasound[c]: hydrocephalus
> > Lazzarini et al., 1987; Herrmann and Sidiropoulos, 1988
> > small cephalometric measurements
> > Viscarello et al., 1991
> > intrauterine growth retardation
> > Lazzarini et al., 1987; Herrmann and Sidiropoulos, 1988

PD 259000 FETAL ASCITES (McKusick No. None)

> Radiograph[d]
> > Barr and MacVicar, 1956
> Ultrasound[d]: fluid-filled abdomen, hydramnios[c]
> > Cederqvist et al., 1977a; Hobbins et al., 1979; Weinraub et al., 1979

PD 259500 FETAL BRAIN DEATH (Intrauterine fetal brain death) (McKusick No. None)

Condition Note: Fetal brain death is the situation where there is death of the brain in utero, but because the heart keeps functioning at least for a while, the fetus remains alive. Because the brain is dead, there are no fetal movements and no variation in heart rate. Due to a lack of swallowing, hydramnios may develop. The cause for the death of the brain may remain undetermined even after delivery.

Zimmer et al., 1992

Ultrasound: absence of fetal movements,[d] fetal heart rate fixed with no beat-to-beat variability, accelerations or response to contraction stress test[d]; no fetal breathing [d]; no fetal response to vibroacoustic stimulation[d]; dilation of the lateral and third ventricles[d]; fetal demise[d]; hydramnios

Zimmer et al., 1992

PD 260000 FETAL DEMISE (Intrauterine fetal death; Fetal death) (McKusick No. None)

Acetylcholinesterase[c]: fast migrating amniotic-fluid isozyme, increased activity in amniotic fluid

Buamah et al., 1980; Dale, 1980; Dale et al., 1981; Hullin et al., 1981; Voigtlander et al., 1981; Crandall et al., 1982; Aitken et al., 1984b; Crandall and Matsumoto, 1984b; Sindic et al., 1984; Wyvill et al., 1984; Raymond and Simpson, 1988; Crandall et al., 1989

fast-migrating isozyme in the amniotic fluid of the surviving twin following the death of the cotwin

Bass et al., 1986; Streit et al., 1989

Comment: One of the twins reported on by Streit and associates (1989) had craniorachischisis.

Alpha-fetoprotein[c]: elevated in maternal serum and amniotic fluid

Seppala and Ruoslahti, 1973; Seppala, 1975; Fisher et al., 1981; Gardner et al., 1981; Haddow et al., 1983; Ryynanen et al., 1983; Aitken et al., 1984b; Crandall and Matsumoto, 1984b; Schnittger and Kjessler, 1984; Sindic et al., 1984; Wyvill et al., 1984; Dyer et al., 1986; Ghosh et al., 1986; Rodriguez et al., 1987b

elevated in maternal serum

Milunsky et al., 1988; Robinson et al., 1988; Streit et al., 1989; Milunsky and Nibiolo, 1995

Comments: Elevation of maternal serum AFP (MSAFP) was found at a higher frequency in mothers who subsequently had an intrauterine fetal death. The elevation of the MSAFP was not on the basis of birth defects or chromosomal abnormalities of the fetuses or to multiple pregnancies. The risk factors include 3.1 times greater likelihood for MSAFP values of 2.0 multiples of the median (MOM) or greater, and 3.6 times greater for 2.5 MOM or greater (Waller et al., 1989).

elevated in amniotic fluid

Crandall et al., 1989; Streit et al., 1989

elevated in maternal serum and amniotic fluid of the surviving twin following the death of the cotwin

Bass et al., 1986

decreased in maternal serum

Gardner et al., 1981; Burton et al., 1983; Davenport and Macri, 1983; Haddow et al., 1987; Milunsky et al., 1988

very low levels (5–9 ng/mL) or undetectable levels (< 5 ng/mL) in maternal serum

Haddow et al., 1987

rapidly declining maternal serum levels
> Taubert et al., 1986

Amniocentesis: elevated amniotic fluid alkaline phosphatase activity[c]
> Jalanko et al., 1983

> increased creatine kinase activity in amniotic fluid[c]
>> Stempel and Lott, 1980

> decreased levels of amniotic fluid trypsin inhibitor[c]
>> Kolho, 1986

> decreased levels of insulin in amniotic fluid[c]
>> Weiss et al., 1984

> presence of S-100 protein in amniotic fluid[c]
>> Sindic et al., 1984

> amniotic fluid contained meconium or was green in color[c]
>> Allen, 1985; Streit et al., 1989

> elevated levels of bilirubin in amniotic fluid[c]
>> Blanc, 1968

> fetal distress cells present in amniotic fluid cell cultures[c]
>> Gosden and Brock, 1978b

Cholinesterase[c]: elevated level of activity in amniotic fluid
> Hullin et al., 1981

Computerized axial tomography (CT scan): air within and distributed throughout the fetus
> Lee and McGahan, 1984

Fetal pyelography[c,d]: lack of excretion of contrast material by fetal kidneys
> Thomas et al., 1963

> *Comment:* The above test was helpful only when contrast material was visualized because of a high false-negative rate.

Maternal blood sampling[c,g]: elevated serum level of human chorionic gonadotropin (hCG)
> Lewis et al., 1995; Milunsky and Nebiolo, 1995

> low or undetectable levels of serum unconjugated estriol (uE_3)
>> Schliefer et al., 1993; Milunsky and Nebiolo, 1995

Maternal history[c]: decreased or absence of fetal movement
> Szymonowicz et al., 1986; Valentin et al., 1986; Streit et al., 1989

Radiograph: intrafetal gas, overlapping or misalignment of cranial bones at the sutures, Deuel's halo sign
> Noonan, 1974

Ultrasound: failure of gestational sac to increase in size, no change in crown-to-rump length or biparietal diameter, absence of fetal heart activity and fetal movement, fetal edema, fetal abdominal gas, hydramnios[c]
> Gottesfeld, 1978; Hassani et al., 1978; Donn et al., 1984; Lee and McGahan, 1984; Abrams et al., 1985a; Bass et al., 1986; Hughes and Miskin, 1986

> absence of fetal heart beat[g]
>> Taubert et al., 1986; Harris et al., 1988

> Spalding's sign
>> Taubert et al., 1986

> *Comment:* Spalding's sign is a halo surrounding the fetus who has died in utero.

> reduced biparietal diameter

Taubert et al., 1986
fetal skull collapse[c]
Shenker et al., 1981
overlapping skull bones[c]
Hughes and Miskin, 1986
reduced crown-to-rump length[c,g]
Harris et al., 1988
generally deformed trunk
Taubert et al., 1986
increased echogenicity of the fetal bowel[c]
Pallante et al., 1985
umbilical vein thrombosis
Abrams et al., 1985a
calcified yolk sac appearing as highly echogenic, floating structure with posterior acoustic shadowing ("comet-tail artifact")[g]
Harris et al., 1988
average daily growth of gestational sac reduced to 0.25 cm/d (normal = 0.12 cm/d)
Bernard and Cooperberg, 1985
oligohydramnios[c]
Dyer et al., 1986; Clement et al., 1987; Striet et al., 1989
hydropic degeneration of the placenta[g]
Harris et al., 1988

PD 261000 FETAL DISTRESS (McKusick No. None)

Alpha-fetoprotein[c]: elevated in maternal serum
Seppala and Ruoslahti, 1973
Ultrasound[d]: tachypnea
Romero et al., 1982b

PD 261500 FETAL HYDANTOIN SYNDROME (Fetal Dilantin syndrome) (McKusick No. 132810)

Syndrome Note: The fetal hydantoin syndrome is the result of in utero exposure to phenytoins, and is characterized by microcephaly, mid-facial hypoplasia, hypoplasia of the distal phalanges, pre- and postnatal growth deficiencies, and mental retardation in some cases. Buehler and co-workers (1990) have presented evidence that fetuses with low activities of epoxide hydrolase are at increased risk for developing the syndrome if they are exposed prenatally to phenytoins (hydantoin).

Amniocentesis[h]: reduced levels of epoxide hydrolase activities in cultured amniotic fluid cells
Buehler et al., 1990
Ultrasound[c,d]: pleural effusion
Nimrod et al., 1986

PD 263500 FETAL HYPOXIA (Hypoxemia; Maternal hypoxia) (McKusick No. None)

Cordocentesis (PUBS)[c]: elevated levels of plasma glutathione S-transferase B_1
Holt et al., 1995

Ultrasound[c,d]: porencephalic cyst, microcephaly, and IUGR in a fetus exposed to severe in utero hypoxia

Goodlin et al., 1984

PD 264100 FETAL MEMBRANES, PREMATURE RUPTURE (Chronic amniotic fluid leakage; Fetal membranes ruptured; Preterm prelabor amniorrhexis) (McKusick No. None)

Instillation of artificial amniotic fluid containing indigo carmine into amniotic cavity; rapid appearance of blue fluid in the vagina

Gembruch and Hansmann, 1988

Ultrasound[c]: oligohydramnios

Gembruch and Hansmann, 1988; Dorfman et al., 1995; Carroll et al., 1996

Comment: In the case reported by Dorfman and co-authors (1995), there was virtually no pocket of amniotic fluid present.

oligohydramnios secondary to chronic amniotic leakage with fetal compression, flattened and distorted left skull and brain, and brain trauma leading to central nervous system (CNS) hemorrhage and right-sided paralysis, infrequent fetal movement

Schmidt and Kubli, 1982; Elejalde et al., 1983

vaginal examination of the mother: nitrazine-positive fluid present

Carroll et al., 1996

amniotic fluid present

Dorfman et al., 1995

PD 265000 FETAL/EMBRYONIC SEX (Embryo sex; Fetal sex; Sex determination) (McKusick No. None)

Amniocentesis: chromosomal analysis of amniotic fluid cells

Schmid, 1977

elevated amniotic fluid testosterone level in male fetuses, lower in female fetuses, significance found only between 15 and 20 weeks of gestation in one study (Carson et al., 1982)

Doran et al., 1980; Wong et al., 1980; Carson et al., 1982; Rodeck et al., 1985

higher fetal plasma testosterone levels in male than female fetuses. Mean values ± standard deviation (SD) were 5.0 ± 5.33 and 1.02 ± 0.03 nmol/L, respectively, ranging from 1.23–28.5 nmol/L in males and 0.51–1.65 nmol/L in females between 15 and 23 weeks of gestation

Rodeck et al., 1985

elevated amniotic fluid follicle-stimulating hormone (FSH) in female fetus

Dodinval and Duvivier, 1980

decreased FSH levels in amniotic fluid of male fetus

Doran et al., 1980; Dalpra et al., 1985

elevated amniotic fluid androstenedione in male fetuses

Carson et al., 1982

testosterone-to-FSH ratio in amniotic fluid greater than 20 in male and less than 20 in female fetuses between 16 and 19 weeks of gestation

Abeliovich et al., 1984

Y-heterochromatin chromosomal probe used to identify male DNA utilizing dot hybridization

Lau et al., 1984

identification of Y-chromosomal DNA by DNA digestion with *Hae*III or *Mbo*I restriction endonucleases, hybridization with probe pS4, and separated and identified on an agarose gel

Hoar et al., 1984

identification of Y chromosome by biotinylated chromosome-specific DNA probe using uncultured amniotic fluid cells

Guyot et al., 1988

Chorionic villus sampling[g]: karyotype of cells derived from cultured chorionic villi or direct preparation of chorionic villi

Gosden et al., 1982; Gustavii, 1983; Lilford et al., 1983; Brambati et al., 1984; Therkelsen et al., 1988

X and Y chromatin assay in biopsy specimen

Kazy et al., 1982

restriction endonuclease digest of DNA isolated from chorionic villi and hybridized with satellite-III derived Y-specific cDNA

Kazy et al., 1982; Simoni et al., 1983; Williams et al., 1983

identification of male DNA by hybridization with Y-chromosome-specific probes, pHY2.1 and 1 WES5, utilizing dot hybridization or Southern blot

Gosden et al., 1984a; Gosden et al., 1984b

female sex determination by four different X-linked RFLPs

Wood et al., 1987

identification of Y repeat sequence and a ubiquitous Alu repeat sequence after PCR

Ivinson et al., 1988

identification of X and Y chromosome by using appropriate X and Y FISH probes

Bischoff et al., 1995b

Maternal blood sampling and isolation of fetal cells by various methods: isolation of nucleated fetal erythrocytes; detection of the Y chromosome by utilization of a 20-bp Y probe

Bianchi et al., 1989

hybridization of fetal cells with a biotinylated Y-specific probe and detecting Y-chromosome fluorescence with fluorescein-labeled avidin[h]

Gray et al., 1988

hybridization of fetal cells by an AAF labeled X-specific probe and a biotinylated Y-specific probe with the AAF labeled probe detected with mouse anti-AAF plus fluorescein-labeled goat antimouse and the biotinylated probe with Texas-red labeled avidin

Gray et al., 1988

Preimplanation embryo biopsy[i]: identification of the Y chromosome by in situ hybridization using a biotinylated Y-specific probe that is detected by a standard streptavidin-linked alkaline phosphatase system

Penketh et al., 1989

polymerase chain reaction to amplify Y-specific sequence from male embryos

Handyside, 1993; Oudejans et al., 1995; Ravia et al., 1995

fluorescent in situ hybridization utilizing X- and Y-specific probes
>> Handyside, 1993; Daryani et al., 1995

Ultrasound[g]: demonstration of fetal labia majora and minora, and occasionally the clitoris; or phallus, scrotum, hydrocele when present, and testes in the scrotum; on occasion voiding may be seen from an erect penis
>> LeLann et al., 1979; Schotten and Giese, 1980; Birnholz, 1983; Plattner et al., 1983; Stephens and Sherman, 1983; Natsuyama, 1984; Dalpra et al., 1985; Elejalde et al., 1985b

Uterine cavity lavage: determination of the presence of X and Y chromosomes by routine cytogenetic techniques and by FISH using specific X and Y probes, and done on cells aspirated by intrauterine lavage
>> Diukman et al., 1993

PD 265250 FETUS PAPYRACEOUS (McKusick No. None)

Acetylcholinesterase[c]: faint isozyme band on gel electrophoresis
>> Winsor et al., 1987

Alpha-fetoprotein[c]: elevated in amniotic fluid
>> Lange et al., 1979; Read et al., 1982a; Winsor et al., 1987

Comments: In the case reported by Winsor and associates (1987), there were no abnormalities in the surviving cotwin either by prenatal ultrasound examination or by physical examination following termination of the pregnancy. The elevation of the AFP and the presence of the acetylcholinesterase isozyme presumably were caused by the dead fetus.

>> rapid decline of maternal serum levels after two of the triplets died at 21 weeks' gestation, reaching normal levels by 31 weeks'
>>> Taubert et al., 1986

>>> *Comments*: The process of resorption that leads to fetus papyraceus is well documented by the death of two of the triplets reported by Taubert and associates (1986). Fetal death occurred at 21 weeks' gestation as determined by ultrasound. Resorption of both fetuses could be seen by ultrasound beginning at 26 weeks of gestation. Maternal serum AFP declined until 31 weeks, when it reached normal levels and stayed there. The dead fetuses were no longer clearly visualized by ultrasound after 31 weeks of gestation. A normal child was born to the parents at 33 weeks.

>> elevated in maternal serum
>>> Brock, 1982; Winsor et al., 1987

Ultrasound[d]: soft tissue mass visualized in the uterine fundus
>> Kurjak and Latin, 1979

Comments: At 20 weeks' gestation, apparently normal twins were detected by ultrasound. Reevaluation at 36 weeks indicated only one fetus. At 38 weeks a healthy male infant and a fetus papyraceous were delivered.

PD 265270 FRAGILE-X SYNDROME (Fragile X-chromosome syndrome; FMR1; Macrotestis, X-linked mental retardation syndrome; Martin–Bell syndrome) (McKusick No. 309550)

Syndrome Note: In developed countries, the fragile-X syndrome is probably the third leading cause of mental retardation in males, exceeded only by the fetal alcohol syndrome and Down syndrome. Estimates of its frequency in males range from 0.19–1.0 per 1000 (Webb et al., 1986). It is inherited as an X-linked recessive disorder, but there may be no expression of the condition in some males who possess the gene (79% penetrance). Carrier females are usually physically normal but may be mentally impaired. The major features of the disorder in expressing males include mental retardation, macrocephaly, large ears and chin, long and narrow face, and macroorchidism.

There is a fragile site on the X chromosome (Xq27-28) that is usually expressed in affected males, most mentally impaired carrier females, and some normal carrier females. The "fragile X chromosome" has led to the name, fragile-X syndrome.

The fragile-X syndrome is produced by expansion of a trinucleotide repeat unit CGG. This unit is located just in front of the fragile-X gene (FMR1). In normal individuals, the number of repeat units varies up to 50 (50XCGG). Individuals who have between 51 and 200 CGG repeats are normal and denoted as premutation carriers. Females who carry the premutation may produce offspring (both males and females) who possess CGG repeats of greater than 200 units, or a full mutation. Males possessing the full mutation have the full syndrome, and normally are retarded; females with the full mutation may have intellectual impairment, or may be perfectly normal. The FMR1 gene is apparently inactivated when the expansion of CGG unit is greater than 200 units.

Prenatal Diagnosis: The most reliable prenatal diagnostic method is a DNA test of fetal tissue or chorionic villi checking for expansion of the CGG trinucleotide repeat segment that is associated with the fragile X gene. This method not only detects pre- and full mutations in the male fetus, and thus predicts if he will be a carrier and a non-expressing male, or will be affected, respectively, but also determines if the female carrier has the pre- or full mutation with the later situation associated with partial expression in some of the resulting female individuals.

Maddelena et al., 1993; Shapiro et al., 1995

Differential Diagnosis: Renpenning syndrome and other X-linked mental retardation disorders

Amniocentesis[i]: direct DNA testing for expansion of the CGG trinucleotide repeat segment of the gene in amniotic fluid cells, detection of the pre- and full mutation in male fetuses

Brown et al., 1993; Maddelena et al., 1993

direct DNA testing for expansion of the CGG trinucleotide repeat segment of the gene in amniotic fluid cells, female fetuses detected with greater than 200 repeat units (full mutation)

Dobkin et al., 1991; Brown et al., 1993; Shapiro et al., 1995

complete methylation of the fragile-X gene

Dobkin et al., 1991

demonstration of the fragile-X chromosome in cultured amniotic fluid cells in male fetuses using various culture media and induction chemicals

Jenkins et al., 1981; Schmidt et al., 1982a; Shapiro et al., 1982b; Nielsen et al., 1983; Hogge et al., 1984; Jenkins et al., 1984; Shapiro et al., 1984; Jenkins et al., 1985; Rocchi et al., 1985; Schmidt, 1985; von Koskull et al., 1985; Jenkins et al., 1986; Shapiro and Wilmot, 1986; Tommerup et al., 1986; Shapiro et al., 1987; Sutherland et al., 1987; Webb et al., 1987; Jenkins et al., 1988; Purvis-Smith et al., 1988; Shapiro et al., 1988; Shapiro et al., 1989; Jenkins et al., 1991

Comments: When non-induced fragile-X chromosomes (fragile-X chromosome found in cell grown in standard culture media) are found, one should not assume the finding to be artifact of tissue culture. Shapiro and colleagues (1995) have identified at least one such case where the mother carried a fragile-X premutation and the female fetus had the full mutation. DNA analysis was done on both mother and fetus.

demonstration of the fragile-X chromosome in cultured amniotic fluid cells in female fetuses using various culture media and induction chemicals

> Venter et al., 1984; Wilson and Marchese, 1984; Jenkins et al., 1985; Schmidt,1985; von Koskull et al., 1985; Jenkins et al., 1986; Shapiro and Wilmot, 1986; Tommerup et al., 1986; Shapiro et al., 1987; Sutherland et al., 1987; Jenkins et al., 1988; Purvis-Smith et al., 1988; Shapiro et al., 1988; Shapiro et al., 1989; Dobkin et al., 1991; Jenkins et al., 1991

linkage between the gene for the fragile-X syndrome and RFLPs

> Shapiro et al., 1987; Shapiro et al., 1988

premutation detected in male fetus

> Brown et al., 1993; Buchanan et al., 1995

Chorionic villus sampling[g,i]: detection of full mutation (200 or more CGG repeat units) in a male fetus by various molecular genetic techniques

> Hirst et al., 1991; Sutherland et al., 1991; Brown et al., 1993; Maddalena et al., 1993; von Koskull et al., 1994

detection of the premutation (50–199 CGG repeats units) in female and male fetuses by various molecular genetic techniques

> Hirst et al., 1991; Brown et al., 1993; Maddalena et al., 1993; Halley et al., 1994; von Koskull et al., 1994

fragile-X chromosome demonstrated in male fetuses by using various media and induction chemicals

> Tommerup et al., 1985; Tommerup, 1986; Jenkins et al., 1988; McKinley et al., 1988a; Purvis-Smith et al., 1988; Shapiro et al., 1989; Jenkins et al., 1991; von Koskull et al., 1994

fragile-X chromosome demonstrated in female fetuses by using various media

> Sutherland et al., 1987; Purvis-Smith et al., 1988; Shapiro et al., 1988; Jenkins et al., 1991

linkage between the fragile-X syndrome gene and various DNA polymorphic markers

> Murphy et al., 1986; Shapiro et al., 1988; Hirst et al., 1991; Jenkins et al., 1991

Cordocentesis (PUBS)[i]: demonstration of the fragile-X chromosome in fetal leukocytes from male fetuses at risk

> Webb et al., 1981b; Shapiro et al., 1982; Webb et al., 1983; Rocchi et al., 1985; Shapiro et al., 1987; Webb et al., 1987; McKinley et al., 1988a; McKinley et al., 1988b; Shapiro et al., 1989

PD 265300 FRIEDREICH ATAXIA (FA; FRDA; Friedreich disease; Hereditofamilial spinal ataxia) (McKusick No. 229300)

Disease Note: Friedreich ataxia is an autosomal recessive spinocerebellar degenerative disorder. This disorder usually presents with ataxia of gait prior to adolescence followed by progressive dysarthria and the development of loss of deep tendon reflexes, impairment of position and vibratory senses, nystagmus, scoliosis, pes cavus, and hammer toe. There is an increased frequency of hypertrophic cardiomyopathy and diabetes in affected individuals.

The gene responsible for Friedreich ataxia has been localized to chromosome 9 (9q13-q21.1). There is tight linkage between several DNA markers (MCT112 and DR47) and the Friedreich ataxia gene.

McKusick, 1990; Wallis et al., 1989

Prenatal Diagnosis: Prenatal diagnosis has been accomplished by linkage of the Friedreich ataxia gene to DNA polymorphisms.

Differential Diagnosis: Abetalipoproteinemia; Ataxia telangiectasia (PD 252500); Familial spastic paraplegia; Metachromatic leukodystrophy (PD 228000); Pseudoarylsulfatase A deficiency (PD 231700); Tay–Sachs disease (PD 233000); Tay–Sachs disease, atypical type (PD 233500)

Amniocentesis[i]: DNA polymorphism linkage to the Friedreich ataxia gene using RFLPs and appropriate probes

Wallis et al., 1989

detection of carrier status in a fetus by polymorphism linkage analysis

Monros et al., 1995

PD 265350 FUKUYAMA TYPE CONGENITAL MUSCULAR DYSTROPHY
(Cerebromuscular dystrophy, Fukuyama type; Fukuyama disease; Muscular dystrophy, congenital progressive, with mental retardation) (McKusick No. 253800)

Condition Note: The condition listed here is noted by cerebral and cerebellar cortical dysplasia (micropolygyria and lissencephaly), and progressive congenital muscular dystrophy. Specific features include generalized hypotonia, weakness present during infancy, marked muscle atrophy, joint contractures, seizures, and psychomotor developmental delay and mental retardation. The clinical course is inexorably progressive, and death usually occurs by age 16. The condition is inherited in an autosomal recessive mode. The gene for the disorder has been localized to 9q31-q33.

Amniocentesis[i]: linkage of the gene to various DNA polymorphic markers

Kondo et al., 1996

PD 265400 GRISCELLI SYNDROME (Chediak–Higashi-like syndrome)
(McKusick No. 214450)

Syndrome Note: The features of this syndrome, which resembles Chediak–Higashi syndrome, are partial albinism; frequent pyogenic infections; and recurrent and acute episodes of fever, neutropenia and thrombocytopenia. There also is hypogammaglobulinemia, deficient antibody production, and no delayed skin hypersensitivity or skin graft refection. The condition differs from Chediak–Higashi syndrome in that there are no giant granules or other abnormalities found in neutrophils, and their bactericidal activity is only moderately reduced. Pigmentary changes are characterized by large clumps of pigment in the hair shafts and an accumulation of melanosomes in melanocytes. This disorder is inherited in an autosomal recessive mode.

Durandy et al., 1993; McKusick, 1994

Prenatal Diagnosis: The diagnosis prenatally has been made by demonstrating pigmentary disturbance in hair shafts and their roots.

Differential Diagnosis: Albinism, oculocutaneous type (PD 194750); Chediak–Higashi syndrome (PD 254400); Hermansky–Pudlak syndrome

Fetal skin biopsy by fetoscopy[i]: large clumps of oval and irregularly distributed melanosomes in hair and hair roots on light microscopic studies
Durandy et al., 1993

PD 265480 HEMATOMA, RETROPLACENTAL (McKusick No. None)

Ultrasound[c]: retroplacental mass
Spirt et al., 1987

PD 265500 HEMATOMA, SUBMEMBRANOUS PLACENTAL (McKusick No. None)

Ultrasound[d]: elevation of the membranes adjacent to the placenta
Spirt et al., 1981

PD 265550 HEMOCHROMATOSIS, NEONATAL (Idiopathic neonatal hemochromatosis; Neonatal giant cell hepatitis) (McKusick No. 231100)

Condition Note: Neonatal hemochromatosis probably is inherited in an autosomal recessive fashion, and is a disorder of iron metabolism where various tissues contain excessive amounts of iron. The massive iron storages in the hepatocytes lead to hepatic fibrosis. Suggested criteria for the diagnosis of this condition include rapid progressive clinical course with death in utero or in the early neonatal period; increased tissue iron deposition in multiple sites, and in particular the liver, pancreas, heart, and endocrine glands with the extra hepatic reticuloendothelial system being unaffected; and no evidence for hemolytic disease, syndromes associated with hemosiderosis, or exogenous iron overload from transfusions.
Wisser et al., 1993; McKusick, 1996

Cordocentesis (PUBS)[c,d]: severe anemia with both low hemoglobin and hematocrit levels, elevated levels of serum glutamic oxalacetic transaminase (SGOT) and serum glutamic pyruvic transaminase (SGPT)
Wisser et al., 1993

Echocardiography [c,d]: dilated venticles, myocardial hypertrophy
Wisser et al., 1993

Ultrasound[c,d]: narrow chest, enlarged abdomen, ascites, short femora, hydrops fetalis, thickened placenta
Wisser et al., 1993

Comments: The fetus reported by Wisser and associates (1993) had had normal ultrasound evaluations at 16 and 28 weeks of gestation. At 35 weeks of gestation, the above findings were discovered. The child was delivered by cesarian section shortly thereafter, and died from respiratory failure in 6 hours. Massive granular iron storage in the hepatocytes and biliary epithelium, and demonstrable iron storage were present in the thyroid parenchyma, pancreatic islet cells and acinar cells on autopsy.

PD 265600 HEMOTHORAX (Fetal hemothorax) (McKusick No. None)

Condition Note: Injuries to the fetus, umbilical cord, or placenta following amniocentesis are relatively uncommon, but are at increased frequency when the procedure is done during the third trimester. Hemothorax is also uncommon and has been reported only in association with amniocentesis.
Achiron and Zakut, 1986

Prenatal Diagnosis: The appearance of a cyst-like mass in the fetal chest following amniocentesis is suggestive of hemothorax.

Differential Diagnosis: Chylothorax (PD 190000); Congenital bronchial cyst (PD 272250); Cystic adenomatoid malformation of the lung (PD 272500); Teratoma, lung (PD 281750)

    Ultrasound[d]: semisolid cyst-like structure in the fetal thorax with poorly defined borders, downward displacement of the diaphragm

        Achiron and Zakut, 1986

    Comments: In the pregnancy reported by Achiron and Zakut (1986), an amniocentesis was done at 31 weeks of gestation to determine lung maturity. Following the procedure a nonstress test revealed a nonreactive pattern with late decelerations. An ultrasound showed the findings described above. The child died after a cesarean section. At autopsy a massive right hemothorax with traumatic laceration of the pulmonary right middle lobe was found.

PD 265700 HUNTINGTON DISEASE (HD; Huntington's chorea; Huntington's disease) (McKusick No. 143100)

Disease Note: Huntington disease is an autosomal dominant degenerative disorder that involves the brain and usually is manifested by midlife. Features include abnormal involuntary movements (choreic movements), personality changes, and dementia. The mean age of onset of symptoms is 37 years, with a range between 5 and 70. Death from Huntington disease occurs from 10–20 years after the onset of symptoms. The gene for the disorder has been mapped to the short arm of chromosome 4 and is linked to a number of DNA polymorphic markers.

    The disease is produced by an expansion of the trinucleotide repeat unit CAG in the Huntington disease gene. In the normal individual, there are up to 35 CAG repeats. In the presymptomatic or affected individual, there are 40 or more repeat units. Individuals with between 35 and 40 may or may not develop the condition. Furthermore, there is an inverse relationship between the number of CAG repeats above 39 and the age of onset of the disease; the larger the repeat size, the earlier the onset.

Prenatal Diagnosis: The carrier status of the fetus can be made by determining the size of the CAG repeat unit. The diagnosis also can be established prenatally by linking of one or more DNA polymorphisms to the Huntington gene using D4S10 and D4595 or other similar probes in a fetus at risk when the family is informative.

        Fahy et al., 1989

Differential Diagnosis: Huntington disease may be confused with psychologic disorders, Benign chorea of late onset, and other neurodegenerative disorders.

    Chorionic villus sampling[g,i]: use of RFLP, restriction endonuclease, appropriate DNA probes; PCR and Southern blotting for linkage analysis in at-risk embryos

        Brock et al., 1988; Thies et al., 1992

PD 265750 HYDROPS FETALIS, IDIOPATHIC (Fetal hydrops; Nonimmune hydrops fetalis) (McKusick No. Unknown; see 236750)

Condition Note: Fetal hydrops, or generalized fetal edema, is a physical finding, not an etiologic diagnosis. When present, efforts should be made to determine its underlying cause. The citations listed under this disorder are reports of idiopathic hydrops fetalis where the etiology was not established.

Prenatal Diagnosis: The presence of generalized edema including edema of the scalp and skin, pleural effusion and ascites is the basis for the diagnosis of hydrops fetalis. Often cystic hygroma is found concurrently with hydrops fetalis.

Prenatal Treatment: None has been established. Thompson and fellow workers (1993) have reported resolution of the hydrops in fetuses where the pleural fluid was drained by pleuroamniotic shunting. The effectiveness of this treatment probably is through improvement of venous return to the heart and/or improvement of cardiac function.

Treatment Modality: Pleuroamniotic shunting of pleural fluid

> Blott et al., 1988a; Nicolaides and Azar, 1990; Thompson et al., 1993

Methods and Findings: Acetylcholinesterase[c]: fast-migrating isozyme on gel electrophoresis

> Crandall et al., 1982; Crandall and Matsumoto, 1984b

Alpha-fetoprotein[c]: elevated in amniotic fluid

> Burck et al., 1981; Crandall and Matsumoto, 1984b; Rodriguez et al., 1987a

elevated in maternal serum

> Rodriguez et al., 1987b

Continuous-wave Doppler evaluation[c,d]: increased peripheral arterial resistance

> Meizner et al., 1987

Cordocentesis (PUBS)[c]: low hematocrit (anemia)

> Murotsuki et al., 1992

Radiograph: straightened fetal trunk with poorly flexed extremities, enlarged fetal abdomen, large placenta, fetal edema, fetal death in third trimester

> Noonan, 1974

Ultrasound: abnormally thickened placenta, increased thickness of scalp and abdominal wall

> Quagliarello et al., 1978; Abrams et al., 1985a

bilateral or multiloculated cystic hygromas arising from the posterior aspect of the neck

> Burck et al., 1981; Spirt et al., 1987

thickening of the skin caused by edema

> Spirt et al., 1987; Hill et al., 1988b

generalized edema

> Broekhuizen et al., 1983b; Curry et al., 1983

pleural effusion[c]

> Lange and Manning, 1981; Quinlan et al., 1983; Abrams et al., 1985a; Meizner et al., 1986c; Spirt et al., 1987; Blott et al., 1988a; Hill et al., 1988b; Rodeck et al., 1988; Thompson et al., 1993

heart failure[c]

> Quinlan et al., 1983

pericardial effusion[c]

> Spirt et al., 1987

hepatomegaly[c]

> Quinlan et al., 1983

ascites[c]
>Quagliarello et al., 1978; Abrams et al., 1985a; Spirt et al., 1987; Hill et al., 1988b

large for gestational age
>Leonard, 1989

large placenta[c]
>Broekhuizen et al., 1983b

hydramnios[c]
>Quagliarello et al., 1978; Lange and Manning, 1981; Quinlan et al., 1983; Abrams et al., 1985a; Blott et al., 1988a

PD 266000 INTERVILLOUS PLACENTAL THROMBUS (McKusick No. None)

Ultrasound[c]: intraplacental sonolucent lesion
Spirt et al., 1987

PD 267000 INTRAUTERINE GROWTH RETARDATION (Fetal growth deficiency; IUGR; Small for gestational age) (McKusick No. None)

Condition Note: Intrauterine growth retardation is where the fetal weight is less than the 10th percentile for gestational age. However, the true fetal weight can only be determined after delivery. Prenatally, fetal size then is an estimate based on various growth parameters such as biparietal diameter, head circumference, abdominal circumference, femur length, and various ratios of these measurements (femur length/abdominal circumference). The determination of fetal size and its appropriateness for gestation is dependent on an accurate gestational age which may not always be available.

Zimmer and Divon (1992) have reviewed the sonographic diagnosis of IUGR. They concluded that the sonographic measurements for IUGR are associated with a high specificity and a somewhat lower sensitivity. These observation imply that the current ultrasound methods are more useful for excluding the possibility of abnormal fetal growth rather than confirming its presence.

The development of fetal blood sampling (cordocentesis) has afforded an opportunity to assess fetal well being (Nicolaides et al., 1986e). Severe intrauterine hypoxic acidosis due to inadequate placental transfer in the absence of fetal abnormalities has been found by this technique (Nicolaides et al., 1986e). Concomitant abnormal blood flow have also been observed by Doppler blood-flow studies (Nicolaides et al., 1986e) in these fetuses. IUGR may be associated with any of the above findings.

Alpha-fetoprotein[c]: elevated in maternal serum
>Wald et al., 1977; Brock et al., 1977; Macri et al., 1978; Brock et al., 1982; Ghosh et al., 1986

Amniocentesis: elevation of catecholamine metabolites (4-hydroxy-3-methoxyphenylglycol; 4-hydroxy-3-methoxy mandelic acid) in amniotic fluid[c]
>Lagercrantz et al., 1980

decreased levels of insulin in amniotic fluid[c]
>Weiss et al., 1984

increase in 3-methyl histidine to creatinine molar ratio in amniotic fluid[c]
>Miodovnik et al., 1982

phosphatidylglycerol present in amniotic fluid[c,d]
>Gross et al., 1981; Gross et al., 1982

fetal distress cells present in amniotic cell culture[c]
> Gosden and Brock, 1978b

Doppler ultrasound[c]: decreased umbilical arterial blood flow
> Reuwer et al., 1987

abnormal utero-placental and fetal velocity wave forms (reduced end-diastolic flow in the arcuate arteries; reverse flow in the fetal aorta and umbilical cord)
> Nicolaides et al., 1986e

in asymmetrical IUGR (where there is relative sparing of brain growth with respect to body height) increase in peripheral vascular resistance
> Rizzo et al., 1987a

Cordocentesis (PUBS)[c]: significantly increased red cell count
> Soothill et al., 1987

Comments: Current data suggest that fetuses with retarded intrauterine growth may often suffer chronic intrauterine hypoxia as a result of inadequate placental transfer. Associated fetal findings (probably also related to placental insufficiencies) are hypercapnia, acidosis, hyperlacticemia, hypoglycemia, and erythroblastosis. These findings further support the notion that prenatal brain damage normally is the result of chronic fetal hypoxia, rather than birth asphyxia (Soothill et al., 1987).

significantly lowered fetal blood oxygen tension (hypoxeimia), low Po_2
> Nicolaides et al., 1986e; Soothill et al., 1987; Economides and Nicolaides, 1989

reduced fetal blood pH
> Nicolaides et al., 1986e; Soothill et al., 1987

reduced fetal blood glucose levels
> Soothill et al., 1987; Economides and Nicolaides, 1989

increased levels of serum lactate
> Nicolaides et al, 1986e; Soothill et al., 1987

increased levels of carbon dioxide in fetal blood
> Niclolaides et al., 1986e; Soothill et al., 1987

Maternal blood sampling[c]: increased maternal plasma glucose disappearance rate (K_t) and 10-minute plasma glucose concentration, decreased fasting and 60-minute plasma glucose concentration following intravenous glucose tolerance test in the mother
> Sokol et al., 1982

reduced levels of insulin-like growth factor-I (IGF-I)
> Chu and Boots, 1995

reduced levels of insulin-like growth factor binding protein-I (IGFBP-I)
> Chu and Boots, 1995

elevated levels of serum hCG
> Lewis et al., 1995

Ultrasound: reduced crown-to-rump length, biparietal diameter, and abdominal area, oligohydramnios[c]
> Tamura et al., 1977; Elias et al., 1980a; Philipson et al., 1983; Geirsson et al., 1985a; Geirsson et al., 1985b; Woo et al., 1985; Nicolaides et al., 1986a; Warsof et al., 1986; Rizzo et al., 1987a

chest circumference less than 5th percentile[c]
> Nimrod et al., 1986

abdominal circumference below the 5th percentile[c]
>Soothill et al., 1987

increased echogenicity of fetal bowel[c]
>Pallante et al., 1995

femur length greater than 2 SD below the mean[c]
>O'Brien and Queenan, 1982; Woo et al., 1985

delay in integration of behavioral patterns (different distribution of fetal breathing and eye movements, and movements in general)[c]
>Rizzo et al., 1987a

reduced or absent fetal movements, or no response to stimulation[c]
>Ianniruberto and Tajani, 1981

determination of advanced placental maturity (Grade III)[c,d]
>Kazzi et al., 1983

reduced total intrauterine, intraamniotic, and placental volumes
>Chinn et al., 1981; Geirsson et al., 1985a; Geirsson et al., 1985b

oligohydramnios[c]
>Gembruch and Hansmann, 1988; Econmides and Nicolaides, 1989

no filling of the fetal bladder after maternal furosemide challenge test[c]
>Gembruch and Hansmann, 1988

filling of the fetal bladder after instillation of amniotic fluid into the amniotic cavity[c]
>Gembruch and Hansmann, 1988

prolonged return to oligohydramnios after instillation of artificial amniotic fluid
>Gembruch and Hansmann, 1988

PD 267250 INTRAUTERINE RESORPTION OF DECEASED COTWIN
(McKusick No. None)

>Ultrasound: cystic mass visualized at 16 weeks of gestation; complete resorption had occurred by 26th week
>>Sabbagha et al., 1980

PD 267300 INTRAUTERINE SEIZURES (McKusick No. Unknown)

Prenatal Diagnosis: Seizures have been observed in 0.5% of all newborns and in up to 20% of neonates admitted to neonatal intensive care units. Forty percent of seizures in infants begin within the first 24 hours of life. The etiology of neonatal and infantile seizure is quite varied. Although 15% of infants with seizures die and 35% of those who survive have permanent handicaps, the worse prognosis is for those with seizures that first occur during the first day of life. In this group one-third die and 50% of the survivors have significant problems. The prognosis for infants with intrauterine seizures is unknown. In many of the neonates where seizures occurred in the first day, the seizures probably were occurring prenatally.
>Conover et al., 1986

Prenatal Diagnosis: Demonstration of seizure-like movements of the fetus should raise the possibility of seizures, particularly if the movements are episodic.

Differential Diagnosis: See Fetal movements, decreased, restricted, or absent in the Index. One case of Hydranencephaly (PD 124000) has also been reported with fetal seizures.

Maternal history: perception of abnormal fetal movements
    Conover et al., 1986
Comments: In the case reported by Conover and associates (1986), a male newborn was found to have multiple anomalies that included narrow palpebral fissures, ocular hypertelorism, clinodactyly, bilateral transverse palmar creases, hypospadias, and micropenis. Despite full support, the neonate died on the third day of life. An autopsy was denied. The karyotype was normal and no diagnosis was established.
Ultrasound[d]: recurrent episodes of rapid, jerking movements of the head and extremities that occurred in unison, lasting 5–10 seconds, and then spontaneously repeating 20–30 seconds later for periods of 5–10 minutes followed by intervals of 5–10 minutes in which there were no fetal movements
    Conover et al., 1986

PD 267435 LITHIUM TOXICITY, FETAL (McKusick No. None)

Condition Note: Lithium treatment frequently is effective for manic-depressive disorder. However, during pregnancy lithium may be toxic to the fetus, and has been associated with increased mortality and morbidity perinatally.
    Physical examination of the mother[c]: increased fundal height
        Krause et al., 1990
Ultrasound[c]: hydramnios
        Krause et al., 1990
Comments: The fetus reported by Krause and associates (1990) developed fetal distress near term and was delivered by cesarean section. At birth he had asphyxia and acidosis; postnatally he had or experienced apnea, cardiac decompensation, respiratory distress, hypoglycemia, thrombocytopenia, diabetes insipidus, hypotonia and seizures. The authors believed that these problems were related to lithium toxicity.

PD 267450 LUPUS ERYTHEMATOSUS (SLE; Systemic lupus erythematosus) (McKusick No 152700)

Disease Note: Active maternal systemic lupus erythematosus (SLE) is associated with high titers of ani-nuclear antibodies and for antibodies to the extractable nuclear antigens, SS-A and SS-B (La). These antibodies may cross the placenta and produce a fetal myocarditis, which in turn may progress to fibrosis of the conduction system, and complete heart block. Fetal death may ensue from subsequent heart failure.
    Buyon et al., 1987; Walkinshaw et al., 1994b
Prenatal Diagnosis: Diagnosis is assumed to be present when there is active SLE in the mother, and evidence of myocarditis and/or complete heart block in the fetus.
Differential Diagnosis: Other autoimmune connective tissue disorders in the mother, such as Sjogren syndrome (PD 198450).
    Romero et al., 1988, p. 418
Prenatal Treatment: At the present time too few cases have been reported to determine the most effective treatment of choice. However, the method reported by Buyon and co-workers (1987) appears to have been successful. In their case, the myocarditis in the fetus whose mother had active SLE was successfully treated by reducing maternal anti-SS-B (La) antibody levels through maternal plasmapheresis and dexamethasone treatments. The therapy resulted in signifi-

cant improvement in the fetal myocarditis but failed to reverse the complete heart block in the fetus.

Treatment Modalities: Intracardiac cardiac pacing by percutaneous transvenous route

Walkinshaw et al., 1994b

Comments: In the case reported by Walkinshaw and co-workers (1994b) at 24 weeks' gestation, intracardiac cardiac pacing was accomplished by passing a pacing wire through a needle that was inserted in the umbilical vein. The pacing wire was lodged in the wall of the right ventricle, the needle removed, and the single chamber pulse generator was implanted subcutaneously in the mother's abdominal wall. For the first 8 hours, the response was excellent with a fetal heart rate of 140 beats per minute. The fetus also became quite active. However, the wire became dislodged and complete heart block returned. During the second attempt at pacing the fetus developed asystole and died.

Maternal medication: dexamethasone

Buyon et al., 1987

corticosteroids, type not stated

Walkinshaw et al., 1994b

Plasmapheresis, maternal blood

Buyon et al., 1987

Comments: In the mother treated by Buyon and associates (1987), the fetus was delivered and was found to have complete atrioventricular dissociation. He had no cutaneous or hematologic signs of SLE, however. No treatment of the heart block was required, and the subsequent growth and development of the child were normal.

Methods and Findings: Echocardiograph[i]: dilation of all four chambers of the heart, significant pericardial effusion, right pleural effusion

Buyon et al., 1987

complete heart block with an atrial rate of 150 beats per minute and a ventricular rate of 40 per minute[d]

Madison et al., 1979

Electocardiography[d]: regular ventricular rate of 60 beats per minute

Berube et al., 1978

Phonocardiogram[d]: complete heart block with an atrial rate of 150 beats per minutes and a ventricular rate of 39 beats per minute

Madison et al., 1979

Ultrasound[i]: fetal bradycardia

Buyon et al., 1987

complete heart block

Walkinshaw et al., 1994b

hydrops fetalis

Walkinshaw et al., 1994b

ascites

Walkinshaw et al., 1994

decreased fetal movement[c]

Buyon et al., 1987; Walkinshaw et al., 1994b

oligohydramnios[c]

Buyon et al., 1987

Method not stated[h]: fetal bradycardia
>   Chameides et al., 1977

PD 267470 MARFAN SYNDROME (McKusick No. 154700)

Chorionic villus sampling[g,i]: linkage between the fibrillin gene and DNA polymorphisms
>   Godfrey et al., 1993
>   directed mutation detection using PCR on cDNA from chorionic villi
>   Godfrey et al., 1993
Ultrasound[i]: significantly increased limb lengths in a fetus at risk
>   Koenigsberg et al., 1981

PD 267475 MARFAN SYNDROME, NEONATAL FORM (Congenital Marfan syndrome) (McKusick No. None; see 154700)

Condition Note: Neonatal Marfan syndrome is a more severe manifestation of Marfan syndrome with marked abnormalities present at birth, and usually with rapid progression of the disease resulting in early death. Features, some of which are those seen in congenital contractural arachnodactyly (Beals syndrome), include crumpled ears, ocular abnormalities, micrognathia, marked arachnodactyly of fingers and toes, contractures of various joints, and cardiovascular abnormalities. The mutations that have produced this severe form of Marfan syndrome have been found in specific regions of the fibrillin-1 (FBN1) gene.
>   Buntinx et al., 1991

Differential Diagnosis: Congenital contractural arachnodactyly; Marfan syndrome (PD 267470)

Chorionic villus sampling[g,i]: detection of a mutation in the FBN1 gene in chorionic villi using appropriate molecular genetic techniques
>   Godfrey et al., 1993; Rantamaki et al., 1995
>   linkage analysis between the FBM1 gene and appropriate DNA markers
>   Godfrey et al., 1993; Wang et al., 1995
>   detection of truncated fibrillin in the media of cultured chorionic villus cells
>   Rantamaki et al., 1995
Echocardiogram[d]: pericardial effusion
>   Lopes et al., 1995
prolapse of the mitral and tricuspid valves
>   Lopes et al., 1995
mitral and tricuspid regurgitation
>   Lopes et al., 1995
dilatation of the aortic root at the level of the sinuses of Valsalva (clover-leaf appearance)
>   Lopes et al., 1995
aortic and pulmonary regurgitation
>   Lopes et al., 1995
>   *Comments:* The father of the fetus reported by Lopes and associates (1995) had typical features of Marfan syndrome. The neonate had multiple abnormalities consistent with Marfan syndrome, and died at 2 months of age from heart failure.

Ultrasound: cardiomegaly[d,i]
    Buntinx et al, 1991; Lopes et al., 1995
Comments: The fetus/neonate reported by Buntinx and co-workers (1991) after birth was found to have crumpled and hypoplastic ears; micrognathia; joint contractures of the elbows, wrists, hips and knees; marked arachnodactyly of the hands and feet; prominent heels; and absence of subcutaneous fat. The neonate died 20 hours after birth. At autopsy there were dysplastic and prolapsed heart valves, long and abnormally inserted chordae tendineae, and severe dilatation and dysplasia of the aortic and pulmonary valves. The latter problems caused failure of the valves leaflets to coapt.
    significant increase in limb lengths in a fetus at risk
        Koenigsberg et al., 1981
    aortic dilation[c,d]
        Buntinx et al., 1991
    growth retardation[d]
        Lopes et al., 1995
    oligohydramnios[c,d]
        Lopes et al., 1995

PD 267750 MATERNAL CHEMOTHERAPY—ACTINOMYCIN D, ISOPHOSPHAMIDE, VINCRISTINE (McKusick No. None)

Maternal history[c,d]: no fetal activity
    Fernandez et al., 1989
Ultrasound[c,d]: cessation of fetal growth, nonoscillating fetal heart rate with late deceleration, oligohydramnios with non-filling of the bladder
    Fernandez et al., 1989
Comments: The mother reported by Fernandez and associates (1989) was diagnosed with rhabdomyosarcoma of the face with bone marrow metastases when she was 23 weeks pregnant. At 23 and 27 weeks of gestation, she was treated with two courses of actinomycin D, isophosphamide, and vincristine. By the second course of treatment, there was oligohydramnios and cessation of fetal growth. The child was delivered at 29 weeks of gestation by cesarean section because of signs of acute fetal hypoxia. Postnatally, the child failed to produce any urine and died at age 7 days. Autopsy findings included bilateral intraventricular hemorrhage, left occipital meningeal hematoma, no discernible renal lesions, and no observed cancer cells. The placenta had large areas of ischemic necrosis, but no observed cancer cells.

PD 267850 MATERNAL HYPERTENSION, TREATMENT OF (McKusick No. None)

Condition Note: Hurst and associates (1995) have reported both a fetus and a neonate with transverse limb defects in both; cleft lip and palate, and abnormal glomenuli and renal tubules in one; and shortened tibiae in the other. Both mothers were hypertensive before their pregnancies, and were taking either prazosin or labetalol at the time of conceptions and throughout the pregnancies. The authors postulated that the defects in the fetuses were caused by hypoxemia secondary to maternal hypotension induced by the antihypertensive drugs that they took.

Maternal report[c]: loss of amniotic fluid
    Hurst et al., 1995
Ultrasound[c]: oligohydramnios, intrauterine death
    Hurst et al., 1995

PD 267865 MATERNAL PHENYLKETONURIA (Maternal PKU) (McKusick No. None; see 261600)

Disease Note: High levels of phenylalanine are toxic to the developing embryo and fetus. Pregnant, untreated phenylketonuric women have a high risk of having offspring with various birth defects including microcephaly, congenital heart defects, and IUGR, and who end up being mentally retarded. When these mothers are treated with a low phenylalanine diet from the beginning and throughout their pregnancies, these problems may be prevented or reduced in severity.
    Levy et al., 1996
Echocardiography [i]: tetralogy of Fallot, coarctation of the aorta, single ventricle heart
    Levy et al., 1996
Ultrasound[i]: nonviability of the pregnancy[g]
    Levy et al., 1996
    congenital heart disease
        Levy et al., 1996
    decreased biparietal diameter
        Levy et al., 1996
    Comments: Of the 39 pregnancies among phenylketonuric women followed by Levy and associates (1996), 33 had ultrasonic evaluations during the second trimester. One of the 33 fetuses had microcephaly (biparietal diameter greater than 2 SD below the mean) at 21 weeks. In addition, 20 of the women had ultrasonic examinations in the third trimester, and three additional fetuses were found to have microcephaly.
    empty gestational sac (blighted ovum)
        Levy et al., 1996

PD 268000 MULTIPLE GESTATION (Monochorionic, monoamniotic twins; Quintuplets; Triplets; Twins) (McKusick No. 276400, 276410)

Twins

    Alpha-fetoprotein[c]: elevated in maternal serum[g]
        Garoff and Seppala, 1973; Gardner et al., 1981; Wald and Cuckle, 1981; Haddow et al., 1983; Ryynanen et al., 1983; Schnittger and Kjessler, 1984; Thom et al., 1984; Ghosh et al., 1986; Scioscia et al., 1987
        elevated in amniotic fluid
            Ryynanen et al., 1983
        Comment: The discordancy between amniotic fluid AFP in the separate sacs of monozygotic and dizygotic twins is greater in dizygotic twins (Drugan et al., 1988).
    Chorionic villus sampling from each sac[g]: karyotyping of villi revealed both 46,XY and 46,XX chromosomal complements
        Mulcahy et al., 1984

Maternal blood sampling: elevation of human placental lactogen (HPL) and hCG in maternal serum[c]

> Dhont et al., 1976; Knight et al., 1981
>> reduced levels of insulin-like growth factor-I (IGF-I)
>>> Chu and Boots, 1995
>> reduced levels of insulin-like growth factor binding protein-I (IGFBP-I)
>>> Chu and Boots, 1995

Radiograph

> Noonan, 1974

Ultrasound[g]: two fetuses identified, two separate sacs delineated

>> Gottesfeld, 1978; Brambati et al., 1984; Filkins et al., 1984; Mulcahy et al., 1984; Erkkola et al., 1985; Pijpers et al., 1989a
> two fetal biparietal diameters
>> Hughes and Miskin, 1986
> cotwin stimulation with response from the second twin[c]
>> Ianniruberto and Tajani, 1981
> intrauterine growth retardation in one or both twins
>> Storlazzi et al., 1987

Monochorionic, monoamniotic twins

Ultrasound[d]: normal amount of amniotic fluid around each fetus, same sex twins, absence of dividing fetal membrane, single placenta

> Rodis et al., 1987

Triplets

Alpha-fetoprotein[c]: elevated in maternal serum

>> Schnittger and Kjessler, 1984; Thom et al., 1984; Taubert et al., 1986; Krantz et al., 1995

Maternal blood drawing[c]: elevated serum levels of free beta hCG

>> Krantz et al., 1995

Ultrasound: identification of three gestational sacs[g]

>> Filkins et al., 1984; Taubert et al., 1986

Quintuplets

Quintuplet Situation Note: The fetuses in a quintuplet pregnancy are at a particular high risk because of premature delivery and complications associated with delivery, normally done by cesarean section. Most quintuplet pregnancies occur because of drug-induced multiple ovulations, and the fetuses have been produced from five different zygotes. Normally, the five fetuses are normal fetuses. Fetal reduction (feticide) is done in part to reduce the pregnancy-associated risks and the risks associated with premature delivery.

Prenatal Treatment: Of the methods used for selected feticide, none seems to be preferred. The method of choice for termination of the fetus is related to the gestational age of the pregnancy, the wishes of the parents, and the experience of the physician doing the procedure (Kanhai et al., 1986).

Treatment Modality: Cardiac puncture with amniocentesis needle under ultrasonic guidance until cardiac activity ceased followed by aspiration of amniotic fluid in the deceased fetus' sac.

>> Kanhai et al., 1986

Methods and Findings: Alpha-fetoprotein[c]: elevated in maternal serum
>> Garoff and Seppala, 1973
> Ultrasound: identification five fetuses
>> Warner et al., 1979; Kanhai et al., 1986

PD 268500 MULTIPLE GESTATION: DISCORDANT TWINS AND TRIPLETS (McKusick No. None)

Situation Note: Discordance between twins or triplets, the situation where one twin or triplet has a significant defect or disorder while the other fetus or fetuses usually are normal, creates a dilemma for the parents and the physicians involved in the case. When there is no definitive treatment for the fetal condition, the parents have three options (Kerenyi and Chitkara, 1981; Redwine and Hays, 1986). The first is to continue the pregnancy and be faced with caring for a defective child. Second, they may elect to have the pregnancy terminated, but in doing so they will end the life of the normal fetus(es). Or third, the parents may elect selected feticide of the abnormal fetus with anticipation of the normal twin or triplets going to term and being healthy at birth. The difficulties for the involved physician(s) is accurate prenatal testing of both twins or each triplet, and when using selected feticide, is there a method that is not injurious to the normal twin or other triplets. Most discordant situations are found in dizygotic twins or triplets, but on occasion the situation arises in monozygotic twins, monozygotic twins plus a dizygotic triplet, or monozygotic triplets, (e.g., acardia [PD 182000]). Most of the latter three situations are listed separately under the title of the condition. A review of selected terminations is presented by Redwine and Hays (1986).

Prenatal Treatment: Of the methods used for selected feticide, none seems to be preferred. The selected method for termination of the fetus is related to the gestational age of the pregnancy, the wishes of the parents, and the experience of the physician doing the procedure.

Treatment Modalities: Amniocentesis with suction of the fetus through the amniocentesis needle[g]
> hemophilia
>> Mulcahy et al., 1984
>> *Comments*: The male twin fetus reported by Mulcahy and associates (1984) was terminated at 10-1/2 weeks of gestation by partially being suctioned through a transabdominal amniocentesis needle.
> Cardiac puncture and exsanguination of abnormal fetus
>> Down syndrome
>>> Kerenyi and Chitkara, 1981
>>> *Comments*: The demise of the fetus reported by Kerenyi and Chitkara (1981) was accomplished after withdrawing 25 cc of blood from the heart of the affected fetus by a needle inserted through the mother's abdomen. The procedure was done at 20 weeks' gestation. Delivery of a normal co-twin occurred at 40 weeks' gestation.
>> Hurler syndrome
>>> Aberg et al., 1978
>>> *Comments*: The procedure performed on the affected fetus reported by Aberg and colleagues (1978) was done at 24 weeks of gestation. Delivery of a normal cotwin occurred at 33 weeks.
> Fetoscopy and injection of sterile air into the umbilical vein of affected fetus

microcephaly of unknown etiology
>Rodeck et al., 1982b
>*Comments*: In the case reported by Rodeck and associates (1982b), 20 cc of air were required at 21 weeks' gestation to cause cardiac arrest. Following the injection, the ultrasound picture was lost ("white-out") because of air in the peripheral circulation of the fetus. Delivery of the other twin occurred at 36 weeks. The microcephalic twin was delivered as a fetus papyraceus.

hemophilia A
>Rodeck et al., 1982b
>*Comments*: The affected male reported by Rodeck and co-workers (1982b) was terminated by injecting 30 cc of sterile air at 21 weeks. A healthy female twin and a fetus papyraceus were delivered at 30 weeks' gestation.

rachischisis
>Rodeck et al., 1982b
>*Comments*: In the fetus reported by Rodeck and co-authors (1982b), 30 cc of sterile air were injected at 15 weeks of gestation. Delivery of a healthy girl and a fetus papyraceus occurred at 38 weeks' gestation.

Intracardiac injection of air producing air embolization
Down syndrome (trisomy 21)
>Redwine and Hays, 1986; Pijpers et al., 1989a
>*Comment*: The diagnosis in the fetus reported by Pijpers and associates (1989a) was confirmed by blood obtained at the time of the procedure in one case.

Tay–Sachs disease
>Petres and Redwine, 1981; Redwine and Petres, 1984; Redwine and
>Hays, 1986

Intracardiac injection of calcium gluconate into affected fetus
thalassemia major
>Antsaklis et al., 1984
>*Comments*: In the induced fetal demise reported by Antsaklis and co-workers (1984), the procedure, done at 24 weeks of gestation, involved first the withdrawal of 40 cc of blood from the heart and then intracardiac injection of 10 mL of calcium gluconate (concentration not stated). Cardiac arrest occurred in 6 minutes.

Intracardiac injection of potassium chloride (26 weeks' gestation): fetus with multiple congenital anomalies
>Still et al., 1989
>*Comments*: The fetus terminated in the report by Still and colleagues (1989) had massive ascites, hydrops fetalis, anencephaly, a single-chambered heart, and absence of kidneys and bladder. The normal cotwin was delivered at 28 weeks. The abnormality in this fetus is listed in this catalog under Anencephaly-single-chambered heart-renal-agenesis (PD 300500).

Sectio parva
Down syndrome
>Beck et al., 1980; Beck et al., 1981
>*Comments*: In the case reported by Beck and associates (1980, 1981), the fetus with Down syndrome was removed from the uterus by

sectio parva in the 22nd week of gestation. A healthy cotwin was delivered at 38 weeks of gestation via cesarean section.

PD 269000 MYOTONIC DYSTROPHY (Congenital myotonic dystrophy; Dystrophia myotonica; Steinert syndrome) (McKusick No. 160900)

Syndrome Note: Myotonic dystrophy is an autosomal dominant disorder with considerable phenotypic variation. Major features include myotonia, muscle weakness, polychromatic cataracts, frontal balding, and intellectual impairment. If a woman is affected, she may give birth to an infant with congenital myotonic dystrophy, a more severe form of the disorder, than is characterized by neonatal hypotonia, respiratory difficulties, mental retardation, and in some cases, early death. The gene for myotonic dystrophy is located at 19q13.2-19q13.3, and the disease is produced by expansion of the trinucleotide CTG in the gene that codes for myotonin protein kinase. The larger the CTG triplet expansion is, the more severely affected is the individual.

> Norman et al., 1989; Lavedan et al., 1991; Gennarelli et al., 1993

Prenatal Diagnosis: The diagnosis can be made by determining the number of repeats of the trinucleotide CTG in the myotonin protein kinase gene.

> Gennarelli et al., 1993

Differential Diagnosis: Congenital myasthenia gravis (PD 254750); Duchenne muscular dystrophy (PD 257000); Myotubular myopathy, X-linked recessive form (PD 269100); Schwartz–Jampel syndrome (PD 271075)

Amniocentesis[i]: genetic linkage with secretor locus; secretor status is determined by examining amniotic fluid

> Insley et al., 1976

increased number of CTG trinucleotides in the myotonin protein kinase gene obtained from amniotic fluid cells

> Stratton and Patterson, 1993

Chorionic villus sampling[i]: increased number of CTG trinucleotides in the myotonin protein kinase gene

> Gennarelli et al., 1993

linkage of the gene to various other genes and DNA polymorphisms

> Norman et al., 1989; Gennarelli et al., 1990; Lavedan et al., 1991

Doppler-based fetal movement detector[c,d]: persistent rapid fetal movements without an accelerated fetal heart rate or uterine contractions

> Hsu et al., 1993a

Maternal history: decreased perception of fetal movement by the mother[d,i]

> Broekhuizen et al., 1983a

Ultrasound[d,i]: distended bowel, poor fetal tone, decreased fetal movements, respiration, and swallowing; hydramnios

> Broekhuizen et al., 1983a; Quinlan et al., 1983

bilateral pleural effusion[c,d]

> Stratton and Patterson, 1993

pericardial effusion[c,d]

> Stratton and Patterson, 1993

ascites[c,d]

> Stratton and Patterson, 1993

no respiratory effort[c,d]

> Stratton and Patterson, 1993

little or no fetal movement[c,d]
> Stratton and Patterson, 1993

hydramnios[c,d]
> Stratton and Patterson, 1993

fetal demise[c,d]
> Stratton and Patterson, 1993

Method not stated: linkage of gene to various RFLPs and genes (CKMM and ApoCII), using probes p alpha 1.4p and D19519, and various restriction endonucleases
> Milunsky and Skare, 1989

PD 269100 MYOTUBULAR MYOPATHY, X-LINKED RECESSIVE FORM
(Centronuclear myopathy, X-linked myotubular myopathy) (McKusick No. 310400)

Condition Note: Three major patterns of inheritance have been described for myotubular myopathies: autosomal dominant, autosomal recessive, and X-linked recessive. The X-linked form of myotubular myopathy may be lethal in the neonatal period. The condition is characterized by hydramnios prenatally; and postnatally, by severe hypotonia with absent deep tendon reflexes; poor respiratory effort; macrocephaly with or without hydrocephalus; an elongated face; and slender, long digits. Muscle pathology consists of small and hypotrophic muscle fibers with centrally placed nuclei that are surrounded by clear areas devoid of myofibrils. The gene for this condition is thought to be located at Xq28, and to code for tyrosine phosphatase.
> Joseph et al., 1995

Prenatal Diagnosis: Hydramnios and/or decreased fetal movements are presumptive evidence for the presence of this condition in the at-risk male fetus.

Differential Diagnosis: Lethal multiple pterygium syndromes (PD 191550, PD 191600, PD 191620); Myotonic dystrophy (PD 269000); Prader–Willi syndrome (PD 193150); Spinal muscular atrophy, type I (PD 271100). For a more extensive differential, see Fetal movements, decreased, restricted, or absent; and Hydramnios in the Index.

Amniocentesis[i]: linkage of the MTM1 gene with DNA markers
> Hu et al., 1996

Ultrasound[d,i]: decreased fetal movements, hydramnios
> Joseph et al., 1995

> poor fetal movements
> Hu et al., 1996

PD 269175 NESIDIOBLASTOSIS, FAMILIAL (Familial neonatal
hyperinsulinemia; Hyperinsulinemia; Nesidioblastosis) (McKusick No. 256450)

Condition Note: Nesidioblastosis is used to describe the morphologic feature of the pancreas where the beta cells have proliferated out of the duct epithelium to form histologically abnormal new islets. The condition normally is associated with persistent neonatal hyperinsulinemia resulting in severe and difficult to control hypoglycemia. Although normally a sporadic condition, nesidioblastosis may be associated with certain syndromes, notably Beckwith–Wiedemann syndrome (PD 187000) or rarely, may be inherited as an autosomal recessive abnormality.
> Bianchi et al., 1992; McKusick, 1995

Prenatal Diagnosis: Based on limited experience, it appears that elevated levels of insulin in the amniotic fluid is presumptive evidence for the diagnosis in the at-risk fetus.

Amniocentesis[d,i]: abnormally low levels of glucose in amniotic fluid
  Bianchi et al., 1992
  elevated levels of insulin in the amniotic fluid
    Bianchi et al., 1992; Aparicio et al., 1993
  elevated levels of C-peptide in the amniotic fluid
    Bianchi et al., 1992; Aparicio et al., 1993
Ultrasound[i]: macrosomia
  Bianchi et al., 1992; Aparicio et al., 1993

PD 269250 NEUROFIBROMATOSIS, TYPE I (McKusick No. 162200)

Chorionic villus sampling[g]: linkage of the neurofibromatosis, type I gene (NF1) to various extra- and intragenic DNA markers
  Upadhyaya et al., 1992; Lazaro et al., 1995
Ultrasound[c,d]: oral mass
  Hoyme et al., 1987
Comments: At birth the child was found to have a tumor filling the oral cavity that turned out to be a congenital gingival granular cell tumor. The infant also was found to have a hypopigmented patch and a cafe-au-lait spot. Her mother exhibited multiple cafe-au-lait spots, Lisch nodules, axillary freckling, and neurofibromas.

  Congenital gingival granular cell tumor previously has not been reported in neurofibromatosis. Thus, further case reporting will be needed to determine if this tumor is associated with neurofibromatosis or if its occurrence in this patient was coincidental.

Method not stated [h]: linkage of gene with various polymorphic DNA markers
  Nelson et al., 1993

PD 269350 NIJMEGEN BREAKAGE SYNDROME (Microcephaly with normal intelligence, immunodeficiency, and lymphoreticular malignancies; Nonsyndromal microcephaly, autosomal recessive, with normal intelligence; Seemanova syndrome II) (McKusick No. 251260)

Chorionic villus sampling[g,i]: radioresistant DNA synthesis following ionizing radiation in cultured chorionic villi
  Jaspers et al., 1990
Method not stated[c,d]: intrauterine growth deficiency
  Der Kaloustian et al., 1996

PD 269500 PATERNITY DETERMINATION (McKusick No. None)

Amniocentesis: HLA typing of cultured amniotic fluid cells
    Pollack et al., 1980b; Roberts and Coleman, 1982; Nora et al., 1983
  chromosomal heteromorphisms: utilization of Q banding and brightly fluorescent region present on 13p arm
    Nora et al., 1983
  detection of a chromosomal rearrangement in the fetus that was previously present in a sibling but not in either the mother or the alleged father
    Hutton et al., 1985

restriction-fragment-length polymorphism disparity between mother and alleged father
                    Hutton et al., 1985
Chorionic villus sampling[g]: DNA testing using 5#AMPFLP systems
                    Strom et al., 1995

PD 269600 PELIZAEUS–MERBACHER DISEASE (McKusick No. 312080)

Disease Note: Pelizaeus–Merbacher disease is an X-linked recessive disorder of myelination. The disease normally begins during infancy and is slowly progressive with affecteds surviving normally to adolescence or young adulthood. Features include pendular eye movements, head shaking, hypotonia, choreoathetosis, ataxia, spasticity, involuntary movements, abnormal pyramidal signs, and microcephaly. The disease is produced by a mutation in the gene coding for myelin proteolipid protein which is a major component of myelin. The gene is located at Xp22.
                    Bridge et al., 1991; McKusick, 1995
Chorionic villus sampling[g,i]: linkage to an intragenic polymorphic marker
                    Bridge et al., 1992
Comment: Bridge and associates (1992) reported a family were a female fetus was found not to carry the abnormal gene causing Pelizaeus–Merbacher disease.

PPD 269700 PLACENTAL INFARCTION SECONDARY TO PLACENTAL ABRUPTION (McKusick No. None)

Maternal blood drawing[c]: low serum levels of hCG
                    Seydel and Eglinton, 1995
Doppler flow studies[c,d]: absence of end-diastolic velocity in the umbilical cord but normal middle cerebral artery flow
                    Seydel and Eglinton, 1995
Comments: At 29 weeks, the fetus reported by Seydel and Eglinton (1995) was delivered. The placenta revealed 90% abruption. Other than for prematurity the child was normal and was sent home at age 6 weeks, physically and neurologically intact.

PD 270000 PLACENTA PREVIA (McKusick No. None)

Ultrasound: placenta covering the internal cervical os
                    Gottesfeld, 1978

PD 271000 PLACENTOMEGALY (McKusick No. None)

Ultrasound[d]: increased placental size, hydramnios
                    Quagliarello et al., 1978

PD 271025 PSEUDOXANTHOMA ELASTICUM (McKusick No. Unknown; see 177850, 177860, 264800, 264810)

Ultrasound: placental calcification that increased significant with increased gestational age, decline in growth velocity, IUGR,[d] no fetal growth during 36–38 weeks' gestation, oligohydramnios[d]
                    Jewel et al., 1993
Comments: In the pregnancy reported by Jewel and co-workers (1993), the mother had pseudoxanthoma elasticum, but the authors did not state

if the condition were one of the dominant or recessive forms. Nor was it stated if the resulting child were affected. The placenta was abnormal, and the authors suggested that the pregnancy problems were the result of abnormal placental vasculature secondary to the maternal condition.

PD 271040 RETINITIS PIGMENTOSA, X-LINKED 2 (Retinitis pigmentosa 2; RP2; X-linked retinitis pigmentosis 2; XLRP2) (McKusick No. 312600)

Disease Note: Retinitis pigmentosa is a progressive degenerative disease of the retina associated with loss of vision and other abnormalities. The condition is inherited with 84% being autosomal recessive, 10% being autosomal dominant, and 6% being X-linked recessive inheritance. Two genes located on the short arm of the X chromosome (Xp11.3-p11.4) have been linked to the X-linked form. The gene for retinitis pigmentosa, X-linked 2 (RPXL2) is located proximal to the marker, DXS7, while retinitis pigmentosa X-linked 3 (RPXL3) (PD 271045) is distal to DXS7, and close to ornithine transcarbamylase (OTC) gene.
> Mingarelli et al., 1992; McKusick, 1996

Amniocentesis[i]: linkage of the RPXL2 gene, and DXS5255 and TIMP loci
> Mingarelli et al., 1992

Chorionic villus sampling[g,i]: linkage of the RPXL2 gene with various DNA markers
> Paola Iampieri et al., 1994

PD 271045 RETINITIS PIGMENTOSA, X-LINKED 3 (Retinitis pigmentosa 3; RP3; X-linked retinitis pigmentosa 3; XLRP3) (McKusick No. 312610)

Disease Note: See Retinitis pigmentosa, X-linked 2 (PD 271040)
Chorionic villus sampling[g,i]: linkage of the RPXL3 gene and orithine transcarbamylase gene
> Mingarelli et al., 1992

linkage of the RPXl3 gene with various DNA markers
> Paola Iampieri et al., 1994

PD 271050 RETINOIC ACID EMBRYOPATHY (Isotretinoin embryopathy) (McKusick No. None; see 243440)

Condition Note: Administration of retinoids during embryogenesis will induce congenital birth defects in a high percentage of cases. Associated anomalies in this embryopathy include hydrocephaly, cerebellar vermis agenesis, microtia, low-set ears, and cardiac defects.
> Van Maldergem et al., 1992

Ultrasound[c,d]: hydrocephaly, congenital heart defect
> Van Maldergem et al., 1992

Comments: In the case published by Van Maldergem and associates (1992), the pregnancy was terminated. At autopsy, the fetus had a number of findings of the retinoic acid embryopathy.

PD 271075 SCHWARTZ–JAMPEL SYNDROME (Chondrodystrophic myotonia; Myotonic myopathy, dwarfism, chondrodystrophy, and ocular and facial abnormalities; Schwartz syndrome; Schwartz–Jampel–Aberfield syndrome) (McKusick No. 255800)

Syndrome Note: Schwartz–Jampel syndrome, an autosomal recessive disorder, has the following major features: myotonia, blepharophimosis, unusual ears, myopia, limited facial movements, microstomia, short stature with dystrophic epiphyseal cartilage, joint contractures, and pectus carinatum. The usual course of the disorder is the onset of progressive myotonia, muscle wasting, and orthopedic problems during infancy. In the other, rarer, form of the condition, onset of the myotonia and skeletal changes occurs in the prenatal or perinatal period.

Smith, 1982; McKusick, 1990; Hunziker et al., 1989

Prenatal Diagnosis: Decreased fetal movements in the at-risk fetus would be presumptive evidence for the diagnosis of this condition.

Differential Diagnosis: Other conditions with altered fetal movements should be considered (see Fetal movements decreased, restricted or absent in the Index).

Ultrasound[i]: decreased fetal movements, virtual absence of movements of the spine and head, scarce movement of the arms and legs, constant flexure of fingers with intermittent extension of the second and fifth digits

Hunziker et al., 1989

anterior bowing and shortening of the femora

Hunziker et al., 1989

PD 271090 SPINAL AND BULBAR MUSCULAR ATROPHY (Bulbospinal muscular atrophy, X-linked; Bulbospinal neuronopathy, X-linked recessive; Kennedy disease) (McKusick No. 313200)

Disease Note: Spinal and bulbar muscular atrophy, an X-linked recessive disorder, is characterized as a late-onset motor neuron disease with slowly progressive muscular weakness of proximal muscles, bulbar problems, and endocrinologic abnormalities including oligo- and azospermia, impotance, gynecomastia, elevated serum gonadotropic hormone levels, and diabetes mellitus. The condition is caused by an expansion of the trinucleotide repeat (CAG) in the first exon of the androgen receptor gene. Determining the number of CAG repeats can confirm the diagnosis.

McKusick, 1996; Yapijakis et al., 1996

Chorionic villus sampling[g,i]: increase number of CAG trinucleotides in at-risk fetuses

Yapijakis et al., 1996

PD 271100 SPINAL MUSCULAR ATROPHY, TYPE I (Amyotonia congenita; Oppenheim disease; Werdnig–Hoffmann disease) (McKusick No. 253300)

Disease Note: The spinal muscular atrophies (SMA) are characterized by progressive weakness without intellectual deterioration, and in most cases, death with time. The weakness is caused by loss of anterior horn cells. Various mechanisms of inheritance occur: autosomal dominant, autosomal recessive, and X-linked dominant. The autosomal recessive, forms are subdivided into SMA type I, type II, and type III with type I having the earliest onset and being the most progressive in the condition's downhill course, while type III (Kugelberg–Welander type) has the latest onset, and the least rapid course. The gene producing all three types of the autosomal recessive forms is the survival motor neuron (SMN) gene located at 5q13. In SMA, type I, onset of the disease may be prenatally or during infancy with death in the neonatal period to the second year of life.

McKusick, 1997

Prenatal Diagnosis: Determination that the fetus probably has the gene has been accomplished by linkage analysis in at-risk fetuses.

Amniography[c,d]: absence of fetal swallowing, hydramnios
White and Steward, 1973
Chorionic villus sampling[g,i]: linkage of the disease gene (SMN) with various DNA markers
Lo Cicero et al., 1994; Matilla et al., 1994; Wirth et al., 1995
Maternal history[c,d]: diminished fetal movements
Kirkinen et al., 1994
Ultrasound[c,d]: no limb movements, elbows and knees fixed in flexion
Kirkinen et al., 1994

PD 271105 SPINAL MUSCULAR ATROPHY, TYPE II (SMA II; Spinal muscular atrophy, infantile chronic form; Spinal muscular atrophy, intermediate type) (McKusick No. 253550)

Disease Note: The spinal muscular atrophies (SMA) are characterized by progressive weakness, no intellectual deterioration, and with time, death. The weakness is caused by loss of anterior horn cells. The autosomal recessive form of SMA is divided into SMA type I, type II, and type III with type II being intermediated between type I which has the earliest onset and is the most rapidly progressive, and type III which has the latest onset and the slow progression. Type II characteristically has onset between 3 and 15 months, and survival is normally beyond 4 years, usually into adolescence or later ages. Affected children seldom walk unaided. The gene producing all three forms of the autosomal recessive types is the survival motor neuron (SMN) gene located at 5q13.
Shagina et al., 1995; McKusick, 1996
Amniocentesis[i]: linkage of the SMN gene with DNA marker
Shagina et al., 1995
Chorionic villus sampling[g,i]: linkage of the SMN gene with various DNA markers
Wirth et al., 1995

PD 271110 SPINAL MUSCULAR ATROPHY, TYPE III
(Kugelberg–Welander syndrome; Muscular atrophy, juvenile; SMA III; Spinal muscular atrophy, mild childhood and adolescent form) (McKusick No. 253400)

Disease Note: Spinal muscular atrophy, type III, has the latest onset and the slowest progression of the SMAs (type I, II, and III). Onset of muscular weakness is usually between 2 and 17 years of age. Proximal muscles are affected first with distal involvement later. Most children learn to walk, and they may survive into the third decade. Intelligence normally is not affected. The gene that results in all three types of SMA is the survival motor neuron gene located at 5q13.
McKusick, 1996
Chorionic villus sampling[g,i]: linkage of SMN gene with various DNA markers
Wirth et al., 1995

PD 271125 STUCK-TWIN PHENOMENON (McKusick No. None)

Condition Note: The stuck-twin phenomenon refers to the situation where one of the twins is "stuck" against the uterine wall because of a combination of oligohydramnios in the affected twin and hydramnios in the cotwin. The condition is not uncommon, occurring in 8% of all twin pregnancies and 35% of monochorionic diamnionic gestations. However, the disorder may be found in dichorionic monozygotic twin as well as dizygotic twin pregnancies. Many but not all cases appear to be associated with the twin transfusion syndrome (PD 115500). Untreated, the situation has a poor prognosis with survival rates for both twins being less than 20%. Premature labor often occurs secondary to uterine distension.

Numerous treatment modalities have been attempted with varying success. Wax and colleagues (1991) have hypothesized that this condition develops when the hydramniotic sac produces increased pressure on the placenta of the stuck twin, resulting in decreased placental and fetal blood flow and oligohydramnios.

Mahony et al., 1990

Prenatal Diagnosis: The diagnosis is made when one of the twins has oligohydramnios, and appears to be fixed in position against the uterine wall, and the cotwin has hydramnios. Zygosity of the twins is not a crucial factor in establishing diagnosis.

Prenatal Treatment: Serial amniocenteses to remove excessive amniotic fluid in the twin with the hydramnios has greatly increased the survival rates in one series (Mahony et al., 1990). This approach appears to be the preferred method of treatment. Treatment is repeated when fluid accumulation becomes moderate to severe (Mahony et al., 1990).

Treatment Modalities: Serial amniocenteses to remove excess amniotic fluid

Mahony et al., 1990

Single amniocentesis to remove excess fluid from the fetus with the hydramnios

Wax et al., 1991

Comments: In this case a single therapeutic amniocentesis was all that was required to correct the disparity between the amniotic fluid volumes of the twins. After birth the diagnosis of twin-to-twin transfusion was established by demonstrating a large-caliber arteriovenous anastomosis in the placenta (Wax et al., 1991)

Methods and Findings: Ultrasound: The stuck twin found to remain relatively fixed in position adjacent to the uterine wall even though there were changes in the maternal position.

Mahony et al., 1990; Wax et al., 1991

severe oligohydramnios in sac of one twin in a diamniotic pregnancy

Mahony et al., 1990; Wax et al., 1991

moderate to severe hydramnios in sac of one twin in a diamniotic pregnancy

Mahony et al., 1990; Wax et al, 1991

increased renal cortical echogenicity in one twin (stuck twin)

Mahony et al., 1990

ascites

Wax et al., 1991

PD 271250 SUBCHORIONIC FIBRIN DEPOSITION, PLACENTAL
(McKusick No. None)

Ultrasound[c]: subchorionic sonolucent lesions in the placenta

Spirt et al., 1987

PD 271500 SUCCENTURIATE LOBE, PLACENTA (Accessory lobe, placenta) (McKusick No. None)

Ultrasound: presence of extra placental tissue or adjacent lobes

Spirt et al., 1981; Spirt et al., 1987

PD 271540 SUPERFETATION TWINNING (Twinning due to superfetation) (McKusick No. 191250)

Condition Note: Superfetation arises as a result of a second ovulation and implantation of a second pregnancy after initiation of an initial pregnancy. The process leads to fraternal twins. In addition to all of the other problems associated with twin pregnancies, there may be significant disparity of size between the twins because one twin may be considerably older than the other. Superfecundation is the more or less simultaneous fertilization of two ova by sperm from different males.

McKusick, 1996

Ultrasound, transvaginal[g]; one intrauterine gestation sac with embryonic echo and embryonic heartbeat at 7 weeks of gestation, twin pregnancies with marked discordant size one month later, disparity in size throughout the pregnancy

Okamura et al., 1992

Comments: Okamura and associates (1992) reported the above cases as superfecundation. We have chosen to use superfetation because it appears that there were at least 2 weeks between fertilization, and presumably the father was the same for both children. The pregnancy resulted in normal and healthy boys at birth, who had no problems during infancy.

PD 271560 THREATEND ABORTION (McKusick No. None)

Condition Note: A threatened abortion is one where the pregnancy is threatened to be lost as indicated by a bloody discharge from the uterus, and sometimes by softening and dilatation of the cervix. The pregnancy may be aborted or it may go to full term without fetal abnormalities.

Ultrasound[g]: crown–rump length smaller than normal for gestational age

Mantoni and Pederson, 1982

PD 271600 TUBEROUS SCLEROSIS (McKusick No. 191100)

Doppler ultrasound[d,i]: increased peak pulmonary artery velocity

Chitayat et al., 1988

Echocardiography[i]: single or multiple rhabdomyomata present in the fetal heart

Crawford et al., 1983; Journel et al., 1986; Platt et al., 1987

Magnetic resonance imaging[d]: hyperdense, well-defined periventricular nodules, and cortical signals suggesting tubers

Werner et al., 1994

Comments: At autopsy of the fetus reported by Werner and co-workers (1994), there were multiple lesions present in the brain that were not seen on MRI, including subependymal nodules, subcortical tubers, and infiltration of the white matter.

Ultrasound: cleft lip[c]

McGillivray et al., 1987; Chitayat et al., 1988

cleft palate[c]

McGillivray et al., 1987; Chitayat et al., 1988

multiple cardiac rhabdomyomata[d,i]

McGillivray et al., 1987; Chitayat et al., 1988

Comments: In the pregnancy reported on by McGillivray and co-workers (1987), at 19 weeks' gestation there were angulation deformities of the lumbar vertebrae that were diagnosed after birth to be hemivertebrae. At 26 weeks, cleft lip and palate were recognized, and finally, at 36 weeks multiple rhabdomyomata of the heart were observed. Hemivertebrae and cleft lip and palate are not usual features of tuberous sclerosis.

narrowing of the right ventricular outflow tract[d,i]
>Chitayat et al., 1988

solid echogenic masses in the right and left ventricles[c,d]
>Schaffer et al., 1986

cardiac tumors
>Werner et al., 1994

angulation deformities of the lumbar vertebrae[c]
>McGillivray et al., 1987

PD 271630 UMBILICAL CORD, TRUE KNOT (True knot) (McKusick No. None)

Condition Note: A true knot of the umbilical cord is seen in 1% of deliveries and in those where there are true knots the mortality rate is 6%.

Ultrasound[d]: cloverleaf pattern of the umbilical cord, tachycardia, decreased heart rate following a oxytocin stress test
>Collins, 1991

PD 271700 UMBILICAL CORD ABNORMALITIES (McKusick No. None)

Condition Note: Abnormalities of the umbilical cord include developmental defects or abnormal position of the umbilical cord.
>Read et al., 1982b

Acetylcholinesterase[c]: presence of fast-migrating amniotic fluid isozyme on gel electrophoresis
>Read et al., 1982b

Alpha-fetoprotein[c]: elevated in amniotic fluid and maternal serum
>Read et al., 1982b

PD 271800 UMBILICAL CORD HEMATOMA (McKusick No. None)

Condition Note: Umbilical cord hematomas are rare complications of pregnancy and amniocentesis, and represent bleeding into the umbilical cord. The incidence of hematomas of the umbilical cord following third trimester amniocentesis is approximately 0.7%. In spontaneous cases, the incidence varies from 1 in 5500 to 1 in 12,699. Bleeding may be from either the umbilical vein or artery (less common). Perinatal mortality in spontaneously arising cord hematomas is about 50%. In cases of umbilical cord lacerations during amniocentesis, ultrasonography immediately following the laceration may show blood spurting from the puncture site (Romero et al., 1982a).

Hematomas of the umbilical cord may also occur as a complication of umbilical vein blood transfusion for a variety of disorders. Keckstein and associates (1990) have reported this complication in 3 of 49 ultrasound-guided transfusions, and in all cases, the bleeding resulted from unexpected movements of the mother or fetus that dislodged the needle from the umbilical vein.
>Sutro et al., 1984; Romero et al., 1988, pp. 396–397

Prenatal Diagnosis: The diagnosis should be suspected whenever there is a thickened and hyperechogenic lesion involving the umbilical cord, particularly if there has been fetal death.

Differential Diagnosis: Hemangioma, umbilical cord (PD 275500); Umbilical cord teratoma; Umbilical cord stricture (PD 271950); Umbilical cord thrombosis (PD 271970)

Ultrasound: 6×8 cm sonolucent, septated intrauterine mass adjacent to the fetal abdomen[d]

Ruvinsky et al., 1981

markedly thickened, sausage-shaped, and extremely echogenic umbilical cord

Sutro et al., 1984

Comments: In the case reported by Sutro and colleagues (1984), the umbilical cord hematoma developed following an amniocentesis at 25 weeks of gestation. The fetus was later found to have trisomy 18. Fetal demise was documented 3 days after the amniocentesis.

hyperechogenic area in the umbilical cord following blood transfusion[d]

Keckstein et al., 1990

bradycardia[d]

Keckstein et al., 1990

fetal demise[d]

Ruvinsky et al., 1981; Sutro et al., 1984

PD 271900 UMBILICAL CORD LACERATION (McKusick No. None)

Ultrasound[d]: intermittent spurts of blood coming from the umbilical cord following a bloody amniocentesis, fetal bradycardia

Romero et al., 1982a

PD 271950 UMBILICAL CORD STRICTURE (McKusick No. None)

Ultrasound[c]: cystic masses present in the posterior neck and spine, collapsed skull

Shenker et al., 1981

PD 271960 UMBILICAL CORD ULCERATION–INTESTINAL ATRESIA ASSOCIATION (McKusick No. None)

Condition Note: An association between umbilical cord ulceration that sometimes is associated with umbilical artery bleeding and intestinal atresia has been reported (Bendon et al., 1991). The mechanism(s) producing these ulcerations and the atresias is unknown.

Prenatal Diagnosis: Not established; the diagnosis should be considered any time there is found substantial blood in the amniotic fluid and the blood is determined to be of fetal origin.

Differential Diagnosis: Hemangioma, umbilical cord (PD 275500); Umbilical cord hematoma (PD 271800); Umbilical cord laceration (PD 271900); Umbilical vein thrombosis (PD 271970)

Amniocentesis[c,d]: bloody amniotic fluid

Bendon et al., 1991

Artificial rupture of fetal membranes[c,d]: bloody amniotic fluid

Bendon et al., 1991

Ultrasound[c,d]: fetal bradycardia followed by fetal demise

Bendon et al., 1991

bowel atresia
>Bendon et al., 1991
hydramnios
>Bendon et al., 1991
>*Comments*: Pathologic findings of the umbilical cord following delivery of the three cases reported by Bendon and associates (1991) included multiple small blood clots along a portion of the umbilical cord, one or more linear umbilical cord ulcerations that exposed a necrotic appearing umbilical artery, blood clots attached to the umbilical arteries, and brown staining of the umbilical cord. All neonates also had intestinal atresia involving different segments of the small intestine.

PD 271970 UMBILICAL VEIN THROMBOSIS (McKusick No. None)

Condition Note: Complete thrombosis of the umbilical vein is a lethal condition for the fetus. Because there is normally only one umbilical vein, thrombosis of the vein prevents placental blood returning to the fetus. As a result, the fetus becomes hypotensive and hypoxic, and dies. When partial thrombotic obstruction occurs, more blood will be pumped into the placenta than is returned to the fetus, resulting in reduced fetal blood volume and increased placental pressure. The latter may lead to fetomaternal hemorrhage. Therefore, anytime there is an unexplained fetal death, a Kleihauer–Betke test should be done on maternal blood to determine if fetomaternal bleeding has occurred. Thrombosis of the umbilical vein has been associated with compression, torsion, trauma, and hematoma of the umbilical cord.
>Hoag, 1986

Prenatal Diagnosis: No definitive method of diagnosis has been reported. Doppler ultrasound studies may be able to show reduced flow in situations of partial obstruction of the umbilical vein or lack of flow in complete obstruction.

Differential Diagnosis: Umbilical cord hematoma (PD 271800); Umbilical cord stricture (PD 271950)

Electrocardiogram[c,d]: fetal bradycardia
>Hoag, 1986
>*Comments*: In the case reported by Hoag (1986), the Kleihauer–Betke test indicated a fetal bleed of approximately 185 mL into the maternal circulation.

Maternal history: decreased fetal movement as perceived by the mother[c,d]
>Hoag, 1986

Maternal nipple stimulation (contraction stress) test[c,d]: variable and late decelerations of the fetal heart
>Hoag, 1986

Ultrasound[d]: echogenic material within the umbilical vein consistent with thrombus, fetal ascites, anasarca
>Abrams et al., 1985a
>no cardiac motion or other signs of life, fetal demise
>>Abrams et al., 1985a; Kristiansen and Nielsen, 1985

PD 271980 VALPROIC ACID EMBRYOPATHY (McKusick No. Unknown; see 311250)

Ultrasound: hydrocephalus
>Palumbos and Stierman, 1989

absence of radius bilaterally, shortened forearm, absent thumb, radial deviation of the hands
> Langer et al., 1994

PD 271990 VANISHING TWIN (McKusick No. None)

Condition Note: The phenomenon of the vanishing twin has been well documented, and the published literature on this topic has been summarized by Sulak and Dodson (1986). From ultrasound studies of first-trimester pregnancies, it would appear that multiple pregnancy rate as indicated by the presence of two or more gestational sacs is not an uncommon occurrence, varying between two and 11% (Sulak and Dodson, 1986). If these pregnancies are evaluated later on or at term, the majority of them have converted to singleton pregnancies, and a normal child is delivered at the appropriate time. The disappearance rate varies depending on the time of ascertainment, with a rate of 71% if the multiple pregnancy were observed before 10 weeks, and 62% if detected between 10 and 15 weeks of gestation. The phenomenon appears to be uncommon after 15 weeks of gestation. The etiology of the vanishing twin is unknown.

Prenatal Diagnosis: Ultrasonographic documentation of the loss of one or more gestational sacs during the first 15 weeks of gestation and survival of one or more cotwins (Sulak and Dodson, 1986) are the basic criteria for the diagnosis of this condition. There also should be documentation of fetal heart motion in two or more separate gestational sacs with a subsequent scan revealing one viable fetus (Landy et al., 1986)

Ultrasound[g]: detection of triplet gestational sacs by 6 weeks, and reduction to a singleton pregnancy by 18 weeks of gestation
> Sulak and Dodson, 1986

presence of two or more gestational sacs
> Landy et al., 1986; Sulak and Dodson, 1986

presence of fetal heart motion in two or more sacs with subsequence loss of one sac, or delivery of one less viable fetus than the number of originally visualized sacs
> Landy et al., 1986

PD 272005 WIEDEMANN–RAUTENSTRAUCH SYNDROME (Neonatal progeroid syndrome; Progeroid syndrome, neonatal) (McKusick No. 264090)

Syndrome Note: The Wiedemann–Rautenstrauch syndrome is a progeroid-like syndrome with onset in the prenatal period. Striking features of this condition including generalized absence of subcutaneous fat, but with paradoxical accumulation of fat in the buttocks, anogenital area, and the flanks. Other features include macrocephaly; sparse scalp hair, eyebrows and eyelashes; ectropion; beaking of the nose; severe growth deficiency of prenatal onset; and mental retardation. Inheritance is autosomal recessive.
> McKusick, 1995

Prenatal Diagnosis: Probably growth deficiency of any type is sufficient for making the diagnosis in the at-risk fetus. Otherwise, there is no direct method for establishing the diagnosis.

Differential Diagnosis: See Intrauterine growth retardation in the Index.

Alpha-fetoprotein[c]: elevated in maternal serum but normal in amniotic fluid
> Hagadorn et al., 1990

Ultrasound: macrocephaly[c]
>McKusick, 1995
>>biparietal and abdominal diameters at the 5th percentile while the femoral length was at the 50th percentile[c]
>>Castineyra et al., 1992
>>biparietal diameter below the 5th percentile, the abdominal diameter between the 3rd and 5th percentile, and the femoral length at the 50th percentile[i]
>>Castineyra et al., 1992
>>oligohydramnios[i]
>>>Hagadorn et al., 1990; Castineyra et al., 1992
>>intrauterine growth retardation[c,d]
>>>Hagadorn et al., 1990

PD 272010 XX MALE (XX male syndrome; XX sex reversal) (McKusick No. 278850)

Condition Note: The XX male is characterized by a normal male phenotype in an individual who has a normal female chromosomal complement (46,XX). The male phenotype is usually the result of the SRY (sex-determining region Y) gene of the Y chromosome being translocated to the X chromosome or an autosome. The translocation may be submicroscopic and its presence detectable only by FISH, or other Y-chromosome probes.
>McKusick, 1994; Olney et al., 1995

Prenatal Diagnosis: The condition should be suspected when there is disparity between the ultrasonic appearance of the external genitalia (male) and the sex chromosome makeup (46,XX) of the fetus. The definity diagnosis is established when the SRY region is shown to be translocated to an X chromosome or an autosome.

Differential Diagnosis: Any of the forms of Congenital adrenal hyperplasia (PD 240950, PD 241000)

Alpha-fetoprotein[c]: low level in maternal serum
>Rao and Atkin, 1988

Amniocentesis[d]: positive SRY gene and the pseudo-autosomal boundary sequence normally located on th p arm of the Y-chromosome as determined by PCR and appropriate probes run on amniotic fluid cell DNA
>Olney et al., 1995
>demonstration of the SRY gene on the distal tip of an Xp by FISH
>Olney et al., 1995
>>*Comments:* In the fetus reported by Olney and associates (1995), a chorionic villus sample showed normal female sex chromosomes (XX). Ultrasound evaluation at 29 weeks' gestation indicated normal male external genital. Amniotic fluid 17-hydroxyprogesterone level was normal. After birth the neonate was physically a male completely normal including normal external male genitalia.

Ultrasound[d]: male appearing genitalia in the light of a normal female chromosomal constitution
>Olney et al., 1995

Chapter 8

Tumors and Cysts[a]

PD 272030 ALLANTOIC CYST (McKusick No. None)

Differential Diagnosis: Omphalocele (PD 144000); Trisomy 18 syndrome (PD 104000)

Ultrasound[c]: cystic umbilical cord mass located several centimeters distal to the umbilicus, omphalocele

Sachs et al., 1982; Fink and Filly, 1983

PD 272050 ARACHNOID CYST (Intracranial arachnoid cyst) (McKusick No. None)

Condition Note: Arachnoid cysts are fluid-filled cavities within the brain or spinal cord that are partly or completely lined by arachnoid membrane. They may be either primary, in which case they are thought to be developmental abnormalities, or secondary as a result of trauma, meningitis, infarction, or bleeding. Arachnoid cysts can be found anywhere in the central nervous system (CNS). Most are asymptomatic and found only at autopsy, whereas others, depending on their size and location, may compress the ventricular system and produce hydrocephalus, or they may lead to mild sensory or motor abnormalities and/or seizures.

Romero et al., 1988, pp. 71–73

Prenatal Diagnosis: Arachnoid cysts, as seen on ultrasound, appear as fluid-filled structures normally located inside the skull. It may be impossible to differentiate these cysts from other intracranial cystic structures. There is no definitive method of diagnosis.

Differential Diagnosis: Aqueductal stenosis (PD 118250) produces an enlargement of the third ventricle, which is oval in shape with posteriorly tapering edges. Agenesis of the corpus callosum (PD 119700) may result in enlargement of the third ventricle, which is higher in location and at the level of the lateral ventricles, and in ventricular atria. Porencephalic cysts (PD 128750) are often associated with ventriculomegaly, and a shift in the midline. Brain tumors are normally found in the brain substance, whereas Arachnoid cysts (PD 272050, PD 272080) most often lie between the skull and brain surface. Other conditions that need to be considered include Dandy–Walker syndrome (PD 121000) and Cystic hygromas (PD 273000).

Diakoumakis et al., 1986; Romero et al., 1988, p. 72

Ultrasound[c,d]: irregular cystic structure in the midline of the brain, hydrocephalus
> Chervenak et al., 1983b
>
> echo-spared area at the level of the midline of the brain in association with hydrocephalus
> Romero et al., 1988, p. 72

PD 272080 ARACHNOID CYST, SUPRASELLAR (McKusick No. None)

Condition Note: Suprasellar arachnoid cysts are arachnoid cysts located in the suprasellar region. If large enough, they may cause obstruction of the foramen of Monro, displacement of the aqueduct posteriorly, and blockage of the basal cisterns. Hydrocephalus frequently develops.
> Diakoumakis et al., 1986

Prenatal Diagnosis: The condition should be considered whenever there is a cystic lesion located in the suprasellar region.

Differential Diagnosis: See Arachnoid cyst (PD 272050)

Ultrasound[d]: rounded midline cystic structure localized in the suprasellar region, enlargement of cyst over 3-week period, hydrocephalus, hydramnios
> Diakoumakis et al., 1986

PD 272100 CAVERNOUS HEMANGIOLYMPHANGIOMA (McKusick No. None)

Condition Note: Cavernous hemangiolymphangioma is a benign tumor composed of both vascular and lymphatic elements. These tumors have the propensity to invade underlying tissues, and to recur locally, features that are not common with pure hemangiomas or lymphangiomas.
> Giacolone et al., 1993

Ultrasound[c,d]: large heterogeneous cystic and solid multiloculated mass located in the posterior abdominal wall
> Giacalone et al., 1993

PD 272120 CHORIOANGIOMA, PLACENTA (Chorioangioma; Hemangioma, placenta; Placental chorioangioma; Placental hemangioma) (McKusick No. None)

Condition Note: Placental chorioangiomas are benign hemangiomas that develop from chorionic mesenchyme. Large clinically significant chorioangiomas are present in 1 in 1000 and 1 in 20,000 births; smaller ones occur as frequently as 1 in 72 placentas examined microscopically. The tumors may range in size from less than 1 cm to greater than 11 cm in diameter. Of clinical significance, there may be shunting of fetal arterial blood through the tumor, leading to decreased oxygenation of fetal blood. If the shunting is great enough, intrauterine growth retardation (IUGR) or even fetal death may occur.
> Rodan and Bean, 1983; Moeschler et al., 1985

Prenatal Diagnosis: Ultrasonographic or amniographic detection of a mass that is attached to the placenta is suggestive of the condition. This tumor should be sought whenever there is an unexplained elevation of the amniotic fluid alpha-fetoprotein (AFP).

Alpha-fetoprotein[c]: elevated in amniotic fluid
> Schnittger et al., 1980; Moeschler et al., 1985

elevated in maternal serum
>Schnittger et al., 1980; Moeschler et al., 1985

Amniography[c]: tumor-like mass identified that appeared to be connected to the umbilical cord; at birth the tumor was found to be located on the placental surface and connected to the umbilical cord
>Schnittger et al., 1980

Ultrasound: cystic area on the fetal surface of the placenta, hydramnios
>Asokan et al., 1978; Spirt et al., 1980; Liang et al., 1982; Quinlan et al., 1983

placental mass that enlarged throughout gestation
>Moeschler et al., 1985

10-cm well-circumscribed solid mass that was contiguous with the placenta[h], fetal demise[h]
>Rodan and Bean, 1983

>*Comments*: The tumor in the above case was in juxtaposition to the attachment of the umbilical cord. Compression of the cord by the tumor was thought to be related to formation of umbilical vessel thromboses, which were found at autopsy and were thought to be the cause of the fetal demise.

hydramnios
>Sweet et al., 1973

PD 272250 CHOROID PLEXUS CYST (Cyst of the choroid plexus) (McKusick No. None)

Condition Note: Cysts of the choroid plexus are relatively common, and have been found in as many as 50% of autopsied brains. They arise from neuroepithelial folds within the choroid plexus. Those that have been discovered during the second trimester frequently regress and have completely disappeared by birth. Choroid plexus cysts are not normally associated with neurologic problems (Romero et al., 1988, pp. 76–77).

In one prospective study, 1 out of 10 fetuses with a choroid plexus cyst had trisomy 18 (Camurri and Ventura, 1989). In another study of 588 infants born at 34 weeks of gestation or less, and below 1.5 kg, 10 (1.7%) were found to have a choroid plexus cyst. None of these ten infants had associated multiple congenital and/or chromosomal abnormalities (Chitayat et al., 1989a). In another series, these cysts measured up to 1.2 cm in diameter but averaged 0.7 cm (Ostlere et al., 1989). Zerres and co-workers (1992) found choroid plexus cysts in 25 of 823 fetuses who also had other congenital anomalies or growth retardation of these 25 cases, five had chromosomal anomalies {four with trisomy 18, one with 46,XX,+t(21;21)}. Six other fetuses who had normal chromosomal constitution had other physical defects.

Prenatal Diagnosis: The detection of a round hypoechogenic cyst inside the choroid plexus, usually located at the level of the atrium of the lateral ventricle, is sufficient to make the diagnosis.

Differential Diagnosis: Papilloma of choroid plexus (PD 278500); Down syndrome (PD 101000); Trisomy 18 syndrome (PD 104000); Subependymal hemorrhages

Ultrasound: cystic structure found within the choroid plexus of the posterior horn of the lateral ventricle
>Campbell and Pearce, 1983; Chudleigh et al., 1984; Farhood et

al., 1987b; Furness, 1987; Camurri and Ventura, 1989; Ostlere et
al., 1989

Comments: Most choroid plexus cysts that are detected between 15 and
20 weeks of gestation are normal variations and have no pathologic significance, particularly if no other fetal abnormalities are noted (Furness, 1987;
Ostlere et al., 1989).

PD 272380 CONGENITAL BRONCHIAL CYST (Bronchiogenic cyst)
(McKusick No. None)

Condition Note: A congenital bronchial cyst is an intrathoracic cystic structure
lined by bronchial epithelium and probably develops by an abnormal budding
of a lung bud from the foregut of the embryo. These cysts may be single or
multiple, and although usually found in the mediastinum, they may be found
elsewhere in the thoracic cavity, pericardium, neck, and other locations.
Reece et al., 1987; Romero et al., 1988, p. 206
Prenatal Diagnosis: The abnormality should be considered whenever there is a
hypoechogenic mass in the intrathoracic area.
Differential Diagnosis: Cystic adenomatoid malformation of lung (PD 272500);
Diaphragmatic cysts of the mediastinum; Diaphragmatic hernia (PD 132000);
Sequestration of lung (PD 193750); Teratoma (lung, PD 281750); Teratoma,
mediastinum (PD 271770); other solid tumors and cysts of the mediastinum
(Romero et al., 1988, p. 206)
Ultrasound[c]: echo-spared mass in right lung
Mayden et al., 1984
unilocular, single, or multiple cysts located intrathoracically
Reece et al., 1987; Romero et al., 1988, p 206
hydrops fetalis
Reece et al., 1987

PD 272400 CONGENITAL GENERALIZED CYSTIC
LYMPHANGIOMATOSIS (McKusick No. None)

Ultrasound: cystic structures of the thoracic wall, pelvis, and lower extremities
that increased in size with time, no movement of the lower extremities[c]
Haeusler et al., 1990

PD 272440 CONGENITAL THORACIC GASTROENTERIC CYST
(Duplication cyst of the foregut; Enteric cyst; Foregut cyst; Intrathoracic cyst;
Reduplication cyst of the alimentary tract) (McKusick No. None)

Ultrasound[d]: tubular, nonpulsatile, and loculated cyst separated by thick septa
and present in the posterior thorax
Hobbins et al., 1979; Newnham et al., 1984

PD 272460 CRANIOPHARYNGIOMA (McKusick No. None)

Magnetic resonance imaging (MRI)[d]: large, slightly heterogeneous mass in
the region of the fetal third ventricle; dilation of the lateral ventricles
Bailey et al., 1990
Ultrasound[d]: 4-cm midline mass near the base of the fetal skull, hydrocepha-
lus, hydramnios
Bailey et al., 1990

PD 272470 CUTANEOUS VASCULAR HAMARTOMATOSIS (Cutaneous widespread vascular hamartomatosis) (McKusick No. None)

Condition Note: A single male fetus was reported by Arienzo and associates (1987) with unusual cutaneous tumors located on the trunk and limbs. Microscopic study of the tumors revealed capillary-like vessels with cavernous dilatation and congestion. The pathologic diagnosis was cutaneous vascular hamartomatosis.

Prenatal Diagnosis: None established.

Differential Diagnosis: Blue rubber bleb nevus syndrome; Cavernous hemangiomas of various locations; Hemangioma, cavernous, of the face (PD 274880); Hemangioma, hepatic, cavernous (PD 274930); Klippel–Trenaunay–Weber syndrome (PD 191530); Maffucci syndrome; Sturge–Weber syndrome

Ultrasound[c]: numerous echo-free subcutaneous–cutaneous masses protruding from the thorax and back ranging in size up to 10 cm, scalp edema, hydramnios

Arienzo et al., 1987

PD 272500 CYSTIC ADENOMATOID MALFORMATION OF LUNG (Adenomatoid hamartoma; Congenital cystic adenomatoid malformation) (McKusick No. None)

Condition Note: Cystic adenomatoid malformation of the lung (CAML) is an intrathoracic hamartoma composed of solid and cystic elements. The condition appears to result from abnormal differentiation of ramifying bronchial buds leading to overgrowth of bronchioles that do not communicate to either alveolar ducts or sacs. The macrocystic type of CAML is noted by lesions containing single or multiple cysts of at least 5 mm in diameter, whereas the microcystic type contains predominantly solid tissue with cysts generally smaller than 5 mm in diameter. The condition is almost always unilobular and is present equally frequently in either lung. If untreated prenatally, these cysts may increase in size to fill the whole hemithorax, and to cause mediastinal shift with compression of the contralateral lung (Nicolaides and Azar, 1990). Associated problems included hydramnios thought to be secondary to esophageal obstruction or excessive fluid produced by the lungs, and hydrops fetalis (25–30% of cases). If untreated prenatally, the condition usually presents in the neonatal period with severe, often fatal, respiratory insufficiency. Prognostic signs for poor outcome after prenatal thoracoamniotic shunting include the presence of (1) associated malformations, (2) bilateral rather than unilateral pleural effusion, and (3) hydrops fetalis and/or hydramnios that did not resolve within 1–3 weeks following shunting (Nicolaides and Azar, 1990).

Nicolaides et al., 1987; Reece et al., 1987; Romero et al., 1988, pp. 198–201

Prenatal Diagnosis: Diagnosis of this condition relies on the demonstration of a nonpulsatile intrathoracic lung tumor that may be cystic or solid in appearance, and often is associated with hydramnios or hydrops fetalis. Diagnosis usually is established postnatally after lobe resection or at autopsy.

Reece et al., 1987; Romero et al., 1988, p. 200

Differential Diagnosis: Congenital bronchial cyst (PD 272380); Diaphragmatic hernia (PD 132000); Hamartoma of the lung; Sequestration of lung (PD 193750); Teratoma, lung (PD 281750); Teratoma, mediastinum (PD 281770)

Prenatal Treatment: The condition has been successfully treated prenatally by placement of a thoracoamniotic shunt into the cyst and removal of the cyst by fetal surgery at 20–32 weeks of gestation. Within 3 weeks of the procedure, the fetal ascites, pleural and pericardial effusions, and hydrops fetalis had resolved in the case reported by Clark and associates (1987). The fetus was born healthy at 37 weeks' gestation. In the case cited by Nicolaides and co-workers (1987), the cyst reduced in size after shunting and the fetus was delivered healthy and in no respiratory distress. However, the cyst reexpanded and the lower lobe of the left lung containing the cyst was removed surgically. In two other cases the cystic adenomatoid malformation was removed surgically at 23 and 27 weeks' of gestation. In the first case, the pregnancy continued to 31 weeks' gestation and the infant did well postnatally. The second fetus was delivered at 28 weeks and died shortly thereafter of respiratory insufficiency (Harrison et al., 1990b). Other cases have been reported (Nicolaides and Azar, 1990).

Treatment Modalities: Thoracoamniotic shunt
> Clark et al., 1987; Nicolaides et al., 1987; Blott et al., 1988b; Nicolaides and Azar, 1990

Fetal surgery with removal of cyst
> Harrison et al., 1990b

Methods and Findings: Alpha-fetoprotein[c]: elevated level in maternal serum
> Albright and Katz, 1989

Ultrasound: scalp edema[c]
> Clark et al., 1987

echo-free cyst located in fetal lung
> Cohen et al., 1983; Mayden et al., 1984; Nicolaides and Azar, 1990

intrathoracic, unilocular cyst
> Clark et al., 1987; Nicolaides et al., 1987; Blott et al., 1988b; Nicolaides and Azar, 1990

echogenic material filling region of the lung or chest
> Johnson et al., 1984a; Reece et al., 1987; Harrison et al., 1990b

unilateral echogenic mass in the thorax
> Albright and Katz, 1989; Harrison et al., 1990b

echodense mass with small peripheral cysts filling one side of the chest[d]
> Reece et al., 1987

multiple large cysts present in the chest[d]
> Romero et al., 1988, p. 200; Harrison et al., 1990b

enlargement of the cyst with time, then reduction in size
> Berry et al., 1995

hydrothorax[c,d]
> Reece et al., 1987

dextroposition of the heart[d]
> Johnson et al., 1984a; Reece et al., 1987; Blott et al., 1988b; Romero et al., 1988, p. 200

mediastinal shift and compression of the lung[c]
> Nicolaides et al., 1987; Blott et al., 1988b; Harrison et al., 1990b; Nicolaides and Azar, 1990l

lateral and posterior displacement of the heart[c]
> Albright and Katz, 1989

mediastinal shift
> Kousseff et al., 1995

flattening of the left hemidiaphragm[c]
    Harrison et al., 1990b
fetal ascites[c]
    Johnson et al., 1984a; Clark et al., 1987; Albright and Katz, 1989;
    Harrison et al., 1990b
enlarged liver[c]
    Albright and Katz, 1989
hydramnios[c,d]
    Johnson et al., 1984a; Reece et al., 1989; Harrison et al., 1990b;
    Kousseff et al., 1995
hydrops fetalis[c]
    Clark et al., 1987; Harrison et al., 1990b; Berry et al., 1995; Kous-
    seff et al., 1995; LeChien and Thomas, 1995
placentomegaly[c]
    Harrison et al., 1990b

PD 273000 CYSTIC HYGROMA (Abdominal cystic hygroma; Cystic
lymphangioma; Lymphangiectasia; Hygroma colli; Nuchal cyst; Nuchal cystic
hygroma; Nuchal lymphangiectasia) (McKusick No. Unknown; see 257350)

Condition Note: Cystic hygromas are developmental tumors of the lymphatic
system, and as such are lymphangiomas. The lymphatic system arises from five
primitive sacs that normally develop connections between themselves as well as
the venous system into which the lymphatic fluid usually drains. Failure to
establish these connections leads to the formation of cystic hygromas that can
be located in the neck, axilla, mediastinum, retroperitoneum, abdominal viscera,
groin, scrotum, or bone. On examination of these structures, the hygromas are
typically multilobular, multicystic masses that vary in size, and are filled with
serous fluid. Microscopically, the cyst walls contain a single layer of epithelium.

Serial ultrasonic evaluations should be performed on a fetus who has a cystic
hygroma. If the cystic structure becomes enlarged or if hydrops fetalis develops,
the prognosis for the fetus is poor. The fetus should be examined for evidence of
pleural and pericardial effusions, ascites, and skin edema (Kozlowski et al., 1988).

The most common cystic hygroma encountered is located in the nuchal area
and, most often is a multiseptated, fluid-filled sac arising from the posterior
aspect of the fetal neck. It is thought that cystic hygromas of the neck occur as
a result of failure of the jugular lymphatic sac, which normally drains the trunk
and left upper extremity, to develop normal connections with the venous system
in the neck. Posterior neck cystic hygromas are frequently found in Turner
syndrome (PD 105000), but also may be seen in Down syndrome (PD 101000),
Giant cystic hygroma of the neck (PD 274250), Hydrops fetalis (PD 265750),
Lethal multiple pterygium syndrome (PD 191550), Lethal multiple pterygium
syndrome, X-linked recessive type (PD 191800), Lethal multiple pterygium syndrome with spinal fusions (PD 191650), Meckel syndrome (PD 192140), Noonan
syndrome (PD 192750), Smith–Lemli–Opitz syndrome (PD 194160), Translocation chromosome 5;7 (PD 101780), Trisomy 18 syndrome (PD 104000), and
Trisomy 22 syndrome (PD 104500). They may also be present as an isolated
finding. When a posterior cystic hygroma of the neck (as well as other cystic
hygromas) is identified, evaluation should include a careful ultrasound assessment of the entire fetus to detect associated anomalies, and a fetal karyotype
(Palumbos et al., 1987; Kozlowski et al., 1988; Shulman et al., 1993).

The general prognosis for the fetus discovered with a nuchal cystic hygroma is not good. In the presentation of 22 fetuses and in a review of the literature on cystic hygromas of the nuchal area, Abramowicz and associates (1989) found that 73% had abnormal karyotypes. Of the affected fetuses who were not terminated, the survival rate was only 2–3%. On the other hand, in some fetuses the cystic hygromas have disappeared with time and the resulting child is totally normal (Baccichetti et al., 1990). In another series of 55 consecutive cases of isolated nuchal cystic hygroma (no concurrent structural anomalies), Shulman and co-workers (1993) found if septation of the cysts were present that there was a higher risk of chromosomal abnormalities (17 of 31 [54.89%] as opposed to 3 of 24 [12.5%]). Among the 35 chromosomally normal cases, 22 women elected to continue their pregnancies. In this latter group, 21 of the fetuses has resolution of their cystic hygroma by the 20th gestational week. Follow-up of all 22 infants showed them to be normal in development and structure except for a single case who had persistence of the cystic hygroma and neck webbing. **Prenatal Diagnosis:** The ultrasonic presence of a thin-walled, multiseptated, frequently asymmetrical fluid-filled mass should raise the possibility of this condition.

Differential Diagnosis: Cystic hygromas need to be distinguished from Encephaloceles (PD 122000); the latter usually do not have well-developed septa, and are associated with skull defects. Singular or multiple large hemangiomas such as found in Klippel–Trenaunay–Weber syndrome (PD 191530) may at times be confused with cystic hygromas. Furthermore, because a number of conditions are associated with nuchal cystic hygroma, as noted above, these specific disorders should be considered.

Abdominal Cystic Hygroma

Condition Note: Abdominal cystic hygromas are uncommon and may be associated with edema of the leg.

Ultrasound: initially, at 19 weeks of gestation, presence of a unilobular hypoechogenic mass that arose from the left pelvis and soft tissue, enlargement of the left leg that contained several hypoechogenic areas, later (22 weeks of gestation) enlarged multilobular retroperitoneal mass, displacement of the left kidney, multiloculated mass arising from the medial aspect of the left thigh
Kozlowski et al., 1988

Neck or Nuchal Cystic Hygroma

Acetylcholinesterase[c]: fast-migrating amniotic fluid isozyme on gel electrophoresis, elevated in amniotic fluid
Voigtlander et al., 1981; Crandall et al., 1982; Crandall and Matsumoto, 1984b; Raymond and Simpson, 1988
Alpha-fetoprotein[c]: elevated in amniotic fluid
Morgan et al., 1975; Voigtlander et al., 1981; Chervenak et al., 1983c; Crandall and Matsumoto, 1984b
Comments: Elevated AFP and the presence of the acetylcholinesterase isozyme may occur with the aspiration of cystic hygroma fluid rather than amniotic fluid.
Amniography[c]: soft tissue defect in the occipital region
Morgan et al., 1975; Balsam and Weiss, 1981

Ultrasound: external fluid-filled or complex cystic mass in the posterior neck region

> Morgan et al., 1975; Adam et al., 1979; Hobbins et al., 1979; O'Brien et al., 1980b; Young et al., 1980; Hill et al., 1983a; Nevin et al., 1983a; Dallapiccola et al., 1984; Redford et al., 1984

posterior cystic neck lesions with or without midline septa or other incomplete septa, or multiseptated, fluid-filled sac with or without hydrops fetalis; normal fetal skull; oligohydramnios,[c] hydramnios,[c] or a normal amniotic fluid volume[c]; frequently, Turner syndrome is present in these fetuses

> O'Brien et al., 1980b; Young et al., 1980; Chervenak et al., 1983c; Gustavii and Edvall, 1984; Carrasco et al., 1985; Marchese et al., 1985a; Rutledge et al., 1986; Palumbos et al., 1987

symmetrical, smooth-walled, echo-free cystic structure in the nuchal region detected at 12th week of gestation[g]

> Gustavii and Edvall, 1984

small, echo-reflecting cystic formation with no internal trabeculae in the occipital region

> Baccichetti et al., 1990

> Comments: The fetus reported by Baccichetti and co-workers (1990) had resolution of the cystic hygroma that was discovered at 13 weeks' gestation. At 20 weeks, the amniotic fluid cell karyotype was normal. After birth the child was also found to be normal.

cystic lesion that lies between the scapula and the lateral aspect of the occiput

> Fiske and Filly, 1982

reduced crown-to-rump length[c,g]

> Tchobroutsky et al., 1985

hydrops fetalis

> Chiba et al., 1990

PD 273500 ENTERIC DUPLICATION CYST OF THE SMALL INTESTINE (McKusick No. None)

Ultrasound[c]: large anterior abdominal cyst that was separate from the bladder

> Spirt et al., 1987

PD 274000 FETAL OVARIAN CYST (Congenital ovarian cyst; includes Serous ovarian cyst; Theca-lutein cyst) (McKusick No. None)

Condition Note: A fetal ovarian cyst is a rare fetal condition of unknown etiology. As a group these cysts are probably the most common cause of abdominal masses in female neonates. Most cases are not associated with other anomalies although there is an increased incidence of hydramnios and juvenile-onset hypothyroidism. The former finding may be related to prenatal compression of the intestines.

> Rizzo et al., 1989

Prenatal Diagnosis: The diagnosis should be considered anytime a cystic mass is present in the fetal lower abdomen, there is normal gastrointestinal and urinary tract anatomy, and the fetus is female. In the majority of cases, the cyst is entirely fluid-filled with well-demarcated borders; occasionally internal septae are seen.

> Rizzo et al., 1989

Differential Diagnosis: Cystic teratoma; Enteric duplication cysts of the small intestine (PD 273500); McKusick–Kaufman syndrome (PD 192080); Mesenteric and Urachal cysts; Sacrococcygeal teratoma (PD 284000); Urethral obstruction malformation sequence (PD 180000)

Amniography[c,d]: displaced colon

Valenti et al., 1975

Ultrasound: lower abdominal cystic mass[d]

Valenti et al., 1975; Jafri et al., 1984; Holzgreve et al., 1985a; Rizzo et al., 1989

Comments: Rizzo and associates (1989) reported on a series of 14 abdominal cystic masses, of which 9 were confirmed postnatally to be ovarian cysts. In one of these cases, the cyst became highly hyperechogenic at 30 weeks, which was felt to be the result of torsion of the cyst with subsequent infarction. Of the nine histologically examined cases, both serous ovarian and theca-lutein cysts were seen. These types could not be distinguished prenatally. In one fetus reported by Jafri and colleagues (1984), the ovarian cyst was a simple follicular cyst lined by a simple squamous to cuboidal epithelium. In another, the cyst was a follicular cyst. Two of the three fetuses reported by Jafri and colleagues (1984) postnatally were found to have hypothyroidism.

two fluid-filled, septated masses in the lower abdomen adjacent to the urinary bladder

Jafri et al., 1984

hydramnios[c,d]

Valenti et al., 1975; Jafri et al., 1984; Holzgreve et al., 1985a; Rizzo et al., 1989

PD 274250 GIANT CYSTIC HYGROMA OF THE NECK (McKusick No. None)

Differential Diagnosis: Cystic hygroma (PD 273000); Hemangioma, cavernous, of the face (PD 274880); Teratoma, neck (PD 283000)

Ultrasound[c,d]: cystic hygroma in the front of the fetal neck containing two cysts, hydramnios

Lyngbye et al., 1986

Comments: At birth the infant reported by Lyngbye and co-workers (1986) had a very large cystic hygroma located primarily in the anterior neck region. The structure was large enough that the infant required intubation after birth. Subsequently, the cyst was reduced in size by surgical means, and the child was able to breathe on his own and had normal growth and development. The hydramnios presumably was secondary to esophageal compression by the cysts, preventing swallowing.

PD 274350 GLIOBLASTOMA MULTIFORME (Anaplastic astrocytoma; Spongioblastoma multiforme) (McKusick No. None)

Condition Note: A glioblastoma multiforme is a grade III or IV astrocytoma, and is usually a rapidly growing tumor confined to the cerebral hemispheres. This type of tumor is composed of a mixture of spongioblasts, astroblasts, and astrocytes. The prognosis for someone with this tumor is consistently poor.

Prenatal Diagnosis: Other than intrauterine tumor biopsy, there is no exact method of making this diagnosis prenatally. A brain tumor should be suspected when there is a combination of hydrocephalus, intracerebral mass, and hydramnios, however.

Differential Diagnosis: Other brain tumors and cysts such as a Teratoma of the brain (PD 281000); Arachnoid cyst (PD 272050); Arachnoid cyst, suprasellar (PD 272080); Choroid plexus cyst (PD 272250); and Posterior fossa cyst (PD 279000); Intracerebral hemorrhage

Ultrasound[c,d]: huge, brightly echogenic mass that largely replaced the right cerebral hemisphere, midline structures of the brain shifted to the left, right lateral ventricle indented by the mass, hydramnios
>Geraghty et al., 1989

Comments: The fetal condition report by Geraghty and associates (1989) was recognized at 33 weeks of gestation. One week later there was central necrosis of the tumor with further dilation of the left lateral ventricle. Labor was induced shortly thereafter, and an infant with an enlarged head (44.6 cm) was delivered who died immediately after birth. A glioblastoma multiforme was found to occupy most of the right cerebral hemisphere.

macrocephaly
>Alvarez et al., 1987; Geraghty et al., 1989

large complex mass with areas of increased echogenicity and echolucency. The mass occupied approximately two-thirds of the intracranial area.
>Alvarez et al., 1987

biparietal diameter and head circumference increased
>Alvarez et al., 1987

falx deviated to one side of the head
>Alvarez et al., 1987

unilateral ventriculomegaly
>Alvarez et al., 1987; Geraghty et al., 1989

bilateral ventriculomegaly
>Alvarez et al., 1987

compression, distortion, and inferior placement of the cerebellar hemispheres
>Alvarez et al., 1987

PD 274500 GOITER (McKusick No. Unknown; see 138800)

Ultrasound[d]: cystic/solid mass in the anterior fetal neck that contained large pulsatile vessels, hydramnios[c]
>Weiner et al., 1980a

PD 274540 HAMARTOMA, CHEST WALL (McKusick No. None)

Ultrasound[c,d]: echogenically heterogeneous mass with hyperechogenic areas located in the upper pole of the left hemithorax
>D'Ercole et al., 1994

dextropositioned heart
>D'Ercole et al., 1994

pleural effusion
>D'Ercole et al., 1994

PD 274580 HEMANGIOENDOTHELIOMA, METASTATIC (McKusick No. None)

Condition Note: All hemangiomas have some recognizable vascular elements. A hemangioendothelioma is a hemangioma with a striking overgrowth of endothelial cells. These types of hemangiomas are rare, usually benign, and when present, most commonly occur in the liver. Most regress spontaneously with no significant residual effect.

Morris and Hertel, 1989

Prenatal Diagnosis: Diagnosis of this tumor has not been made prenatally, and most likely would require an in utero biopsy.

Differential Diagnosis: Other cystic tumors should be included in the differential of a cystic mass, including Congenital bronchial cyst (PD 272380); Cutaneous vascular hamartomatosis (PD 272470); Cystic adenomatoid malformation of the lung (PD 272500); Cystic hygroma (PD 273000); Giant cystic hygroma of the neck (PD 274250); Hemangioendothelioma, neck (PD 274600); Hemangioma, atrium (PD 274750); Hemangioma, cavernous, of the face (PD 274880); Hemangioma, neck (PD 275000); Mesenchymal hamartoma of the liver (PD 276620); Neuroblastoma of the neck with metastatic spread (PD 277500); Neuroblastoma, thoracic (PD 277750); Teratoma, brain (PD 281000); Teratoma, lung (PD 281750); Teratoma, neck (PD 283000); and Teratoma, sacrococcygeal (PD 284000)

Physical examination of the mother[c,d]: inappropriate increase in the fundal height for gestation

Morris and Hertel, 1989

Ultrasound[c,d]: massive hydrops fetalis, diffuse soft tissue calcifications

Morris and Hertel, 1989

Comments: The fetus reported by Morris and Hertel (1989) at autopsy had widespread malignant vascular neoplasm involving the retroperitoneal area, mediastinum, chest and abdominal wall, diaphragm, esophagus, stomach, and bones, particularly the long bones of the lower extremities.

PD 274600 HEMANGIOENDOTHELIOMA, NECK (McKusick No. None)

Condition Note: In all hemangiomas there is some recognizable vascular element. In hemangiomas of the hemangioendothelial type, the vascular component is present as well as a striking overgrowth of endothelial cells.

Prenatal Diagnosis: A hemangioma should be considered in any mass arising from the neck of the fetus. However, a posterior nuchal mass, particularly if it is echogenic, will more likely be a cystic hygroma. There is no specific prenatal method for differentiating hemangiomas from other tumors of the neck or hemangioendotheliomas from other types of hemangiomas short of a tumor biopsy and histologic evaluation.

Differential Diagnosis: Cystic hygroma (PD 273000); Giant cystic hygroma of the neck (PD 274250); Hemangioma, neck (PD 275000); Teratoma, neck (PD 283000)

Doppler ultrasound[c]: nuchal mass demonstrated arterial and venous pulsations

McGahan and Schneider, 1986

Ultrasound[c]: large, well-demarcated echogenic mass arising from the posterior aspect of the fetal neck and extending down over the back

McGahan and Schneider, 1986

hydrops fetalis, heart enlargement,[d] pericardial effusion,[d] ascites[d]

McGahan and Schneider, 1986

Comments: The fetus reported on by McGahan and Schneider (1986) was delivered at 28 weeks because his condition deteriorated. He died from high-output failure on the third day following birth. An autopsy showed the tumor to have a prominence of multiple vascular channels lined with a large number of endothelial cells. These findings were consistent with a hemangioendothelioma.

PD 274750 HEMANGIOMA, ATRIUM (McKusick No. None; see 140800)

Condition Note: Primary cardiac tumors are rare in fetuses, infants, and children. When present, they are most often benign rhabdomyomas either with or without association of Tuberous sclerosis (PD 271600), teratomas, and fibromas. Atrial hemangiomas are rarely seen, and when recognized may be successfully resected after birth.

> Leithiser et al., 1986

Prenatal Diagnosis: An atrial hemangioma should be considered whenever a cardiac mass is detected in the fetus. However, at this time there is no definitive method of prenatal diagnosis of this tumor.

Differential Diagnosis: Other cardiac tumors should be considered in the differential diagnosis, including fibromas; Rhabdomyoma, heart (PD 280500); and teratomas.

> Ultrasound[c,d]: hydrops fetalis, scalp edema, pulsatile liver, hyperdynamic cardiac contractions
> > Platt et al., 1981
> pericardial effusion
> > Platt et al., 1981; Leithiser et al., 1986
> lobulated pericardial mass arising from the right atrial wall
> > Leithiser et al., 1986
> ascites
> > Platt et al., 1981; Leithiser et al., 1986

PD 274880 HEMANGIOMA, CAVERNOUS, OF THE FACE (Cavernous hemangioma) (McKusick No. None; see 140850)

Condition Note: Hemangiomas are among the most common tumors of childhood. Most involve the skin, appear before the age of 6 months, and after an initial rapid growth, regress, disappearing by 5 or 6 years of age. Most hemangiomas are benign but can cause life-threatening situations or grotesque deformities if located in vital areas or they become excessively large. Cavernous hemangiomas are characterized by widely dilated nonseptated vascular spaces lined by flat endothelial cells and supported by fibrous tissue. Because thrombi may form within the vascular lumina, platelet trapping, thrombocytopenia, hypofibrinogenemia, and hemolysis may occur. Calcification within the tumor may be present. Hemangiomas are rarely encountered in the fetus.

> Meizner et al., 1985

Prenatal Diagnosis: The diagnosis should be suspected whenever a solid facial or cervical tumor is detected by ultrasound, especially if there are very small and widely scattered calcifications giving rise to a homogeneous echogenic pattern.

Differential Diagnosis: Branchial cleft cyst; Cystic hygroma (PD 273000); Encephalocele (PD 122000); Goiter (PD 274500); Hydrops fetalis (PD 265750); Mesenchymal sarcoma; Teratoma, hypopharyngeal (PD 281500); Teratoma, neck (PD 283000); Teratoma, pharyngeal (PD 283500); Thyroglossal duct cyst

> Meizner et al., 1985

> Ultrasound[d]: round, multiple internal homogeneous echogenic regions

protruding from the cheek just below the zygomatic arch, puffiness of eyelids, widely opened mouth, no swallowing movements, hydramnios
>Meizner et al., 1985

Comments: In the case reported by Meizner and co-authors (1985), the multiple internal homogeneous echogenic areas were believed to be produced from the multiple calcified areas within the tumor. No explanation of the hydramnios or the subsequent death of the fetus was established.

spherical soft tissue mass located anterior to the left ear which was moderately hyperechoic and had a hyperechoic rim and small internal hypoechoic spaces placed peripherally in a spoke-wheel configuration, tiny pulsations within hypoechoic spaces, increase in size with gestational age
>Pennell and Baltarowich, 1986

PD 274910 HEMANGIOMA, HEPATIC (Hemangioma, liver) (McKusick No. None)

Condition Note: Like most hemangiomas, hepatic hemangiomas are normally benign tumors that often spontaneously resolve during the first few years of life. Occasionally because of intratumor vascular shunting, high-output failure may occur which in turn may lead to hydrops fetalis, and fetal demise (see Hemangioma, hepatic, cavernous [PD 274930]).

Hemangioma is the most common of the benign hepatic tumors, but the diagnosis is rarely made either pre- or postnatally. The explanation for lack of diagnosis postnatally is related to the benign nature of the tumor, and the fact that the tumor normally regresses with time.
>Dreyfus et al., 1996

Pulse doppler ultrasound[a]: vascular tumor attached to the liver
>Dreyfus et al., 1996

Ultrasound[d]: complex mass attached to the left lobe of the liver, and composed of thick septa with disseminated peripheral calcification
>Dreyfus et al., 1996

PD 274930 HEMANGIOMA, HEPATIC, CAVERNOUS (Hemangiomas, liver, cavernous (McKusick No. None)

Condition Note: Cavernous hemangiomas of the liver are highly vascular tumors that if large enough may cause high-output cardiac failure. The failure in turn may cause hydrops fetalis, and ultimately fetal demise.
>Nakamoto et al., 1983

Auscultation[c,d]: absence of fetal heart tones
>Nakamoto et al., 1983

Maternal examination[c]: uterus large for gestational age
>Nakamoto et al., 1983

Ultrasound[c,d]: large hyperechogenic solid mass occupying most of the liver, ascites, hydrops fetalis, no fetal movement, no fetal heart beats, hydramnios
>Nakamoto et al., 1983

Comments: At autopsy, the fetus reported by Nakamoto and co-workers (1983) had multiple large vascular tumors occupying the liver. Cavernous hemangiomas were diagnosed by histologic examination. In addition, there were cardiomegaly with right atrial and ventricular dilation, and right and left ventricular hypertrophy, all of which indicated high-output cardiac failure.

PD 275000 HEMANGIOMA, NECK (McKusick No. None; see 140850)

Differential Diagnosis: Cystic hygroma (PD 273000); Giant cystic hygroma of the neck (PD 274250); Hemangioendothelioma, neck (PD 274600); Teratoma, neck (PD 283000)

    Radiograph[c,d]: hyperextended head, large neck mass, hydramnios
        Griscom, 1974

PD 275500 HEMANGIOMA, UMBILICAL CORD (McKusick No. None)

Condition Note: Hemangiomas of the umbilical cord and/or placentas have an incidence of about 1%. Because of shunting of blood that may occur within the tumor, maternal and fetal complications may occur. Whenever markedly elevated levels of amniotic fluid AFP are encountered with no obvious fetal defects, a hemangioma of the umbilical cord should be considered. The amniotic fluid AFP level was 151 standard deviations (SD) above the mean in one case (Morrone et al., 1988).

Prenatal Diagnosis: The finding of an umbilical cord mass through which the umbilical vessels pass is suggestive, but not diagnostic, of an umbilical cord hemangioma.

Differential Diagnosis: Chorioangioma, placenta (hemangioma of the placenta) (PD 272120); Umbilical cord abnormalities (PD 271700); Umbilical cord hematoma (PD 271800); Umbilical cord laceration (PD 271900)

    Acetylcholinesterase[c]: faintly positive, fast migrating amniotic fluid isoenzyme on gel electrophoresis
        Morrone et al., 1988
    Alpha-fetoprotein[c]: elevated in amniotic fluid
        Barson et al., 1980; Read et al., 1982b
      elevated in maternal serum
        Barson et al., 1980; Read et al., 1982
    Doppler flow analysis[c]: fetal blood flow through the mass that was attached to the umbilical cord
        Morrone et al., 1988
    Maternal physical examination[c,d]: vaginal bleeding several hours after spontaneous rupture of the fetal membranes, fetal distress
        Dombrowski et al., 1987

    Comments: In the case reported by Dombrowski and associates (1987), there was spontaneous and massive fetal hemorrhage from a ruptured umbilical hemangioma leading to severe fetal distress and depression. After delivery by an emergency cesarean section, blood was found to be oozing from an umbilical hematoma located approximately 3 cm from the abdominal insertion of the cord.

PD 275600 HEPATOBLASTOMA, FETAL TYPE (McKusick No. Undetermined; see 191170)

    Ultrasound[c]: discrete mass detected in the liver, hydramnios
        Terespolsky and Weksberg, 1995

    Comments: In the fetus cited by Terespolsky and Weksberg (1995), there was premature delivery at 31 weeks' gestation. She had a dysmorphic and coarse facies, hypertrichosis, depressed nasal bridge, anteverted nares and micrognathia; asymmetric right ventricular hypertrophy; and extensive hepatosplenomegaly. Subsequently, she developed symmetric biventricular hypertrophy, and had resection of the left lobe of the liver that contained a fetal type hepatoblastoma. The tumor recurred, and the infant subsequently died.

PD 276250 LACRIMAL DUCT CYST (Amniotocele; Benign dacryocystocele; Dacryocystocele; Mucocele) (McKusick No. None)

Condition Note: The nasolacrimal duct is formed from a fold of ectoderm that becomes buried in the subcutaneous tissue of the nasooptic fissure. The latter fissure lies between the maxillary and the lateral nasal processes. Canalization of the duct begins in the middle of the third intrauterine month and proceeds medially and caudally to both ends with the average age of patency of the entire duct being eight months of gestation. Nonpatency of the nasolacrimal duct later than this time usually results from a thin mucosal membrane obstructing the duct near the nasal end, resulting in a dacryocystocele located inferomedial to the orbit. The condition usually is benign, because the membrane normally ruptures spontaneously prior to or after birth. The main prenatal significance of the cyst is its possible confusion with other conditions.
> Davis et al., 1987

Prenatal Diagnosis: The condition should be suspected whenever a hypoechogenic mass is located medially and inferiorly to the eye.

Differential Diagnosis: Anterior encephalocele (PD 122000); Hemangioma cavernous, of the face (PD 274880); Teratoma, mouth (PD 282000)
> Davis et al., 1987

Ultrasound[d]: hypoechoic mass located medially and inferiorly to the eye, hydramnios
> Davis et al., 1987

PD 276300 LYMPHANGIOMA, AXILLARY (McKusick No. None)

Ultrasound[c,d]: septated cystic mass present in the left axilla and extending from the apex of the axilla down the chest wall to approximately the level of the xyphoid, humerus raised to and fixed in 90° abduction
> Kaufman et al., 1996

PD 276500 MECONIUM PSEUDOCYST (McKusick No. None)

Amniography[d]: faint calcification within the wall of an intraabdominal cyst
> McGahan and Hanson, 1983

Ultrasound[d]: large anechoic mass in the midabdomen, hydramnios[c]
> McGahan and Hanson, 1983

complex cystic mass with hyperechoic rim
> Spirt et al., 1987

PD 276580 MELANOMA (Congenital malignant melanoma; Congenital melanoma; Fetal malignant melanoma; Primary congenital malignant melanoma) (McKusick No. Unknown; see 155600)

Condition Note: As of 1987 there were seven reported cases of congenital malignant melanoma, three primary in the fetus and four secondary to maternal disease. In all seven cases, the infant died shortly after birth or during infancy; maternal death occurred only when the disease was primary in the mother.

Campbell et al., 1987; Schneiderman et al., 1987

Prenatal Diagnosis: There have been too few cases to establish diagnostic criteria.

Differential Diagnosis: Teratomas (PD 281000, PD 281200, PD 281500, PD 281750, PD 281770, PD 282000, PD 283000, PD 283500, PD 284000) and other tumors such as hemangiomas and hamartomas that are frequently localized to the surface of the fetus

Ultrasound[c,d]: complex solid and cystic mass present over the upper fetal spine that appeared to be growing around the vertebral bodies rather than originating from them, hydrocephalus with the lateral ventricular width/hemispheric width ratio being 0.79 (normal = 0.26–0.34), shortened femora, humeri, and tibiae, oligohydramnios.

Campbell et al., 1987; Schneiderman et al., 1987

Comments: The fetus reported by Campbell and associates (1987) and Schneiderman and co-workers (1987) was delivered at 33 weeks and died within minutes. On examination, there was a 14 × 10 cm darkly pigmented lobulated and cystic mass on the back extending from the midcervical region to the upper lumbar area. On histologic examination, the tumor was a malignant melanoma arising from a congenital nevus. There also were widespread metastases to the spinal and cerebellar meninges, lung, liver, and placenta.

PD 276620 MESENCHYMAL HAMARTOMA OF THE LIVER (McKusick No. None)

Condition Note: This tumor is one of several rare, pathologically distinctive mass lesions of the liver. It occurs almost exclusively in children and has no malignant potential. It may, however, be of a size to necessitate surgical resection.

Foucar et al., 1983

Maternal blood sampling[c,d]: elevated human chorionic gonadotropin (beta-subunit) in the maternal serum (117,557 mIU/mL; normal = 4,000–5,000 mIU/mL)

Foucar et al., 1983

Ultrasound[c,d]: large hypoechoic masses that appeared to replace the liver parenchyma, reduced biparietal diameter for fetal gestation, oligohydramnios, and markedly thickened placenta

Foucar et al., 1983

Comments: The fetus reported on by Foucar and associates (1983) was delivered as a stillborn at 34 weeks. The liver, which weighed 200 g, filled the abdomen and contained three large thin-walled cysts. The placenta had prominent dilation of vessels with multiple thromboses.

complex multicystic, well-circumscribed mass in fetal abdomen that contained echolucencies surrounded by multiple echodense membranes and appeared to arise inferiorly from the left lobe of the liver

Hirata et al., 1990

increased abdominal circumference

Hirata et al., 1990

hydramnios [c,d]

Hirata et al., 1990

PD 276750 MESOBLASTIC NEPHROMA (Leiomyomatous hamartoma; Mesenchymal hamartoma) (McKusick No. None)

Ultrasound[c,d]: solid mass in the region of the right renal bed
Giulian, 1984
solid renal mass in the lower part of the kidney with loss of normal architecture, distension of the superior minor calyx
Haddad et al., 1996
hydramnios
Giulian, 1984; Haddad et al., 1996

PD 277000 MOLAR PREGNANCY (Gestational trophoblastic disease; Hydatidiform mole) (McKusick No. 231090)

COMPLETE

Condition Note: Complete hydatidiform mole is produced by a conception with two sets of paternal chromosomes (androgenic). About 90% of complete moles are homozygous; that is, there are identical paired chromosomes, indicating development by duplication of a haploid set. The others represent dispermy with fertilization of an anucleate egg or loss of the female pronucleus prior to pronuclear fusion.
McKusick, 1995
Alpha-fetoprotein[c]: low level in maternal serum
Gardner et al., 1981; Davenport and Macri, 1983
Amniofetography: clusters of contrast medium
Noonan, 1974
Maternal blood sampling[c,g]: elevated levels of human chorionic gonadotropin (hCG) in the maternal serum
Zaragoza et al., 1995
Ultrasound[g]: uterus filled with multiple white spicules that were more dense at the area of implantation; no fetus, fetal heart, or fetal movement identified; uterus filled with multiple cystic structures
Gottesfeld, 1978; Wittmann et al., 1981b; Spirt et al., 1987
anechoic spaces within the placenta
Vejerslev et al., 1986
uterus filled with echogenic material with multiple sonolucent spaces
Spirt et al., 1987
increased placental mass
Vejerslev et al., 1986

PARTIAL

Condition Note: Partial hydatidiform mole is associated with triploidy which normally has arisen by fertilization of an egg by two sperm. The placentae in these situations are usually large with some areas of molar degeneration.
Ultrasound[c]: oligohydramnios
Herrmann and Sidiropoulos, 1988

PD 277450 NEUROBLASTOMA, ADRENAL (McKusick No. 256700)

Ultrasound[c,d]: mixed cystic and solid mass present in the superior aspect of the kidney in the adrenal gland region
Giulian et al., 1986

cystic or thinly septated cystic mass at the upper pole of the kidney
Dreyfus et al., 1994

PD 277500 NEUROBLASTOMA, NECK, WITH METASTATIC SPREAD
(McKusick No. 256700)

Ultrasound[c,d]: solid mass in the region of the neck, edema of the fetal scalp
and body, tachycardia, large placenta, hydramnios
Gadwood and Reynes, 1983
Comments: The fetus reported by Gadwood and Reynes (1983) was stillborn at 32 weeks. An autopsy showed widespread metastatic neuroblastoma.

PD 277750 NEUROBLASTOMA, THORACIC (McKusick No. 256700)

Ultrasound[c,d]: paraspinal mass with high-level peripheral echogenicity and
central hypoechogenicity, reduced circumference of the abdomen
de Filippi et al., 1986

PD 278000 NUCHAL BLEB, FAMILIAL (Cystic hygroma, familial) (McKusick No. 257350)

Alpha-fetoprotein (AFP)[c]: elevated in amniotic fluid
Bieber and Petres, 1978; Bieber et al., 1979
Amniography[i]: occipital and nuchal saccular structure, hydramnios, fetal
scalp edema
Bieber and Petres, 1978
Ultrasound[i]: occipital and nuchal saccular structure, ascites hydramnios
Bieber and Petres, 1978
cystic hydroma
Bieber and Petres, 1978; Watson et al., 1990a
hydrops fetalis
Bieber and Petres, 1978; Watson et al., 1990a

PD 278250 OMPHALOMESENTERIC DUCT CYST (Omphalomesenteric cyst) (McKusick No. None)

Condition Note: The omphalomesenteric duct is the embryonic communication
between the embryonic gut and the yolk sac. The duct is normally obliterated
by the 16th week of gestation. An omphalomesenteric duct cyst then results
from the persistence and dilatation of a segment of the omphalomesenteric duct.
When present, the cyst is usually located near the insertion of the umbilical cord
at the fetus. Normally, these cysts are benign, although they may be as large as
6 cm in diameter.
Rosenberg et al., 1986; Romero et al., 1988, pp. 391-392
Prenatal Diagnosis: No definitive method of diagnosing this specific condition
has been set forth. The condition should be considered any time there is a
hypoechogenic lesion in the umbilical cord.
Differential Diagnosis: Allantoic cyst (PD 270000); Hemangioma, umbilical cord
(PD 275500); Umbilical cord hematoma (PD 271800)
Doppler ultrasound[c]: no blood flow through the umbilical cord mass
Rosenberg et al., 1986

Ultrasound[c]: an echoic mass that was contained within the umbilical cord, no increase in size of cyst with time
>> Rosenberg et al., 1986

PD 278500 PAPILLOMA OF CHOROID PLEXUS (McKusick No. 260500)

Ultrasound[h]: mass projecting into lateral ventricle, hydrocephalus with ventricular enlargement
>> Sabbagha et al., 1981

PD 279000 POSTERIOR FOSSA CYST (McKusick No. None)

Prenatal Diagnosis: Presence of a cyst-like lesion in the posterior fossa is suggestive of a posterior fossa cyst.
Differential Diagnosis: Arachnoid cyst in the posterior fossa; Dandy–Walker cyst (PD 121000)
>> Ultrasound: posterior fossa cyst, enlarged fluid-filled lateral ventricles
>>> Lee and Newton, 1976; Hatjis et al., 1981a
>>> *Comments*: The exact types of cysts in the cases presented by Lee and Newton (1976) and Hatjis and colleagues (1981a) were not stated.

PD 280000 RENAL CYSTS, CALCIFIED (McKusick No. None)

Radiograph[d]
>> Russell, 1973

PD 280250 RETINOBLASTOMA (RB1) (McKusick No. 180200)

Procedure and time of testing not stated: linkage of the retinoblastoma gene Rb-1 with esterase D (EsD) gene/*Apal* and 9D11/*Mspl*
>> Buchanan et al., 1989
>> *Comments*: In the family reported on by Buchanan and associates (1989), a father and his son had both been affected with retinoblastoma. Linkage data indicated a recombination between EsD and 9D11 in the fetus with a probability of the fetus possessing the retinoblastoma gene being approximately 85%. The pregnancy was continued, and although the child had normal retinal findings at birth and at 3 weeks of age, a tumor had developed by 6 weeks. Subsequently, multiple bilateral tumors grew.

PD 280500 RHABDOMYOMA, HEART (McKusick No. None)

Auscultation[c,d]: short runs of tachycardia
>> Hoadley et al., 1986
Echocardiograph[c]: interventricular septal cardiac mass, fetal hydrops, hydramnios
>> DeVore et al., 1982a; Kleinman et al., 1982
>> masses in the apex of the left ventricle, interventricular septum, and ventricular outflow tract; premature atrial beats[d]
>> Hoadley et al., 1986
Ultrasound[d]: echogenic intracardiac masses, fetal tachycardia, hydrops fetalis, pleural effusion, ascites, hydramnios
>> Dennis et al., 1985

PD 280750 RHABDOMYOSARCOMA, EMBRYONAL (McKusick No. Unknown; see 268210, 268220)

Condition Note: Rhabdomyosarcomas are one of the most prevalent soft tissue tumors in children. These tumors are divided into alveolar, botryoid, embryonal, and pleomorphic subtypes, and may develop within or outside of muscle any-where in the body at any age. Embryonal rhabdomyosarcoma in general have the best prognosis of the subtypes, but all types have a generally poor prognosis when they occur before the age of 1 year.

> Steele et al., 1988; Hart et al., 1990

Prenatal Diagnosis: Any mass that is attached or associated with muscle should be considered a rhabdomyosarcoma until determined otherwise. Definite diagnosis may be made prenatally by fetal biopsy.

Ultrasound[c]: soft tissue mass attached to the left thigh and extending to the left calf; deformity of the left thigh, calf, and foot

> Steele et al., 1988; Hart et al., 1990

PD 280850 SEMINAL VESICULAR CYST (McKusick No. None)

Condition Note: The seminal vesicles are sacculated pouch-like structures attached to the posterior part of the urinary bladder. The duct from each seminal vesicle joins the ipsilateral ductus deferens to form the ejaculatory duct. Rarely, obstruction of seminal vesicle duct occurs, and leads to a seminal vesicular cyst.

> Hammadeh et al., 1994

Ultrasound[c]: cyst behind the bladder, hyperechogenic left kidney, ureterocele

> Hammadeh et al., 1994

> *Comments:* In the child reported by Hammadeh and co-workers (1994), there was no functioning left kidney after birth. By the age of 2 months, a left retrovesical cyst was found, and at 8 months was removed. The diagnosis was established by histologic examination of the cyst.

PD 281000 TERATOMA, BRAIN (Intracranial teratoma) (McKusick No. None)

Amniocentesis[c,d]: partial duplication and inversion of chromosome No. 1 (46,XX,inv dup(1)(qterq21::p35qter) in amniotic fluid cells

> Hecht et al., 1984

> *Comments:* In the postpartum period of the fetus reported by Hecht and associates (1984), a tumor was found that had a mosaic chromosome constitution. In half of the tumor cells, there was the same chromosomal abnormality as found in the amniotic fluid cells; in the other half there was a normal constitution. Skin fibroblasts from the child had a normal 46,XX chromosome make-up.

Computerized tomography (CT) scan[c,d]: no recognizable bone in the area of the left orbit, osseous defect involving the left lateral face

> Hecht et al., 1984

Radiograph[d]: enlargement of the fetal skull, extensive bony defect of the fetal skull, orbit, and frontal-parietal regions

> Vinters et al., 1982; Hecht et al., 1984

Ultrasound[d]: cystic solid area within the fetal head, increased biparietal diameter, distortion of facial features, hydramnios

> DeVore and Hobbins, 1979; Hoff and Mackay, 1980; Vinters et al., 1982; Crade, 1982; Hecht et al., 1984; Chervenak et al., 1985b
> large cystic lesion in the right parietal area that was 1.5–2 times the size of the fetal head
> Saul, 1982

hydrocephalus
> Chervenak et al., 1985b; Lipman et al., 1985

enlarged fetal head[c]
> Lipman et al., 1985

increased biparietal diameter
> Lipman et al., 1985

gross distortion of normal cerebral architecture, or no recognizable normal brain parenchyma
> Lipman et al., 1985

hyperechoic, multicystic mass
> Lipman et al., 1985

solid tumor involving the right temporal lobe and the posterior fossa, and extending through the skull into the neck
> Lipman et al., 1985

> *Comments:* In two of three fetuses reported by Lipman and associates (1985), ultrasonic evaluation during the second trimester revealed no abnormalities.

obliteration of the 3rd ventricle by a tumor mass
> Lipman et al., 1985

calcification present in the tumor mass as indicated by multiple areas of low-level echoes, and discrete hyperechoic densities with acoustic shadowing
> Lipman et al., 1985

enlarged lateral ventricles
> Lipman et al., 1985

hydrops fetalis
> Lipman et al., 1985

hydramnios[c]
> Lipman et al., 1985

PD 281200 TERATOMA, HEART (Intrapericardial teratoma) (McKusick No. None)

Ultrasound[d]: large pericardial effusion[c]; solid, heterogeneous mass about 2 cm in diameter that was present in the pericardial space and attached to the left part of the heart
> Alegre et al., 1990

Echocardiography[d]: abrupt movements of the right atrial wall that suggested slight cardiac tampanade[c]
> Alegre et al., 1990

PD 281500 TERATOMA, HYPOPHARYNGEAL (McKusick No. None)

Alpha-fetoprotein[c,d]: elevated in amniotic fluid
> Hashimoto et al., 1985

Ultrasound[c,d]: hydramnios
> Hashimoto et al., 1985

PD 281750 TERATOMA, LUNG (McKusick No. None)

Ultrasound[c,d]: fluid or fluid-containing structure present in one hemithorax, displacement of the heart, ascites
> Spirt et al., 1987

PD 281770 TERATOMA, MEDIASTINAL (Mediastinal teratoma) (McKusick No. None)

Condition Note: Mediastinal teratomas are uncommon, representing only 7% of all germ-cell tumors in childhood. Approximately 10% of teratomas are found in the mediastinal area. When these tumors are present in newborns, they may cause respiratory distress. Mediastinal teratomas are malignant in about 15% of cases.

Weinraub et al., 1989

Prenatal Diagnosis: A mediastinal teratoma should be suspected whenever a mass is present in the mediastinum, particularly if it is a mixed cystic and solid structure.

Differential Diagnosis: Congenital bronchial cyst (PD 272380); Cystic adenomatoid malformation of lung (PD 272500); Diaphragmatic hernia (PD 132000); Hamartoma, chest wall (PD 274540); Hamartoma of the lung; Sequestration of lung (PD 193750); Teratoma, lung (PD 281750)

Ultrasound[c,d]: multilocular cystic tumor in the anterosuperior mediastinum, hydrops fetalis, hydrops placentae, ascites, pleural effusion, hypoplastic lungs, hydramnios

Weinraub et al., 1989

Comments: In the fetus reported on by Weinraub and associates (1989), fetal demise occurred at about 30 weeks of gestation. An autopsy found a 4.5 × 3.5 × 3.8 cm teratoma in the anterior superior part of the mediastinum extending cranially to the upper part of the thyroid. The authors speculated that the hydrops fetalis resulted from compression of venous return.

PD 282000 TERATOMA, MOUTH (Epignathus; Teratoma, oropharynx) (McKusick No. None)

Acetylcholinesterase[c]: fast-migrating isozyme present in amniotic fluid
Smart et al., 1990

Alpha-fetoprotein[c]: elevated in amniotic fluid
Burck et al., 1981; Smart et al., 1990

Radiograph[c]: displacement of the mandible
Saul, 1982

Ultrasound: solid cystic mass originating from the mouth, calcified area within the mass, hydramnios[c,d]
Kang et al., 1978; Burck et al., 1981; Saul, 1982; Chervenak et al., 1985b

complex mass with large cystic component anterior to fetal face
Spirt et al., 1987

mass protruding from the face involving the right orbital and nasal regions
Smart et al., 1990

hydramnios[c]
Smart et al., 1990

PD 283000 TERATOMA, NECK (McKusick No. None)

Differential Diagnosis: Cystic hygroma (PD 273000); Giant cystic hygroma of the neck (PD 274250); Hemangioma, cavernous, of the face (PD 274880); Teratoma of the thyroid (PD 284500); Teratoma of the pharynx (PD 283500)

Ultrasound: displacement of the fetal head associated with a large cervical mass, hydramnios

> Schoenfeld et al., 1978; Patel et al., 1982; Spirt et al., 1987

cyst-like structure on the right side of the neck

> Hill et al., 1988a

Comment: The fetus reported on by Hill and associates (1988a) also had trisomy 20 mosaicism in amniotic fluid cells.

PD 283500 TERATOMA, PHARYNGEAL (McKusick No. None)

Alpha-fetoprotein[c,d]: elevated in amniotic fluid

> Anderson et al., 1984

Comment: Teratomas of the oropharynx should be considered in the differential diagnosis of unexplained elevation of amniotic fluid AFP.

Ultrasound[c,d]: hydramnios

> Anderson et al., 1984

PD 284000 TERATOMA, SACROCOCCYGEAL (McKusick No. None)

Acetylcholinesterase[c]: presence of fast-migrating amniotic fluid isozyme on gel electrophoresis

> Hecht et al., 1982; Holzgreve et al., 1984; Holzgreve et al., 1985b

Alpha-fetoprotein[c]: elevated in amniotic fluid

> Verma et al., 1979; Holzgreve et al., 1984; Holzgreve et al., 1985b

Comment: Amniotic fluid AFP levels have been found to be normal in other reported cases (Holzgreve et al., 1985b; Sherowsky et al., 1985; Szabo et al., 1985a).

elevated in maternal serum

> Hecht et al., 1982; Brock et al., 1983a

Amniography: soft tissue mass with a smooth encapsulated outline

> Verma et al., 1979; Balsam and Weiss, 1981

Maternal history[c,d]: decreased fetal movement

> Spahr et al., 1980

Ultrasound: soft tissue mass attached to the lower pole of the fetal spine (sacrococcygeal region) in an otherwise normal fetal spine; the mass may be partly cystic; hydramnios[c]

> DeVore and Hobbins, 1979; Verma et al., 1979; Balsam and Weiss, 1981; Hecht et al., 1982; Brock et al., 1983a; Hill et al., 1983a; Holzgreve et al., 1984; Holzgreve et al. 1985b; Sherowsky et al., 1985; Szabo et al., 1985a; Spirt et al., 1987; Hill et al., 1988

large complex mass posterior to sacrum

> Spirt et al., 1987

a tumor mass protruding into the pelvis and abdomen with displacement of the abdominal wall ventrally and the viscera and diaphragm cranially, hypoplastic lungs[c]

> Holzgreve et al., 1985b

hydronephrosis,[c] hydroureter,[c] dilated bowel[c]

> Chervenak et al., 1985b

ascites[c]

> Spirt et al., 1987

hydramnios[c,d]

> Spahr et al., 1980

PD 284500 TERATOMA, THYROID (McKusick No. None)

Ultrasound[c]: pleural effusion
    Nicolaides and Azar, 1990
hydrops fetalis
    Nicolaides and Azar, 1990
hydramnios
    Nicolaides and Azar, 1990
    Comments: The case reported by Nicolaides and Azar (1990) had pleural effusion which was treated by a pleuroamniotic shunt at 33 weeks of gestation. The fetus was delivered at 34 weeks and survived.

PD 284700 TERATOMA, TONGUE (Lingual teratoma) (McKusick No. None)

Ultrasound[c]: anterior neck mass which almost doubled in size from 19 to 29 weeks gestation, marked fetal head deflexion, hydramnios
    Kuller et al., 1995
    Comments: Following delivery by cesarean section at 29 weeks, the neonate reported by Kuller and associates (1995) required a tracheostomy because of oral airway obstruction by the teratoma. The teratoma subsequently was removed surgically. It was attached to the base of the tongue.

PD 285000 TUMOR, LUNG (McKusick No. None)

Differential Diagnosis: Congenital bronchial cyst (PD 272380); Cystic adenomatoid malformation of lung (PD 272500); Diaphragmatic hernia (PD 132000); Hamartoma of the lung; Sequestration of lung (PD 193750); Teratoma, mediastinum (PD 281770)

Ultrasound[d]: cystic fluid-filled areas within the lung, enlarged lung, displaced heart, fetal ascites, hydrops fetalis, hydramnios
    Garrett et al., 1975a

PD 287000 TUMOR, THYROID (McKusick No. Unknown; see 188550)

Radiograph[c,d]
    Russell, 1973

PD 295000 VON HIPPEL–LINDAU SYNDROME (von Hippel–Lindau disease) (McKusick No. 193300)

Syndrome Note: von Hippel–Lindau syndrome is an autosomal dominant cancer syndrome with variable expression. Features include retinal, cerebellar and spinal hemangiomas and hemangioblastomas; renal cell carcinoma; pheochromocytoma; other hemangiomas; hypertension; renal cysts; and other problems related to the function and location of the tumors. The gene, mutations in which cause this disorder, is located at 3p26-p25. A number of different types of mutations located in various locations within the gene have been identified.
    Payne et al., 1992, McKusick, 1996
Chorionic villus sampling[g,i]: linkage of the gene with various DNA polymorphic markers
    Payne et al., 1992

Chapter 9

Multiple Congenital Anomalies of Unknown Etiology—Single Case Reports

Chapter Note: In this chapter, there are included single case reports where the fetuses/neonates have multiple congenital anomalies of unknown etiology, and where a syndrome name has not been assigned. The name of each entry is based on one or more (normally three) prominent features of the case. Entries are listed in alphabetical order of the first feature.

PD 300125 AGNATHIA–HEART BLOCK–SITUS INVERSUS (McKusick No. None)

Condition Note: Abdulla and Charters (1975) reported hydramnios in a pregnancy where the fetus had bradycardia (56 beats/min). At birth the neonate was found to have a cleft of both the upper and lower lips, cleft palate, absence of the mandible, severe microstomia and microglossia, low-set left ear, complete absence of the right ear and auditory canal, complete atrial-ventricular dissociation (3rd degree heart block), dextrocardia, ventricular septal defect, agenesis of the right lung, only partial division of the left lung, complete situs inversus of the abdominal viscera with incomplete rotation of the gut and partial failure of fixation of the colon. The neonate died shortly after birth. The central nervous system was normal. Chromosomal studies also were normal.

Amniogram[c,d]: absence of contrast medium in the fetal gut
Abdulla and Charters, 1975
Ultrasound [c,d]: bradycardia, hydramnios
Abdulla and Charters, 1975

PD 300250 AMELIA–ENCEPHALOCELE–OMPHALOCELE (McKusick No. None)

Ultrasound: severe hydrocephalus with lemon sign, bilateral cleft lip and palate, kyphoscoliosis of the thoracic spine, omphalocele, single umbilical artery, bilateral amelia of the arms, shortened femora, shortened lower limbs, bilateral clubfeet
Froster et al., 1996a
Comments: After termination of the pregnancy, the fetus was found to have, in addition to the above findings, an anterior encephalocele, elongated and dysplastic diencephalon that had foci of gliosis and calcification, absence of the frontal bones, cystic replacement of right eye, eventration of the liver and bowel, ventricular heart defect, bifid ureter on the left, abnormal

fibulae and bilateral oligodactyly (three toes on the right, two on the left). Chromosomal studies failed.

PD 300500 ANENCEPHALY–SINGLE–CHAMBERED HEART–RENAL AGENESIS (McKusick No. None)

Condition Note: Still and co-workers (1989) reported one twin who had multiple anomalies including anencephaly, single-chamber heart, abnormalities of the upper limb (specific defects not listed), and absence of kidneys and bladder. In addition there was hydrops fetalis and massive ascites. Feticide of the abnormal twin was accomplished by intracardiac injection of potassium chloride. Delivery occurred 10 days later. After delivery and at autopsy, additional findings included hypoplastic ovaries, adrenal glands, pancreas and liver; and absence of uterus, vagina, ureters, and one lung.

Treatment Modalities: Withdrawal of ascitic fluid by amniocentesis needle
Still et al., 1989
intracardiac injection of potassium chloride (KCl) solution until cardiac arrest occurred
Still et al, 1989

Methods and Findings: Ultrasound[c,d]: anencephaly, single-chambered heart, renal agenesis, bladder agenesis, massive ascites, hydrops fetalis in one twin
Still et al., 1989

Comment: In the above fetus, Still and co-workers (1989) did not report the chromosomal constitution of the fetus.

PD 301500 ASCITES–CLEFT LIP/PALATE–ABSENT TOES–HYDRAMNIOS (McKusick No. None)

Condition Note: Hersh and Weisskopf (1983) reported a fetus with ascites and hydramnios who after delivery had facial flattening, ocular hypertelorism, dysplastic and low-set ears, unilateral cleft lip and palate, short neck and chest, ventricular septal defect, laryngeal atresia and tracheomalacia, massive fetal ascites, and absence of all except the great toes. The child died postnatally.
Ultrasound[c,d]: ascites, hydramnios
Hersh and Weisskopf, 1983

PD 301550 ASCITES–OCULAR HYPERTELORISM–OMPHALOCELE (McKusick No. None)

Condition Note: Hersh and Weisskopf (1983) cited a fetus with ascites and hydramnios who postnatally had microphthalmia, epicanthal folds, a broad nasal bridge with ocular hypertelorism, dysplastic and low-set ears, long philtrum, thin upper lip, micrognathia, webbed neck, ventricular septal defect, omphalocele, and excessive fetal lobulations of the kidney.
Ultrasound[c,d]: ascites, hydramnios
Hersh and Weisskopf, 1983

PD 330000 HAMARTOMA–VERTICAL MOUTH–HYPOPLASTIC KIDNEY (McKusick No. None)

Condition Note: Tromans and associates (1984) reported a fetus where a 19-week ultrasound evaluation revealed a grossly misshapen skull, dilatation of the lateral ventricles, splaying of the lumbar vertebrae, and oligohydramnios. Maternal serum alpha-fetoprotein (AFP) was also elevated. An ectopic pregnancy was discovered at laparotomy following failed induction with prostaglandin and oxytocin. After delivery, the fetus had a sac-shaped hamartoma attached to the occipital region without an underlying cranial bone defect, low-ears, flat nasal bridge with telecanthus, epicanthal folds, short philtrum, a vertical mouth, incomplete rotation of the bowel and a hypoplastic left kidney. The brain and spine were normal.

Ultrasound[c]: grossly misshapen skull, splaying of the lumbar spine, lateral ventricular dilatation, oligohydramnios

Tromans et al., 1984

Alpha-fetoprotein[c]: elevated in maternal serum

Tromans et al., 1984

PD 345000 LOWER BODY POLE DEFICIENCY, SEVERE (McKusick No. None)

Condition Note: Rossi and co-workers (1995) reported a newborn with severe deficiency of the lower half of the body. Defects in the neonate included diaphragmatic hernia, single necrotic kidney and ureter, hypoplastic bladder and obliterated intestine, abnormal ribs and upper vertebrae, marked deficiency or absence of vertebrae below T4, minute but contracted legs, syndactyly of toes, and a single umbilical artery. The child died in the immediate postnatal period. The karyotype was normal. No history of maternal diabetes was obtained.

Ultrasound [c,d]: ahydramnios

Rossi et al., 1995

PD 355000 MICROCEPHALY–ARTHROGRYPOSIS–ABSENT DUCTUS VENOSUS (McKusick No. None)

Condition Note: Jorgensen and Andolf (1994) reported four fetuses, each of whom had absence of the ductus venosus. The fourth case they reported had microcephaly, arthrogryposis, and absent ductus venosus at autopsy. A prenatal cord blood karyotype was normal. The neonate died immediately after birth.

Ultrasound[c,d]: small biparietal diameter, abnormal intracranial structures, no fetal movement

Jorgensen and Andolf, 1994

PD 360000 PHOCOMELIA–FEMOROTIBIAL SYNOSTOSIS (McKusick No. None)

Condition Note: Delooz and co-authors (1992) cited a case which had bilateral upper extremity phocomelia, flexion contractures of both knees, and complete bony femorotibial synostosis. There was also bilateral absence of the humeri, radii, and ulnae with both hands attached directly to the shoulders. In addition there were bilateral synostosis of the proximal ends of the fourth and fifth metacarpals, absence of the first metacarpal on the right hand, complete cutaneous syndactyly of the fourth and fifth toes on the right foot, and fusion of metatarsals 4 and 5 on the right. Bone marrow examination was normal, and no structural anomalies of the megakaryocytes were seen. The pregnancy of this fetus was terminated at around 23 weeks of gestation.

Ultrasound: bilateral absence of the humeri, ulnae and radii with hands attached to the shoulders, hypoplastic lower limbs with fixed 90° flexion of the knees

Delooz et al., 1992

References

Abbott, C.M., McMahon, C.J., Whitehouse, D.B. and Povey, S.: Prenatal diagnosis of alpha-1-antitrypsin deficiency using polymerase chain reaction. Lancet 2:763, 1988.

Abbott, C.M., Lovegrove, J.U., Whitehouse, D.B., Hopkinson, D.A. and Povey, S.: Prenatal diagnosis of alpha-1-antitrypsin deficiency by PCR of linked polymorphisms: A study of 17 cases. Prenat. Diagn. 12:235, 1992.

Abdulla, U. and Charters, D.W.: Congenital heart block diagnosed antenally associated with multiple fetal abnormality. Br. Med. J. 2:263, 1995.

Abeliovich, D., Leiberman, J.R., Teuerstein, I. and Levy, J.: Prenatal sex diagnosis: Testosterone and FHS levels in mid-trimester amniotic fluids. Prenat. Diagn. 4:347, 1984.

Aberg, A., Mitelman, F., Cantz, M. and Gehler, J.: Cardiac puncture of fetus with Hurler's disease avoiding abortion of unaffected co-twin. Lancet 2:990, 1978.

Abramowicz, J.S., Warsof, S.L., Lochner, D., Doyle, L., Smith, D. and Levy, D.L.: Congenital cystic hygroma of the neck diagnosed prenatally: Outcome with normal and abnormal karyotype. Prenat. Diagn. 9:321, 1989.

Abrams, S.L. and Filly, R.A.: Congenital vertebral malformations: Prenatal diagnosis using ultrasonography. Radiology. 155:762, 1985.

Abrams, S.L., Callen, P.W. and Filly, R.A.: Umbilical vein thrombosis: Sonographic detection in utero. J. Ultrasound Med. 4:283, 1985a.

Abrams, S.L., Callen, P.W., Anderson, R.L. and Stephens, J.D.: Anencephaly with encephalocele in craniopagus twins: Prenatal diagnosis by ultrasonography and computed tomography. J. Ultrasound Med. 4:485, 1985b.

Abramson, A., Chitkara, U. and Berkowitz, R.L.: A technique for mid-trimester termination of pregnancies with severe oligohydramnios. J. Ultrasound Med. 4:551, 1985.

Abuelo, D.N. and Barsel-Bowers, G.: Two male infants with amniotic fluid 45,XO karyotypes. Am. J. Hum. Genet. 43(Suppl.):A224, 1988.

Abuelo, D.N., Canick, J.A., Tint, G.S., Salen, G., Batta, A.K. and Kelley, R.I.: The Smith–Lemli–Opitz syndrome, problems of prenatal diagnosis and management. Am. J. Med. Genet. 52:371, 1994.

Abuelo, D.N., Tint, G.S., Kelley, R., Batta, A.K., Shefer, S. and Salen, G.: Prenatal detection of the cholesterol biosynthetic defect in the Smith–Lemli–Opitz syndrome by the analysis of amniotic fluid sterols. Am. J. Med. Genet. 56:281, 1995.

Achiron, R. and Zakut, H.: Fetal hemothorax complicating amniocentesis—Antenatal sonographic diagnosis. Acta Obstet. Gynecol. Scand. 65:869, 1986.

Achiron, R., Malinger, G., Zaidel, L. and Zakut, H.: Prenatal sonographic diagnosis of endocardial fibroelastosis secondary to aortic stenosis. Prenat. Diagn. 8:73, 1988.

Adam, A.H., Robinson, H.P., Pont, M., Hood, V.D. and Gibson, A.A.M.: Prenatal diagnosis of fetal lymphatic system abnormalities by ultrasound. J. Clin. Ultrasound 7:361, 1979.

Adinolfi, A., Adinolfi, M. and Lessof, M.H.: Alpha-feto-protein during development and in disease. J. Med. Genet. 12:138, 1975.

Adinolfi, M., Sherlock, J., Tutschek, B., Halder, A., Delhanty, J.D.A. and Rodeck, C.H.: Detection and analysis of fetal cells in transcervical samples using fluorescent in situ hybridization (FISH) and PCR amplication of unique fetal DNA sequence. Am. J. Hum. Genet. 57(Suppl.):A32, 1995.

Adzick, N.S., Harrison, M.R., Glick, P.L., Nakayama, D.K., Manning, F.A. and deLorimier, A.A.: Diaphragmatic hernia in the fetus: Prenatal diagnosis and outcome in 94 cases. Pediatr. Surg. 20:357, 1985.

Agarwala, B.N.: Fetal tachycardia without fetal distress. Hosp. Pract. 20:53, 1985.

Aikawa, J., Noro, T., Narisawa, K. and Tada, K.: Prenatal diagnosis in a new peroxisomal disease by the W-particle separation method. J. Inher. Metab. Dis. 17:621, 1994.

Aitken, D.A., May, H.M. and Ferguson-Smith, M.A.: Amniotic band disruption syndrome associated with elevated amniotic AFP and normal acetylcholinesterase gel test. Prenat. Diagn. 4:443, 1984a.

Aitken, D.A., Morrison, N.M. and Ferguson-Smith, M.A.: Predictive value of amniotic acetylcholinesterase analysis in the diagnosis of fetal abnormality in 3700 pregnancies. Prenat. Diagn. 4:329, 1984b.

Aitken, D.A., Yaqoob, M. and Ferguson-Smith, M.A.: Microvillar enzyme analysis in amniotic fluid and the prenatal diagnosis of cystic fibrosis. Prenat. Diagn. 5:119, 1985.

Akhunov, V.S., Gargaun, S.S. and Krasnopolskaya, X.D.: First-trimester enzyme exclusion of Farber disease using a micromethod with [^{3}H]ceramide. J. Inher. Metab. Dis. 18:616, 1995.

Albrechtsen, M., Bock, E. and Norgaard-Pedersen, B.: Glial fibrillary acidic protein in amniotic fluids from pregnancies with fetal neural tube defects. Prenat. Diagn. 4:405, 1984.

Albright, S.G. and Katz, V.L.: Alpha-fetoprotein findings in a case of cystic adenomatoid malformation of the lung. Clin. Genet. 35:75, 1989.

Alegre, M., Torrents, M., Carreras, E., Mortera, C., Cusi, V. and Carrera, J.M.: Prenatal diagnosis of intrapericardial teratoma. Prenat. Diagn. 10:199, 1990.

Alexander, E., Jr., and Davis, C.H.: Intra-uterine fracture of the infant's skull. J. Neurosurg. 30:446, 1969.

Alford, R.L., Redman, J.B., O'Brien, W.E. and Caskey, C.T.: Lesch–Nyhan syndrome: Carrier and prenatal diagnosis. Prenat. Diagn. 15:329, 1995.

Al-Gazali, L.I., Donnai, D. and Mueller, R.F.: Hirschsprung's disease, hypoplastic nails, and minor dysmorphic features: A distinct autosomal recessive syndrome? J. Med. Genet. 25:758, 1988.

Al-Gazali, L.I., Abdel Raziq, A., Al-Shather, W. Shahzadi, R and Azhar, N.: Meckel syndrome and Dandy–Walker malformation. Clin. Dysmorph. 5:73–76, 1996.

Alkalay, A.L., Gonzalez, C.L., Chou, P.J., Medearis, A.L., Austin, E., Pomerance, J.J. and Young, L.W.: Radiological case of the month. Am. J. Dis. Child. 141:89, 1987a.

Alkalay, A.L., Pomerance, J.J. and Rimoin, D.L.: Fetal varicella syndrome. J. Pediatr. 111:320, 1987b.

Allan, L.D., Tynan, M., Campbell, S. and Anderson, R.H.: Normal fetal cardiac anatomy—A basis for the echocardiographic detection of abnormalities. Prenat. Diagn. 1:131, 1981a.

Allan, L.D., Tynan, M., Campbell, S. and Anderson, R.H.: Identification of congenital cardiac malformations by echocardiography in midtrimester fetus. Br. Heart J. 46:358, 1981b.

Allan, L.D., Desai, G. and Tynan, M.J.: Prenatal echocardiographic screening for Ebstein's anomaly for mothers on lithium therapy. Lancet 2:875, 1982.

Allan, L.D., Crawford, D.C. and Tynan, M.J.: Pulmonary atresia in prenatal life. J. Am. Coll. Cardiol. 8:1131, 1986.

Allen, R.: The significance of meconium in midtrimester genetic amniocentesis. Am. J. Obstet. Gynecol. 152:413, 1985.

Allen R.C., Nachtman, R.G., Rosenblatt, H.M. and Belmont, J.W.: Application of carrier testing to genetic counseling for X-linked agammaglobulinemia. Am. J. Hum. Genet. 54:25, 1994.

Allison, F., Barnes, I.C.S. and Bennett, M.J.: The oxidation of octanoic acid by cultured amniotic fluid cells: The effect of cell type and passage number. Prenat. Diagn. 8:383, 1988.

Almeida, M.R., Alves, I.L., Sakaki, Y., Costa, P.P. and Saraiva, M.J.M.: Prenatal diagnosis of familial amyloidotic polyneuropathy: Evidence for an early expression of the associated transthyretin methionine 30. Hum. Genet. 85:623, 1990.

Al Saadi, A.: Cystic hygroma cells as source for prenatal diagnosis. Am. J. Hum. Genet. 45(Suppl.):A252, 1989.

Altenburger, K.M., Jedziniak, M., Roper, W.L. and Hernandez, J.: Congenital complete heart block associated with hydrops fetalis. J. Pediatr. 91:618, 1977.

Alter, P.A.: Intrauterine diagnosis of hemoglobinopathies. Semin. Perinatol. 4:189, 1980.

Alter, B.P.: Prenatal diagnosis of hematologic diseases, 1986 update. Acta Haematol. 78:137, 1987.

Alter, B.P. and Nathan, D.G.: Antenatal diagnosis of haematological disorders. Clin. Haematol. 7:195, 1978.

Alter, B.P., Modell, C.B., Fairweather, D., Hobbins, J.C., Mahoney, M.J., Frigoletto, F.D., Sherman, A.S. and Nathan, D.G.: Prenatal diagnosis of hemoglobinopathies: A review of 15 cases. N. Engl. J. Med. 295:1437, 1976.

Alter, B.P., Orkin, S.H., Forget, B.G. and Nathan, D.G.: Prenatal diagnosis of hemoglobinopathies: The New England approach. Ann. N.Y. Acad. Sci. 344:151, 1980.

Alvarez, M., Chitkara, U., Lynch, L., Mehalek, K.E., Heller, D. and Berkowitz, R.L.: Prenatal diagnosis of fetal brain tumors. Fetal Ther. 2:203, 1987.

Amato, M., Howald, H. and von Muralt, G.: Fetal ventriculomegaly, agenesis of the corpus callosum and chromosomal translocation—Case report. J. Perinat. Med. 14:271, 1986.

Ampola, M.G., Mahoney, M.J., Nakamura, E. and Tanaka, K.: Prenatal therapy of a patient with vitamin-B_{12}–responsive methylmalonic acidemia. N. Engl. J. Med. 293:313, 1975.

Anderson, C.W. and Cordero, L.: Changes in amniotic fluid optical density at 450 mu in Rh-sensitized patients after maternal hydrocortisone treatment. Am. J. Obstet. Gynecol. 137:820, 1980.

Anderson, A.: Some clinical implications of recombinant DNA technology with emphasis on prenatal diagnosis of hemoglobinopathies. Clin. Biochem. 17:112, 1984.

Anderson, R.L., Simpson, G.F., Sherman, S., Dedo, H.H. and Golbus, M.S.: Fetal pharyngeal teratoma—Another cause of elevated amniotic fluid alpha-fetoprotein. Am. J. Obstet. Gynecol. 150:432, 1984.

Anhalt, H., Parker, B., Paranjpe, D.V., Neely, E.K., Silverman, F.N. and Rosenfeld, R.G.: Novel spinal dysplasia in two generations. Am. J. Med. Genet. 56:90, 1995.

Anneren, G., Esscher, T., Larsson, L., Olsen, L. and Pahlman, S.: S-100 protein and neuron-specific enolase in amniotic fluid as markers of abdominal wall and neural tube defects in the fetus. Prenat. Diagn. 8:323, 1988.

Anneren, G., Andersson, T., Lindgren, P.G. and Kjartansson, S.: Ectrodactyly–ectodermal dysplasia–clefting syndrome (EEC): The clinical variation and prenatal diagnosis. Clin. Genet. 40:257, 1991.

Antich, J., Manzanares, R., Camarasa, F., Krauel, X., Vila, J. and Cusi, V.: Schinzel–Giedion syndrome: Report of two sibs. Am. J. Med. Genet. 59:96, 1995.

Antonarakis, S.E., Copeland, K.L., Carpenter, R.J., Jr., Carta, C.A., Hoyer, L.W., Caskey, C.T., Toole, J.J. and Kazazian, H.H., Jr.: Prenatal diagnosis of haemophilia A by factor VIII gene analysis. Lancet 1:1407, 1985.

Anton-Lamprecht, I.: Prenatal diagnosis of genetic disorders of the skin by means of electron microscopy. Hum. Genet. 59:392, 1981.

Anton-Lamprecht, I.: Prenatal diagnosis of epidermolysis bullosa hereditaria: A review. Semin. Dermatol. 3:229, 1984.

Anton-Lamprecht, I. and Arnold, M.-L.: Prenatal diagnosis of severe genetic disorder of the skin. In: *Pediatric Dermatology.* Happle, R. and Grosshans, E., (Eds.), Berlin: Springer-Verlag, 1987a.

Anton-Lamprecht I. and Arnold M.-L.,: Prenatal diagnosis of inherited epidermolyses. Curr. Probl. Dermatol. 16:146, 1987b.

Anton-Lamprecht, I., Rauskolb, R., Jovanovic, V., Kern, B., Arnold, M.-L. and Schenck, W.: Prenatal diagnosis of epidermolysis bullosa dystrophica, Hallopeau–Siemens with electron microscopy of fetal skin. Lancet. 2:1077, 1981.

Anton-Lamprecht, I., Arnold, M.-L., Rauskolb, R., Schinzel, A., Schmid, W. and Schnyder, U.W.: Prenatal diagnosis of anhidrotic ectodermal dysplasia. Hum. Genet. 62:180, 1982.

Antsaklis, A., Politis, J., Karagiannopoulos, C. and Kaskarelis, D.: Selective survival of only the healthy fetus following prenatal diagnosis of thalassaemia major in binovular twin gestation. Prenat. Diagn. 4:289, 1984.

Anyane-Yeboa, K., Kasznica, J., Malin, J. and Maidman, J.: Hermann–Opitz syndrome: Report of an affected fetus. Am. J. Med. Genet. 27:467, 1987.

Aparicio, L., Carpenter, M.W., Schwartz, R. and Gruppuso, P.A.: Prenatal diagnosis of familial neonatal hyperinsulinemia. Acta Paediatr. 82:683, 1993.

Applegarth, D.A., Levy, H.L., Shih, V.E., McGillivray, B., Wong, J.T., Toone, J.R. and Kirby, L.T.: Prenatal diagnosis of non-ketotic hyperglycinemia. Prenat. Diagn. 6:257, 1986.

Apuzzio, J.J., Ganesh, V., Landau, I. and Pelosi, M.: Prenatal diagnosis of conjoined twins. Am. J. Obstet. Gynecol. 148:343, 1984.

Apuzzio, J.J., Diamond, N., Ganesh, V. and Deposito, F.: Difficulties in the prenatal diagnosis of Jarcho–Levin syndrome. Am. J. Obstet. Gynecol. 156:916, 1987.

Arab, H. Siegel-Bartelt, J., Wong, P.Y. and Doran, T.: Maternal serum beta human chorionic gonadotropin (MSHOG) combined with maternal serum alpha-fetoprotein (MSAFP) appears superior for prenatal screening for Down syndrome (DS) than either test alone. Am. J. Hum. Genet. 43(Suppl.):A225, 1988.

Aramaki, S., Lehotay, D., Nyhan, W.L., Macleod, P.M. and Sweetman, L.: Methylcitrate in maternal urine during a pregnancy with a fetus affected with propionic acidaemia. J. Inher. Metab. Dis. 12:86, 1989.

Archer, I.M., Kingston, H.M. and Harper, P.S.: Prenatal diagnosis of Hunter syndrome. Prenat. Diagn. 4:195, 1984.

Ardinger, H.H., Williamson, R.A. and Grant, S.: Association of neural tube defects with omphalocele in chromosomally normal fetuses. Am. J. Med. Genet. 27:135, 1987.

Arienzo, R., Ricco, C.S. and Romeo, F.: A very rare fetal malformation: The cutaneous widespread vascular hamartomatosis. Am. J. Obstet. Gynecol. 157:1162, 1987.

Armstrong, D.H., Murata, Y., Martin, C.B., Jr., and Ikenoue, T.: Antepartum detection of congenital complete fetal heart block: A case report. Am. J. Obstet. Gynecol. 126:291, 1976.

Arnold, M.-L. and Anton-Lamprecht, I.: Prenatal diagnosis of epidermal disorders. Curr. Probl. Dermatol. 16:120, 1987.

Arnold, M.-L., Rauskolb, R., Anton-Lamprecht, I., Schinzel, A. and Schmid, W.: Prenatal diagnosis of anhidrotic ectodermal dysplasia. Prenat. Diagn. 4:85, 1984.

Arnon J. and Ornoy A.: Clinical teratology counseling and consultation case report: Outcome of pregnancy after failure of early induced abortions. Teratology. 51:120, 1995.

Asensio, S.H., Figueroa-Longo, J.G. and Pelegrina, I.A.: Intrauterine exchange transfusion. Am. J. Obstet. Gynecol. 95:1129, 1966.

Ash, K.M., Mibashan, R.S. and Nicolaides, K.H.: Diagnosis and treatment of feto-maternal hemorrhage in a fetus with homozygous von Willebrand's disease. Fetal. Ther. 3:189, 1988.

Ashkenazy, M., Lurie, S., Ben-Itzhak, I., Appelman, Z. and Caspi, B.: Unilateral congenital short femur: A case report. Prenat. Diagn. 10:67, 1990.

Ashwood, E.R., Cheng, E. and Luthy, D.A.: Maternal serum alpha-fetoprotein and fetal trisomy-21 in women 35 years and older: Implications for alpha-fetoprotein screening programs. Am. J. Med. Genet. 26:531, 1987.

Asokan, S., Chadalavada, K., Gardi, R. and Sastry, V.: Prenatal diagnosis of placental tumor by ultrasound. J. Clin. Ultrasound 6:180, 1978.

Auerbach, A.D.: Prenatal diagnosis in twenty-seven pregnancies at risk for Fanconi anemia. Am. J. Hum. Genet. 36(Suppl.):184S, 1984.

Auerbach, A.D., Adler, B. and Chaganti, R.S.K.: Fanconi anemia: Pre- and postnatal diagnosis and carrier detection by a cytogenetic method. Am. J. Hum. Genet. 32(Suppl.):61A, 1980.

Auerbach, A.D., Adler, B. and Chaganti, R.S.K.: Prenatal and postnatal diagnosis and carrier detection of Fanconi anemia by a cytogenetic method. Pediatrics 67:128, 1981.

Auerbach, A.D., Sagi, M. and Adler, B.A.: Fanconi anemia: Prenatal diagnosis in 30 fetuses at risk. Pediatrics. 76:794, 1985.

Auerbach, A.D., Min, Z., Ghosh, R., Pergament, E., Verlinsky, Y., Nicolas, H. and Boue, J.: Clastogen-induced chromosomal breakage as a marker for first trimester prenatal diagnosis of Fanconi anemia. Hum. Genet. 73:86, 1986.

Aughton, D.J., Lang, M.J., Riggs, T.W., Milad, M. and Biesecker, L.: Dizygotic twins concordant for truncus arteriosus. Proc. Greenwood Genet. Cent. 9:105, 1990.

Aula, P., Rapola, J., Autio, S., Raivio, K. and Karjalainen, O.: Prenatal diagnosis and fetal pathology of I-cell disease (mucolipidosis type II). J. Pediatr. 87:221, 1975.

Aula, P., Rapola, J., von Koskull, H. and Ammala, P.: Prenatal diagnosis and fetal pathology of aspartylglucosaminuria. Am. J. Med. Genet. 19:359, 1984.

Aula, P., Mattila, K. Piiroinen, O., Ammala, P. and Von Koskull, H.: First-trimester prenatal diagnosis of aspartylglucosaminuria. Prenat. Diagn. 9:617, 1989.

Aulehla-Scholz, C., Miny, P., Holzgreve, W., Epplen, J.T. and Horst, J.: A pitfall in the prenatal diagnosis of beta-thalassaemia by RFLP. Prenat. Diagn. 9:140, 1989a.

Aulehla-Scholz, C., Spiegelberg, R., Miny, P., Holzgreve, W., Eigel, A., Dworniczak, B. and Horst, J.: Direct sequencing of amplified DNA in prenatal diagnosis of beta-thalassaemia. Lancet 1:326, 1989b.

Avni, E.F., Thoua, Y., Lalmand, B., Didier, F., Droulle, P. and Schulman, C.C.: Multicystic dysplastic kidney: Natural history from in utero diagnosis and postnatal followup. J. Urol. 138:1420, 1987a.

Avni, E.F., Thoua, Y., Van Gansbeke, D., Matos, C., Didier, F., Droulez, P. and Schulman, C.C.: Development of the hypodysplastic kidney: Contribution of antenatal US diagnosis. Radiology 164:123, 1987b.

Aylsworth, A.S., Seeds, J.W., Guilford, W.B., Burns, C.B. and Washburn, D.B.: Prenatal diagnosis of a severe deforming type of osteogenesis imperfecta. Am. J. Med. Genet. 19:707, 1984.

Aylsworth, A.S., Miller, C.G. and Mesrobian, H.G.J.: Familial recurrence of the prune belly phenotype. Proc. Greenwood Genet. Cent. 10:52, 1991.

Ayme, S., Julian, C., Gambarelli, D., Mariotti, B., Luciani, A., Sudan, N., Maurin, N., Philip, N., Serville, F., Carles, D., Rolland, M. and Giraud, F.: Fryns syndrome: Report on 8 new cases. Clin. Genet. 35:191, 1989.

Ayme, S., Gambarelli, D., Luciani, A. and Philip, N.: Walker–Warburg and cerebro-oculomuscular syndromes: Should we split or lump them? Proc. Greenwood Genet. Cent. 9:75, 1990.

Babay, Z.A., Lange, I.R, Elliott, P.D. and Hwang, W-S.: A case of varix dilatation of the umbilical vein and review of the literature. Fetal Diagn. Ther. 11:221, 1996.

Baccichetti, C., Lenzini, E., Suma, V., Benini, F. and Marini, A.: Spontaneous resolution of cystic hygroma in a 46,XX normal female. Prenat. Diagn. 10:399, 1990.

Bach, G. and Zlotogora, J.: Hunter syndrome: Early prenatal diagnosis in maternal serum. Am. J. Hum. Genet. 36(Suppl.):184S, 1984.

Bach, G. and Zlotogora, J.: Prenatal diagnosis of Hunter syndrome. Clin. Genet. 28:412, 1985.

Bacino, C.A., Schreck, R., Fischel-Ghodsian, N., Pepkowitz, S., Prezant, T.R. and Graham, J.M., Jr.: Clinical and molecular studies in full trisomy 22: Further delineation of the phenotype and review of the literature. Am. J. Med. Genet. 56:359, 1995.

Bader, P.I. and Bixler, D.: A severe form of Pfeiffer syndrome. Proc. Greenwood Genet. Cent. 9:106, 1990.

Bader, P.I. and Lewis, W.: "Spur-linked" dwarfism identified as hypophosphatasia. Dysmorph. Clin. Genet. 2:124, 1988.

Baggot, P.J., Chrismas, J.T. and Markello, T.C.: Fetal microcephaly due to microlissencephaly. Am. J. Hum. Genet. 57(Suppl.):A275, 1995.

Baier, W. and Harzer, K.: Sulfatides in prenatal metachromatic leukodystrophy. J. Neurochem. 41:1766, 1983.

Bailey, W., Freidenberg, G.R., James, H.E., Hesselink, J.R. and Jones, K.L.: Prenatal diagnosis of a craniopharyngioma using ultrasonography and magnetic resonance imaging. Prenat. Diagn. 10:623, 1990.

Bakay, B., Francke, U., Nyhan, W.L. and Seegmiller, J.E.: Experience with detection of heterozygous carriers and prenatal diagnosis of Lesch–Nyhan disease. Adv. Exp. Med. Biol. 76A:351, 1977.

Baker, S. and Dann, L.G.: Peptidases in amniotic fluid: Low values in cystic fibrosis. Lancet 1:716, 1983.

Bakker, E., Hofker, M.H., Goor, N., Mandel, J.L., Wrogemann, K., Davies, K.E., Kunkel, L.M., Willard, H.F., Fenton, W.A., Sandkuyl, L., Majoor-Krakauer, D., Essen, A.J.V., Jahoda, M.G.J., Sachs, E.S., van Ommen, G.J.B. and Pearson, P.L.: Prenatal diagnosis and carrier detection of Duchenne muscular dystrophy with closely linked RFLPs. Lancet 1:655, 1985.

Bakker, E., Bonten, E.J., Veenema, H., den Dunnen, J.T., Grootscholten, P.M., van Ommen, G.J.B. and Pearson, P.L.: Prenatal diagnosis of Duchenne muscular dystrophy: A three-year experience in a rapidly evolving field. J. Inher. Metab. Dis. 12:(Suppl. 1)174, 1989a.

Bakker, E., Bonten, E.J., den Dunnen, J.T., Veenema, H., Grootscholten, P.M., van Ommen, G.J.B. and Pearson, P.L.: Carrier detection and prenatal diagnosis of Duchenne/Becker muscular dystrophy (D/BMD) by DNA analysis. Prog. Clin. Biolog. Res. 306:51, 1989b.

Balcar, I., Grant, D.C., Miller, W.A. and Bieber, F.A.: Antenatal detection of Down syndrome by sonography. Am. J. Roentgenogr. 143:29, 1984.

Balci, S., Ercal, M.D., Onol, B., Caglar, M., Dogan, A. and Dogruel, N.: Familial short rib syndrome, type Beemer, with pyloric stenosis and short intestine, one case diagnosed prenatally. Clin. Genet. 39:298, 1991.

Baldinger, S., Pierpont, M.E. and Wenger, D.A.: Pseudodeficiency of arylsulfatase A a counseling dilemma. Clin. Genet. 31:70, 1987.

Bale, A., Bialer, M., Gailani, M. and Dokras, A.: Prenatal symptomatic and preimplantation diagnosis of Gorlin syndrome. Am. J. Hum. Genet. 53(Suppl.):1381, 1993.

Balfour, R.P. and Laurence, K.M.: Raised serum AFP levels and fetal renal agenesis. Lancet. 1:317, 1980.

Balsam, D. and Weiss, R.R: Amniography in prenatal diagnosis. Radiology. 141:379, 1981.

Bamforth, J.S., Leonard, C.O., Chodirker, B.N., Chitayat, D., Gritter, H.L., Evans, J.A., Keena, B., Pantzar, T., Fiedman, J.M. and Hall, J.G.: Congenital diaphragmatic hernia, coarse facies, and acral hypoplasia: Fryns syndrome. Am. J. Med. Genet. 32:93, 1989.

Bamforth, F.J., Johnson, J.L., Davidson, A.G.F., Wong, L.T.K., Lockitch, G. and Applegarth, D.A.: Biochemical investigation of a child with molybdenum cofactor deficiency. Clin. Biochem. 23:537, 1990.

Bamforth, J.S., Kaurah, P., Byrne, J. and Ferreira, P.: Adams Oliver syndrome: A family with extreme variability in clinical expression. Am. J. Med. Genet. 49:393, 1994.

Bang, J., Bock, J.E. and Trolle, D.: Ultrasound-guided fetal intravenous transfusion for severe Rhesus haemolytic disease. Br. Med. J. 284:373, 1982.

Bankier, A., Fortune, D., Duke, J. and Sillence, D.O.: Fibrochondrogenesis in male twins at 24 weeks gestation. Am. J. Med. Genet. 38:95, 1991.

Banna, M., Omojola, M.F., Toi, A. and deSa, D.J.: The cloverleaf skull. Br. J. Radiol. 53:730, 1980.

Baraitser, M., Rodeck, C. and Garner, A.: A new craniosynostosis/mental retardation syndrome diagnosed by fetoscopy. Clin. Genet. 22:12, 1982.

Baranov, V.S., Gorbunova, V.N., Ivaschenko, T.E., Shwed, N.Y., Osinovskaya, N.S., Kascheeva, T.K., Lebedev, V.M., Mikhailov, A.V, Vakharlovsky, V.G. and Kuznetzova, T.V.: Five year's experience of prenatal diagnosos of cystic fibrosis in the former U.S.S.R. Prenat. Diagn. 12:575, 1992.

Bar-Hava, I., Bronshtein, M. and Drugan, A.: Changing dysmorphology of trisomy 18 midtrimester. Fetal Diagn. Ther. 8:171, 1993.

Barkai, G., Reznik, H., Ries, L., Chaki, R. and Goldman, B.: High serum levels of beta subunit human chorionic gonadotropin in trisomy X. Prenat. Diagn. 11:922, 1991.

Barr, J.S. and MacVicar, J.: Dystocia due to foetal ascites. J. Obstet. Gynaecol. Br. Commonw. 63:890, 1956.

Barr, M., Jr., Heidelberger, K.P. and Comstock, C.H.: Craniomicromelic syndrome: A newly recognized lethal condition with craniosynostosis, distinct facial anomalies, short limbs, and intrauterine growth retardation. Am. J. Med. Genet. 58:348, 1995.

Barrett, I.J., Kalousek, D.K., Telenius, A. and Howard-Peebles, P.H.: Cell lineages involved in CVS mosaicism and pregnancy outcome. Am. J. Hum. Genet. 57(Suppl.):A275, 1995.

Barry, C.W., Gustashaw, K., Golden, W.L., Johnson, W.E. and Jassani, M.: Prenatal diagnosis of Turner syndrome by cells cultured from cystic hygromas. Am. J. Hum. Genet. 37(Suppl.):A211, 1985.

Bars, J.O., Aleck, K.A., Finberg, H.J. and Grebe, T.A.: Unusual presentation of two-generation velo-cardio-facial syndrome: Hydronephrosis diagnosed on prenatal ultrasound. Am. J. Hum. Genet. 57(Suppl.):A82, 1995.

Barsel-Bowers, G. and Abuelo, D.: Genetic counseling for nuchal cysts diagnosed prenatally. Am. J. Hum. Genet. 39(Suppl.):A174, 1986.

Barsel-Bowers, G., Abuelo, D.N., Richardson, A. and Goldstein, A.: Genetic counseling for patients with low MSAFP. Am. J. Hum. Genet. 45(Suppl.):A119, 1989.

Barson, A.J., Donnai, P., Ferguson, A., Donnai, D. and Read, A.P.: Haemangioma of the cord: Further cause of raised maternal serum and liquor alpha-fetoprotein. Br. Med. J. 281:1252, 1980.

Barss, V.A., Benacerraf, B.R., Greene, M.F. and Frigoletto, F.D.: Use of a small-gauge needle for intrauterine fetal transfusions. Am. J. Obstet. Gynecol. 155:1057, 1986.

Bartley, J.A., Golbus, M.S., Filly, R.A. and Hall, B.D.: Prenatal diagnosis of dysplastic kidney disease. Clin. Genet. 11:375, 1977.

Bartsch, O., Meinecke, P. and Kamin, G.: Fryns syndrome: Two further cases without lateral diaphragmatic defects. Clin. Dysmorph. 4:352, 1995.

Bass, H.N., Oliver, J.B. and Srinivasan, M.: Persistently elevated AFP and AChE in amniotic fluid from a normal fetus following demise of its twin. Prenat. Diagn. 6:33, 1986.

Baty, B.J., Drayna, D., Leonard, C.O. and White, R.: Prenatal diagnosis of factor VIII deficiency to help with the management of pregnancy and delivery. Lancet 1:207, 1986.

Baty, B.J., Cubberley, D., Morris, C. and Carey, J.: Prenatal diagnosis of distal arthrogryposis. Am. J. Med. Genet. 29:501, 1988.

Baumgarten, A., Schoenfeld, M., Mahoney, M.J., Greenstein, R.M. and Saal, H.M. Prospective screening for Down syndrome using maternal serum AFP. Lancet 1:1280, 1985.

Bawle, E.V. and Black, V.: Nonimmune hydrops fetalis in Noonan's syndrome. Am. J. Dis. Child. 140:758, 1986.

Baxi, L.V., Yeh, M.-N., Blanc, W.A. and Schullinger, J.N.: Antepartum diagnosis and management of in utero intestinal volvulus with perforation. N. Engl. J. Med. 308:1519, 1983.

Bean, W.J., Calonje, M.A., Aprill, C.N. and Geshner, J.: Anal atresia: A prenatal ultrasound diagnosis. J. Clin. Ultrasound. 6:111, 1978.

Beaudet, A.L., Buffone, G.J., Fernbach, S.D., Greenberg, F. and Carpenter, R.J.: Automated analysis of amniotic fluid alkaline phosphatase as a fetal marker and for prenatal diagnosis of cystic fibrosis. Am. J. Hum. Genet. 37(Suppl.):A211, 1985.

Beck, L., Terinde, R. and Dolff, M.: Zwillingsschwangerschaft mit freier Trisomie 21 eines Kindes; Sectio parva mit Entfernug des Kranken und spatere Geburt des gesunden Kindes. Geburtsh. Frauenheilkd. 40:397, 1980.

Beck, L., Terinde, R., Rohrborn, G., Claussen, U., Gebauer, H.J. and Rehder, H.: Twin pregnancy, abortion of one fetus with Down's syndrome by sectio parva, the other delivered mature and healthy. Europ. J. Obstet. Gynecol. Reprod. Biol. 12:267, 1981.

Beck, M., Braun, S., Coerdt, W., Merz, E., Young, E., and Sewell, A.C.: Fetal presentation of Morquio disease type A. Prenat. Diagn. 12:1019, 1992.

Beeson, D. and Golbus, M.S.: Decision making: Whether or not to have prenatal diagnosis and abortion for X-linked conditions. Am. J. Med. Genet. 20:107, 1985.

Belhassen, B., Pauzner, D., Blieden, L., Sherez, J., Zinger, A., David, M., Muhlbauer, B. and

Laniado, S.: Intrauterine and postnatal atrial fibrillation in the Wolff–Parkinson–White syndrome. Circulation. 66:1124, 1982.

Bellingham, A.J. and Lestas, A.N.: Prenatal diagnosis of triose phosphate isomerase deficiency. Lancet. 1:230, 1990.

Bellingham, A.J., Williams, L.H.P., Lestas, A.N. and Nicolaides, K.H.: Prenatal diagnosis of a red-cell enzymopathy: Triose phosphate isomerase deficiency. Lancet 2:419, 1989.

Bellus, G.A., Escallon, C.S., de Luna, R.O., Shumway, J.B., Blakemore, K.J., McIntosh, I. and Francomano, C.A.: First-trimester prenatal diagnosis in couple at risk for homozygous achondroplasia. Lancet 344:1512, 1994.

Belmont, J.W., Hawkins, E., Hejtmancik, J.F. and Greenberg, F.: Two cases of severe lethal Smith–Lemli–Opitz syndrome. Am. J. Med. Genet. 26:65, 1987.

Benacerraf, B.R. and Frigoletto, F.D., Jr.: Sonographic sign for the detection of early fetal ascites in the management of severe isoimmune disease without intrauterine transfusion. Am. J. Obstet. Gynecol. 152:1039, 1985.

Benacerraf, B.R. and Frigoletto, F.D., Jr.: In utero treatment of a fetus with diaphragmatic hernia complicated by hydrops. Am. J. Obstet. Gynecol. 155:817, 1986.

Benacerraf, B.R., Frigoletto, F.D., Jr., and Bieber, F.R.: The fetal face: Ultrasound examination. Radiology 153:495, 1984.

Benacerraf, B.R., Barss, V.A. and Labods, L.A.: A sonographic sign for the detection in the second trimester of the fetus with Down's syndrome. Am. J. Obstet. Gynecol. 151:1078, 1985.

Benacerraf, B.R., Greene, M.F. and Barss, V.A.: Prenatal sonographic diagnosis of congenital hemivertebra. J. Ultrasound Med. 5:257, 1986a.

Benacerraf, B.R., Frigoletto, F.D., Jr., and Green, M.F.: Abnormal facial features and extremities in human trisomy syndromes: Prenatal US appearance. Radiology. 159:243, 1986b.

Benacerraf, B.R., Frigoletto, F.D., Jr. and Wilson, M.: Successful midtrimester thoracentesis with analysis of the lymphocyte population in the pleural effusion. Am. J. Obstet. Gynecol, 155:398, 1986c.

Benacerraf, B.R., Gelman, R. and Frigoletto, F.D., Jr.: Sonographic identification of second-trimester fetuses with Down syndrome. N. Engl. J. Med. 317:1317, 1987.

Benacerraf, B.R., Nadel, A. and Bromley, B.: Identification of second trimester fetuses with autosomal trisomy by use of a sonographic scoring index. Radiology. 193:135, 1994.

Ben-Ami, M., Shalev, E., Romano, S. and Zuckerman, H.: Midtrimester diagnosis of endocardial fibroelastosis and atrial septal defect: A case report. Am. J. Obstet. Gynecol. 155:662, 1986.

Bendon, R.W., Siddiqi, T., Soukup, S. and Srivastava, A.: Prenatal detection of triploidy. J. Pediatr. 112:149, 1988.

Bendon, R.W., Tyson, R.W., Baldwin, V.J. , Cashner, K.A., Mimouni, F. and Miodovnik, M.: Umbilical cord ulcertion and intestinal atresia: A new association? Am. J. Obstet. Gynecol. 164:582, 1991.

Benke, P. and Strassberg, R.: Prenatal study of X-linked aqueductal stenosis. J. Med. Genet. 17:158, 1980.

Benn, P., Craffey, A., Horne, D., Cusick, W. and Smeltzer, J.: An association between trisomy 16 (and other fetal aneuploidy) in women with grossly elevated second trimester maternal serum human chorionic gonadotropin. Am. J. Hum. Genet. 57(Suppl.):A275, 1995.

Ben-Neriah, Z., Yagel, S. and Ariel, I.: Renal anomalies in Marden–Walker syndrome: A clue for prenatal diagnosis. Am. J. Med. Genet. 57:417, 1995.

Bennett, M.J., Curnock, D.A., Enggel, P.C., Shaw, L., Gray, R.G.F., Hull, D., Patrick, A.D. and Pollitt, R.J.: Glutaric aciduria type II: Biochemical investigation and treatment of a child diagnosed prenatally. J. Inherit. Metab. Dis. 7:57, 1984.

Bennett, M.J., Allison, F., Lowther, G.W., Gray, R.G.F., Johnston, D.I., Fitzsimmons, J.S., Manning, N.J. and Pollitt, R.J.: Prenatal diagnosis of medium-chain acyl-coenzyme A dehydrogenase deficiency. Prenat. Diagn. 7:135, 1987.

Bennett, M.J., Gibson, K.M., Sherwood, W.G., Divry, P., Rolland, M.O., Elpeleg, O.N., Rinaldo, P. and Jakobs, C.: Reliable prenatal diagnosis of Canavan disease (aspartoacylase deficiency): Comparison of enzymatic and metabolite analysis. J. Inher. Metab. Dis. 16:831, 1993.

Ben-Yishay, M., Turolla, L., Nakagawa, S., Sachs, G.S., Sato, M., Madan, S. and Nitowsky, H.M.: Low maternal serum alpha fetoprotein (MS-AFP): Pregnancy outcomes following genetic amniocentesis. Am. J. Hum. Genet. 43(Suppl.):A226, 1988.

Ben-Yoseph, Y., Mitchell, D.A. and Nadler, H.L.: First trimester prenatal evaluation for I-cell disease by N-acetyl-glucosamine 1-phosphotransferase assay. Clin. Genet. 33:38, 1988.

Benzie, R.J. and Doran, T.A.: The "fetoscope"—A new clinical tool for prenatal genetic diagnosis. Am. J. Obstet. Gynecol. 121:460, 1975.

Benzie, R., Doran, T.A., Escoffery, W., Gardner, H.A., Hoar, D.I., Hunter, A., Malone, R., Miskin, M. and Rudd, N.L.: Prenatal diagnosis of hypophosphatasia. Birth Defects. 12(6):271, 1976.

Beratis, N., Sklower, S., Wilbor, L. and Matalong, R.: Sanfilippo B syndrome in Greece and prenatal diagnosis. Am. J. Hum. Genet. 36(Suppl.):6S, 1984.

Berkeley, A.S., Killackey, M.A. and Cederqvist, L.L.: Elevated maternal serum alpha-fetoprotein levels associated with breakdown in fetal-maternal-placental barrier. Am. J. Obstet. Gynecol. 146:859, 1983.

Berkowitz, R.L. and Hobbins, J.C.: Intrauterine transfusion utilizing ultrasound. Obstet. Gynecol. 57:33, 1981.

Berkowitz, R.L., Glickman, M.G., Smith, G.J.W., Siegel, N.J., Weiss, R.M., Mahoney, M.J. and Hobbins, J.C.: Fetal urinary tract obstruction: What is the role of surgical intervention in utero? Am. J. Obstet. Gynecol. 144:367, 1982.

Berkowitz, R.L., Chitkara, U., Goldberg, J.D., Wilkins, I., Chervenak, F.A. and Lynch, L.: Intrauterine intravascular transfusions for severe red blood cell isoimmunization: Ultrasound-guided percutaneous approach. Am. J. Obstet. Gynecol. 155:574, 1986a.

Berkowitz, R.L., Chitkara, U., Goldberg, J.D., Wilkins, I. and Chervenak, F.A.: Intravascular transfusion in utero: The percutaneous approach. Am. J. Obstet. Gynecol. 154:622, 1986b.

Berlin, B.M., Shephard, B.A., Elias, E.R., Lazar, E.C. and Bianchi, D.W.: Abnormal serum triple screen and cri-du-chat syndrome. Am. J. Hum. Genet. 57(Suppl.):A343, 1995.

Bernard, K.G. and Cooperberg, P.L.: Sonographic differentiation between blighted ovum and early viable pregnancy. Am. J. Roentg. 144:597, 1985.

Bernier, F.P., Martyn, P., Elliott, P.D., Simrose, B. and Harder, J.: Fetal lung mass associated with significant mediastinal shift: A pulmonary sequestration with good outcome. Am. J. Hum. Genet. 57(Suppl.):A343, 1995.

Bernstein, R., Koo, G.C. and Wachtel, S.S.: Abnormality of the X chromosome in human 46,XY female siblings with dysgenetic ovaries. Science. 207:768, 1980.

Berry, M.N. and Lamm, F.: Unexplained markedly elevated amniotic fluid alpha-fetoprotein (AFAFP) values. Am. J. Hum. Genet. 57(Suppl.):A275, 1995.

Berry, S.M., Gosden, C., Snijders, R.J.M. and Nicolaides, K.H.: Fetal holoprosencephaly: Associated malformations and chromosomal defects. Fetal Diagn. Ther. 5:92, 1990.

Berry, D., Jackson, C., Linn, K., Thomas,. R. and Filkins, K.: Positive outcomes following the prenatal diagnosis of congenital cystic adenomatoid malformation of the lung (CCAML). Am. J. Hum. Genet. 57(Suppl.):A275, 1995.

Bertrand, J.M., Dubois, P., Battisti, O., Langhendries, J.P. and Withofs, L.: Successful treatment of intrauterine supraventricular tachycardia and hydrops fetalis with digoxin. Eur. J. Pediatr. 145:449, 1986.

Berube, S., Lister, G., Jr., Toews, W.H., Creasy, R.K. and Heymann, M.A.: Congenital heart block and maternal systemic lupus erythematosus. Am. J. Obstet. Gynecol. 130:595, 1978.

Besancon, A.-M., Belon, J.P., Castelnau, L., Dumez, Y. and Poenaru, L.: Prenatal diagnosis of atypical Tay–Sachs disease by chorionic villi sampling. Prenat. Diagn. 4:365, 1984.

Besancon, A.-M., Castelnau, L., Nicolesco, H., Dumez, Y. and Poenaru, L.: Prenatal diagnosis of glycogenosis type II (Pompe's disease) using chorionic villi biopsy. Clin. Genet. 27:479, 1985.

Besley, G.T.N.: The use of natural and artificial substrates in the prenatal diagnosis of Krabbe's disease. J. Inherit. Metab. Dis. 1:115, 1978.

Besley, G.T.N., Ferguson-Smith, M.E., Frew, C., Morris, A. and Gilmore, D.H.: First trimester diagnosis of Gaucher disease in a fetus with trisomy 21. Prenat. Diagn. 8:471, 1988.

Besley, G.T.N., Broadhead, D.M., Nevin, N.C., Nevin, J. and Dornan, J.C.: Prenatal diagnosis of mucolipidosis II by early amniocentesis. Lancet. 1:1164, 1990.

Besley, G.T.N., Broadhead, D.M. and Ellis, P.M.: First-trimester diagnosis of Hunter syndrome (MPS II). Prenat. Diagn. 12:72, 1992.

Bevis, D.C.A.: Composition of liquor amnii in haemolytic disease of newborn. Lancet. 2:443, 1950.

Bevis, D.C.A.: The antenatal prediction of haemolytic disease of the newborn. Lancet. 1:395, 1952.

Bevis, D.C.A.: Blood pigments in haemolytic disease of the newborn. J. Obstet. Gynecol. Brit. Commonw. 63:68, 1956.

Bharathur, R., Ragam, K., Delacruz, A., Bircsak, M., Haider, M. and Lee, M.L.: Amniotic fluid beta hCG levels associated with Down syndrome and other chromosome abnormalities. Am. J. Hum. Genet. 43(Suppl.):A226, 1988.

Bialer, M.G., Gailani, M.R., McLaughlin, J.A., Petrikovsky, B. and Bale, A.E.: Prenatal diagnosis of Gorlin syndrome. Lancet 344:477, 1994.

Bianchi, D.W., Flint, A.F., Pizzimenti, M.F. and Latt, S.A.: Demonstration of fetal gene sequences in nucleated erythrocytes isolated from maternal blood. Am. J. Hum. Genet. 45(Suppl.):A252, 1989.

Bianchi, C., Corbella, E., Beccaria, L., Bolla, P. and Chiumello, G.: A case of familial nesidioblastosis: Prenatal diagnosis of foetal hyperinsulinism. Acta Paediatr. 81:853, 1992.

Bick, D.P., Balkite, E.A., Baumgarten, A., Hobbins, J.C. and Mahoney, M.J.: Occurrence of amniotic fluid acetylcholinesterase in association with congenital skin disorders. Am. J. Hum. Genet. 37(Suppl.):A213, 1985.

Bick, D.P., Balkite, E.A., Baumgarten, A., Hobbins, J.C. and Mahoney, M.J.: The association of congenital skin disorders with acetylcholinesterase in amniotic fluid. Prenat. Diagn. 7:543, 1987.

Bick, D.P., Schwanzel-Fukuda, M., Pfaff, D.W., Schorderet, D.F., Price, P.A., Campbell, L., Huff, R.W. and Moore, C.M.: Prenatal diagnosis and investigation of a fetus with chondrodysplasia punctata, ichthyosis and Kallmann syndrome due to an Xp deletion: Evidence for a neuronal migration defect in Kallmann syndrome. Am. J. Hum. Genet. 45(Suppl.):A252, 1989.

Bick, D.P., Schorderet, D.F., Price, P.A., Campbell, L., Huff, R.W., Shapiro, L.J. and Moore, C.M.: Prenatal diangosis and investigation of a fetus with chondrodysplasia punctata, ichthyosis, and Kallmann syndrome due to an Xp deletion. Prenat. Diagn. 12:19, 1992.

Bidwell, J.K. and Nelson, A.: Prenatal ultrasonic diagnosis of congenital duplication of the stomach. J. Ultrasound Med. 5:589, 1986.

Bieber, F.R. and Petres, R.E.: Raised amniotic fluid alpha-fetoprotein in a case of nuchal bleb. Lancet. 2:374, 1978.

Bieber, F.R., Petres, R.E., Bieber, J.M. and Nance, W.E.: Prenatal detection of a familial nuchal bleb simulating encephalocele. Birth Defects. 15(5A):51, 1979.

Bieber, F.R., Krauss, C.M., Nickerson, K., Sandstrom, M.McH. and Stryker, J.M.: Percutaneous umbilical blood sampling (PUBS) for rapid fetal chromosome analysis in high risk pregnancies. Am. J. Hum. Genet. 41(Suppl.):A266, 1987.

Bingol, N., Fuchs, M., Pagan, M., Pearl, M. and Stone, R.K.: In utero ultrasound diagnosis of achondrogenesis, type II (Langer–Saldino type). Am. J. Hum. Genet. 41:A48, 1987.

Birnholz, J.C.: Determination of fetal sex. N. Engl. J. Med. 309:942, 1983.

Birnholz, J.C. and Frigoletto, F.D.: Antenatal treatment of hydrocephalus. N. Engl. J. Med. 304:1021, 1981.

Bischoff, F.Z., Lewis, D.E., Nguyen, D., Murrell, S., Schober, W., Scott, J., Simpson, J.L. and Elias, S.: Detection of XY/XXY mosaicism in fetal cells in maternal blood: Is analysis of fetal cells in maternal blood more sensitive than invasive analysis? Am. J. Hum. Genet. 57(Suppl.):A113, 1995a.

Bischoff, F.Z., Nguyen, D., Simpson, J.L. and Elias, S.: Rapid fluorescence in situ hybridization

(FISH) for the identification of fetal sex using chorionic villi sampling (CVS) transport media: A useful method in the development of protocols for the isolation and analysis of fetal cells from maternal blood. Am. J. Hum. Genet. 57(Suppl.):A121, 1995b.

Bjaler, M.G., Nada, M.A., Vianey-Saban, C., Roe, C.R., Mathieu, M., McGlynn, J.A., Ding, J.H., Mandon, G. and Slonim, A.E.: Prenatal diagnosis of very long chain acyl-CoA dehydrogenase (VLCAD) deficiency. Am. J. Hum. Genet. 57(Suppl.):A275, 1995.

Bjornstahl, H., Kullendorff, C.-M. and Westgren, M.: Gastroschisis diagnosed in utero by ultrasound. Acta Obstet. Gynecol. Scand. 62:283, 1983.

Blaakaer, J.: Ultrasonic diagnosis of fetal ascites and toxoplasmosis. Acta Obstet. Gynecol. Scand. 65:653, 1986.

Black, S.H., Chambers, S. Soenksen, D. Roberts, J. and Schulman, J.D.: Cystic nuchal abnormalities identified by sonography in the first trimester in three fetuses with trisomy 18. Am. J. Hum. Genet. 43:A226, 1988.

Blackwell, D.E., Spinnato, J.A., Hirsch, G., Giles, H.R. and Sackler, J.: Antenatal ultrasound diagnosis of holoprosencephaly: A case report. Am. J. Obstet. Gynecol. 143:848, 1982.

Blagowidow, N., Mennuti, M.T., Huff, D.S., Eagle, R.C. and Zackai, E.H.: A possible X-linked lethal disorder characterized by brain, eye, and urogenital malformations. Am. J. Hum. Genet. 34(Suppl.):A53, 1986.

Blanc, W.A.: The future of antepartum morphologic studies. In: *Diagnosis and Treatment of Fetal Disorders.* Adamsons, K., (Ed.), New York: Springer-Verlag, 1968.

Blanchet-Bardon, C. and Dumez, Y.: Prenatal diagnosis of harlequin fetus. Semin. Dermatol. 3:225, 1984.

Blanchet-Bardon, C., Dumez, Y., Labbe, F., Lutzner, M.A., Puissant, A., Benrion, R. and Bernheim, A.: Prenatal diagnosis of harlequin fetus. Lancet 1:132, 1983.

Blau, K., Rattenbury, J.M., Pryse-Davies, J., Clark, P. and Sandler, M.: Prenatal detection of hypophosphatasia: Cytological and genetic considerations. J. Inher. Metab. Dis. 1:37, 1978.

Blau, N., Niederwieser, A., Curtius, H.C., Kierat, L., Leimbacher, W., Matasovic, A., Binkert, F., Lehmann, H., Leupold, D., Guardamagna, O., Ponzone, A., Schmidt, H., Coskun, T., Ozalp, I., Giugliani, R., Biasucci, G. and Giovannini, M.: Prenatal diagnosis of atypical phenylkeonuria. J. Inher. Metab. Dis. 12(Suppl. 2):295, 1989.

Blott, M., Nicolaides, K.H. and Greenough, A.: Pleuroamniotic shunting for decompression of fetal pleural effusions. Obstet. Gynecol. 71:798, 1988a.

Blott, M., Nicolaides, K.H. and Greenough, A.: Postnatal respiratory function after chronic drainage of fetal pulmonary cyst. Am. J. Obstet. Gynecol. 159:858, 1988b.

Blouquit, Y., Beuzard, Y., Varnavides, L., Chabret, C., Dumez, Y., John, P.N., Rodeck, C. and White, J.M.: Antenatal diagnosis of haemoglobinopathies by Biorex chromatography of haemoglobin. Br. J. Haematol. 50:7, 1982.

Blumenthal, S., Jacobs, J.C., Steer, C.M. and Williamson, S.W.: Congenital atrial flutter: Report of a case documented by intra-uterine electrocardiogram. Pediatrics 41:659, 1968.

Bobrow, M., Evans, C.J., Noble, J. and Patel, C.: Cellular content of amniotic fluid as predictor of central nervous system malformations. J. Med. Genet. 15:97, 1978.

Boccacci, M., Massa, A. and Tentori, L.: Application of cellulose acetate electrophoresis to globin chain separation for antenatal diagnosis of beta thalassemia. Clin. Chim. Acta. 116:137, 1981.

Bocian, M., Karp, L.E., Mohandas, T., Sarti, D., Lachman, R. and Wisot, A.: Intrauterine diagnosis of triploidy: The use of radiologic and ultrasonographic techniques in conjunction with amniocentesis. Am. J. Med. Genet. 1:323, 1978.

Bock, J.E.: Intra-uterine transfusion in the management of pregnant women with severe Rhesus isoimmunization. Acta Obstet. Gynecol. Scand. 53:20(Suppl.), 1976.

Boehm, C.D., Antonarakis, S.E., Phillips, J.A., III, Stetten, G. and Kazazian, H.H., Jr.: Prenatal diagnosis using DNA polymorphisms: Report on 95 pregnancies at risk for sickle-cell disease or beta-thalassemia. N. Engl. J. Med. 308:1054, 1983.

Boehm, C.D., Dowling, C.E., Scott, A.F., Saiki, R.S., Erlich, H.A. and Kazazian, H.H.: General usefulness of the polymerase chain reaction technique to prenatal diagnosis of hemoglobin-opathies. Am. J. Hum. Genet. 41(Suppl.):A94, 1987.

Boehmer, S.M., Hildebrandt, R.J. and McCorquodale, M.M.: Difficulties in genetic counseling and assessing risk: Couple with 2 consecutive, unrelated trisomies plus a paternal 13;14 translocation. Am. J. Hum. Genet. 57(Suppl.):A343, 1995.

Bofinger, M.K. and Saldana, L.R.: Kniest syndrome: Prenatal sonographic findings. Am. J. Hum. Genet. 45(Suppl.):A253, 1989.

Bofinger, M.K., Opitz, J.M., Soukup, S.W., Ekblom, L.S., Phillips, S., Daniel, A. and Greene, E.W.: A familial MCA/MR syndrome due to translocation t(10;16)(q26;p13.1): Report of six cases. Am. J. Med. Genet. 38:1, 1991.

Bogart, M.H.: Prenatal screening for Down's syndrome. Br. Med. J. 303:55, 1991.

Bogart, M.H., Pandian, M.R. and Jones, O.W.: Abnormal maternal serum chorionic gonadotropin levels in pregnancies with fetal chromosome abnormalities. Prenat. Diagn. 7:623, 1987.

Boles, R.G., Teebi, A.S., Nielson, K.A. and Meyn, M.S.: Pseudo-trisomy 13 syndrome with upper limb shortness and radial hypoplasia. Am. J. Med. Genet. 44:638, 1992.

Boman, H. and Schneider, J.A.: Prenatal diagnosis of nephropathic cystinosis. Acta Paediatr. Scand. 70:389, 1981.

Bombard, A.T., Sachs, G., Nakagawa, S., Carter, S.M., Cohen, B.L., Runowicz, C.D., Eluma, F.O. and Nitowsky, H.M.: Unusual maternal serum oncofetal antigen screening results as a risk factor for abdominal pregnancy: An unreported relationship. Am. J. Hum. Genet. 53(Suppl.):1383, 1993.

Boogert, A., Aarnoudse, J.G., De Bruijn, H.W.A. and Gouw, A.: False-negative amniotic fluid acetylcholinesterase in a case of meningo-encephalocele. Prenat. Diagn. 9:133, 1989.

Booth, C.W., Gerbie, A.B. and Nadler, H.L.: Intrauterine detection of Gm₁ gangliosidosis, type 2. Pediatrics. 52:521, 1973.

Booth, P., Nicolaides, K.H., Greenough, A. and Gamsu, H.R.: Pleuro-amniotic shunting for fetal chylothorax. Early Hum. Develop. 15:365, 1987.

Borlum, K.G.: Amniotic band syndrome in second trimester associated with fetal malformations. Prenat. Diagn. 4:311, 1984.

Borochowitz, Z., Jones, K.L., Silbey, R., Adomian, G., Lachman, R. and Rimoin, D.L.: A distinct lethal neonatal chondrodysplasia with snail-like pelvis: Schneckenbecken dysplasia. Am. J. Med. Genet. 25:47, 1986.

Borochowitz, Z., Lachman, R., Adomian, G.E., Spear, G., Jones, K. and Rimoin, D.L.: Achondrogenesis type I: Delineation of further heterogeneity and identification of two distinct subgroups. J. Pediatr. 112:23, 1988.

Borregaard, N., Bang, J., Berthelsen, J.G., Johansen, K.S., Koch, C., Philip, J., Rasmussen, K., Schwartz, M., Therkelsen, A.J. and Valerius, N.H.: Prenatal diagnosis of chronic granulomatosis disease. Lancet. 1:114, 1982.

Borresen, A.L. and van der Hagen, C.B.: Metachromatic leukodystrophy II: Direct determination of arylsulphatase A activity in amniotic fluid. Clin. Genet. 4:442, 1973.

Borresen, A.L., Hellerud, C., Moller, P., Sovid, O. and Berg, K.: Prenatal diagnosis of glycerol-kinase deficiency associated with a DNA deletion on the short arm of the X-chromosome. Clin. Genet. 32:254, 1987.

Boue, J., Vignal, P., Aubry, J.P., Aubry, M.C. and MacAleese, J.: Ultrasound movement patterns of fetuses with chromosome anomalies. Prenat. Diagn. 2:61, 1982.

Boue, J., Chalmers, R.A., Tracey, B.M., Watson, D., Gray, R.G.F., Keeling, J.W., King, G.S., Pettit, B.R., Lindenbaum, R.H., Rocchiccioli, F. and Saudubray, J.-M.: Prenatal diagnosis of dysmorphic neonatal-lethal type II glutaricaciduria. Lancet 1:846, 1984.

Boue, J., Oberle, I., Heilig, R., Mandel, J.L., Moser, A., Moser, H., Larsen, J.W., Jr., Dumez, Y. and Boue, A.: First trimester prenatal diagnosis of adrenoleukodystrophy by determination of very long chain fatty acid levels and by linkage analysis to a DNA probe. Hum. Genet. 69:272, 1985.

Bovicelli, L., Rizzo, N., Orsini, L.F. and Michelacci, L.: Prenatal diagnosis of the prune belly syndrome. Clin. Genet. 18:79, 1980.

Bovicelli, L., Rizzo, N., Orsini, L.F. and Calderoni, P.: Ultrasonic real-time diagnosis of fetal hydrothorax and lung hypoplasia. J. Clin. Ultrasound. 9:253, 1981.

Bovicelli, L., Picchio, F.M., Pilu, G., Baccarani, G., Orsini, L.F., Rizzo, N., Alampi, G.,

Benenati, P.M. and Hobbins, J.C.: Prenatal diagnosis of endocardial fibroelastosis. Prenat. Diagn. 4:67, 1984.

Bovicelli, L., Rizzo, N., Montacuti, V., Morandi, R., Vullo, C., Toffoli, C. and Venturoli, A.: Transabdominal chorionic villus sampling: Analysis of 350 consecutive cases. Prenat. Diagn. 8:495, 1988.

Bowie, J.D. and Clair, M.R.: Fetal swallowing and regurgitation: Observation of normal and abnormal activity. Radiology. 144:877, 1982.

Bowman, J.M.: The management of Rh-isoimmunization. Obstet. Gynecol. 52:1, 1978.

Bowman, J.M. and Manning, F.A.: Intrauterine fetal transfusions: Winnipeg 1982. Obstet. Gynecol. 61:203, 1983.

Bowman, J.M., Lewis, M. and de Sa, D.J.: Hydrops fetalis caused by massive maternofetal transplacental hemorrhage. J. Pediatr. 104:769, 1984.

Boyd, J.J., Bowman, J.M., McInnis, A.C. and Kiernan, M.K.: Fetal diaphragmatic hernia detected at intra-uterine transfusion. Can. Med. Assoc. J. 100:1105, 1969.

Boyd, P.A., Keeling, J.W. and Lindenbaum, R.H.: Fraser syndrome (cryptophthalmos-syndactyly syndrome): A review of eleven cases with postmortem findings. Am. J. Med. Genet. 31:159, 1988.

Bozon, D., Maire, I., Vialle, A., Mandon, G., Guibaud, P. and Gilly, R.: Prenatal diagnosis of cystic fibrosis: Experience of two complementary methods. J. Inher. Metab. Dis. 12(Suppl. 2):305, 1989.

Bradley, L.A., Horwitz, J.A., Dowman, A.C., Ponting, N.R. and Peterson, L.M.: Triple marker screening for fetal Down syndrome. Int. Pediatr. 9:168, 1994.

Brady, R.O., Uhlendorf, B.W. and Jacobsen, C.B.: Fabry's disease: Antenatal detection. Science. 172:174, 1971.

Brady, K., Stephan, M., Duff, P., Stone, I.K. and Jordan, G.: Successful intervention for fetal ascites with obstructive uropathy secondary to hydrocolpos. Proc. Greenwood Genet. Cent. 8:180, 1989.

Brady, A.F., Pandva, P.P., Yuksel, B., Greenough, A., Patton, M.A. and Nicolaides, K.H.: The outcome of the livebirths of pregnancies associated with nuchal translucency >3.5 mm and normal karyotypes. Am. J. Hum. Genet. 57(Suppl.):A276, 1995.

Brahman, S., Jenna, R. and Wittennauer, H.T.: Sonographic in utero appearance of kleeblatt-schadel syndrome. J. Clin. Ultrasound 7:481, 1979.

Brambati, B. and Simoni, G.: Diagnosis of fetal trisomy 21 in first trimester. Lancet 1:586, 1983.

Brambati, B., Oldrini, A., Simoni, G., Terzoli, G.L., Romitti, L., Rossella, F. and Ferrari, M.: First trimester fetal karyotyping in twin pregnancy. J. Med. Genet. 21:58, 1984.

Braunstein, G.D., Ziel, F.H., Allen, A., Van de Velde, R. and Wade, M.E.: Prenatal diagnosis of placental steroid sulfatase deficiency. Am. J. Obstet. Gynecol. 126:716, 1976.

Brennan, J.N., Diwan, R.V., Rosen, M.G. and Bellon, E.M.: Fetofetal transfusion syndrome: Prenatal ultrasonographic diagnosis. Radiology. 143:535, 1982.

Bresson, J.L., Arbez-Gindre, F., Peltie, J. and Gouget, A.: Pallister Killian-mosaic tetrasomy 12 P syndrome another prenatally diagnosed case. Prenat. Diagn. 11:271, 1991.

Bridge, P.J., MacLeod, P.M. and Lillicrap, D.P.: Carrier detection and prenatal diagnosis of Pelizaeus–Merzbacher disease using a combination of anonymous DNA polymorphisms and the proteolipid protein (PLP) gene cDNA. Am. J. Med. Genet. 38:616, 1991.

Brock, D.J.H.: Mechanisms by which amniotic-fluid alpha-fetoprotein may be increased in fetal abnormalities. Lancet 2:345, 1976.

Brock, D.J.H.: The use of amniotic fluid AFP action limits in diagnosing open neural tube defects. Prenat. Diagn. 1:11, 1981.

Brock, D.J.H.: Impact of maternal serum alpha-fetoprotein screening on antenatal diagnosis. Br. Med. J. 285:365, 1982.

Brock, D.J.H. Amniotic fluid alkaline phosphatase isozymes in early prenatal diagnosis of cystic fibrosis. Lancet. 2:941, 1983.

Brock, D.J.H.: Prenatal diagnosis of cystic fibrosis using monoclonal antibodies specific for the isoenzymes of alkaline phosphatase. Am. J. Hum. Genet. 36(Suppl.):186S, 1984a.

Brock, D.J.H.: Amniotic fluid alkaline phosphatase isoenzymes in the early prenatal diagnosis of cystic fibrosis. J. Med. Genet. 21:140, 1984b.

Brock, D.J.H.: A comparative study of microvillar enzyme activities in the prenatal diagnosis of cystic fibrosis. Prenat. Diagn. 5:129, 1985.

Brock, D.J.H. and Barron, L.: First-trimester prenatal diagnosis of hypophosphatasia: Experience with 16 cases. Prenat. Diagn. 11:387, 1991.

Brock, D.J.H. and Hayward, C.: Prenatal diagnosis of cystic fibrosis by methylumbelliferylguanidinobenzoate protease titration in amniotic fluid. Prenat. Diagn. 3:1, 1983.

Brock, D.J.H. and Sutcliffe, R.G.: Alpha-fetoprotein in the antenatal diagnosis of anencephaly and spina bifida. Lancet 2:197, 1972.

Brock, D.J.H., Bolton, A.E. and Monaghan, J.M.: Prenatal diagnosis of anencephaly through maternal serum-alpha fetoprotein measurement. Lancet. 2:923, 1973.

Brock, D.J.H., Barron, L., Jelen, P., Watt, M. and Scrimgeour, J.B.: Maternal serum-alphafetoprotein measurements as an early indicator of low birthweight. Lancet. 2:267, 1977.

Brock, D.J.H., Barron, L., Watt, M., Scrimgeour, J.B. and Keay, A.J.: Maternal plasma alphafetoprotein and low birthweight: A prospective study throughout pregnancy. Br. J. Obstet. Gynaecol. 89:348, 1982.

Brock, D.J.H., Richmond, D.H. and Liston, W.A.: Normal second-trimester amniotic fluid alphafetoprotein and acetylcholinesterase associated with fetal sacrococcygeal teratoma. Prenat. Diagn. 3:343, 1983a.

Brock, D.J.H., Hayward, C. and Gosden, C.: Amniotic fluid GGTP in prenatal diagnosis of cystic fibrosis: A word of warning. Lancet. 1:1099, 1983b.

Brock, D.J.H., Bedgood, D., Hayward, C., Carbarns, N.J. and Gosden, C.: Amniotic fluid microvillar enzyme activities in the early detection of fetal abnormalities. Prenat. Diagn. 4:261, 1984a.

Brock, D.J.H., Bedgood, D. and Hayward, C.: Prenatal diagnosis of cystic fibrosis by assay of amniotic fluid microvillar enzymes. Hum. Genet. 65:248, 1984b.

Brock, D.J.H., Barron, L. and Bedgood, D.: Prenatal diagnosis of cystic fibrosis using a monoclonal antibody specific for intestinal alkaline phosphatase. Prenat. Diagn. 4:421, 1984c.

Brock, D.J.H., Barron, L., Bedgood, D. and Rodeck, C.: Distinguishing hygroma and amniotic fluid. Prenat. Diagn. 5:363, 1985a.

Brock, D.J.H., Barron, L., Bedgood, D. and Hayward, C.: Prospective prenatal diagnosis of cystic fibrosis. Lancet. 1:1175, 1985b.

Brock, D.J.H., Barron, L. and van Heyningen, V.: Prenatal diagnosis of neural-tube defects with a monoclonal antibody specific for acetylcholinesterase. Lancet. 1:5, 1985c.

Brock, D.J.H., McIntosh, I., Curtis, A. and Millan, F.A.: Use of the polymerase chain reaction in prenatal exclusion testing for Huntington's disease. Am. J. Hum. Genet. 43(Suppl.):A79, 1988.

Brocker-Vriends, A.H.J.T., Briet, E., Kanhal, H.H.H., Bakker, E., Dreesen, J.C.F.M., Leschot, N.J., van de Kamp, J.J.P. and Pearson, P.L.: First trimester prenatal diagnosis of haemophilia A: Two years' experience. Prenat. Diagn. 8:411, 1988.

Broekhuizen, F.F., de Elejalde, M., Elejalde, R. and Hamilton, P.R.: Neonatal myotonic dystrophy as a cause of hydramnios and neonatal death: A case report and literature review. J. Reprod. Med. 28:595, 1983a.

Broekhuizen, F.F., Elejalde, R. and Hamilton, P.R.: Early-onset preeclampsia, triploidy and fetal hydrops. J. Reprod. Med. 28:223, 1983b.

Brons, J.T.J., Van Geijn, H.P., Wladimiroff, J.W., Van Der Harten, J.J., Kwee, M.L., Sobotka-Plojhar, M. and Arts, N.F.T.: Prenatal ultrasound diagnosis of the Holt-Oram syndrome. Prenat. Diagn. 8:175, 1988.

Brook, J.D., Harley, H.G., Walsh, K.V., Rundle, S.A., Siciliano, M.J., Harper, P.S. and Shaw, D.J.: Identification of new DNA markers close to the myotonic dystrophy locus. J. Med. Genet. 28:84, 1991.

Brown, B.I.: Prenatal diagnosis of glycogen storage disease. Am. J. Hum. Genet. 36:186S, 1984.

Brown, B.I. and Brown, D.H.: Branching enzyme activity of cultured amniocytes and chorionic villi: Prenatal testing for type IV glycogen storage disease. Am. J. Hum. Genet. 44(Suppl.):378, 1989.

Brown, R.M. and Brown, G.K.: Prenatal diagnosis of pyruvate dehydrogenase E1alpha subunit deficiency. Prenat. Diagn. 14:435, 1994.

Brown, R. and Robertson, E.G.: Fetal heart monitoring during intrauterine transfusion. J. Obstet. Gynaecol. Br. Commonw. 80:116, 1973.

Brown, M.S., Kovanen, P.T., Goldstein, J.L., Eeckels, R., Vandenberghe, K., van den Berghe, H., Fryns, J.P. and Cassiman, J.J.: Prenatal diagnosis of homozygous familial hypercholesterolaemia: Expression of a genetic receptor disease in utero. Lancet. 1:526, 1978.

Brown, T., Anand, A., Ritchie, L.D., Clewley, J.P. and Reid, T.M.S.: Intrauterine parvovirus infection associated with hydrops fetalis. Lancet. 2:1033, 1984.

Brown, J., Gunn, T.R., Mora, J.D. and Mok, P.M.: The prenatal ultrasonographic diagnosis of cardiomegaly due to tricuspid incompetence. Pediatr. Radiol. 16:440, 1986.

Brown, W.T., Houck, G.E., Jeziorowska, A., Levinson, F.N., Ding, X., Dobkin, C., Zhong, N., Henderson, J., Brooks, S.S. and Jenkins, E.C.: Rapid fragile X carrier screening and prenatal diagnosis using a nonradioactive PCR test. J. Am. Med. Assoc. 270:1569, 1993.

Brown, G.K., Otero, L.J., LeGris, M. and Brown, R.M.: Pyruvate dehydrogenase deficiency. J. Med. Genet. 31:875, 1994.

Brown, S., Jackey, P.E., Lien, J.M. and Warburton, D.: A small deletion in the putative "critical region" in chromosome 13q32 in a fetus with isolated holoprosencephaly. Am. J. Hum. Genet. 57(Suppl.):A109, 1995.

Brugman, S.M., Bjelland, J.J., Thomasson, J.E., Anderson, S.F. and Giles, H.R.: Sonographic findings with radiologic correlation in meconium peritonitis. J. Clin. Ultrasound. 7:305, 1979.

Bruinse, H.W., Vermeulen-Meiners, C. and Wit, J.M.: Fetal treatment for thyrotoxicosis in non-thyrotoxic pregnant women. Fetal Ther. 3:152, 1988.

Brumfield, C.G., Lin, S., Conner, W., Cosper, P., Davis, R.O. and Owen, J.: Pregnancy outcome following genetic amniocentesis at 11–14 versus 16–19 weeks' gestation. Obstet. Gynecol. 88:114, 1996.

Bruno, M., Iskra, L., Dolfin, G. and Farina, D.: Congenital pleural effusion: Prenatal ultrasonic diagnosis and therapeutic management. Prenat. Diagn. 8:157, 1988.

Brusilow, S.W. and Horwich, A.L.: The urea cycle enzymes. In: *The Metabolic Basis of Inherited Disease.* 6th ed. Scriver, C.R., Beudet, A.L., Sly, W.S. and Valle, D. (Eds.), New York: McGraw Hill, 1989, p. 629.

Bryant, E.M. and Hoehn, H.: Adherent amniotic-fluid cells and neural-tube defects. Lancet. 1:1203, 1977.

Buamah, P.K., Evans, L. and Ward, A.M.: Amniotic fluid acetylcholinesterase isoenzyme patterns in the diagnosis of neural tube defects. Clin. Chim. Acta. 103:147, 1980.

Buchanan, P.D., Kahler, S.G., Sweetman, L. and Nyhan, W.L.: Pitfalls in the prenatal diagnosis of propionic acidemia. Clin. Genet. 18:177, 1980.

Buchanan, J.A., Jacky, P.B., Houwen, R.H.J. and Ray, P.N.: DNA-based diagnosis for familial retinoblastoma: 3 cases in 2 families, with recombination and paternal origin of mutation. Am. J. Hum. Genet. 45(Suppl.):A254, 1989.

Buchanan, J.A., Klock, R.J., Doran, K., Kennedy, D. and Wyatt, P.: Prenatal test for fragile X syndrome reveals apparent FMR1 gene contraction. Am. J. Hum. Genet. 57(Suppl.):A276, 1995.

Bucholz, R. and Mauldin, D.: Prenatal diagnosis of intrauterine fetal fracture: A case report. J. Bone Joint Surg. [Am.] 60A:712, 1978.

Buehler, B.A., Delimont, D., van Waes, M. and Finnell, R.H.: Prenatal prediction of risk of the fetal hydantoin syndrome. N. Engl. J. Med. 322:1567, 1990.

Bui, T.-H., Marsk, L. and Eklof, O.: Prenatal diagnosis of chondroectodermal dysplasia with fetoscopy. Prenat. Diagn. 4:155, 1984.

Buis-Liem, T.N., Ottenkamp, J., Meerman, R.H. and Verwey, R.: The concurrence of fetal supraventricular tachycardia and obstruction of the foramen ovale. Prenat. Diagn. 7:425, 1987.

Bundy, A.L., Saltzman, D.H., Pober, B., Fine, C., Emerson, D., and Doubilet, P.M.: Antenatal sonographic findings in trisomy 18. J. Ultrasound Med. 5:361, 1986a.

Bundy, A.L., Saltzman, D.H., Emerson, D., Fine, C., Doubilet, P. and Jones, T.B.: Sonographic features associated with cleft palate. J. Clin. Ultrasound. 14:486, 1986b.

Bunge, S., Steglich, C., Lorenz, P., Beck, M., Xu, S., Hopwood, J.J. and Gal, A.: Prenatal diagnosis and carrier detection in mucopolysaccharidosis type II by mutation analysis. A 47,XXY male heterozygous for a missense point mutation. Prenat. Diagn. 14:777, 1994.

Buntinx, I.M., Willems, P.J., Spitaels, S.E., Van Reempst, P.J., De Paepe, A.M. and Dumon, J.E.: Neonatal Marfan syndrome with congenital arachnodactyly, flexion contractures, and severe cardiac valve insufficiency. J. Med. Genet. 28:267, 1991.

Burck, U., Held, K.R., Kitschke, H-J. and Carstensen, M.: Congenital malformation syndromes and elevation of amniotic fluid alpha$_1$-fetoprotein. Teratology. 24:125, 1981.

Burrows, P.E., Stannard, M.W., Pearrow, J., Sutterfield, S. and Baker, M.L.: Early antenatal sonographic recognition of thanatophoric dysplasia with cloverleaf skull deformity. Am. J. Roentgenol. 143:841, 1984.

Burt, B., Boelter, W., Hoffman, E., Crandall, B. and Spector, E.: Carrier detection and prenatal diagnosis of Duchenne muscular dystrophy (DMD) using DNA probes and antibodies. Am. J. Hum. Genet. 45(Suppl.):A254, 1989.

Burton, B.K.: Positive amniotic fluid acetycholinesterase: Distinguishing between open spina bifida and ventral wall defects. Am. J. Obstet. Gynecol. 155:984, 1986.

Burton, B.K.: Outcome of pregnancy in patients with unexplained elevations of maternal serum alpha-fetoprotein (MSAFP). Am. J. Hum. Genet. 41(Suppl.):A268, 1987.

Burton, B.K., Sowers, S.G. and Nelson, L.H.: Maternal serum alpha-fetoprotein screening in North Carolina: Experience with more than twelve thousand pregnancies. Am. J. Obstet. Gynecol. 146:439, 1983.

Bussel, J.B., Berkowitz, R.L., McFarland, J.G., Lynch, L. and Chitkara, U.: Atenatal treatment of neonatal alloimmune thrombocytopenia. N. Engl. J. Med. 319:1374, 1988.

Buyon, J.P., Swersky, S.H., Fox, H.E., Bierman, F.Z. and Winchester, R.J.: Intrauterine therapy for presumptive fetal myocarditis with acquired heart block due to systemic lupus erythematosus. Arthritis. Rheum. 30:44, 1987.

Cacheux, V., Milesi-Fluet, C., Tachdjian, G., Druart, L., Bruch, J.F., His, B.L., Uzan, S. and Nessmann, C.: Detection of 47,XYY trophoblast fetal cells in maternal blood by fluorescence in situ hybridization after using immunomagnetic lymphocyte depletion and flow cytometry sorting. Fetal Diagn. Ther. 7:190, 1992.

Cadkin, A.V. and Sabbagha, R.E.: Ultrasonic diagnosis of abnormal pregnancy. Clin. Obstet. Gynecol. 20:265, 1977.

Callahan, J.W., Archibald, A., Skomorowski, M.-A., Shuman, C. and Clarke, J.T.R.: First trimester prenatal diagnosis of Tay–Sachs disease using the sulfated synthetic substrate for hexosaminidase A. Clin. Biochem. 23:533, 1990.

Callen, P.W., Filly, R.A., Creasy, R.K. and Parer, J.T.: Ultrasonography in the evaluation of intrauterine transfusion. Obstet. Gynecol. 53:656, 1979.

Callen, P.W., Bolding, D., Filly, R.A. and Harrison, M.R.: Ultrasonographic evaluation of fetal paranephric pseudocysts. J. Ultrasound Med. 2:309, 1983.

Callen, D.F., Korban, G., Dawson, G., Gugasyan, L., Krumins, E.J.M., Eichenbaum, S., Petrass, J., Purvis-Smith, S., Smith, A., den Dulk, G. and Martin, N.: Extra embryonic/fetal karyotypic discordance during diagnostic chorionic villus sampling. Prenat. Diagn. 8:453, 1988.

Camaschella, C., Alfarano, A., Gottardi, E., Travi, M., Primignani, P., Cappio, F.C. and Saglio, G.: Prenatal diagnosis of fetal hemoglobin Lepore–Boston disease on maternal peripheral blood. Blood. 75:2102, 1990.

Camera, G., Dodero, D. and De Pascale, S.: Prenatal diagnosis of thanatophoric dysplasia at 24 weeks. Am. J. Med. Genet. 18:39, 1984.

Campbell, S.: Early prenatal diagnosis of neural tube defects by ultrasound. Clin. Obstet. Gynecol. 20:351, 1977.

Campbell, S. and Pearce, J.M.: Ultrasound visualization of congenital malformations. Br. Med. Bull. 39:322, 1983.

Campbell, S., Johnstone, F.D., Holt, E.M. and May, P.: Anencephaly: Early ultrasonic diagnosis and active management. Lancet. 2:1226, 1972.

Campbell, S., Pryse-Davies, J., Coltart, T.M., Seller, M.J. and Singer, J.D.: Ultrasound in the diagnosis of spina bifida. Lancet. 1:1065, 1975.

Campbell, S., Rodeck, C., Thoms, A., Little, D. and Roberts, A.: Early diagnosis of exomphalos. Lancet. 1:1098, 1978.

Campbell, S., Tsannatos, C. and Pearce, J.M.: The prenatal diagnosis of Joubert's syndrome of familial agenesis of the cerebellar vermis. Prenat. Diagn. 4:391, 1984.

Campbell, W.A., Storlazzi, E., Vintzileos, A.M., Wu, A., Shneiderman, H. and Nochimson, D.J.: Fetal malignant melanoma: Ultrasound presentation and review of the literature. Obstet. Gynecol. 70:434, 1987.

Camurri, L. and Ventura, A.: Choroid plexus cysts: A prenatal indication for fetal trisomy 18. Am. J. Hum. Genet. 45(Suppl.):A254, 1989.

Cangany, N.S., Vance, G.H., Heerema, N.A., Perry, M. and Sumners, J.: Pallister–Killian syndrome (PKS) with diaphragmatic hernia (DH) and Dandy Walker malformtion (DWM). Am. J. Hum. Genet. 59(Suppl.):A84, 1995.

Canick, J.A., Knight, G.J., Palomaki, G.E., Haddow, J.E., Cuckle, H.S. and Wald, N.J.: Low second trimester maternal serum unconjugated estriol in Down syndrome pregnancies. Am. J. Hum. Genet. 41:A269, 1987.

Canick, J.A., Stevens, L.D., Abell, K.B., Panizza, D.S., Osathanondh, R., Knight, G.J., Palomaki, G.E. and Haddow, J.E.: Second trimester maternal serum unconjugated estriol and human chorionic gonadotropin in pregnancies affected with fetal trisomy 18, anencephaly, and open spina bifida. Am. J. Hum. Genet. 45(Suppl.):A255, 1989.

Canick, J.A., Palomaki, G.E. and Osathanondh, R.: Prenatal screening for trisomy 18 in the second trimester. Prenat. Diagn. 10:546, 1990.

Canty, T.G., Leopold, G.R. and Wolf, D.A.: Maternal ultrasonography for the antenatal diagnosis of surgically significant neonatal anomalies. Ann. Surg. 194:353, 1981.

Cao, A., Furbetta, M., Angius, A., Ximenes, A., Rosatelli, C., Tuveri, T., Scalas, M.T., Falchi, A.M., Angioni, G. and Caminiti, F.: Haematological and obstetric aspects of antenatal diagnosis of beta-thalassaemia: Experience with 200 cases. J. Med. Genet. 19:81, 1982.

Cao, A., Falchi, A.M., Tuveri, T., Scalas, M.T., Monni, G. and Rosatelli, C.: Prenatal diagnosis of thalassemia major by fetal blood analysis: Experience with 1000 cases. Prenat. Diagn. 6:159, 1986.

Carbarns, N.J.B., Gosden, C. and Brock, D.J.H.: Microvillar peptidase activity in amniotic fluid: Possible use in the prenatal diagnosis of cystic fibrosis. Lancet. 1:329, 1983.

Careilli, M.P., Lamb, A.N., Estabrooks, L.L. and Ward, B.E.: Prenatal interphase FISH analysis of amniocytes: Longitudinal study of accuracy and detection rates. Am. J. Hum. Genet. 57(Suppl.):A50, 1995.

Carey, W.F. and Pollard, A.C.: Microvillar enzymes in amniotic fluid: Considerations for the prenatal diagnosis of cystic fibrosis. Med. J. Aust. 144:68, 1986.

Carey, J.C., Golbus, M.S., Filly, R.A., Hall, J.G., Sillence, D.O. and Hsia, Y.T.: Prenatal diagnosis of a previously undescribed heritable chondrodystrophy. March of Dimes Birth Defects Conference Abstract, 1979.

Carey, W.F., Hopwood, J.J., Poulos, A., Petersons, D., Nelson, P.V., Muller, V., Harrison, R. and Pollard, A.C.: Prenatal diagnosis of lysosomal storage diseases. Review of experience in 145 patient referrals over a period of eight years. Med. J. Aust. 140:203, 1984.

Carey, W.F., Robertson, E.F., Van Crugten, C., Poulos, A. and Nelson P.V.: Prenatal diagnosis of Zellweger's syndrome by chorionic villus sampling—And a caveat. Prenat. Diagn. 6:227, 1986.

Carey, W.F., Poulos, A. Sharp, P., Nelson, P.V., Robertson, E.F., Hughes, J.L. and Gill, A.: Pitfalls in the prenatal diagnosis of peroxisomal beta-oxidation defects by chorionic villus sampling. Prenat. Diagn. 14:813, 1994.

Carlson, D.E. and Platt, L.D.: The association of isolated early second trimester fetal ventriculomegaly and Down syndrome: An indication for placental biopsy. Am. J. Hum. Genet. 53(Suppl.):1388, 1993.

Carlson, D.H., Hamburger, R. and Yeransian, J.: Cephalothoracopagus syncephalus: Prenatal roentgenographic diagnosis. Pediatr. Radiol. 3:50, 1975.

Carlson, E.E., Platt, L.D., Medearis, A.L. and Horenstein, J.: The prediction of autosomal trisomies by prenatal ultrasound detection of the triad: Polyhydramnios, abnormal hand posturing, and any other anomaly. Am. J. Hum. Genet. 43(Suppl.):A227, 1988.

Carmi, R., Hershkovich, A., Abeliovich, D. and Potashnik, R.: Maple syrup urine disease—Prenatal diagnosis and heterozygotes detection. Am. J. Hum. Genet. 39(Suppl.):A251, 1986.

Carpenter, R.J., Jr., Strasburger, J.F., Garson, A., Jr., Smith, R.T., Deter, R.L. and Engelhardt, H.T., Jr.: Fetal ventricular pacing for hydrops secondary to complete atrioventricular block. J. Am. Coll. Cardiol. 8:1434, 1986.

Carr, R.F., Ochs, R.H., Ritter, D.A., Kenny, J.D., Fridey, J.L. and Ming, P.L.: Fetal cystic hygroma and Turner's syndrome. Am. J. Dis. Child. 140:580, 1986.

Carrasco, C.R., Stierman, E.D., Harnsberger, H.R. and Lee, T.G.: An algorithm for prenatal ultrasound diagnosis of congenital CNS abnormalities. J. Ultrasound Med. 4:163, 1985.

Carroll, S.G., Philpott-Howard, J. and Nicolaides, K.H.: Amniotic fluid gram stain and leukocyte count in the prediction of intrauterine infection in preterm prelabour amniorrhexis. Fetal Diagn. Ther. 11:1, 1996.

Carson, D.J., Okuno, A., Lee, P.A., Stetten, G., Didolkar, S.M. and Migeon, C.J.: Amniotic fluid steroid levels: Fetuses with adrenal hyperplasia, 46,XXY fetuses, and normal fetuses. Am. J. Dis. Child. 136:218, 1982.

Caruso, U., Cerone, R., Schiaffino, M.C., Minniti, G., Romano, C., Gatti, R., Filocamo, M. and Colombo, J.P.: Prenatal diagnosis of argininemia: Experience on two pregnancies in the same family. Int. Pediatr. 9(Suppl. 2):77, 1994.

Case, J.T.: Anencephaly successfully diagnosed before birth. Surg. Gyn. Obstet. 24:312, 1917.

Cash, L., McCorquodale, M.M. and Lenke, R.R.: Genetic amniocentesis vs. fetal tissue karyotyping. Am. J. Hum. Genet. 43(Suppl.):A228, 1988.

Caspi, B., Elchalal, U., Lancet, M. and Chemke, J.: Prenatal diagnosis of cystic fibrosis: Ultrasonographic appearance of meconium ileus in the fetus. Prenat. Diagn. 8:379, 1988.

Castineyra, G., Panal, M., Presas, H.L., Goldschmidt, E. and Sanchez, J.M.: Two sibs with Wiedemann–Rautenstrauch syndrome: Possibilities of prenatal diagnosis by ultrasound. J. Med. Genet. 29:434, 1992.

Cayea, P.D., Balcar, I., Alberti, O. Jr. and Jones, T.B.: Prenatal diagnosis of semilobar holoprosencephaly. Am. J. Roentgenogr. 142:401, 1984.

Cayea, P.D., Bieber, F.R., Ross, M.J., Davidoff, A., Osathanondh, R. and Jones, T.B.: Sonographic findings in otocephaly (synotia). J. Ultrasound Med. 4:377, 1985.

Cazenave, J., Forestier, F., Bessieres, M.H., Broussin, B. and Begueret, J.: Contribution of a new PCR assay to the prenatal diagnosis of congenital toxoplasmosis. Prenat. Diagn. 12:119, 1992.

Ceccherini, I, Lituania, M., Cordone, M.S., Perfumo, F., Gusmano, R., Callea, F., Archidiacono, N. and Romeo, G.: Autosomal dominant polycystic kidney disease: Prenatal diagnosis by DNA analysis and sonography at 14 weeks. Prenat. Diagn. 9:751, 1989.

Cederqvist, L.L., Williams, L.R., Symchych, P.S. and Saary, Z.I.: Prenatal diagnosis of fetal ascites by ultrasound. Am. J. Obstet. Gynecol. 128:229, 1977a.

Cederqvist, L.L., Zervoudakis, I.A., Ewool, L.C., Senterfit, L.B. and Litwin, S.D.: Prenatal diagnosis of congenital rubella. Br. Med. J. 1:615, 1977b.

Cervetti, T.A., Shulman, L.P., Emerson, D.S. and Phillips, O.P.: Frequency of fetal aneuploidy in women with elevated maternal serum alpha-fetoprotein levels and normal ultrasound. Am. J. Hum. Genet. 57(Suppl.):A276, 1995.

Chadefaux, B., Augereau, C., Rabier, D., Rocchiccioli, F., Boue, J., Oury, F.F. and Kamoun, P.: Prenatal diagnosis of propionic acidemia in chorionic villi by direct assay of propionyl CoA carboxylase. Prenat. Diagn. 8:161, 1988a.

Chadefaux, B., Rabier, D. and Kamoun, P.: Pitfalls in the prenatal diagnosis of argininosuccinuria. Am. J. Med. Genet. 30:999, 1988b.

Chadefaux, B., Rabier, D., Bonnefont, J.P., Jakobs, C., Dumez, Y. and Kamoun, P.: Prenatal diagnosis of propionic acidemia: Amniocentesis at the 11th week of pregnancy. Prenat. Diagn. 9:448, 1989a.

Chadefaux, B. Rabier, D., Dumez, Y., Oury, J.F. and Kamoun, P.: Eleventh week amniocentesis for prenatal diagnosis of metabolic diseases. Lancet 1:849, 1989b.

Chalmers, R.A., Tracey, B.M., King, G.S., Pettit, B., Rocchiccioli, F., Saudubray, J.-M., Gray, R.G.F., Boue, J., Keeling, J.W. and Lindenbaum, R.H.: The prenatal diagnosis of glutaric aciduria type II, using quantitative GC-MS. J. Inher. Metab. Dis. 8(Suppl. 2):145, 1985.

Chalmers, R.A., Mistry, J., Penketh, R. and McFadyen, I.R.: First trimester prenatal diagnosis of 3-hydroxy-3-methylglutaric aciduria. J. Inher. Metab. Dis. 12(Suppl. 2):283, 1989a.

Chalmers, R.A., Tracey, B.M., Mistry, J. Stacey, T.E. and McFadyen, I. R.: Prenatal diagnosis of 3-hydroxy-3-methylglutaric aciduria by GC-MS and enzymology on cultured amniocytes and chorionic villi. J. Inher. Metab. Dis. 12:286, 1989b.

Chalmers, R.A., Mistry, J., Docherty, P.W. and Stratton, D.: First trimester prenatal exclusion of biotinidase deficiency. J. Inher. Metab. Dis. 17:751, 1994.

Chameides, L., Truex, R.C., Vetter, V., Rashkind, W.J., Galioto, F.M., Jr., and Noonan, J.A.: Association of maternal systemic lupus erythematosus with congenital complete heart block. N. Engl. J. Med. 297:1204, 1977.

Chan, D.P.C.: Thoracoomphalpagus diagnosed before delivery. Med. J. Aust. 1:480, 1976.

Chan, T., Potter, R.T. and Liu, L.: Congenital intraventricular trifascicular block. Am. J. Dis. Child. 125:82, 1973.

Chang, J.C. and Kan, Y.W.: A sensitive new prenatal test for sickle-cell anemia. N. Engl. J. Med. 307:30, 1982.

Chang, J.C., Golbus, M.S. and Kan, Y.W.: Antenatal diagnosis of sickle cell anaemia by sensitive DNA assay. Lancet. 1:1463, 1982.

Chang, H.J., Clark, R.D. and Bachman, H.: The phenotype of 45,X/46,XY mosaicism: An analysis of 92 prenatally diagnosed cases. Am. J. Hum. Genet. 46:156, 1990.

Charles, A.G. and Blumenthal, L.S.: Promethazine hydrochloride therapy in severely Rh-sensitized pregnancies. Obstet. Gynecol. 60:627, 1982.

Charles, A., Moulinasse, R. and Versailles, L.: Harlequin fetus and micromelia. Prenat. Diagn. 9:709, 1989.

Chatterjee, M.S., Weiss, R.R., Verma, U.L., Tejani, N.A. and Macri, J.: Prenatal diagnosis of conjoined twins. Prenat. Diagn. 3:357, 1983.

Chehab, F.F., Doherty, M., Cai, S., Kan, Y.W., Cooper, S. and Rubin, E.M.: Detection of sickle cell anaemia and thalassaemias. Nature. 329:293, 1987.

Chemke, J., Nisani, R., Kassif, R., Lancet, M., Beiser, R. and Hurwitz, N.: Prenatal diagnosis of severe congenital malformations associated with elevated amniotic fluid alpha-fetoprotein. Clin. Genet. 15:351, 1979.

Chemke, J., Voss, R., Hertz, B., Peretz, H., Legum, C. and Caspi, B.: Prenatal diagnosis of cystic fibrosis using DNA probes, microvillar enzymes, and ultrasonography. Am. J. Hum. Genet. 41(Suppl.):A270, 1987.

Chen, H. and Gonzalez, E.: Amniotic band sequence and its neurocutaneous manifestations. Am. J. Med. Genet. 28:661, 1987.

Chen, S.-H., Horowitz, S. and Scott, C.R.: The prenatal detection of a fetus with deficiency of adenosine deaminase (ADA) activity. Am. J. Hum. Genet. 32(Suppl.):38A, 1980.

Chen, H., Blumberg, B., Immken, L., Lachman, R., Rightmire, D., Fowler, M., Bachman, R. and Beemer, F.A.: The Pena–Shokeir syndrome: Report of five cases and further delineation of the syndrome. Am. J. Med. Genet. 16:213, 1983.

Chen, H., Immken, L., Lachman, R., Yang, S., Rimoin, D.L., Rightmire, D., Eteson, D., Stewart, F., Beemer, F.A., Opitz, J.M., Gilbert, E.F., Langer, L.O., Shapiro, L.R. and Duncan, P.A.: Syndrome of multiple pterygia, camptodactyly, facial anomalies, hypoplastic lungs and heart, cystic hygroma, and skeletal anomalies: Delineation of a new entity and review of lethal forms of multiple pterygium syndrome. Am. J. Med. Genet. 17:809, 1984.

Chen, H., Blackburn, W.R. and Wertelecki, W.: Fetal akinesia and multiple perinatal fractures. Am. J. Med. Genet. 55:472, 1995.

Chervenak, F.A. and McCullough, L.B.: Perinatal ethics: A practical method of analysis of obligations to mother and fetus. Obstet. Gynecol. 66:442, 1985.

Chervenak, F.A., Romero, R., Berkowitz, R.L., Mahoney, M.J., Tortora, M., Mayden, K. and Hobbins, J.C.: Antenatal sonographic findings of osteogenesis imperfecta. Am. J. Obstet. Gynecol. 143:228, 1982.

Chervenak, F.A., Blakemore, K.J., Isaacson, G., Mayden, K. and Hobbins, J.C.: Antenatal sonographic findings of thanatophoric dysplasia with cloverleaf skull. Am. J. Obstet. Gynecol. 146:984, 1983a.

Chervenak, F.A., Berkowitz, R.L., Romero, R., Tortora, M., Mayden, K., Duncan, C., Mahoney, M.J. and Hobbins, J.C.: The diagnosis of fetal hydrocephalus. Am. J. Obstet. Gynecol. 147:703, 1983b.

Chervenak, F.A., Isaacson, G., Blakemore, K.J., Breg, W.R., Hobbins, J.C., Berkowitz, R.L., Tortora, M., Mayden, K. and Mahoney, M.J.: Fetal cystic hygroma: Cause and natural history. N. Engl. J. Med. 309:822, 1983c.

Chervenak, F.A., Duncan, C., Ment, L.R., Hobbins, J.C., McClure, M., Scott, D. and Berkowitz, R.L.: Outcome of fetal ventriculomegaly. Lancet. 2:179, 1984a.

Chervenak, F.A., Tortora, M., Mayden, K., Mesologites, T., Isaacson, G., Mahoney, J.J. and Hobbins, J.C.: Antenatal diagnosis of median cleft face syndrome: Sonographic demonstration of cleft lip and hypertelorism. Am. J. Obstet. Gynecol. 149:94, 1984b.

Chervenak, F.A., Isaacson, G., Mahoney, M.J., Tortora, M., Mesologites, T. and Hobbins J.C.: The obstetric significance of holoprosencephaly. Obstet. Gynecol. 63:115, 1984c.

Chervenak, F.A., Isaacson, G., Mahoney, M.J., Berkowitz, R.L., Tortora, M. and Hobbins, J.C.: Diagnosis and management of fetal cephalocele. Obstet. Gynecol. 64:86, 1984d.

Chervenak, F.A., Jeanty, P., Cantraine, F., Chitkara, U., Venus, I., Berkowitz, R.L. and Hobbins, J.C.: The diagnosis of fetal microcephaly. Am. J. Obstet. Gynecol. 149:512, 1984e.

Chervenak, F.A., Farley, M.A., Walters, L., Hobbins, J.C. and Mahoney, M.J.: When is termination of pregnancy during the third trimester morally justifiable? N. Eng. J. Med. 310:501, 1984f.

Chervenak, F.A., Tortora, M. and Hobbins, J.C.: Antenatal sonographic diagnosis of clubfoot. J. Ultrasound Med. 4:49, 1985a.

Chervenak, F.A., Isaacson, G., Touloukian, R., Tortora, M., Berkowitz, R.L. and Hobbins, J.C.: Diagnosis and management of fetal teratomas. Obstet. Gynecol. 66:666, 1985b.

Chervenak, F.A., Isaacson, G., Hobbins, J.C., Chitkara, U., Tortora, M. and Berkowitz, R.L.: Diagnosis and management of fetal holoprosencephaly. Obstet. Gynecol. 66:322, 1985c.

Chervenak, F.A., Hobbins, J.C., Wertheimer, I., O'Neal, J.P. and Mahoney, M.J.: The natural history of ventriculomegaly in a fetus without obstructive hydrocephalus. Am. J. Obstet. Gynecol. 152:574, 1985d.

Chervenak, F.A., Rosenberg, J., Brightman, R.C., Chitkara, U. and Jeanty, P.: A prospective study of the accuracy of ultrasound in predicting fetal microcephaly. Obstet. Gynecol. 69:908, 1987.

Chessa, L., Antonozzi, I., Fiorilli, M., Arslanian, A., Prudente, S., Piombo, G., Bianco, G. and Ferraggiana, T.: Histopathologic findings in a fetus with prenatally diagnosed ataxia telangiectasia. Am. J. Hum. Genet. 53:1539, 1993.

Chiba, Y., Kobayashi, H., Kanzaki, T. and Murakami, M.: Quantitative analysis of cardiac function in non-immunological hydrops fetalis. Fetal Diagn. Ther. 5:175, 1990.

Chinn, D.H., Filly, R.A. and Callen, P.W.: Prediction of intrauterine growth retardation by sonographic estimation of total intrauterine volume. J. Clin. Ultrasound 9:175, 1981.

Chitayat, D., Hahm, S.Y.E., Marion, R.W., Sachs, G.S., Goldman, D., Hutcheon, R.G., Weiss, R., Cho, S. and Nitowsky, H.M.: Further delineation of the McKusick–Kaufman hydrometrocolpos–polydactyly syndrome. Am. J. Dis. Child. 141:1133, 1987.

Chitayat, D., McGillivray, B.C., Diamant, S., Wittmann, B.K. and Sandor, G.G.S.: Role of prenatal detection of cardiac tumours in the diagnosis of tuberous sclerosis—Report of two cases. Prenat. Diagn. 8:577, 1988.

Chitayat, D., Creighton, S., Whitfield, M. and Poskitt, K.J.: Choroid plexus cyst in newborns: A benign finding. Am. J. Hum. Genet. 45(Suppl.):A256, 1989a.

Chitayat, D., McGillivray, B.C., Solimano, A. and Norman, M.G.: Severe arthrogryposis associated with maternal myasthenia gravis. Teratology. 39:445, 1989b.

Chitayat, D., Chemke, J., Gibson, K.M., Mamer, O.A., Kronick, J.B., McGill, J.J., Rosenblatt, B., Sweetman, L. and Scriver, C.R.: 3-Methylglutaconic aciduria: A marker for as yet unspecified disorders and the relevance of prenatal diagnosis in a "new" type ("type 4"). J. Inher. Metab. Dis. 15:204, 1992.

Chitayat, D., Gruber, H., Mullen, B.J., Pauzner, D., Costa, T., Lachman, R. and Rimoin, D.L.: Hydrops–ectopic calcification–moth-eaten skeletal dysplasia (Greenberg dysplasia): Prenatal diagnosis and further delineation of a rare genetic disorder. Am. J. Med. Genet. 47:272, 1993a.

Chitayat, D., Toi, A, Sermer, M., Ritchie, S., Wilson, S.R., and Cole, W.: Pregnancy in a patient with OI type III. Proof of autosomal dominant inheritance and prenatal U/S findings indistinguishable from OI type II. Am. J. Hum. Genet. 53(Suppl.):1390, 1993b.

Chitayat, D., Hodgkinson, K., Luke, A., Winsor, E., Rose, T. and Kalousek, D.: Prenatal diagnosis and fetopathological findings in five fetuses with trisomy 9. Am. J. Hum. Genet. 56:247, 1995a.

Chitayat, D., Moola, S., Toi, A., Conacher, S., Strasberg, P., Bar-Levi, F., Semer, M., Farrell, S., Cytrynbaum, C., Siegel-Bartel, T.J. and Van Allen, M.: Fetal meconium peritonitis: Etiology and prognosis. Am. J. Hum. Genet. 57(Suppl.):A276, 1995b.

Chitayat, D., Toi, A., Babul, R., Levin, A., Michaud, J., Summers, A., Rutka, J., Blaser, S. and Becker, L.E.: Prenatal diagnosis of retinal nonattachment in the Walker–Warburg syndrome. Am. J. Med. Genet. 56:351, 1995c.

Chitkara, U., Gergely, R.Z., Gleicher, N., Kerenyi, T.D., Longhi, R.: Persistent supraventricular tachycardia in utero. Diagn. Gynecol. Obstet. 2:291, 1980.

Chitty, L.S., Hall, C.M. and Baraitser, M.: Two brothers with deafness, femoral epiphyseal dysplasia, short stature and developmental delay. Clin. Dysmorph. 5:17, 1996.

Chodirker, B.N., Harman, C.R. and Greenberg, C.R.: Spontaneous resolution of a cystic hygroma in a fetus with Turner syndrome. Prenat. Diagn. 8:291, 1988.

Chow, C.W., Borg, J., Billson, V.R. and Lake, B.D.: Fetal tissue involvement in the late infantile type of neuronal ceroid lipofuscinosis. Prenat. Diagn. 13:833, 1993.

Christensen, E.: Prenatal diagnosis of glutaryl-CoA dehydrogenase deficiency: Experience using first-trimester chorionic villus sampling. Prenat. Diagn. 14:333, 1994.

Christensen, E. and Brandt, N.J.: Prenatal diagnosis of 5,10-methylenetetrahydrofolate reductase deficiency. N. Engl. J. Med. 313:50, 1985.

Christiano, A.M., Pulkkinen, L., McGrath, J.A. and Uitto, J.: Mutation-based prenatal diagnosis of Herlitz junctional epidermolysis bullosa. Prenat. Diagn. 17:343, 1997.

Christodoulou, J., Teo, S.H., Hammond, J., Sim, K.G., Hsu, B.Y.L., Stanley, C.A., Watson, B., Lau, K.C. and Wilcken, B.: First prenatal diagnosis of the carnitine transporter defect. Am. J. Med. Genet. 66:21, 1996.

Christomanou, H. and Cap, C.: Prenatal monitoring for Wolman's disease in a pregnancy at risk: First case in the Federal Republic of Germany. Hum. Genet. 57:440, 1981.

Christopher, C.R., Spinelli, A. and Severt, D.: Ultrasonic diagnosis of prune-belly syndrome. Obstet. Gynecol. 59:391, 1982.

Chu, D.C. and Boots, L.R.: Retrospective study of maternal serum insulin-like growth factor-I (IGF-I) and its binding proteins (IGFBP-1, IGFBP-3) in various complicated pregnancies in the second trimester. Am. J. Hum. Genet. 57(Suppl.):A277, 1995.

Chubb, I.W., Pilowsky, P.M., Springell, H.J. and Pollard, A.C.: Acetylcholinesterase in human amniotic fluid: An index of fetal neural development? Lancet. 1:688, 1979.

Chudleigh, P., Pearce, J.M. and Campbell, S.: The prenatal diagnosis of transient cysts of the fetal choroid plexus. Prenat. Diagn. 4:135, 1984.

Chueh, J., Chen, E., Wohlferd, M.M. and Golabi, M.: Prenatal diagnosis of Simpson–Golabi–Behmel syndrome: A new family with three severely affected males and elevated maternal serum alpha fetoprotein associated with cystic hygroma. Am. J. Hum. Genet. 53(Suppl.): 1393, 1993.

Claass, A.H.W., Kleijer, W.J., Van Diggelen, O.P., Van Der Veer, E. and Sips, H.J.: Prenatal detection of cystic fibrosis: Comparative study of maltase and alkaline phosphatase activities in amniotic fluid. Prenat. Diagn. 6:419, 1986.

Claiborne, A.K., Blocker, S.H., Martin, C.M. and McAlister, W.H.: Prenatal and postnatal sonographic delineation of gastrointestinal abnormalities in a case of the VATER syndrome. J. Ultrasound Med. 5:45, 1986.

Clair, M.R., Rosenberg, E.R., Ram, P.C. and Bowie, J.D.: Prenatal sonographic diagnosis of meconium peritonitis. Prenat. Diagn. 3:65, 1983.

Clark, B.A. and Bissonnette, J.M.: Fetomaternal hemorrhage during chorionic villus sampling: Detection by hemoglobin F and alpha-fetoprotein analysis. Am. J. Med. Genet. 45:A256, 1989.

Clark, S.L., Vitale, D.J., Minton, S.D., Stoddard, R.A. and Sabey, P.L.: Successful fetal therapy for cystic adenomatoid malformation associated with second-trimester hydrops. Am. J. Obstet. Gynecol. 157:294, 1987.

Clark, R.D., Smith, M., Pandolfo, M., Fausel, R.E. and Bustillo, A.M.: Trisomy due to t(11q23.3;22q11.2) translocation and tuberous sclerosis in a liveborn infant: Is neural cell adhesion molecule a candidate gene for tuberous sclerosis? Proc. Greenwood Genet. Cent. 8:162, 1989.

Clark, B.A., Ashmead, G.G., Crowe, C.A., Foster, A., Stewart, J., Weiser, J.J. and Sanford Hanna J.S.: Triple mosaic aneuploidy at amniocentesis and phenotypically normal pregnancy outcome. Am. J. Hum. Genet. 57(Suppl.):A277, 1995.

Clarke, C.A., Bradley, J., Elson, C.J., and Donohoe, W.T.A.: Intensive plasmapheresis as a therapeutic measure in Rhesus-immunised women. Lancet. 1:793, 1970.

Clarke, O.W., et al.: Ethical issues related to prenatal genetic testing. Arch. Fam. Med. 3:633, 1994.

Clement, D., Schifrin, B.S. and Kates, R.B.: Acute oligohydramnios in postdate pregnancy. Am. J. Obstet. Gynecol. 157:884, 1987.

Clementi, M., Notari, L. and Tenconi, R.: Lethal multiple pterygium syndrome: Importance of fetal physical examination. Am. J. Med. Genet. 57:119, 1995.

Clements, P.R., Taylor, J.A. and Hopwood, J.J.: Biochemical characterization of patients and prenatal diagnosis of sialic acid storage disease for three families. J. Inher. Metab. Dis. 11:30, 1988.

Clewell, W.H., Johnson, M.L., Meier, P.R., Newkirk, J.B., Hendee, R.W., Bowes, W.A., Jr., Zide, S.L., Hecht, F., Henry, G. and O'Keefee, D.: Placement of ventriculoamniotic shunt for hydrocephalus in a fetus. N. Engl. J. Med. 305:955, 1981.

Coates, P.M., Cortner, J.A., Mennuti, M.T. and Wheeler, J.E.: Prenatal diagnosis of Wolman disease. Am. J. Med. Genet. 2:397, 1978.

Cobellis, G., Iannoto, P., Stabile, M., Lonardo, F., Della Bruna, M. Caliendo, E. and Ventruto, V.: Prenatal ultrasound diagnosis of macroglossia in the Wiedemann–Beckwith syndrome. Prenat. Diagn. 8:79, 1988.

Cochrane, D.D. and Myles, S.T.: Management of intrauterine hydrocephalus. J. Neurosurg. 57:590, 1982.

Cohen, R.A., Moskowitz, P.S. and McCallum W.D.: Sonographic diagnosis of cystic adenomatoid malformation in utero. Prenat. Diagn. 3:139, 1983.

Cohen, J. M., Weinreb, J.C., Lowe, T.W. and Brown, C.: MR imaging of a viable full-term abdominal pregnancy. Am. J. Roentgenol. 145:407, 1985.

Cole, C.G., Coyne, A., Hart, K.A., Sheridan, R., Walker, A., Johnson, L., Hodgson, S. and Bobrow, M.: Prenatal testing for Duchenne and Becker muscular dystrophy. Lancet. 1:262, 1988.

Collins, J.H.: First report: Prenatal diagnosis of a true knot. Am. J. Obstet. Gynecol. 165:1898, 1991.

Colley, N. and Hooker, J.G.: Prenatal diagnosis of pelvic kidney. Prenat. Diagn. 9:361, 1989.

Colley, N., Knott, P.D. and Gould, S.J.: Misdiagnosis of omphalocele associated with Edwards syndrome and congenital heart disease. Prenat. Diagn. 7:377, 1987.

Colwill, J.R., Machin, G.A., Popkin, J.S. and Styles, S.M.: Acute second trimester EPH (edema/proteinuria/hypertension) gestosis as an indicator of fetal anomaly. Birth Defects. 23(1):179, 1987.

Comas, A.P. and Castro, J.M.G.: Prenatal diagnosis of OFCTAD dysplasia or Jarcho Levin syndrome. Birth Defects. 15(5A):39, 1979.

Comas, C., Martinez Crespo, J.M., Puerto, B., Borrell, A. and Fortuny, A.: Bilateral renal agenesis and cytomegalovirus infection in a case of Fraser syndrome. Fetal Diagn. Ther. 8:285, 1993.

Comstock, C.H.: The antenatal diagnosis of diaphragmatic anomalies. J. Ultrasound Med. 5:391, 1986.

Comstock, C.H. and Boal, D.B.: Enlarged fetal cisterna magna: Appearance and significance. Obstet. Gynecol. 66:25S, 1985.

Connor, J.M., Aitken, D.A., Maatouk, J.A.H., Graham, G.W. and Gracey, E.: Reduced activity of enzymes bound to the microvillar membrane function of amniotic fluid from pregnancies with cystic fibrosis. Am. J. Hum. Genet. 43(Suppl.):A229, 1988.

Conover, W.B., Yarwood, R.L., Peacock, M.D. and Thomas, B.A.: Antenatal diagnosis of fetal seizure activity with use of real-time ultrasound. Am. J. Obstet. Gynecol. 155:846, 1986.

Conradi, N.G., Uvebrant, P., Hokegard, K.-H., Wahlstrom, J. and Mellqvist, L.: First-trimester diagnosis of juvenile neuronal ceroid lipofuscinosis by demonstration of fingerprint inclusions in chorionic villi. Prenat. Diagn. 9:283, 1989.

Cook, J.A. and Bennett, C.: A child with oligo-syndactyly and 'apple peel' bowel atresia. Clin. Dysmorph. 4:79, 1995.

Cooper, C., Mahony, B.S., Bowie, J.D. and Pope, I.I.: Prenatal ultrasound diagnosis of ambiguous genitalia. J. Ultrasound Med. 4:433, 1985.

Cooper, A., Thornley, M. and Wraith, J.E.: First-trimester diagnosis of Hunter syndrome: Very low iduronate sulphatase activity in chorionic villi from a heterozygous female fetus. Prenat. Diagn. 11:731, 1991.

Cooperberg, P.L. and Carpenter, C.W.: Ultrasound as an aid in intrauterine transfusion. Am. J. Obstet. Gynecol. 128:239, 1977.

Cooperberg, P.L., Romalis, G. and Wright, V.: Megacystis (prune-belly syndrome): Sonographic demonstration in utero. J. Can. Assoc. Radiol. 30:120, 1979.

Corney, G., Whitehouse, D.B. and Hopkinson, D.A.: Prenatal diagnosis of alpha-1-antitrypsin deficiency by fetal blood sampling. Prenat. Diagn. 7:101, 1987.

Corson, V.L., Sanders, R.C., Johnson, T.R.B., Jr., and Winn, K.J.: Mid-trimester fetal ultrasound: Diagnostic dilemmas. Prenat. Diagn. 3:47, 1983.

Cosper, P., Finley, S.C., Davis, R.O., Brumfield, C.G., Goldenberg, R.L. and Finley, W.H.: Non-immunologic hydrops fetalis and chromosomal aberrations. Am. J. Hum. Genet. 43(Suppl.):A229, 1988.

Coss, L.N., Hogge, W.A., Kochmar, S.J., Surti, U., McPherson, E.W., Lazebnik, N. and Hill, L.M.: Isolated abdominal situs inversus associated with an unbalanced 1 : 15 translocation. Am. J. Hum. Genet. 57(Suppl.):A86, 1995.

Cossu, P., Pirastu, M., Nucaro, A., Figus, A., Balestrieri, A., Borrone, C., Giacchino, R., Devoto, M., Monni, G. and Cao, A.: Prenatal diagnosis of Wilson's disease by analysis of DNA polymormorphism. N. Engl. J. Med. 327:57, 1992.

Couillin, P., Boue, J., Nicolas, H., Cheruy, C. and Boue, A.: Prenatal diagnosis of congenital adrenal hyperplasia (21-OH deficiency type) by HLA typing. Prenat. Diagn. 1:25, 1981.

Couvreur, J., Thulliez, P., Daffos, F., Aufrant, C., Bompard, Y., Gesquiere, A. and Desmonts, G.: In utero treatment of toxoplasmic fetopathy with the combination pyrimethamine–sulfadiazine. Fetal Diagn. Ther. 8:45, 1993.

Cove, D.H. and Johnston, P.: Fetal hyperthroidism: Experience of treatment in four siblings. Lancet. 1:430, 1985.

Cox, D.W. and Billingsley, G.D.: Restriction enzyme MaeIII for prenatal diagnosis of alpha-antitrypsin deficiency. Lancet. 2:741, 1986.

Cox, D.W. and Mansfield, T.: Prenatal diagnosis of alpha$_1$-antitrypsin deficiency and estimates of fetal risk for disease. J. Med. Genet. 24:52, 1987.

Cox, R.P., Hutzler, J. and Dancis, J.: Antenatal diagnosis of maple-syrup urine disease. Lancet. 2:212, 1978.

Cox, D.W., Mansfield, T., Sifers, R., Ward, P. and Hejtmancik, J.F.: Prenatal diagnosis of alpha$_1$-antitrypsin deficiency in seven families. Am. J. Hum. Genet. 37(Suppl.):A149, 1985.

Crade, M.: Ultrasonic demonstration in utero of an intracranial teratoma. J. Am. Med. Assoc. 247:1173, 1982.

Crandall, B.F. and Matsumoto, M.: Amniotic fluid AFP: Experience with 40,000 pregnancies. Am. J. Hum. Genet. 36(Suppl.):186S, 1984a.

Crandall, B.F. and Matsumoto, M.: Routine amniotic fluid alpha-fetoprotein measurement in 34,000 pregnancies. Am. J. Obstet. Gynecol. 149:744, 1984b.

Crandall, B.F., Lebherz, T.B. and Freihube, R.: Neural tube defects: Maternal serum screening and prenatal diagnosis. Pediatr. Clin. North Am. 25:619, 1978.

Crandall, B.F., Kasha, W. and Matsumoto, M.: Prenatal diagnosis of neural tube defects: Experiences with acetylcholinesterase gel electrophoresis. Am. J. Med. Genet. 12:361, 1982.

Crandall, B.F., Matsumoto, M. and Perdue, S.: Amniotic fluid (AF)-AFP in Down syndrome (DS) and other chromosome abnormalities. Am. J. Hum. Genet. 41(Suppl.):A271, 1987.

Crandall, B.F., Matsumoto, M. and Perdue, S.: Amniotic fluid-AFP in Down syndrome and other chromosome abnormalities. Prenat. Diagn. 8:255, 1988.

Crandall, B.F., Hanson, F.W. and Tennant, F.: Acetylcholinesterase (AChE) electrophoresis and early amniocentesis. Am. J. Hum. Genet. 45(Suppl.):A257, 1989.

Crane, J.P. and Beaver, H.A.: Midtrimester sonographic diagnosis of mandibulofacial dysostosis. Am. J. Med. Genet. 25:251, 1986.

Crane, J.P. and Heise, R.L.: New syndrome in three affected siblings. Pediatrics. 68:235, 1981.

Crane, J.P., Beaver, H.A. and Cheung, S.W.: Antenatal ultrasound findings in fetal triploidy syndrome. J. Ultrasound Med. 4:519, 1985.

Crawford, C.S.: Antenatal diagnosis of fetal cardiac abnormalities. Ann. Clin. Lab. Sci. 12:99, 1982.

Crawford, D.C., Garrett, C., Tynan, M., Neville, B.G. and Allan, L.D.: Cardiac rhabdomyomata as a marker for the antenatal detection of tuberous sclerosis. J. Med. Genet. 20:303, 1983.

Creech, G.R., Bialer, M.G., Hogge, W.A. and Atkin, J.F.: Pitfalls of prenatal diagnosis: Meckel syndrome versus Bardet–Biedl syndrome. Am. J. Hum. Genet. 43(Suppl.):A230, 1988.

Cremer, M., Schachner, M., Cremer, T., Schmidt, W. and Voigtlander, T.: Demonstration of astrocytes in cultured amniotic fluid cells of three cases with neural-tube defect. Hum. Genet. 56:365, 1981.

Cremin, B.J. and Shaff, M.I.: Congenital syphilis diagnosis in utero. Br. J. Radiol. 48:939, 1975.

Cremin, B.J. and Shaff, M.I.: Ultrasonic diagnosis of thanatophoric dwarfism in utero. Radiology 124:479, 1977.

Crowe, C., Jassani, M. and Dickerman, L.: The prenatal diagnosis of Warburg syndrome. Am. J. Hum. Genet. 37(Suppl.):A214, 1985.

Crowe, C., Jassani, M. and Dickerman L.: The prenatal diagnosis of the Walker–Warburg syndrome. Prenat. Diagn. 6:177, 1986.

Crowley, D.: Combined two-dimensional (2-D) and M-mode echocardiographic evaluation of fetal arrhythmia. Pediatr. Res. 14:442, 1980.

Cuckle, H.S. and Wald, N.J.: Amniotic fluid alpha-fetoprotein levels in Down syndrome. Lancet. 2:290, 1986.

Cuckle, H.S., Wald, N.J. and Lindenbaum, R.H.: Maternal serum alpha-fetoprotein measurement: A screening test for Down syndrome. Lancet. 1:926, 1984.

Cuckle, H.S., Wald, N.J., Lindenbaum, R.H. and Jonasson, J.: Amniotic fluid AFP levels and Down syndrome. Lancet. 1:290, 1985.

Cullen, M., Green, A., Scioscia, M., Mahoney, M., and Hobbins, J.: Ultrasound in the diagnosis of aneuploidy during the first trimester. Am. J. Hum. Genet. 43(Suppl.):A230, 1988.

Cullen, M.T., Athanassiadis, A.P., Grannum, P., Green J.J. and Hobbins, J.C.: In utero intravesicular pressure and the prune belly syndrome. Fetal Ther. 4:73, 1989.

Curry, C.J.R., Fluskey, L., Holland J. and Winter, S.C.: Nonimmune fetal hydrops: A clinical analysis of 19 cases. Proc. Greenwood Genet. Cent. 2:111, 1983.

Curry, C.J.R., Jensen, K., Holland, J., Miller, L. and Hall, B.D.: The Potter sequence: A clinical analysis of 80 cases. Am. J. Med. Genet. 19:679, 1984.

Curry, C.J.R., Carey, J.C., Holland, J.S., Chopra, D., Fineman, R., Golabi, M., Sherman, S., Pagon, R.A., Allanson, J., Shulman, S., Barr, M., McGravey, V., Dabiri, C., Schimke, N., Ives, E. and Hall, B.D.: Smith–Lemli–Opitz syndrome—type II: Multiple congenital anomalies with male pseudohermaphroditism and frequent early lethality. Am. J. Med. Genet. 26:45, 1987.

Curry, C.J.R., Smith, J.C., O'Lague, P., Workman, L.A. and Golbus, M.S.: The prenatal diagnosis of autosomal dominant hypophosphatasia. Am. J. Hum. Genet. 43(Suppl.): A230, 1988.

Curtis, A., Strain, L., Mennie, M. and Brock, D.J.H.: Confirmation of prenatal diagnosis of cystic fibrosis by DNA typing of fetal tissues. J. Med. Genet. 25:79, 1988.

Curtis, D., Blank, C.E., Parsons, M.A. and Hughes, H.N.: Carrier detection and prenatal diagnosis in Norrie disease. Prenat. Diagn. 9:735, 1989a.

Curtis, A., Strain, L., McIntosh, I., Barron, L., Holloway, S. and Brock, D.J.H.: Prenatal diagnosis of cystic fibrosis: A comprehensive approach. Am. J. Hum. Genet. 45(Suppl.): A257, 1989b.

Cuthbertson, G., Weiner, C.P., Giller, R.H. and Grose, C.: Prenatal diagnosis of second-trimester congenital varicella syndrome by virus-specific immunoglobulin. J. Pediatr. 111:592, 1987.

Daffos, F., Capella-Pavlovsky, M. and Forestier, F.: Fetal blood sampling via the umbilical cord using a needle guided by ultrasound. Prenat. Diagn. 3:271, 1983a.

Daffos, F., Capella-Pavlovsky, M. and Forestier, F.: A new procedure for fetal blood sampling in utero: Preliminary results of fifty-three cases. Am. J. Obstet. Gynecol. 146:985, 1983b.

Daffos, F., Forestier, F., Muller, J.Y., Reznikoff-Etievant, M.F., Habibi, B., Capella-Pavlovsky, M., Maigret, P. and Kaplan, C.: Prenatal treatment of alloimmune thrombocytopenia. Lancet. 2:632, 1984a.

Daffos, F., Forestier, F., Grangeot-Keros, L., Pavlovsky, M.C., Lebon, P., Chartier, M. and Pillot, J.: Prenatal diagnosis of congenital rubella. Lancet. 2:1, 1984b.

Daffos, F., Forestier, F., Capella-Pavlovsky, M., Thulliez, P., Aufrant, C., Valenti, D. and Cox, W.L.: Prenatal management of 746 pregnancies at risk for congenital toxoplasmosis. N. Engl. J. Med. 318:271, 1988a.

Daffos, F., Forestier, F., Mac Aleese, J., Aufrant, C., Mandelbrot, L., Cabanis, E.A., Iba-Zizen, M.T., Alfonso, J.M. and Tamraz, J.: Fetal curarization for prenatal magnetic resonance imaging. Prenat. Diagn. 8:311, 1988b.

Dahl, H.H.M., Wake, S., Cotton, R.G.H. and Danks, D.M.: The use of restriction fragment length polymorphisms in prenatal diagnosis of dihydropteridine reductase deficiency. J. Med. Genet. 25:25, 1988.

Dale, G.: Amniotic fluid acetylcholinesterase. Lancet. 2:975, 1980.

Dale, G., Archibald, A., Bonham, J.R. and Lowdon, P.: Diagnosis of neural tube defects by estimation of amniotic fluid acetylcholinesterase. Br. J. Obstet. Gynaecol. 88:120, 1981.

Dallapiccola, B., Zelante, L., Perla, G. and Villani, G.: Prenatal diagnosis of recurrence of cystic hygroma with normal chromosomes. Prenat. Diagn. 4:383, 1984.

Dalpra, L., Castagni, M., Nocera, G., Tibiletti, M.G., Riboni, G. and Agosti, S.: The use of amniotic FSH levels in resolving a discrepancy between fetal chromosomal and phenotypic sex. Prenat. Diagn. 5:419, 1985.

Danpure, C.J., Jennings, P.R., Penketh, R.J., Wise, P.J., Cooper, P.J. and Rodeck, C.H.: Fetal liver alanine: Glyoxylate aminotransferase and the prenatal diagnosis of primary hyperoxaluria type I. Prenat. Diagn. 9:271, 1989a.

Danpure, C.J., Cooper, P.J., Jennings, P.R., Wise, P.J., Penketh, R.J. and Rodeck, C.H.: Enzymatic prenatal diagnosis of primary hyperoxaluria type 1: Potential and limitations. J. Inher. Metab. Dis. 12(Suppl. 2):286, 1989b.

Darras, B.T., Harper, J.F. and Francke, U.: Prenatal diagnosis and detection of carriers with DNA probes in Duchenne's muscular dystrophy. N. Engl. J. Med. 316:985, 1987.

Daryani, Y.P., Penna, L.K. and Patton, M.A.: The detection of cells of fetal origin in cervical washing samples. Am. J. Hum. Genet. 57(Suppl.):A277, 1995.

Das, S., Whitney, S., Taylor, J., Chen E., Levinson, B., Vulpe, C., Gitschier, J. and Packman, S.: Prenatal diagnosis of Menkes disease by mutation analysis. J. Inher. Metab. Dis. 18:364, 1995.

Dash, S., Panourgias, J. and Karababa, P.: Prenatal diagnosis of thalassaemia by haemoglobin chromatography on Biorex: An evaluation of the method. Prenat. Diagn. 4:11, 1984.

Davenport, D.M. and Macri, J.N.: The clinical significance of low maternal serum alpha-fetoprotein. Am. J. Obstet. Gynecol. 146:657, 1983.

Davidson, J.M., Johnson, T.R.B., Rigdon, D.T. and Thompson, B.H.: Gastroschisis and ompha-locele: Prenatal diagnosis and perinatal management. Prenat. Diagn. 4:355, 1984.

Davidson, K.M., Richards, D.S., Schatz, D.A. and Fisher, D.A.: Successful in utero treatment of fetal goiter and hypothyroidism. N. Engl. J. Med. 324:543, 1991.

Davies, G.A.L., Gadi, I.K., Diamond, T. and Papenhausen, P.: Discordant maternal serum and amniotic fluid alpha-fetoprotein results in mosaic trisomy 16 pregnancies. Am. J. Hum. Genet. 57(Suppl.):A278, 1995.

Davis, L.E., Tweed, G.V., Chin, T.D.Y. and Miller, G.L.: Intrauterine diagnosis of cytomeg-alovirus infection: Viral recovery from amniocentesis fluid. Am. J. Obstet. Gynecol. 109:1217, 1971.

Davis, P., Gosden, C. and Brock, D.J.H.: Acetylcholinesterase, blood-stained amniotic fluids, and prenatal diagnosis of neural-tube defects. Lancet. 1:1303, 1979.

Davis, W.K., Mahony, B.S., Carroll, B.A. and Bowie, J.D.: Antenatal sonographic detection of benign dacrocystoceles (lacrimal duct cysts). J. Ultrasound Med. 6:461, 1987.

Davis, G.K., Farquhar, C.M., Allan, L.D., Crawford, D.C. and Chapman, M.G.: Structural cardiac abnormalities in the fetus: Reliability of prenatal diagnosis and outcome. Br. J. Obstet. Gynaecol. 97:27, 1990.

Deacon, J.S., Machin, G.A., Martin, J.M.E., Nicholson, S., Nwankwo, D.C. and Wintemute, R.: Investigation of acephalus. Am. J. Med. Genet. 5:85, 1980.

De Boer, M., Bolscher, B.G.J.M., Sijmons, R.H., Scheffer, H., Weening, R.S. and Roos, D.: Prenatal diagnosis in a family with X-linked chronic granulomatous disease with the use of the polymerase chain reaction. Prenat. Diagn. 12:773, 1992.

Decoret, E., Sibony, O., Vuillard, E., Bedu, A., Faure, O., Mandelbrot, L., Muller, F., Oury, J.F. and Blot, P.: Prenatal diagnosis of an in utero fetal gastrointestinal bleeding. Fetal Diagn. Ther. 9:252, 1994.

de Crespigny, L.C., Robinson, H.P., Quinn, M., Doyle, L., Ross, A. and Cauchi, M.: Ultrasound-guided fetal blood transfusion for severe Rhesus isoimmunization. Obstet. Gynecol. 66:529, 1985.

de Elejalde, M.M. and Elejalde, B.R.: Visualization of the fetal face by ultrasound. J. Craniofac. Genet. Dev. Biol. 4:251, 1984.

de Elejalde, M.M. and Elejalde, B.R.: Ultrasonographic visualization of the fetal eye. J. Craniofac. Genet. Dev. Biol. 5:319, 1985a.

de Elejalde, M.M. and Elejalde, B.R.: Visualization of the fetal spine: A proposal of a standard system to increase reliability. Am. J. Med. Genet. 21:445, 1985b.

de Filippi, G., Canestri, G., Bosio, U., Derchi, L.E. and Coppi, M.: Thoracic neuroblastoma: Antenatal demonstration in a case with unusual postnatal radiographic findings. Br. J. Radiol. 59:704, 1986.

Defoort, P. and Thiery, M.: Antenatal diagnosis of congenital chylothorax by gray scale sonography. J. Clin. Ultrasound 6:47, 1978.

de Gennes, J.L., Daffos, F. Dairou, F., Forestier, F., Capella-Pavlosky, M., Truffert, J., Gaschard, J.C. and Darbois, Y.: Direct fetal blood examination for prenatal diagnosis of homozygous familial hypercholesterolemia. Arteriosclerosis 5:440, 1985.

de Jong, G. and Muller, L.M.M.: Perinatal death in two sibs with infantile cortical hyperostosis (Caffey disease). Am. J. Med. Genet. 59:134, 1995.

Del Junco, D., Greenberg, F., Darnule, A., Contant, C., Weyland, B., Schmidt, D., Faucett, A., Rose, E. and Alpert, E.: Statistical analysis of maternal age, maternal serum alpha fetoprotein, β human chorionic gonadotropin, and unconjugated estriol for Down syndrome screening in midtrimester. Am. J. Hum. Genet. 45(Suppl.):A257, 1989.

Delooz, J., Moerman, P., Van Den Berghe, K. and Fryns, J.P.: Tetraphocomelia and bilateral femorotibial synostosis. A severe variant of the thrombocytopenia–absent radii (TAR) syndrome? Genet. Counsel. 3:91, 1992.

Delozier-Blanchet, C.D., Pellegrini, B., Hahnemann, J.M and Vejersley, L.O.: Uniparental disomy and feto-placental discrepancies on chorionic villus sampling. Am. J. Hum. Genet. 57(Suppl.):A51, 1995.

Delprado, W.J. and Baird, P.J.: Cephalothoracopagus syncephalus: A case report with previously unreported anatomical abnormalities and chromosomal analysis. Teratology. 29:1, 1984.

Demers, S.I., Phaneuf, D. and Tanguay, R.M.: Hereditary tyrosinemia type I: Strong association with haplotype 6 in French Canadians permits simple carrier detection and prenatal diagnosis. Am. J. Hum. Genet. 55(Suppl.):327, 1994.

Dempsey, P.J. and Koch, H.J.: In utero diagnosis of the Dandy–Walker syndrome: Differentiation from extra-axial posterior fossa cyst. J. Clin. Ultrasound. 9:403, 1981.

Dennis, M.A., Appareti, K., Manco-Johnson, M.L., Clewell, W. and Wiggins, J.: The echocardiographic diagnosis of multiple fetal cardiac tumors. J. Ultrasound Med. 4:327, 1985.

Dennis, N.R., Fairhurst, J. and Moore, I.E.: Lethal syndrome of slender bones, intrauterine fractures, characteristic facial appearance, and cataracts, resembling Hallermann–Streiff syndrome in two sibs. Am. J. Med. Genet. 59:517, 1995.

D'Ercole, C., Boubli, L., Potier, A., Borrione, C.L., Leclaire, M. and Blanc, B.: Fetal chest wall hamartoma: A case report. Fetal Diagn. Ther. 9:261, 1994.

Der Kaloustian, V.M., Kleijer, W., Booth, A., Auerbach, A.D., Mazer, B., Elliott, A.M., Abish, S., Usher, R., Watters, G., Vekemans, M. and Eydoux, P.: Possible new variant of Nijmegen breakage syndrome. Am. J. Med. Genet. 65:21, 1996.

Desai, P.K., Astrin, K.H., Thung, S.N., Gordon, R.E., Short, M.P., Coates, P.M. and Desnick, R.J.: Cholesteryl ester storage disease: Pathologic changes in an affected fetus. Am. J. Med. Genet. 26:689, 1987.

de Sierra, T.M., Ashmead, G. and Bilenker, R.: Prenatal diagnosis of short rib (polydactyly) syndrome with situs inversus. Am. J. Med. Genet. 44:555, 1992.

Desmonts, G., Daffos, F., Forestier, F., Capella-Pavlovsky, M., Thulliez, P. and Chartier, M.: Prenatal diagnosis of congenital toxoplasmosis. Lancet. 1:500, 1985.

Desnick, R.J., Krivit, W. and Sharp, H.L.: In utero diagnosis of Sandhoff's disease. Biochem. Biophys. Res. Commun. 51:20, 1973.

Desnick, R.J., Grabowski, G.A. and Hirschhorn, K.: Prenatal metabolic diagnosis: A compendium. In: *Human Prenatal Diagnosis.* Filkins, K. and Russo, J.F. (Eds.), New York: Marcel Dekker, 1985. p. 59.

Desnick, R. J., Schuette, J.L., Golbus, M.S., Jackson, L., Lubs, H.A., Ledbetter, H., Mahoney, M.J., Pergament, E., Simpson, J.L., Zachary, J.M., Fowler, S.E., Rhoads, G.G. and De La Cruz, F.: First-trimester biochemical and molecular diagnoses using chorionic villi: High accuracy in the U.S. collaborative study. Prenat. Diagn. 12:357, 1992.

Deter, R.L., Hadlock, F.P., Gonzales, E.T. and Wait, R.B.: Prenatal detection of primary megaureter using dynamic image ultrasonography. Obstet. Gynecol. 56:759, 1980.

Devi, A.S., Eisenfeld, L., Uphoff, D. and Greenstein, R.: New syndrome of hydrocephalus, endocardial fibroelastosis, and cataracts (HEC syndrome). Am. J. Med. Genet. 56:62, 1995.

DeVore, G.R. and Hobbins, J.C.: Diagnosis of structural abnormalities in the fetus. Clin. Perinatol. 6:293, 1979.

DeVore, G.R., Hakim, S., Kleinman, C.S. and Hobbins, J.C.: The in utero diagnosis of an interventricular septal cardiac rhabdomyoma by means of real-time-directed, M-mode echocardiography. Am. J. Obstet. Gynecol. 143:967, 1982a.

DeVore, G.R., Donnerstein, R.L., Kleinman, C.S., Platt, L.D. and Hobbins, J.C.: Fetal echocardiography: II, The diagnosis and significance of a pericardial effusion in the fetus using real-time-directed M-mode ultrasound. Am. J. Obstet. Gynecol. 144:693, 1982b.

Devriendt, K., Deloof, E., Moerman, P., Legius, E., Vanhole, C., de Zegher, F., Proesmans,

W. and Devlieger, H.: Diaphragmatic hernia in Denys–Drash syndrome. Am. J. Med. Genet. 57:97, 1995.

Dewbury, K.C., Aluwihare, A.P.R., Birch, S.J. and Freeman, N.V.: Prenatal ultrasound demonstration of a choledochal cyst. Br. J. Radiol. 53:906, 1980.

Dhermy, D., Feo, C. Garbarz, M., Lecomte, M.C., Bournier, O., Chaveroche, I., Gautero, H., Boivin, P., Daffos, F. and Forestier, F.: Prenatal diagnosis of hereditary elliptocytosis with molecular defect of spectrin. Prenat. Diagn. 7:471, 1987.

Dhillon, H.K., Yeung, C.K., Duffy, P.G. and Ransley, P.G.: Cowper's glands cysts—A cause of transient intra-uterine bladder outflow obstruction? Fetal Diagn. Ther. 8:51, 1993.

Dhont, M., Thiery, M. and Vandekerckhove, D.: Hormonal screening for detection of twin pregnancies. Lancet. 2:861, 1976.

Diakoumakis, E.E., Weinberg, B. and Mollin, J.: Prenatal sonographic diagnosis of a suprasellar arachnoid cyst. J. Ultrasound Med. 5:529, 1986.

Diament, M.J., Fine, R.N., Ehrlich, R. and Kangarloo, H.: Fetal hydronephrosis: Problems in diagnosis and management. J. Pediatr. 103:435, 1983.

Dickerman, L.H., Jassani, M.J., Golden, W.L. and Rush, P.W.: Ultrasound dating in association with low MSAFP values and autosomal abnormality. Am. J. Hum. Genet. 41(Suppl.): A273, 1987.

Dickerman, L.H., Lewis, S.M. and Golden, W.L.: Elevated MSAFP as well as low MSAFP significantly increases risk for chromosomal abnormalities. Am. J. Hum. Genet. 43(Suppl.):A231, 1988.

Didolkar, S.M., Hall, J., Phelan, J., Gutberlett, R. and Hill, J.L.: The prenatal diagnosis and management of a hepatoomphalocele. Am. J. Obstet. Gynecol. 141:221, 1981.

Diehn, T.N., Netzloff, M.L. and Storto, P.D.: Alobar holoprosencephaly and multiple anomalies in a stillborn with ring chromosome 18. Am. J. Hum. Genet. 57(Suppl.):A344, 1995.

DiMaio, M.S., Bryke, C.R., Mahoney, M.J. and Yang-Feng, T.: Antenatal diagnosis of a fetus with 45,X/48,XYYY mosaicism. Am. J. Hum. Genet. 43(Suppl.):A231, 1988.

Di Natale, P., Pannone, N., D'Argenio, G., Gatti, R., Ricci, R. and Lombardo, C.: First-trimester prenatal diagnosis of Sanfilippo C disease. Prenat. Diagn. 7:603, 1987.

Dinno, N.D., Yacoub, U.A., Kadlec, J.F. and Garver, K.L.: Midtrimester diagnosis of osteogenesis imperfecta, type II. Birth Defects. 18(3A):125, 1982.

Diukman, R., Ishai, D., Abramovici, H., Cogan, S. and Amiel, A.: A new method for first trimester prenatal diagnosis by uterine cavity lavage, cytogenetic analysis and fluorescent in situ hybridization (FISH). Am. J. Hum. Genet. 53(Suppl.):1398, 1993.

Dobkin, C.S., Ding, X-H., Jenkins, E.C., Krawczun, M.S., Brown, W.T., Goonewardena, P., Willner, J., Benson, C., Heitz, D. and Rousseau, F.: Prenatal diagnosis of fragile X syndrome. Lancet. 338:957, 1991.

Dodinval, P. and Duvivier, J.: Diagnostic prenatal du sexe par dosage de la testosterone et de la F.S.H. amniotiques. J. Genet. Hum. 28:207, 1980.

Dombrowski, M.P., Budev, H., Wolfe, H.M., Sokol, R.J. and Perrin, E.: Fetal hemorrhage from umbilical cord hemangioma. Obstet. Gynecol. 70:439, 1987.

Dommergues, M., Petitjean, J., Aubry, M.C., Delezoide, A.L., Narcy, F., Fallet-Bianco, C., Freymuth, F., Dumez, Y. and Lebon, P.: Fetal enteroviral infection with cerebral ventriculomegaly and cardiomyopathy. Fetal Diagn. Ther. 9:77, 1994.

Donald, I.: Sonar: A new diagnostic echo-sounding technique in obstetrics and gynaecology. Proc. Roy. Soc. Med. 55:637, 1962.

Donald, I.: Ultrasonics in diagnosis (sonar). Proc. Roy. Soc. Med. 62:442, 1969.

Donald, I., MacVicar, J., Brown, T.G.: Investigation of abdominal masses by pulsed ultrasound. Lancet. 1:1188, 1958.

Donn, S.M., Barr, M., Jr., and McLeary, R.D.: Massive intracerebral hemorrhage in utero: Sonographic appearance and pathologic correlation. Obstet. Gynecol. 63:28S, 1984.

Donnai, D.: Fetal hydrops: Mechanisms and syndromes. Proc. Greenwood Genet. Cent. 8:108, 1989.

Donnai, D. and Winter, R.M.: Disorganisation: A model for 'early amnion rupture'? J. Med. Genet. 26:421, 1989.

Donnai, P., Donnai, D., Harris, R., Stephens, R., Young, E. and Campbell, S.: Antenatal diagnosis of Niemann–Pick disease in a twin pregnancy. J. Med. Genet. 18:359, 1981.

Donnenfeld, A.E. and Mennuti, M.T.: Second trimester diagnosis of fetal skeletal dysplasias. Obstet. Gynecol. Surv. 42:199, 1987.

Donnenfeld, A.E., Dunn, L.K. and Rose, N.C.: Discordant amniotic band sequence in monozygotic twins. Am. J. Med. Genet. 20:685, 1985.

Donnenfeld, A.E., Gussman, D., Mennuti, M.T. and Zackai, E.H.: Evaluation of an unknown fetal skeletal dysplasia: Prenatal findings in hypochondrogenesis. Am. J. Hum. Genet. 39(Suppl.):A252, 1986.

Donnenfeld, A.E., Conard, K.A., Roberts, N.S., Borns, P.F. and Zackai, E.H.: Melnick–Needles syndrome in males: A lethal multiple congenital anomalies syndrome. Am. J. Med. Genet. 27:159, 1987.

Donnenfeld, A.E., Wiseman, B., Lavi, E. and Weiner, S.: Prenatal diagnosis of thrombocytopenia absent radius syndrome by ultrasound and cordocentesis. Prenat. Diagn. 10:29, 1990.

Dooley, T., Fairbanks, L.D., Simmonds, H.A., Rodeck, C.H., Nicolaides, K.H., Soothill, P.W., Stewart, P., Morgan, G. and Levinsky, R.J.: First trimester diagnosis of adenosine deaminase deficiency. Prenat. Diagn. 7:561, 1987.

Doran, T.A., Wong, P.Y., Allen, L.C. and Falk, M.: Amniotic fluid testosterone and follicle-stimulating hormone assay in the prenatal determination of fetal sex. Am. J. Obstet. Gynecol. 136:309, 1980.

Dorfman, S.A., Robins, R.M., Jewell, W.H., St. Louis, L. and Evans, M.I.: Second trimester selective termination of a twin with ruptured membranes: Elimination of fluid leakage and preservation of pregnancy. Fetal Diagn. Ther. 10:186, 1995.

Douglas, D.L.: Gastroschisis and alpha-fetoprotein. Lancet. 1:42, 1977.

Dowman, C., Vnencak-Jones, C., McClure, M., and Kaplan, G.: Incidence of cystic fibrosis mutations in pregnancies with echogenic bowel. Am. J. Hum. Genet. 53(Suppl.):1400, 1993.

Dozy, A.M., Forman, E.N., Abuelo, D.N., Barsel-Bowers, G., Mahoney, M.J., Forget, B.G. and Kan, Y.W.: Prenatal diagnosis of homozygous alpha-thalassemia. J. Am. Med. Assoc. 241:1610, 1979.

Dreyfus, M., Neuhart, D., Baldauf, J-J, Casanova, R., Becmeur, F. and Ritter, J.: Prenatal diagnosis of cystic neuroblastoma. Fetal Diagn. Ther. 9:269, 1994.

Dreyfus, M., Baldauf, J-J., Dadoun, K., Becmeur, F., Berrut, F. and Ritter, J.: Prenatal diagnosis of hepatic hemangioma. Fetal Diagn. Ther. 11:57, 1996.

Drinkwater, B.M., Crino, J.P., Etzel, F.K., Ogburn, J. and Hecht, J.T.: Severe infantile cortical hyperostosis (Caffey's disease) is siblings evidence for autosomal recessive inheritance. Am. J. Hum. Genet. 57(Suppl.):A344, 1995.

Driscoll, M.C., Lerner, N., Anyane-Yeboa, K., Maidman, J., Warburton, D., Schaefer-Rego, K., Hsu, R., Ince, C., Malin, J., Pallai, M., Mears, J.G. and Bank, A.: Prenatal diagnosis of sickle hemoglobinopathies: The experience of the Columbia University Comprehensive Center for sickle cell disease. Am. J. Hum. Genet. 40:548, 1987.

Driscoll, D.A., Salvin, J., Sellinger, B., Budarf, M.L., McDonald-McGinn, D.M., Zackai, E.H. and Emanuel, B.S.: Prevalence of 22q11 microdeletions in DiGeorge and velocardiofacial syndromes: Implications for genetic counselling and prenatal diagnosis. J. Med. Genet. 30:813, 1993a.

Driscoll, D.A. Sellinger, B., Budarf, M.L., Emanuel, B.S., Miller, R.C., Donnenfeld, A.E. and Reeser, S.L.: Prenatal diagnosis of cat eye syndrome by fluorescence in situ hybridization (FISH). Am. J. Hum. Genet. 53(Suppl.):1401, 1993b.

Drugan, A., Sokol, R.J., Syner, F., Ager, J., Zador, I. and Evans, M.I.: Clinical interpretation of amniotic fluid alpha-fetoprotein (AF-AFP) and acetylcholinesterase (ACHE) in twin pregnancies. Am. J. Hum. Genet. 43(Suppl.):A232, 1988.

Drugan, A., Krause, B., Canady, A., Zador, I.E., Sacks, A.J. and Evans, M.I.: The natural history of prenatally diagnosed cerebral ventriculomegaly. J. Am. Med. Assoc. 261:1785, 1989a.

Drugan, A., Johnson, M.P., Dvorin, E., Moody, J., Krivchenia, E.L., Schwartz, D. and Evans, M.I.: Aneuploidy with neural tube defects: Another reason for complete evaluation in patients with suspected ultrasound anomalies or elevated maternal serum alpha-fetoprotein. Fetal Ther. 4:88, 1989b.

Dubart, A., Goossens, M., Beuzard, Y., Monplaisir, N., Testa, U., Basset, P. and Rosa, J.: Prenatal diagnosis of hemoglobinopathies: Comparison of the results obtained by isoelectric focusing of hemoglobins and by chromatography of radioactive globin chains. Blood. 56:1092, 1980.

Dubbins, P.A., Kurtz, A.B., Wapner, J.R. and Goldberg, B.B.: Renal agenesis: Spectrum of in utero findings. J. Clin. Ultrasound. 9:189, 1981.

Dubel, J.R., Finwick, R. and Hejtmancik, J.F.: Denaturing gradient gel electrophoresis of the alpha 1-antitrypsin gene: Application to prenatal diagnosis. Am. J. Med. Genet. 41:39, 1991.

Duckett, D.P., Roberts, E., McKeever, P. and Young, I.D.: Prenatal diagnosis of trisomy for the distal two-thirds of the long arm of chromosome 14(q21-qter). Prenat. Diagn. 10:261, 1990.

Dumesic, D.A., Silverman, N.H., Tobias, S. and Golbus, M.S.: Transplacental cardioversion of fetal supraventricular tachycardia with procainamide. N. Engl. J. Med. 307:1128, 1982.

Dumoulin, R., Divry, R., Mandon, G. and Mathieu, M.: A new case of prenatal diagnosis of isovaleric acidemia. Prenat. Diagn. 11:921, 1991.

Dungan, S., Hogge, W.A., Dilks, S.A., Hogge, J.S. and Ferguson, J.E.: Diagnosis, management, and longitudinal evaluation of prenatally detected myelomeningocele (MMC). Am. J. Hum. Genet. 45(Suppl.):A258, 1989.

Dunn, H.P.: Antenatal diagnosis of congenital heart block. J. Obstet. Gynaecol. Br. Commonw. 67:1006, 1960.

Dunn, V. and Glasier, C.M.: Ultrasonographic antenatal demonstration of primary megaureters. J. Ultrasound Med. 4:101, 1985.

Dunnill, M.G.S., Rodeck, C.H., Richards, A.J., Atherton, D., Lake, B.D., Petrou, M., Eady, R.A.J. and Pope, F.M.: Use of type VII collagen gene (COL7A1) markers in prenatal diagnosis of recessive dystrophic epidermolysis bullosa. J. Med. Genet. 32:749, 1995.

Duran, M., Schutgens, R.B.H., Ketel, A., Heymans, H., Berntssen, M.W.J., Ketting, D. and Wadman, S.K.: 3-Hydroxy-3-methylglutaryl coenzyme A lyase deficiency: Postnatal management following prenatal diagnosis by analysis of maternal urine. J. Pediatr. 95:1004, 1979.

Durand, P., Gatti, R., Borrone, C., Costantino, G., Cavalier, S., Filocamo, M. and Romeo, G.: Detection of carriers and prenatal diagnosis for lucosidosis in calabria. Hum. Genet. 51:195, 1979.

Durandy, A., Griscelli, C., Dumez, Y., Oury, J.F., Henrion, R., Briard, M.L. and Frezal, J.: Antenatal diagnosis of severe combined immunodeficiency from fetal cord blood. Lancet. 1:852, 1982a.

Durandy, A., Dumez, Y., Guy-Grand, D., Oury, C., Henrion, R. and Griscelli, C.: Prenatal diagnosis of severe combined immunodeficiency. J. Pediatr. 101:995, 1982b.

Durandy, A., Cerf-Bensussan, N., Dumez, Y. and Griscelli, C.: Prenatal diagnosis of severe combined immunodeficiency with defective synthesis of HLA molecules. Prenat. Diagn. 7:27, 1987.

Durandy, A., Breton-Gorius, J., Guy-Grand, D., Dumez, C. and Griscelli, C.: Prenatal diagnosis of syndormes associating albinism and immune deficiencies (Chediak–Higashi syndrome and variant). Prenat. Diagn.13:13, 1993.

Dyer, S.N., Burton, B.K. and Nelson, L.H.: Elevated maternal serum alpha-fetoprotein (MSAFP) and oligohydramnios: Poor prognosis for pregnancy outcome. Am. J. Hum. Genet. 39(Suppl.):A253, 1986.

Eady, R.A.J., Gunner, D.B., Garner, A. and Rodeck, C.H.: Prenatal diagnosis of oculocutaneous albinism by electron microscopy of fetal skin. J. Invest. Dermatol. 80:210, 1983.

Eady, R.A.J., Gunner, D.B., Carbone, L.D.L., Bricarelli, F.D., Gosden C.M. and Rodeck, C.H.: Prenatal diagnosis of bullous ichthyosiform erythroderma: Detection of tonofilament clumps in fetal epidermal and amniotic fluid cells. J. Med. Genet. 23:46, 1986.

Economides, D.L. and Nicolaides, K.H.: Blood glucose and oxygen tension levels in small-for-gestational-age fetuses. Am. J. Obstet. Gynecol. 160:385, 1989.

Edwards, R.J., Watts, D.C. and Watts, R.L.: Creatine kinase estimation in pure fetal blood samples for the prenatal diagnosis of Duchenne muscular dystrophy. Prenat. Diagn. 4:267, 1984.

Edwards, M.T., Smith, W.L., Hanson, J. and Yousef, M.A.: Prenatal sonographic diagnosis of triploidy. J. Ultrasound Med. 5:279, 1986.

Edwards, M.J., Rawnsley, E. and Graham, J.M.: Posterior nuchal cystic hygroma and lethal multiple pterygia. Proc. Greenwood Genet. Cent. 8:156, 1989a.

Edwards, A., Gibbs, R.A., Nguyen, P.-N., Ansorge, W. and Caskey, C.T.: Automated DNA sequencing methods for detection and analysis of mutations: Applications to the Lesch–Nyhan syndrome. Trans. Assoc. Am. Phys. 102:185, 1989b.

Edwards, S.J., Fowlie, A., Cust, M.P., Liu, D.T.Y., Young, I.D. and Dixon, M.J.: Prenatal diagnosis in Treacher Collins syndrome using combined linkage analysis and ultrasound imaging. J. Med. Genet. 33:603, 1996.

Egeblad, H., Bang, J. and Northeved, A.: Ultrasonic identification and examination of fetal heart structures. J. Clin. Ultrasound 3:95, 1975.

Eiben, B., Hammans, W., Hansen, S., Trawicki, W., Osthelder, B., Stelzer, A., Jaspers, K.-D. and Goebel, R.: On the complication risk of early amniocentesis versus standard amniocentesis. Fetal Diagn. Ther. 12:140, 1997.

Eisensmith, R.C., Goltsov, A.A. and Woo, S.L.C.: Simple, rapid, and highly informative PCR-based procedure for prenatal diagnosis and carrier screening of phenylketonuria. Prenat. Diagn. 14:1113, 1994.

Elejalde, B.R. and de Elejalde, M.M.: Prenatal diagnosis of perinatally lethal osteogenesis imperfecta. Am. J. Med. Genet. 14:353, 1983.

Elejalde, B.R. and de Elejalde, M.M.: Thanatophoric dysplasia: Fetal manifestations and prenatal diagnosis. Am. J. Med. Genet. 22:669, 1985.

Elejalde, B.R., de Elejalde, M.M. and Machinton, S.: Ultrasonographic determination of intrauterine central nervous system trauma. Wis. Med. J. 82:21, 1983.

Elejalde, B.R., de Elejalde, M.M., Booth, C., Kaye, C. and Hollison, L.: Prenatal diagnosis of Weyers syndrome (deficient ulnar and fibular rays with bilateral hydronephrosis). Am. J. Med. Genet. 21:439, 1985a.

Elejalde, B.R., de Elejalde, M.M. and Heitman, T.: Visualization of the fetal genitalia by ultrasonography: A review of the literature and analysis of its accuracy and ethical implications. J. Ultrasound Med. 4:633, 1985b.

Elejalde, B.R., de Elejalde, M.M. and Pansch, D.: Prenatal diagnosis of Jeune syndrome. Am. J. Med. Genet. 21:433, 1985c.

Elias, S., Gerbie, A.B. and Simpson, J.L.: Amniocentesis for prenatal diagnosis in twin gestation. Clin. Genet. 17:300, 1980a.

Elias, S., Mazur, M., Sabbagha, R., Esterly, N.B. and Simpson, J.L.: Prenatal diagnosis of harlequin ichthyosis. Clin. Genet. 17:275, 1980b.

Elias, S., Simpson, J.L., Emerson, D. and Holbrook, K.A.: Ultrasound directed fetal skin sampling: A potentially safer method than fetoscopy for the prenatal diagnosis of genodermatosis. Am. J. Hum. Genet. 43(Suppl.):A232, 1988.

El Khazen, N., Faverly, D., Vamos, E., Van Regemorter, N., Flament-Durand, J., Carton, B. and Cremer-Perlmutter, N.: Lethal osteopetrosis with multiple fractures in utero. Am. J. Med. Genet. 23:811, 1986.

Elliott, J.P.: Massive fetomaternal hemorrhage treated by fetal intravascular transfusion. Obstet. Gynecol. 78:520, 1991.

Elliott, J.P., Garite, T.J., Freeman, R.K., McQuown, D.S. and Patel, J.M.: Ultrasonic prediction of fetal macrosomia in diabetic patients. Obstet. Gynecol. 60:159, 1982.

Elliott, J.P., Foley, M.R. and Finberg, H.J.: In utero fetal cardiac resuscitation: A case report. Fetal Diagn. Ther. 9:226, 1994.

Ellis, W.G., Schneider, E.L., McCulloch, J.R., Suzuki, K. and Epstein, C.J.: Fetal globoid cell leukodystrophy (Krabbe disease): Pathological and biochemical examination. Arch. Neurol. 29:253, 1973.

Ellsworth, R.M., Haik, B.G. and Weiss, R.A.: Norrie disease. In: Buyse, M.L. (Ed.), *Birth Defects Encyclopedia.* Dover, Massachusetts: Blackwell Scientific, 1990.

Elpeleg, O.N., Shaag, A., Anikster, Y. and Jakobs, C.: Prenatal detection of Canavan disease (aspartoacylase deficiency) by DNA analysis. J. Inher. Metab. Dis. 17:664, 1994.

Elrad, H., Mayden, K.L., Ahart, S., Giglia, R. and Gleicher, N.: Prenatal ultrasound diagnosis of choledochal cyst. J. Ultrasound Med. 4:553, 1985.

Emerson, D.S., Dungan, J.S., Shulman, L.P., Phillips, O.P., Grevengood, C., Gross, S., Elias, S.: Prenatal diagnosis of cartilage-hair hypoplasia syndrome. Am. J. Hum. Genet. 53(Suppl.):1403, 1993.

Emery, A.E.H., Burt, D., Dubowitz, V., Rocher, I., Donnai, D., Harris, R. and Donnai, P.: Antenatal diagnosis of Duchenne muscular dystrophy. Lancet. 1:847, 1979.

Enders, G. and Jonatha, W.: Prenatal diagnosis of intrauterine rubella. Infection. 15:162, 1987.

Eng, C.M., Slaugenhaupt, S.A., Blumenfeld, A., Axelrod, F.B., Gusella, J.F. and Desnick, R.J.: Prenatal diagnosis of familial dysautonomia by analysis of linked CA-repeat polymorphisms on chromosome 9q31-q33. Am. J. Med. Genet. 59:349, 1995.

Epstein, B.S.: Radiographic identification of arthrogryposis multiplex congenita in utero. Radiology. 77:108, 1961.

Epstein, C.J., Brady, R.O., Schneider, E.L., Bradley, R.M. and Shapiro, D.: In utero diagnosis of Niemann–Pick disease. Am. J. Hum. Genet. 23(Suppl.):533, 1971.

Erdl, R., Schmidtke, K., Jakobeit, M., Nerlich, A. and Schramm, T.: Pena–Shokeir phenotype with major CNS-malformations: Clinicopathological report of two siblings. Clin. Genet. 36:127, 1989.

Erkkola, R., Ala-Mello, S., Piironinen, O., Kero, P. and Sillanpaa, M.: Growth discordancy in twin pregnancies: A risk factor not detected by measurements of biparietal diameter. Obstet. Gynecol. 66:203, 1985.

Escobar, L.F., Weaver, D.D., Bixler, D., Hodes, M.E. and Mitchell, M.: Urorectal septum malformation sequence: Report of 5 cases and embryological analysis. Am. J. Dis. Child. 141:1020, 1987.

Escobar, L.F., Bixler, D., Padilla, L.-M. and Weaver, D.D.: Fetal craniofacial morphometrics: In utero evaluation at 16 weeks' gestation. Obstet. Gynecol. 72:674,1988.

Escobar, L.F., Bixler, D., Weaver, D.D., Padilla, L.-M. and Golichowski, A.: Bone dysplasias: The prenatal diagnostic challenge. Am. J. Med. Genet. 36:488, 1990.

Eto, Y., Tahara, T., Koda, N. and Yamaguchi, S.: Prenatal diagnosis of metachromatic leukodystrophy: A diagnosis with amniotic fluid by DEAE-Sepharose column chromatography and its confirmation by kidney lipid analysis. J. Inher. Metab. Dis. 5:77, 1982.

Evans, M.I., Zador, I.E., Qureshi, F., Budev, H., Quigg, M.H. and Nadler, H.L.: Ultrasonographic prenatal diagnosis and fetal pathology of Langer mesomelic dwarfism. Am. J. Med. Genet. 31:915, 1988.

Evans, M.I., Johnson, M.P., Dvorin, E., Moody, J., Krivchenia, E.I. and Drugan, A.: Aneuploidy with neural tube defects: Another reason for complete evaluation in patients with suspected ultrasound anomalies or elevated maternal serum alpha-fetoprotein. Am. J. Hum. Genet. 45(Suppl.):A258, 1989.

Evans, M.I., Krivchenia, E.L., Johnson, M.P., Quintero, R., King, M., Pegoraro, E. and Hoffman, E.P.: In utero fetal muscle biopsy (IUFMB) alters diagnosis and carrier risks in Duchenne and Becker muscular dystrophy. Am. J. Hum. Genet. 53(Suppl.):1405, 1993.

Evans, J.A., MacDonald, K., Harman, C.R. and Chodirker, B.N.: Fetal anomalies associated with very high maternal serum alpha-fetoprotein levels. Am. J. Hum. Genet. 57(Suppl.): A279, 1995a.

Evans, M.I., Krivchenia, E.L., Johnson, M.P., Quintero, R.A., King, M., Pegoraro, E. and Hoffman, E.P.: In utero fetal muscle biopsy alters diagnosis and carrier risks in Duchenne and Becker muscular dystropy. Fetal Diagn. Ther. 10:71, 1995b.

Evans, J., MacDonald, K., Harman, C. and Chodirker, B.: Breus mole and large chorioangiomata: Two unusual placental anomalies associated with high maternal serum alphafetoprotein. Proc. Greenwood Genet. Cent. 15:111, 1996.

Eydoux, P., Choiset, A., Le Porrier, N., Thepot, F., Szpiro-Tapia, S., Alliet, J., Ramond, S., Viel, J.F., Gautier, E., Morichon, N. and Girard-Orgeolet, S.: Chromosomal prenatal diagnosis: Study of 936 cases of intrauterine abnormalities after ultrasound assessment. Prenat. Diagn. 9:255, 1989.

Ezaki, M., Sugiyama, K., Wada, Y. and Suzumori, K.: The first trimester prenatal diagnosis of Pompe's disease at risk. Jpn. J. Hum. Genet. 32:267, 1987.

Fahy, M., Robbins, C., Bloch, M., Turnell, R.W. and Hayden, M.R.: Different options for prenatal testing for Huntington's disease using DNA probes. J. Med. Genet. 26:353, 1989.

Fairweather, D.V.I., Tacchi, D., Coxon, A., Hughes, M.I., Murray, S., Walker, W.: Intrauterine transfusion in Rh-isoimmunization. Brit. Med. J. 4:189, 1967.

Fairweather, D.V.I., Whyley, G.A. and Millar, M.D.: Six years' experience of the prediction of severity in Rhesus haemolytic disease. Br. J. Obstet. Gynaecol. 83:698, 1976.

Falik-Borenstein, T.C., Holmes, S.A., Borochowitz, Z., Levin, A., Rosenmann, A. and Spritz, R.A.: DNA-based carrier detection and prenatal diagnosis of tyrosinase-negative oculocutaneous albinism (OCA1A). Prenat. Diagn. 15:345, 1995.

Fan, Y-S, and Farrell, S.D.: Prenatal diagnosis of interstitial deletion of 17(p11.2p11.2) Smith–Magenis syndrome. Am. J. Med. Genet. 49:253, 1994.

Farag, T.I., Al-Awadi, S.A., El-Badramany, M.H., and Usha, R. and El-Ghanem, M.: Second family with "apple peel" syndrome affecting four siblings: Autosomal recessive inheritance confirmed. Am. J. Med. Genet. 47:119, 1993.

Farhood, A.I., Morris, J.H. and Bieber, F.R.: Transient cysts of the fetal choroid plexus: Morphology and histogenesis. Am. J. Hum. Genet. 41(Suppl.):A275, 1987a.

Farhood, A.I., Morris, J.H. and Bieber, F.R.: Transient cysts of the fetal choroid plexus: Morphology and histogenesis. Am. J. Hum. Genet. 27:977, 1987b.

Farrall, M., Law, H.Y., Rodeck, C.H., Warren, R., Stanier, P., Super, M., Lissens, W., Scambler, P., Watson, E., Wainwright, B. and Williamson, R.: First-trimester prenatal diagnosis of cystic fibrosis with linked DNA probes. Lancet. 1:1402, 1986.

Farrant, P.: Ultrasound diagnosis of fetal urinary obstructions. In: Non-invasive Diagnosis of Kidney Disease, Karger Continuing Education Series, vol. 3. Lubec, G. (Ed.). Basel: S. Karger, A.G, 1983, p. 297.

Farrell, S.A.: Intrauterine death in megacystis-microcolon-intestinal hypoperistalsis syndrome. J. Med. Genet. 25:350, 1988.

Farrell, S.A. and Geddie, W.: Fetus in fetu with complex host twin anomalies. Am. J. Hum. Genet. 45(Suppl.):A259, 1989.

Farrell, D.F., Sumi, S.M., Scott, C.R. and Rice, G.: Antenatal diagnosis of Krabbe's leukodystrophy: Enzymatic and morphological confirmation in an affected fetus. J. Neurol. Neurosurg. Psychiatry. 41:76, 1978.

Farrell, S.A., Toi, A., Leadman, M.L., Davidson, R.G. and Caco, C.: Prenatal diagnosis of retinal detachment in Walker–Warburg syndrome. Am. J. Med. Genet. 28:619, 1987.

Farrell, S.A., Sue-Chue-Lam, A., Miskin, M. and Fan, Y.S.: Prenatal diagnosis of trisomy 10 following observation of fetal nuchal edema. Am. J. Hum. Genet. 53(Suppl.):1406, 1993.

Faucett, W.A., Greenberg, F., Rose, E., Alpert, E., Bancalari, L., Kardon, N.B., Mizjewski, G., Knight, G. and Haddow, J.E.: Congenital deficiency of alpha-fetoprotein. Am. J. Hum. Genet. 45(Suppl.):A259, 1989.

Feingold, M., Cetrulo, C.L., Newton, E.R., Weiss, J., Shakr, C. and Shmoys, S.: Serial amniocenteses in the treatment of twin-to-twin transfusion complicated with acute polyhydramnios. Acta Genet. Med. Gemellol. (Roma). 35:107, 1986.

Fejgin, M., Zeitune, M., Amiel, A. and Beyth, Y.: Elevated maternal serum alpha-fetoprotein level and sex chromosome aneuploidy. Prenat. Diagn. 10:414, 1990.

Feldman, E., Shalev, E., Weiner, E., Cohen, H. and Zuckerman, H.: Microphthalmia—Prenatal ultrasonic diagnosis: A case report. Prenat. Diagn. 5:205, 1985.

Feldman, G.L., O'Brien, W.E., Durtschi, B., Gardner, P., Williamson, R. and Beaudet, A.L.: Prenatal diagnosis of cystic fibrosis (CF) using the polymerase chain reaction (PCR) for detection of the KM-19 polymorphism. Am. J. Hum. Genet. 43(Suppl.):A83, 1988a.

Feldman, G.L., Williamson, R., Beaudet, A.L. and O'Brien, W.E.: Prenatal diagnosis of cystic fibrosis by DNA amplification for detection of KM-19 polymorphism. Lancet. 2:102, 1988b.

Feldman, G.L., Lewiston, N., Fernbach, S.D., O'Bien, W.E., Williamson, R., Wainwright, B.J.

and Beaudet, A.L.: Prenatal diagnosis of cystic fibrosis by using linked DNA in 138 pregnancies at 1-in-4 risk. Am. J. Med. Genet. 32:238, 1989.

Fellous, M., Boue, J., Malbrunot, C., Sasportes, M., Cong, N.V., Marcelli, A., Rebourcet, R., Hubert, C., Demenais, F., Elston, R.C., Namboodiri, K.K., Kaplan, E.B. and Fellous, M.: A five-generation family with sacral agenesis and spina bifida: Possible similarities with the mouse T-locus. Am. J. Med. Genet. 12:465, 1982.

Fensom, A.H. and Benson, P.F.: Assay of galactose-1-phosphate uridyl transferase in cultured amniotic cells for prenatal diagnosis of galactosaemia. Clin. Chim. Acta. 62:189, 1975.

Fensom, A.H. and Benson, P.F.: Recent advances in the prenatal diagnosis of the mucopolysaccharidoses. Prenat. Diagn. 14:1, 1994.

Fensom, A.H., Benson, P.F., Blunt, S., Brown, S.P. and Coltart, T.M.: Amniotic cell 4-methylumbelliferyl-alpha-glucosidase activity for prenatal diagnosis of Pompe's disease. J. Med. Genet. 13:148, 1976.

Fensom, A.H., Neville, B.R.G., Moser, A.E., Benson, P.F., Moser, H.W. and Dulaney, J.T.: Prenatal diagnosis of Farber's disease. Lancet. 2:990, 1979.

Fensom, A.H., Benson, P.F., Chalmers, R.A., Tracey, B.M., Watson, D., King, G.S., Pettit, B.R. and Rodeck, C.H.: Experience with prenatal diagnosis of propionic acidemia and methylmalonic aciduria. J. Inher. Metab. Dis. 7(Suppl. 2):127, 1984.

Fensom, A.H., Marsh, J., Jackson, M., McGuire, V.M., Vimal, C., Nicolaides, K. and Sheridan, R.: First-trimester diagnosis of metachromatic leucodystrophy. Clin. Genet. 34:122, 1988.

Ferec, C., Verlingue, C., Audrezet, M.P., Guillermit, H., Quere, I., Raguenes, O. and Mercier, B.: Prenatal diagnosis of cystic fibrosis in different European populations: Application of denaturing gradient gel electrophoresis. Fetal Diagn. Ther. 8:341, 1993.

Fernandez, H., Diallo, A., Baume, D. and Papiernik, E.: Anhydramnios and cessation of fetal growth in a pregnant mother with polychemotherapy during the second trimester. Prenat. Diagn. 9:681, 1989.

Ferrari, M., Rajnoldi, A.C., Crema, A., Pietri, S. and Travi, M.: Prenatal diagnosis of thalassaemia and fetal red cell microcytosis. Prenat. Diagn. 2:143, 1982.

Ferre, M.M., Keene, C.L., Jewell, A.J. and Stetka, D.G.: Prenatal diagnosis of 46,XX,i(18q) associated with holoprosencephaly and cyclopia. Am. J. Hum. Genet. 53(Suppl.):1568, 1993.

Figuera, L.E., Ramirez-Duenas, M.P., Gallegos-Arreola, M.P. and Cantu, J.M.: Spondyloepimetaphyseal dysplasia (SEMD) Shohat type. Am. J. Med. Genet. 51:213, 1994.

Fileni, A., Colosimo, C., Jr., Mirk, P., De Gaetano, A.M. and Di Rocci, C.: Dandy–Walker syndrome: Diagnosis in utero by means of ultrasound and CT correlations. Neuroradiology. 24:233, 1983.

Filion, R., Grignon, A. and Boisvert, J.: Antenatal diagnosis of ipsilateral multicystic kidney in identical twins. J. Ultrasound Med. 4:211, 1985.

Filkins, K. and Russo, J.: Prenatal diagnosis of thrombocytopenia absent radius syndrome using ultrasound and fetoscopy. Prenat. Diagn. 4:139, 1984.

Filkins, K., Russo, J., Brown, T., Schmerler, S. and Searle, B.: Genetic amniocentesis in multiple gestations. Prenat. Diagn. 4:223, 1984.

Filkins, K., Russo, J. and Flowers, W.K. III: Third trimester ultrasound diagnosis of intestinal atresia following clinical evidence of polyhydramnios. Prenat. Diagn. 5:215, 1985.

Filly, R.A. and Golbus, M.S.: Ultrasonography of the normal and pathologic fetal skeleton. Radiol. Clin. North Am. 20:311, 1982.

Filly, R.A., Golbus, M.S., Carey, J.C. and Hall, J.G.: Short-limbed dwarfism: Ultrasonographic diagnosis by mensuration of fetal femoral length. Radiology. 138:653, 1981.

Filly, R.A., Chinn, D.H. and Callen, P.W.: Alobar holoprosencephaly: Ultrasonographic prenatal diagnosis. Radiology. 151:455, 1984.

Fineman, R.M. and Gordis, D.M.: Jewish perspective on prenatal diagnosis and selective abortion of affected fetuses, including some comparisons with prevailing Catholic beliefs. Am. J. Med. Genet. 12:355, 1982.

Fink, I.J. and Filly, R.A.: Omphalocele associated with umbilical cord allantoic cyst: Sonographic evaluation in utero. Radiology. 149:473, 1983.

Firgaira, F.A., Cotton, R.G.H., Danks, D.M., Fowler, K., Lipson, A. and Yu, J.S.: Prenatal determination of dihydropteridine reductase in a normal fetus at risk for malignant hyper-phenylalaninemia. Prenat. Diagn. 3:7, 1983.

Firshein, S.I., Hoyer, L.W., Lazarchick, J., Forget, B.G., Hobbins, J.C., Clyne, L.P., Pitlick, F.A., Muir, W.A., Merkatz, I.R. and Mahoney, M.J.: Prenatal diagnosis of classic hemophilia. N. Engl. J. Med. 300:937, 1979.

Fischbeck, K.H. and Ritter, A.W.: Prenatal diagnosis of Duchenne's muscular dystrophy. N. Engl. J. Med. 317:1097, 1987.

Fisher, N.L., Luthy, D.A., Peterson, A., Williamson, R. and Karp, L.: Amniotic fluid alpha fetoprotein from midtrimester genetic amniocenteses in women at low risk for neural tube defects. Am. J. Hum. Genet. 32(Suppl.):105A, 1980.

Fisher, N.L., Luthy, D.A., Peterson, A., Karp, L.E., Williamson, R. and Cheng, E.: Prenatal diagnosis of neural tube defects: Predictive value of AF-AFP in a low-risk population. Am. J. Med. Genet. 9:201, 1981.

Fisher, R.A., Mather, J.M., Zipple, N.J., Shanahan, R.H., Schehr, A.B., Suppnick, C.T. and Peabody, C.K.: MSAFP screening for chromosome abnormalities: Results of a 2 1/2 year study. Am J. Hum. Genet. 43(Suppl.):A233, 1988.

Fiske, C.E. and Filly, R.A.: Ultrasound evaluation of the normal and abnormal fetal neural axis. Radiol. Clin. North Am. 20:285, 1982.

Fitzgerald, E.J., Toi, A. and Cochlin, D.L.: Conjoined twins: Antenatal ultrasound diagnosis and a review of the literature. Br. J. Radiol. 58:1053, 1985.

Fleisher, L.D., Harris, C.J., Mitchell, D.A. and Nadler, H.L.: Citrullinemia: Prenatal diagnosis of an affected fetus. Am. J. Hum. Genet. 35:85, 1983.

Fletcher, J.C.: Prenatal diagnosis of the hemoglobinopathies: Ethical issues. Am. J. Obstet. Gynecol. 135:53, 1979.

Fletcher, J.C.: Ethical considerations in and beyond experimental fetal therapy. Semin. Perinatol. 9:130, 1985.

Fletcher, J.C.: Moral problems and ethical guidance in prenatal diagnosis: Past, present, and future. In: Milunsky, A. (Ed.), *Genetic Disorders and the Fetus: Diagnosis, Prevention, and Treatment,* 2nd ed. New York: Plenum Press, 1986, p. 819.

Fletcher, J.C., Berg, K., Tranoy, K.E.: Ethical aspects of medical genetics. Clin. Genet. 27:199, 1985.

Fontaine, F., Vasseur, F., Savary, J.B., Menais, M., Roussel, M. and Deminatti, M.M.: Useful-ness of linked DNA probes for prenatal diagnosis of cystic fibrosis: Report of a case in a 1:4 risk pregnancy. Ann. Genet. 31:102, 1988.

Forest, M.G. and Dorr, H.G.: Prenatal treatment of congenital adrenal hyperplasia due to 21-hydroxylase deficiency: European experience in 253 pregnancies at risk. Clin. Courier. 11(11):2, 1993.

Forest, M.G., Betuel, H., Couillin, P., Boue, A., David, M., Floret, D., Francois, R., Guibaud, P., Plauchu, H. and Rappaport, R.: Prenatal diagnosis of congenital adrenal hyperplasia (CAH) due to 21-hydroxylase deficiency by steroid analysis in the amniotic fluid of mid-pregnancy: Comparison with HLA typing in 17 pregnancies at risk for CAH. Prenat. Diagn. 1:197, 1981.

Forest, M.G., Betuel, H. and David, M.: Prenatal treatment in congenital adrenal hyperplasia due to 21-hydroxylase deficiency: Up-date 88 of the French multicentric study. Endocr. Res. 15:277, 1989.

Forestier, F., Daffos, F. and Capella-Pavlovsky, M.: Premier diagnostic prenatal d'une hemo-phillie a par ponction directe du cordon ombilical. Presse Med. 12:2462, 1983.

Forestier, F., Daffos, F., Sole, Y. and Rainaut, M.: Prenatal diagnosis of hemophilia by fetal blood sampling under ultrasound guidance. Haemostasis 16:346, 1986.

Forrest, S.M., Dry, P.J. and Cotton, R.G.H.: Use of the chemical cleavage of mismatch method for prenatal diagnosis of alpha-1-antitrypsin deficiency. Prenat. Diagn. 12:133, 1992.

Fost, N.: Guiding principles for prenatal diagnosis. Prenat. Diagn. 9:335, 1989.

Foster, M.A., Nyberg, D.A., Mahony, B.S., Mack, L.A., Marks, W.M. and Raabe, R.D.: Meconium peritonitis: Prenatal sonographic findings and their clinical significance. Radiol-ogy. 165:661, 1987.

Foster, J.W., Dominguez-Steglich, M.A., Guioli, S., Kwok, C., Weller, P.A., Stevanovic, M., Weissenbach, J., Mansour, S., Yourng, I.D., Goodfellow, P.N., Brook, J.D. and Schafer, A.J.: Campomelic dysplasia and autosomal sex reversal caused by mutations in an SRY-related gene. Nature. 372:525, 1994.

Foucar, E., Williamson, R.A., Yiu-Chiu, V., Varner, M.W. and Kay, B.R.: Mesenchymal hamartoma of the liver identified by fetal sonography. Am. J. Roentgenol. 140:970, 1983.

Fowler, B., Borresen, A.L. and Boman, N.: Prenatal diagnosis of homocystinuria. Lancet. 2:875, 1982.

Fowler, B., Giles, L., Sardharwalla, I.B., Donnai, P. and Clayton, J.K.: First trimester diagnosis of methylmalonic aciduria. Prenat. Diagn. 8:207, 1988.

Fox, J.E., Hack, A.M., Fenton, W.A., Golbus, M.S., Winter, S.C. and Rosenberg, L.E.: Prenatal diagnosis of ornithine transcarbamylase (OTC) deficiency using DNA polymorphisms. Am. J. Hum. Genet. 37(Suppl.):A217, 1985.

Fox, J., Hack, A.M., Fenton, W.A., Golbus, M.S., Winter, S., Kalousek, F., Rozen, R., Brusilow, S.W. and Rosenberg, L.E.: Prenatal diagnosis of ornithine transcarbamylase deficiency with use of DNA polymorphisms. N. Engl. J. Med. 315:1205, 1986.

Francannet, C., Vanlieferinghen, P., Dechelotte, P., Urbain, M.F., Campagne, D. and Malpuech, G.: Ladd syndrome in five members of a three-generation family and prenatal diagnosis. Genet. Counsel. 5:85, 1994.

Fraser, I.D., Bennett, M.O., Bothamley, J.E., Airth, G.R., Lehane, D., McCarthy, M. and Roberts, F.M.: Intensive antental plasmapheresis in severe Rhesus isoimmunisation. Lancet. 1:6, 1976.

Freda, V.J.: The Rh problem in obstetrics and a new concept of its management using amniocentesis and spectrophotometric scanning of amniotic fluid. Am. J. Obstet. Gynecol. 92:341, 1965.

Freda, V.J. and Adamsons, K.: Exchange transfusion in utero. Am. J. Obstet. Gynecol. 89:817, 1964.

Freeman, R.W. and Harbison, R.D.: Analysis of maternal alpha-fetoprotein: A comparison of three radioimmunoassays. Teratogenesis Carcinog. Mutagen. 3:407, 1983.

Freeman, R.K., McQuown, D.S., Secrist, L.J. and Larson, E.J.: The diagnosis of fetal hydrocephalus before viability. Obstet. Gynecol. 49:109, 1977.

Freeman, S.B., Priest, J.H., Fernhoff, P.M., MacMahon, W.C. and Elsas II, L.J.: Prenatal ascertainment of triploidy by maternal serum alpha-fetoprotein screening. Am. J. Hum. Genet. 43(Suppl.):A234, 1988.

Freeman, S.B., Priest, J.H., MacMahon, W.C., Fernhoff, P.M. and Elsas, L.J.: Prenatal ascertainment of triploidy by maternal serum alpha-fetoprotein screening. Prenat. Diagn. 9:339, 1989.

Freiberg, A.S., Blumberg, B., Lawce, H. and Mann, J.: XX/XY chimerism encountered during prenatal diagnosis. Prenat. Diagn. 8:423, 1988.

Friedman, D.M.: Fetal echocardiography and Doppler blood flow studies. In: Filkins, K. and Russo, J.F. (Eds.), *Human Prenatal Diagnosis.* New York: Marcel Dekker, 1985, p. 271.

Friedman, J.M. and Santos-Ramos, R.: Natural history of X-linked aqueductal stenosis in the second and third trimester of pregnancy. Am. J. Obstet. Gynecol. 150:104, 1984.

Friedman, J.M., Wilson, R.D. and Norman, M.D.: Prenatal diagnosis of an unrecognized familial multiple congenital anomaly syndrome. Proc. Greenwood Genet. Cent. 8:179, 1989.

Friedrich, U., Hansen, K.B., Hauge, M., Hagerstrand, I., Kristoffersen, K., Ludvigsen, E., Merrild, U., Norgaard-Pedersen, B., Petersen, G.B. and Therkelsen, A.J.: Prenatal diagnosis of polycystic kidneys and encephalocele (Meckel syndrome). Clin. Genet. 15:278, 1979.

Frigoletto, F.D., Birnholz, J.C., Rothchild, S.B., Finberg, H.J. and Umansky, I.: Intrauterine transfusion with the use of phased array ultrasonography: A new technique. Am. J. Obstet. Gynecol. 131:273, 1978.

Frigoletto, F.D., Jr., Birnholz, J.C., Driscoll, S.G. and Finberg, H.J.: Ultrasound diagnosis of cystic hygroma. Am. J. Obstet. Gynecol. 136:962, 1980.

Frigoletto, F.D., Jr., Umansky, I., Birnholz, J., Acker, D., Easterday, C.L., Harris, G.B.C. and

Griscom, N.T.: Intrauterine fetal transfusion in 365 fetuses during fifteen years. Am. J. Obstet. Gynecol. 139:781, 1981.

Froehlich, L.A. and Fujikura, T.: Significance of a single umbilical artery. Report from the collaborative study of cerebral palsy. Am. J. Obstet. Gynecol. 94:274, 1966.

Froster, U.G., Briner J., Zimmermann, R., Huch, R. and Huch, A.: Bilateral brachial amelia, facial clefts, encephalocele, orbital cyst and omphalocele: A recurrent fetal malformation pattern coming into focus. Clin. Dysmorph. 5:171, 1996a.

Froster, U.G., Wallner, S.J., Reusche, E., Schwinger, E. and Rehder, H.: VACTERL with hydrocephalus and branchial arch defects: Prenatal, clinical, and autopsy findings in two brothers. Am. J. Med. Genet. 62:169, 1996b.

Frydman, M., Weinstock, A.L., Cohen, H.A., Savir, H. and Varsano, I.: Autosmal recesive Peters anomaly, typical facial appearance, failure to thrive, hydrocephalus, and other anomalies: Further delineation of the Krause–Kivlin syndrome. Am. J. Med. Genet. 40:34, 1991.

Fryer, A.: Filippi syndrome with mild learning difficulties. Clin. Dysmorph. 5:35, 1996.

Fryns, J.P., Vandenberghe, K., van Assche, F.A., Cassiman, J.J. and van den Berghe, H.: Prenatal diagnosis of Meckel syndrome. J. Genet. Hum. 28:89, 1980.

Fryns, J.P., van den Berghe, K., van Assche, A. and van den Berghe, H.: Prenatal diagnosis of campomelic dwarfism. Clin. Genet. 19:199, 1981.

Fryns, J.P., van den Berghe, K., Moerman, F., Kleczkowska, A. and van den Berghe H.: Tetraploidy with hydrops fetalis, cystic nuchal hygroma and 90,XX karyotype. Clin. Genet. 31:158, 1987.

Fryns, J.P., Kleczkowska, A. and van den Berghe, H.: De novo 3q/7q translocation and associated interstitial 7q35 deletion. Clin. Genet. 33:60, 1988.

Fryns, J.P., Moerman, F., Van den Berghe, H. and Ayme, S.: The syndrome of diaphragmatic hernia, distal limb hypoplasia and coarse face ("Fryns syndrome"): Prevalance, clinical variability, etiology, survival and prenatal diagnosis. Proc. Greenwood Genet. Cent. 9:91, 1990.

Fryns, J.P., Kleczkowska, A., Moerman, P. and Vandenberghe, K.: Hereditary hydronephrosis and the short arm of chromosome 6. Hum. Genet. 91:514, 1993.

Fuchs, F. and Riis, P.: Antenatal sex determination. Nature. 177:330, 1956.

Fuhrmann, W.: Maternal serum alpha-fetoprotein screening for neural tube defects. Prenat. Diagn. 5:77, 1985.

Fuhrmann, W., Fuhrmann-Rieger, A., Jovanovic, V. and Render, H.: A new autosomal recessive skeletal dysplasia syndrome—Prenatal diagnosis and histopahtology. Prog. Clin. Biol. Res. Skel. Dysplas. 104:519, 1982.

Fuhrmann, W., Wendt, P. and Weitzel, H.K.: Maternal serum-AFP as screening test for Down syndrome. Lancet. 2:413, 1984.

Fukao, T., Wakazono, A., Song, X-Q, Yamaguchi, S., Zacharias, R., Donlan, M.A. and Orii, T.: Prenatal diagnosis in a family with mitochondrial acetoacetyl-coenzyme A thiolase deficiency with the use of the polymerase chain reaction followed by the heteroduplex detection method. Prenat. Diagn. 15:363, 1995.

Fukao, T., Song, X-Q., Watanabe, H., Hirayama, K., Sakazaki, H., Shintaku, H., Imanaka, M., Orii, T. and Kondo, N.: Prenatal diagnosis of succinyl-coenzyme A : 3-ketoacid coenzyme A transferase deficiency. Prenat. Diagn. 16:471, 1996.

Furbetta, M., Angius, A., Falchi, A.M., Tuveri, T., Tannoia, N., Pertosa, A.P. and Cao, A.: Prenatal diagnosis of thalassaemia major resulting from Lepore/beta-thalassaemia genotype. J. Med. Genet. 18:476, 1981.

Furness, M.E.: Choroid plexus cysts and trisomy 18. Lancet. 2:693, 1987.

Gadwood, K.A. and Reynes, C.J.: Prenatal sonography of metastatic neuroblastoma. J. Clin. Ultrasound 11:512, 1983.

Gadziala, N.A., Kawada, C.Y., Doherty, F.J. and Koza, D.J.: Intrauterine decompression of megalocystis during the second trimester of pregnancy. Am. J. Obstet. Gynecol. 144:355, 1982.

Gagne, R.: Prenatal diagnosis of hereditary tyrosinemia. N. Engl. J. Med. 310:855, 1984.

Gagne, R., Lescault, A., Grenier, A., Laberge, C., Melancon, S.B. and Dallaire, L.: Prenatal diagnosis of hereditary tyrosinaemia: Measurement of succinylacetone in amniotic fluid. Prenat. Diagn. 2:185, 1982a.

Gagne, R., Lescault, A., Grenier, A. and Laberge, C.: Prenatal diagnosis of hereditary tyrosinaemia confirmed. Prenat. Diagn. 2:323, 1982b.

Gagne, R., Grenier, A., Lescault, A., Laberge, C., Melancon, S. and Dallaire, L.: The prenatal diagnosis of hereditary tyrosinemia by succinylacetone measurement in amniotic fluid: A four year experience. Am. J. Hum. Genet. 36(Suppl.):188S, 1984.

Gal, A., Wirth, B., Kaariainen, H., Lucotte, G., Landais, P., Gillessen-Kaesbach, G., Muller-Wiefel, D.E. and Zerres, K.: Childhood manifestation of autosomal dominant polycystic kidney disease: No evidence for genetic heterogeneity. Clin. Genet. 35:13, 1989.

Game, K., Friedman, J.M., Paradice, B. and Norman, M.G.: Fetal growth retardation, hydrocephalus, hypoplastic multilobed lungs, and other anomalies in 4 sibs. Am. J. Med. Genet. 33:276, 1989.

Ganshirt, D., Garritsen, H.S.P. and Holzgreve, W.: Fetal cells in maternal blood. Obstet. Gynecol. 7:103, 1995.

Garber, A., Shohat, M. and Sarti, D.: Megacystis–microcolon–intestinal hypoperistalsis syndrome in two male siblings. Prenat. Diagn. 10:377, 1990.

Garcia-Castro, J.M., Isales-Forsythe, C.M., Levy, H.L., Shih, V.E., Lao-Velez, C.R., Gonzalez-Rios, M.D.C. and Reyes de Torres, L.C.R.: Prenatal diagnosis of glycine encephalopathy. N. Engl. J. Med. 306:1425, 1982a.

Garcia-Castro, J.M., Isales-Forsythe, C.M., Levy, H.L., Shih, V.E., Lao-Velez, C.R., Gonzalez-Rios, M.C. and Reyes de Torres, L.C.: Prenatal diagnosis of nonketotic hyperglycinemia. N. Engl. J. Med. 306:79, 1982b.

Garcia-Munoz, M.J., Belloque, J., Merinero, B., Perez-Cerda, C., Sanz, P. and Ugarte, M.: Non-ketotic hyperglycinaemia glycine/serine ratio in amniotic fluid—An unreliable method for prenatal diagnosis. Prenat. Diagn. 9:473, 1989.

Garcia Silva, M.T., De Castro, J., Stibler, H., Simon, R., Chasco Yrigoyen, A., Mateos, F., Ferrer, I., Madero, S., Velasco, J.M. and Guttierrez-Larraya, F.: Prenatal hypertrophic cardiomyopathy and pericardial effusion in carbohydrate-deficient glycoprotein syndrome. J. Inher. Metab. Dis. 19:257, 1996.

Gardner, S., Burton, B.K. and Johnson, A.M.: Maternal serum alpha-fetoprotein screening: A report of the Forsyth County Project. Am. J. Obstet. Gynecol. 140:250, 1981.

Garoff, L. and Seppala, M.: Alpha fetoprotein and human placental lactogen levels in maternal serum in multiple pregnancies. J. Obstet. Gynaecol. Br. Commonw. 80:695, 1973.

Garrett, W.J. and Robinson, D.E.: Fetal heart size measured in vivo by ultrasound. Pediatrics. 46:25, 1970.

Garrett, W.J., Kossoff, G. and Lawrence, R.: Gray scale echography in the diagnosis of hydrops due to fetal lung tumor. J. Clin. Ultrasound 3:45, 1975a.

Garrett, W.J., Kossoff, G. and Osborn, R.A.: The diagnosis of fetal hydronephrosis, megaureter and urethral obstruction by ultrasonic echography. Br. J. Obstet. Gynaecol. 82:115, 1975b.

Garver, K.L., Blitzer, M.G., Ibezim, G., Marchese, S.G., Pegram, D.L., Hagins, A.M. and Zhang, Y.: Evaluation of inorganic pyrophosphate in amniotic fluid as a mode of prenatal diagnosis of osteogenesis imperfecta. Prenat. Diagn. 4:109, 1984.

Gasparini, P., Novelli, G., Savoia, A., Dallapiccola, B. and Pignatti, P.F.: First-trimester prenatal diagnosis of cystic fibrosis using the polymerase chain reaction: Report of eight cases. Prenat. Diagn. 9:349, 1989.

Gatti, R., Lombardo, C., Filocamo, M., Borrone, C. and Porro, E.: Comparative study of 15 lysosomal enzymes in chorionic villi and cultured amniotic fluid cells. Early prenatal diagnosis in seven pregnancies at risk for lysosomal storage diseases. Prenat. Diagn. 5:329, 1985.

Gatti, R.A., Peterson, K.L., Novak, J., Chen, X., Yang-Chen, L., Liang, T., Lange, E. and Lange, K.: Prenatal genotyping of ataxia–telangiectasia. Lancet. 342:376, 1993.

Ged, C., Moreau-Gaudry, F., Taine, L., Hombrados, I., Calvas, P., Colombies, P. and De

Verneuil, H.: Prenatal diagnosis in congenital erythropoietic porphyria by metabolic measurement and DNA mutation analysis. Prenat. Diagn. 16:83, 1996.

Geirsson, R.T., Patel, N.B. and Christie, A.D.: Efficacy of intrauterine volume, fetal abdominal area, and biparietal diameter measurements with ultrasound in screening for small-for-dates babies. Br. J. Obstet. Gynaecol. 92:929, 1985a.

Geirsson, R.T., Patel, N.B. and Christie, A.D.: Intrauterine volume, fetal abdominal area, and biparietal diameter measurements with ultrasound in the prediction of small-for-dates babies in a high-risk obstetric population. Br. J. Obstet. Gynaecol. 92:936, 1985b.

Gelman-Kohan, Z., Nisani, R., Chemke, J., Appelman, Z., Rappaport, S. and Hegesh, E.: Prenatal detection of recurrent SLOS type 2. Am. J. Hum. Genet. 47(Suppl.):A57, 1990.

Gembruch, U. and Hansmann, M.: Artificial instillation of amniotic fluid as a new technique for the diagnostic evaluation of cases of oligohydramnios. Prenat. Diagn. 8:33, 1988.

Gembruch, U., Hansmann, M. and Fodisch, H.J.: Early prenatal diagnosis of short rib–polydactyly (SRP) syndrome type I (Majewski) by ultrasound in a case at risk. Prenat. Diagn. 5:357, 1985.

Gembruch, U., Niesen, M., Hansmann, M. and Knopfle, G.: Listeriosis: A cause of non-immune hydrops fetalis. Prenat. Diagn. 7:277, 1987.

Gembruch, U., Niesen, M., Kehrberg, H. and Hansmann, M.: Diastrophic dysplasia: A specific prenatal diagnosis by ultrasound. Prenat. Diagn. 8:539, 1988.

Gembruch, U., Chatterjee, M., Bald, R., Eldering, G., Gocke, H., Urban, A.E. and Hansmann, M.: Prenatal diagnosis of aortic atresia by colour doppler flow mapping. Prenat. Diagn. 10:211, 1990a.

Gembruch, U., Steil, E., Redel, D.A. and Hansmann, M.: Prenatal diagnosis of a left ventricular aneurysm. Prenat. Diagn. 10:203, 1990b.

Gendall, P.W. and Kozlowski, K.: Oto–palato–digital syndrome type II: Report of two related cases. Pediatr. Radiol. 22:267, 1992.

Gennarelli, M., Novelli, G., Grovannucci Uzielli, M.L., Pietropolli, A. and Dallapiccola, B.: Rapid prenatal diagnosis of myotonic dystrophy in the second trimester using polymerase chain reaction. J. Med. Genet. 27:662, 1990.

Gennarelli, M., Cobo, A., Fattorini, C., Martorell, L., Carrera, M., Novelli, G., Baiget, M. and Dallapiccola, B.: Prognostic assessment of pregnancies at risk for myotonic dystrophy based on the CTG expansion. Am. J. Hum. Genet. 53(Suppl.):1410, 1993.

Genuardi, M., Chiurazzi, P., Capelli, A. and Neri, G.: X-linked VACTERL with hydrocephalus: The VACTERL-H syndrome. Birth Defects. 29(1):235, 1993a.

Genuardi, M., Dionisis-Vici, C., Sabetta, G., Mignozzi, M., Rizzoni, G., Cotugno, G. and Neri, M.E.M.: Cerebro-reno-digital (Meckel-like) syndrome with Dandy–Walker malformation, cystic kidneys, hepatic fibrosis, and polydactyly. Am. J. Med. Genet. 47:50, 1993b.

Geraghty, A.V., Knott, P.D. and Hanna, H.M.: Prenatal diagnosis of fetal glioblastoma multiforme. Prenat. Diagn. 9:613, 1989.

Gershoni-Baruch, R., Ludatscher, R.M., Lichtig, C., Sujov, P. and Machoul, I.: Cerebro-oculo-facio-skeletal syndrome: Further delineation. Am. J. Med. Genet. 41:74, 1991.

Gewolb, I.H., Freedman, R.M., Kleinman, C.S. and Hobbins, J.C.: Prenatal diagnosis of a human pseudoacardiac anomaly. Obstet. Gynecol. 61:657, 1983.

Ghosh, A., Woo, J.S.K., Wan, C.W. and Wong, V.C.W.: Simple ultrasonic diagnosis of osteogenesis imperfecta type II in early second trimester. Prenat. Diagn. 4:235, 1984.

Ghosh, A., Tang, M.H.Y., Tai, D., Nie, G. and Ma, H.K.: Justification of maternal serum alphafetoprotein screening in a population with low incidence of neural tube defects. Prenat. Diagn. 6:83, 1986.

Ghosh, A., Tang, M.H.Y., Liang, S.T., Ma, H.K., Chan, V. and Chan, T.K.: Ultrasound evaluation of pregnancies at risk for homozygous alpha-thalassaemia-1. Prenat. Diagn. 7:307, 1987.

Giacolone, P.L., Boulot, P., Marty, M., Deschamps, F., Laffargue, F. and Viala, J.L.: Fetal hemangiolymphangioma: A case report. Fetal Diagn. Ther. 8:338, 1993.

Gibbs, D.A., McFadyen, I.R., Crawford, M.d'A., de Muinck Keizer, E.E., Headhouse-Benson,

C.M., Wilson, T.M. and Farrant, P.H.: First-trimester diagnosis of Lesch–Nyhan syndrome. Lancet. 2:1180, 1984.

Gibbs, D.A., Headhouse-Benson, C.M. and Watts, R.W.E.: Family studies of the Lesch–Nyhan syndrome: The use of a restriction fragment length polymorphism (RFLP) closely linked to the disease gene for carrier state and prenatal diagnosis. J. Inher. Metab. Dis. 9:45, 1986.

Gibson, K.M., Baumann, C., Ogier, H., Rossier, E., Vollmer, B. and Jakobs, C.: Pre- and postnatal diagnosis of succinic semialdehyde dehydrogenase deficiency using enzyme and metabolite assays. J. Inher. Metab. Dis. 17:732, 1994.

Gilbert, F., Mulivor, R., Calderon, A., Lalatta, F., Wilkins, I., Chitkara, U., Guttenberg, M. and Dische, R.: Prospective prenatal diagnosis of cystic fibrosis. Am. J. Hum. Genet. 37(Suppl.):A218, 1985.

Giles, L., Cooper, A., Fowler, B., Sardharwalla, I.B. and Donnai, P.: Krabbe's disease: First trimester diagnosis confirmed on cultured amniotic fluid cells and fetal tissues. Prenat. Diagn. 7:329, 1987.

Giles, L., Cooper, A., Fowler, B., Sardharwalla, I.B. and Donnai, P.: First trimester prenatal diagnosis of Sandhoff's disease. Prenat. Diagn. 8:199, 1988.

Gill, R.W., Trudinger, B.J., Garrett, W.J., Kossoff, G. and Warren, P.S.: Fetal umbilical venous flow measured in utero by pulsed Doppler and B-mode ultrasound. Am. J. Obstet. Gynecol. 139:720, 1981.

Giulian, B.B.: Prenatal ultrasonographic diagnosis of fetal renal tumors. Radiology. 152:69, 1984.

Giulian, B.B. and Alvear, D.T.: Prenatal ultrasonographic diagnosis of fetal gastroschisis. Radiology. 129:473, 1978.

Giulian, B.B., Chang, C.C.N. and Yoss, B.S.: Prenatal ultrasonographic diagnosis of fetal adrenal neuroblastoma. J. Clin. Ultrasound. 14:225, 1986.

Gleicher, N. and Elkayam, U.: Intrauterine dysrhythmias. In: Elkayam, U. and Gleicher, N. (Eds.), *Cardiac Problems in Pregnancy: Diagnosis and Management of Maternal and Fetal Disease.* New York: A.R. Liss, 1982a, p. 555.

Gleicher, N. and Elkayam, U.: Intrauterine congestive heart failure. In: Elkayam, U. and Gleicher, N. (Eds.), *Cardiac Problems in Pregnancy: Diagnosis and Management of Maternal and Fetal Disease.* New York: A.R. Liss, 1982b, p. 565.

Glendon, G., Toi, A., Babul, R., Bandler, L. and Chitayat, D.: Prenatal diagnosis of brachydactyly B by fetal ultrasound. Am. J. Hum. Genet. 53(Suppl.):1413, 1993.

Glick, P.L., Harrison, M.R. and Filly, R.A.: Antepartum diagnosis of meconium peritonitis. N. Engl. J. Med. 309:1392, 1983.

Godfrey, M., Vandemark, N., Wang, M., Velinov, M., Wargowski, D., Tsipoiuras, P., Han, J., Becker, J., Robertson, W., Droste, S. and Rao, V.H.: Prenatal diagnosis and a donor splice site mutation in fibrillin in a family with Marfan syndrome. Am. J. Hum. Genet. 53:472, 1993.

Golabi, M., Sago, H., Chen, E., Conte, W.J., Cox, V.A. and Lebo, R.V: True trisomy 2 mosaicism in amniocytes and newborn liver associated with multiple system abnormalities. Am. J. Hum. Genet. 57(Suppl.):A91, 1995.

Golbus, M.S., Hall, B.D., Filly, R.A. and Poskanzer, L.B.: Prenatal diagnosis of achondrogenesis. J. Pediatr. 91:464, 1977.

Golbus, M.S., Stephens, J.D., Mahoney, M.J., Hobbins, J.C., Haseltine, F.P., Caskey, C.T. and Banker, B.Q.: Failure of fetal creatine phosphokinase as a diagnostic indicator of Duchenne muscular dystrophy. N. Engl. J. Med. 300:860, 1979.

Golbus, M.S., Sagebiel, R.W., Filly, R.A., Gindhart, T.D. and Hall, J.G.: Prenatal diagnosis of congenital bullous ichthyosiform erythroderma (epidermolytic hyperkeratosis) by fetal skin biopsy. N. Engl. J. Med. 302:93, 1980.

Golbus, M.S., Simpson, T.J., Koresawa, M., Appelman, Z. and Alpers, C.E.: The preantal determination of glucose-6-phosphatase acitivity by fetal liver biopsy. Prenat. Diagn. 8:401, 1988.

Goldberg, J.D., Chervenak, F.A., Lipman, R.A. and Berkowitz, R.L.: Antenatal sonographic diagnosis of arthrogryposis multiplex congenita. Prenat. Diagn. 6:45, 1986.

Goldfine, C., Miller, W.A. and Haddow, J.E.: Amniotic fluid gel cholinesterase density ratios in fetal open defects of the neural tube and ventral wall. Br. J. Obstet. Gynaecol. 90:238, 1983.

Goldfine, C., Knight, G.J., Haddow, J.E. and Palomaki, G.E.: Amniotic fluid acetylcholinesterase measurements: Comparing immunochemical and polyacrylamide gel techniques. Prenat. Diagn. 9:167, 1989.

Goldstein, D.J.: "Spur-limbed" dwarfism identified as hypophosphatase. Dysmorph. Clin. Genet. 2:127, 1988.

Goldstein, D.J., Nichols, W.C. and Mirkin, L.D.: Short-limbed osteochondrodysplasia with osteochondral spurs of knee and elbow joints (spur-limbed dwarfism). Dysmorph. Clin. Genet. 1:12, 1987.

Gollop, T.R. and Eigier, A.: Ellis-van Creveld syndrome: Early prenatal diagnosis with ultrasound. Rev. Brasil. Genet. 9:555, 1986a.

Gollop, T.R. and Eigier, A.: Ultrasonographic diagnosis of fetal hydrops caused by cytomegalovirus infection. Rev. Brasil. Genet. 9:703, 1986b.

Gollop, T.R. and Eigier, A.: Prenatal ultrasound diagnosis of diastrophic dysplasia at 16 weeks. Am. J. Med. Genet. 27:321, 1987.

Gollop, T.R., Eigier, A., and Neto, G.J.: Prenatal diagnosis of thalidomide syndrome. Prenat. Diagn. 7:295, 1987.

Gompertz, D., Goodey, P.A., Thom, H., Russell, G., MacLean, M.W., Ferguson-Smith, M.E. and Ferguson-Smith, M.A.: Antenatal diagnosis of propionicacidaemia. Lancet. 1:1009, 1973.

Gompertz, D., Goodey, P.A., Thom, H., Russell, G., Johnston, A.W., Mellor, D.H., MacLean, M.W., Ferguson-Smith, M.E. and Ferguson-Smith, M.A.: Prenatal diagnosis and family studies in a case of propionicacidaemia. Clin. Genet. 8:244, 1975.

Goodlin, R.C. and Lowe, E.W.: Unexplained hydramnios associated with a thanatophoric dwarf. Am. J. Obstet. Gynecol. 118:873, 1974.

Goodlin, R.C., Heidrick, W.P., Papenfuss, H.L. and Kubitz, R.L.: Fetal malformations associated with maternal hypoxia. Am. J. Obstet. Gynecol. 149:228, 1984.

Goodman, S.I., Mace, J.W., Turner, B. and Garrett, W.J.: Antenatal diagnosis of argininosuccinic aciduria. Clin. Genet. 4:236, 1973.

Goodman, S.I., Wise, G., Halpern, B., Ryan, E. and Whelan, D.: Antenatal diagnosis of glutaric acidemia. Am. J. Hum. Genet. 31(Suppl.):49A, 1979.

Goodship, J., Curtis, A., Cross, I., Brown, J., Emslie, J., Wolstenholme, J., Bhattacharya, S. and Burn, J.: A submicroscopic translocation t(4;10), responsible for recurrent Wolf–Hirschhorn syndrome identified by allele loss and fluorescent in situ hybridisation. J. Med. Genet. 29:451, 1992.

Goossens, M., Dumez, Y., Kaplan, L., Lupker, M., Chabret, C., Henrion, R. and Rosa, J.: Prenatal diagnosis of sickle-cell anemia in the first trimester of pregnancy. N. Engl. J. Med. 309:831, 1983.

Gorlin, R.J., Cohen, M.M., Jr. and Levin, L.S.: *Syndromes of the Head and Neck,* 3rd ed. New York: Oxford University Press, 1990.

Gosden, C.M. and Brock, D.J.H.: Morphology of rapidly adhering amniotic-fluid cells as an aid to the diagnosis of neural-tube defects. Lancet. 1:919, 1977.

Gosden, C. and Brock, D.J.H.: Combined use of alpha fetoprotein and amniotic fluid cell morphology in early prenatal diagnosis of fetal abnormalities. J. Med. Genet. 15:262, 1978a.

Gosden, C. and Brock, D.J.H.: Amniotic fluid cell morphology in early antenatal prediction of abortion and low birth weight. Br. Med. J. 2:1186, 1978b.

Gosden, C. and Brock, D.J.H.: Prenatal diagnosis of exstrophy of the cloaca. Am. J. Med. Genet. 8:95, 1981.

Gosden, J.R., Mitchell, A.R., Gosden, C.M., Rodeck, C.H. and Morsman, J.M.: Direct vision chorion biopsy and chromosome-specific DNA probes for determination of fetal sex in first-trimester prenatal diagnosis. Lancet. 2:1416, 1982.

Gosden, C.M., Brock, D.J.H., Hayward, C. and Carbarns, N.J.B.: Prenatal diagnosis of cystic fibrosis by measurement of microvillar peptidase activity in amniotic fluid. Clin. Genet. 24:302, 1983.

Gosden, J.R., Gosden, C.M., Christie, S., Morsman, J.M. and Rodeck, C.H.: Rapid fetal sex determination in first trimester prenatal diagnosis by dot hybridization of DNA probes. Lancet. 1:540, 1984a.

Gosden, J.R., Gosden, C.M., Christie, S., Cooke, H.J., Morsman, J.M. and Rodeck, C.H.: The use of cloned Y chromosome-specific DNA probes for fetal sex determination in first trimester prenatal diagnosis. Hum. Genet. 66:347, 1984b.

Gottesfeld, K.R.: Ultrasound in obstetrics. Clin. Obstet. Gynecol. 21:311, 1978.

Goyert, G.L., Blitz, D., Gibson, P., Seabolt, L., Olszewski, M., Wright, D.J. and Schwartz, D.B.: Prenatal diagnosis of duplication cyst of the pylorus. Prenat. Diagn. 11:483, 1991.

Goyert, G.L., Charfoos, D.A., Ward, B.E., Gold, R.B., Gersen, S.L., Bronsteen, R.A. and Wright, D.J.: Prenatal identification of a tetraploid fetus using FISH. Am. J. Hum. Genet. 53(Suppl.):1414, 1993.

Grabowski, G.A., Kruse, J.R., Goldberg, J.D., Chockkalingam, K., Gordon, R.E., Blakemore, K.J., Mahoney, M.J. and Desnick, R.J.: First-trimester prenatal diagnosis of Tay–Sachs disease. Am. J. Hum. Genet. 36:1369, 1984.

Grace, K., Martel, M. and Kardon, N.: A case of trisomy 5 mosaicism: Expansion of phenotype and example of variability with prenatally diagnosed chromosome mosaicism. Am. J. Hum. Genet. 57(Suppl.):A344, 1995.

Graff, G., Chemke, J. and Lancet, M.: Familial recurring thanatophoric dwarfism: A case report. Obstet. Gynecol. 39:515, 1972.

Graham, M.: Congenital short femur: Prenatal sonographic diagnosis. J. Ultrasound Med. 4:361, 1985.

Graham, G.W., Aitken, D.A. and Connor, J.M.: Undetectable maternal serum PAPP-A in Cornelia de Lange syndrome. J. Med. Genet. 25:641, 1988.

Graham, G.W., Aitken, D.A. and Connor, J.M.: Prenatal diagnosis by enzyme analysis in 15 pregnancies at risk for the Lesch–Nyhan syndrome. Prenat. Diagn. 16:647, 1996.

Grange, D.K., Arya, S., Opitz, J.M., Laxova, R., Herrmann, J. and Gilbert, E.F.: The short umbilical cord. Birth Defects. 23(1):191, 1987.

Grange, G., Favre, R. and Gasser, B.: Endovaginal sonographic diagnosis of craniorachischisis at 13 weeks of gestation. Fetal Diagn. Ther. 9:391, 1994.

Grannum, P.A., Copel, J.A., Plaxe, S.C., Scioscia, A.L. and Hobbins, J.C.: In utero exchange transfusion by direct intravascular injection in severe erythroblastosis fetalis. N. Engl. J. Med. 314:1431, 1986.

Grannum, P.A.T., Copel, J.A., Moya, F.R., Scioscia, A.L., Robert, J.A., Winn, H.N., Coster, B.C., Burdine, C.B. and Hobbins, J.C.: The reversal of hydrops fetalis by intravascular intrauterine transfusion in severe isoimmune fetal anemia. Am. J. Obstet. Gynecol. 158:914, 1988.

Gray, J., Pinkel, D., Yu, L.-C., Collins, C., Fuscoe, I., Tenjin, H., Tenjin, T. and Golbus, M.: Fluorescence in situ hybridization (FISH) applied to prenatal diagnosis. Am. J. Hum. Genet. 43(Suppl.):A235, 1988.

Gray, D.L., Ball, R., Bauer, J., Crawford, A., Babb, S., Beaver, H., Guckenberger, S. and Hsieh, C.-L.: Identification and characterization of de novo bisatellited marker chromosomes in three prenatal cases. Am. J. Hum. Genet. 57(Suppl.):A344, 1995a.

Gray, R.G.F., Green, A., Cole, T., Davidson, V., Giles, M., Schutgens, R.B.H. and Wanders, R.J.A.: A misdiagnosis of X-linked adrenoleucodystrophy in cultured chorionic villus cells by the measurement of very long chain fatty acids. Prenat. Diagn. 15:486, 1995b.

Grebner, E.E. and Jackson, L.G.: Prenatal diagnosis for Tay–Sachs disease using chorionic villus sampling. Prenat. Diagn. 5:313, 1985.

Grebner, E.E. and Wenger, D.A.: A simple, reliable prenatal test for Tay–Sachs disease using sulfated substrate and chorionic villi. Am. J. Med. Genet. 34:A11, 1986.

Grebner, E.E. and Wenger, D.A.: Use of 4-methylumbelliferyl-6-sulpho-2-acetamido-2-deoxy-beta-d-glucopyranosi for prenatal diagnosis of Tay–Sachs disease using chorionic villi. Prenat. Diagn. 7:419, 1987.

Grebner, E.E., Wapner, R.J., Barr, M.A. and Jackson, L.G.: Prenatal Tay–Sachs diagnosis by chorionic villi sampling. Lancet. 2:286, 1983.

Grebner, E.E., Wapner, R. and Jackson, L.: Prenatal diagnosis for Tay–Sachs disease using chorionic villus sampling (CVS). Am. J. Hum. Genet. 36(Suppl.):189S, 1984.

Green, J.R., Lentze, M.J., Rossi, E., Sidiropoulos, D. and Schubiger, G.: Prenatal diagnosis of cystic fibrosis: False negative result with the 4-methylumbelliferyl-p-guanidinobenzoate assay for proteases in amniotic fluid. Eur. J. Pediatr. 139:35, 1982.

Greenberg, F., Carpenter, R.J. and Ledbetter, D.H.: Cystic hygroma and hydrops fetalis in a fetus with trisomy 13. Clin. Genet. 24:389, 1983.

Greenberg, F., Stein, F., Gresik, M.V., Finegold, M.J., Carpenter, R.J., Riccardi, V.M. and Beaudet, A.L.: The Perlman familial nephroblastomatosis syndrome. Am. J. Med. Genet. 24:101, 1986.

Greenberg, F., Gresik, M.V., Carpenter, R.J., Law, S.W., Hoffman, L.P. and Ledbetter, D.H.: The Gardner–Silengo–Wachtel or genito-palato-cardiac syndrome: Male pseudohermaphroditism with micrognathia, cleft palate, and conotruncal cardiac defect. Am. J. Med. Genet. 26:59, 1987.

Greenberg, F., Courtney, K.B., Wessels, R.A., Huhta, J., Carpenter, R.J., Rich, D.C. and Ledbetter, D.H.: Prenatal diagnosis of deletion 17p13 associated with DiGeorge anomaly. Am. J. Med. Genet. 31:1, 1988a.

Greenberg, C.R., Trevenen, C.L. and Evans, J.A.: The BOR syndrome and renal agenesis— Prenatal diagnosis and further clinical delineation. Prenat. Diagn. 8:103, 1988b.

Greenberg, C.R., Rimoin, D.L., Gruber, H.E., DeSa, D.J.B., Reed, M. and Lachman, R.S.: A new autosomal recessive lethal chondrodystrophy with congenital hydrops. Am. J. Med. Genet. 29:623, 1988c.

Greenberg, F., Copeland, K. and Gresik, M.V.: Expanding the spectrum of the Perlman syndrome. Am. J. Med. Genet. 29:773, 1988d.

Greenberg, C.R., Evans, J.A., McKendry-Smith, S., Redekopp, S., Haworth, J.C., Mulivor, R. and Chodirker, B.N.: Infantile hypophosphatasia: Localization within chromosome region 1p36.1-34 and prenatal diagnosis using linked DNA markers. Am. J. Hum. Genet. 46:286, 1990.

Greenblatt, A.M., Beretsky, I., Lankin, D.H. and Phelan, L.: In utero diagnosis of crossed renal ectopia using high-resolution real-time ultrasound. J. Ultrasound Med. 4:105, 1985.

Gregersen, N., Winter, V., Jensen, P.K.A., Holmskov, A., Kolvraa, S., Andresen, B.S., Christensen, E., Bross, P., Lundemose, J.B. and Gregersen, M.: Prenatal diagnosis of medium-chain acyl-CoA dehydrogenase (MCAD) deficiency in a family with a previous fatal case of sudden unexpected death in childhood. Prenat. Diagn. 15:82, 1995.

Grevengood, C., Dalton, J.D., Dungan, J.S., Park, V.M., Tharapel, A.T., Martens, P., Ward, J.C., Shulman, L.P., Simpson, J.L. and Elias, S.: Prenatal detection of a de novo supernumary marker chromosome as der(2)(p13q12) in a fetus with abnormal facies, single umbilical artery and diaphragmatic hernia. Am. J. Hum. Genet. 53(Suppl.):1796, 1993.

Griscom, N.T.: Possible radiologic approaches to fetal diagnosis and therapy. Clin. Perinatol. 1:435, 1974.

Grix, A., Jr.: VATER association with hydrocephalus. Proc. Greenwood Genet. Cent. 8:216, 1989.

Gross, T.L., Sokol, R.J., Wilson, M.V., Kuhnert, P.M. and Hirsch, V.: Amniotic fluid phosphatidylglycerol: A potentially useful predictor of intrauterine growth retardation. Am. J. Obstet. Gynecol. 140:277, 1981.

Gross, T.L., Sokol, R.J., Wilson, M.V. and Zador, I.E.: Using ultrasound and amniotic fluid determinations to diagnose intrauterine growth retardation before birth: A clinical model. Am. J. Obstet. Gynecol. 143:265, 1982.

Gross, S.J., Shulman, L.P., Tolley, E.A., Emerson, D.S., Felker, R.E., Simpson, J.L. and Elias, S.: Isolated fetal choroid plexus cysts and trisomy 18: A review and meta-analysis. Am. J. Obstet. Gynecol. 172:83, 1995.

Grosse-Wilde, H., Valentine-Thon, E., Vogeler, U., Passarge, E., Lorenzen, F., Sippell, W.G., Bidlingmaier, F. and Knorr, D.: HLA-A,B,C,DR typing and 17-OHP determination for second trimester prenatal diagnosis of 21-hydroxylase deficient CAH. Prenat. Diagn. 8:131, 1988.

Gruber, A., Zeitune, M. and Fejgin, M.: Failure to diagnose Lesch–Nyhan syndrome by first trimester chorionic villus sampling. Prenat. Diagn. 9:452, 1989.

Gruenewald, S.M., Crocker, E.F., Walker, A.G. and Trudinger, B.J.: Antenatal diagnosis of urinary tract abnormalities. Correlation of ultrasound appearance with postnatal diagnosis. Am. J. Obstet. Gynecol. 148:278, 1984.

Guibaud, S., Bonnet, M., Khalil, F., Combet, A., Thoulon, J.M. and Dumont, M.: Glucose concentration in amniotic fluid from anencephalic pregnancies. Lancet. 1:661, 1978.

Gualandri, V., Lalatta, F., Orsini, G.B., Zorzoli, A., Bertagnoli, L. and Gallicchio, R.: Diagnostic prenatal d'un cas de repetition familiale d'agenesie unilaterale du diaphragme. J. Genet. Hum. 31:125, 1983.

Guion-Almeida, M.L. and Richieri-Costa, A.: Acrocallosal syndrome: Report of a Brazilian girl. Am. J. Med. Genet. 43:938, 1992.

Guntheroth, W.G., Cyr, D.R., Mack, L.A., Benedetti, T., Lenke, R.R. and Petty, C.N.: Hydrops from reciprocating atrioventricular tachycardia in a 27-week fetus requiring quinidine conversion. Obstet. Gynecol. 66:29S, 1985.

Guo, W., Mason, J.S., Stone, C.G., Jr., Morgan, S.A., Madu, S.I., Baldini, A., Lindsay, E.A., Biesecker, L.G., Copeland, K.C., Horlick, M.N.B., Pettigrew, A.L., Zanaria, E. and McCabe, E.R.B.: Diagnosis of X-linked adrenal hypoplasia congenita by mutation analysis of the DAX1 Gene. J. Am. Med. Assoc. 274:324, 1995.

Gustavii, B.: First-trimester chromosomal analysis of chorionic villi obtained by direct vision technique. Lancet. 2:507, 1983.

Gustavii, B. and Edvall, H.: First-trimester diagnosis of cystic nuchal hygroma. Acta Obstet. Gynecol. Scand. 63:377, 1984.

Guyot, B., Bazin, A., Sole, Y., Julien, C., Daffos, F. and Forestier, F.: Prenatal diagnosis with biotinylated chromosome specific probes. Prenat. Diagn. 8:485, 1988.

Hackeloer, B.J.: The value of combined real-time and compound scanning in the detection of fetal heart disease. Contrib. Gynecol. Obstet. 6:115, 1979.

Haddad, B., Haziza, J., Touboul, C., Abdellilah, M., Uzan, S. and Paniel, B.J.: The congenital mesoblastic nephroma: A case report of prenatal diagnosis. Fetal Diagn. Ther. 11:61, 1996.

Haddow, J.E., Kloza, E.M., Smith, D.E. and Knight, G.J.: Data from an alpha-fetoprotein pilot screening program in Maine. Obstet. Gynecol. 62:556, 1983.

Haddow, J.E., Hill, L.E., Palomaki, G.E. and Knight, G.J.: Very low versus undetectable maternal serum alpha-fetoprotein values and fetal death. Prenat. Diagn. 7:401, 1987.

Haddow, J.E., Foss, K.C., Knight, G.J., Blitzer, M.G. and Fenske, M.: The significance of very faint pseudocholinesterase bands in amniotic fluid samples analyzed by gel electrophoresis. Am. J. Hum. Genet. 45:A260, 1989.

Hadi, H.A. and Wade, A.: Prenatal diagnosis of unilateral proximal femoral focal deficiency in diabetic pregnancy: A case report. Am. J. Perinatol. 10:285, 1993.

Hadlock, F.P., Deter, R.L., Carpenter, R., Gonzalez, E.T. and Park, S.K.: Sonography of fetal urinary tract anomalies. Am. J. Roentgenol. 137:261, 1981.

Haentjens-Verbeke, K., Dufour, P., Vinatier, D., Tordjeman, N., Monnier, J.C. and Manessier, L.: Anti-TJa alloimmunization (anti-PP1P). Fetal Diagn. Ther. 11:120, 1996.

Haeusler, M.C.H., Hofmann, H.M.H., Hoenigl, W., Karpf, E.F. and Rosenkranz, W.: Congenital generalized cystic lymphangiomatosis diagnosed by prenatal ultrasound. Prenat. Diagn. 10:617, 1990.

Hagadorn, J.I., Wilson, W.G., Hogge, W.A., Callicott, J.H. and Beale, E.F.: Neonatal progeroid syndrome: More than one disease? Am. J. Med. Genet. 35:91, 1990.

Hagberg, B.A., Blennow, G., Kristiansson, B. and Stibler, H.: Carbohydrate-deficient glycoprotein syndromes: Peculiar group of new disorders. Pediatr. Neurol. 9:255, 1993.

Hage, M.L., Wall, L.L. and Killam, A.: Expectant management of abdominal pregnancy: A report of two cases. J. Reprod. Med. 33:407, 1988.

Hahnel, R., Hahnel, E., Wysocki, S.J., Wilkinson, S.P. and Hockey, A.: Prenatal diagnosis of X-linked ichthyosis. Clin. Chim. Acta 120:143, 1982.

Hahnemann, N.: Early prenatal diagnosis: A study of biopsy techniques and cell culturing from extraembryonic membranes. Clin. Genet. 6:294, 1974.

Hahnemann, N. and Mohr, J.: Genetic diagnosis in the embryo by means of biopsy from extraembryonic membranes. Bull. Eur. Soc. Hum. Genet. 2:23, 1968.

Hajdu, J., Bardoczy, Z., Papp, Z., Szabo, M. and Veress, L.: Elevated MSAFP levels and congenital heart defects: Are there associations? Am. J. Med. Genet. 58:292, 1995.

Hajianpour, M.J., Penabad, E. and Warren, R.J.: Borderline elevated maternal serum alpha-fetoprotein in a twin pregnancy concordant for Klinefelter syndrome. Am. J. Hum. Genet. 45(Suppl.):A277, 1989.

Hajra, A.K., Datta, N.S., Jackson, L.G., Moser, A.B., Moser, H.W., Larsen, J.W., Jr., and Powers, J.: Prenatal diagnosis of Zellweger cerebrohepatorenal syndrome. N. Engl. J. Med. 312:445, 1985.

Hall, J.G.: The lethal multiple pterygium syndrome. Am. J. Med. Genet. 17:803, 1984.

Hall, J.G.: Analysis of Pena Shokeir phenotype. Am. J. Med. Genet. 25:99, 1986.

Hall, B.D.: Penoscrotal transposition and the VATER association. Clin. Res. 40:56A, 1992.

Hallak, M., Neerhof, M.G., Perry, R., Nazir, M. and Huhta, J.C.: Fetal supraventricular tachycardia and hydrops fetalis: Combined intensive, direct, and transplacental therapy. Obstet. Gynecol. 78:523, 1991.

Halley, D.J.J., Keijzer, W., Jaspers, N.G.J., Niermeijer, M.F., Kleijer, W.J., Boue, J., Boue, A. and Bootsma, D.: Prenatal diagnosis of xeroderma pigmentosum (group C) using assay of unscheduled DNA synthesis and postreplication repair. Clin. Genet. 16:137, 1979.

Halley, D., Van Den Ouweland, A., Deelen, W., Verma, I. and Oostra, B.: Strategy for reliable prenatal detection of normal male carriers of the fragile X syndrome. Am. J. Med. Genet. 51:471, 1994.

Hamel, B.C.J., Happle, R., Steylen, P.M., Kollee, L.A.A., Stekhoven, J.H., Nijhuis, J.G., Rauskolb, R. and Anton-Lamprecht, I.: False-negative prenatal diagnosis of restrictive dermopathy. Am. J. Med. Genet. 44:824, 1992.

Hamilton, E.G.: Intrauterine transfusion: Safeguard or peril. Obstet. Gynecol. 50:255, 1977.

Hammadeh, M.Y., Dhillon, H.K., Duffy, P.G. and Ransley, P.G.: Antenatally diagnosed seminal vesicular cyst. Fetal Diagn. Ther. 9:62, 1994.

Handyside, A.H.: Preimplantation diagnosis. Teratology. 48:17A, 1993.

Hansen, M., Lucarelli, M.J., Whiteman, D.A.H. and Mulliken, J.B.: Treacher Collins syndrome: Phenotypic variability in a family including an infant with arhinia and uveal colobomas. Am. J. Med. Genet. 61:71, 1996.

Harding, A.E., Holt, I.J., Sweeney, M.G. Brockington, M. and Davis, M.B.: Prenatal diagnosis of mitochondrial DNA$^{8993T>G}$ disease. Am. J. Hum. Genet. 50:629, 1992.

Harger, J.H., Doshi, N., Marchese, S., Hinkle, R.S. and Garver, K.L.: Increased amniotic fluid alpha-fetoprotein due to a holoacardium amorphous twin. Clin. Genet. 19:257, 1981.

Harman, C.R., Bowman, J.M., Menticoglou, S.M., Pollock, J.M. and Manning, F.A.: Profound fetal thrombocytopenia in Rhesus disease: Serious hazard at intravascular transfusion. Lancet. 2:741, 1988.

Harman, C.R., Menticoglou, S.M., Bowman, J.M. and Manning, F.A.: Current technique of intraperitoneal transfusion: Do not throw away the renografin. Fetal Ther. 4:78, 1989.

Harmon, J.V., Osathanondh, R. and Holmes, L. B.: Symmetrical terminal transverse limb defects: Report of a twenty-week fetus. Teratology. 51:237, 1995.

Harper, P.S., Laurence, K.M., Parkes, A., Wusteman, F.S., Kresse, H., von Figura, K., Ferguson-Smith, M.A., Duncan, D.M., Logan, R.W., Hall, F. and Whiteman, P.: Sanfilippo A disease in the fetus. J. Med. Genet. 11:123, 1974.

Harris, R.D., Nyberg, D.A., Mack, L.A. and Weinberger, E.: Anorectal atresia: Prenatal sonographic diagnosis. Am. J. Roentgenol. 149:395, 1987.

Harris, R.D., Vincent, L.M. and Askin, F.B.: Yolk sac calcification: A sonographic finding associated with intrauterine embryonic demise in the first trimester. Radiology. 166:109, 1988.

Harrison, N.A.: "Missed beats" in a fetus, a case report. S. Afr. Med. J. 57:330, 1980.

Harrison, M.R., Filly, R.A., Parer, J.T., Faer, M.J., Jacobson, J.B. and de Lorimier, A.A.: Management of the fetus with a urinary tract malformation. J. Am. Med. Assoc. 246:635, 1981.

Harrison, M.R., Golbus, M.S. and Filly, R.A. (Eds.). *The Unborn Patient: Prenatal Diagnosis and Treatment.* Orlando: Grune & Stratton, 1984.

Harrison, M.R., Adzick, N.S., Nakayama, D.K. and deLorimier, A.A.: Fetal diaphragmatic hernia: Fatal but fixable. Semin. Perinatol. 9:103, 1985.

Harrison, M.R. Adzick, N.S., Longaker, M.T., Goldberg, J.D., Rosen, M.A., Filly, R.A., Evans, M.I. and Golbus, M.S.: Successful repair in utero of a fetal diaphragmatic hernia after removal of herniated viscera from the left thorax. N. Engl. J. Med. 322:1582, 1990a.

Harrison, M.R., Adzick, N.S., Jennings, R.W., Duncan, B.W., Rosen, M.A., Filly, R.A., Goldberg, J.D., DeLorimier, A.A. and Golbus, M.S.: Antenatal intervention for congenital cystic adenomatoid malformation. Lancet. 336:965, 1990b.

Harrison, K., Keisenger, K., Anyane-Yeboa, K. and Brown, S.: Maternal uniparental disomy of chromosome 2 in a baby with trisomy 2 mosaicism in amniotic fluid culture. Am. J. Med. Genet. 58:147, 1995.

Harrod, M.J.E., Friedman, J.M., Jimenez, J., Santos-Ramos, R., Byrne, J.B., Dev, V.G. and Weinberg, A.G.: Rapidly adhering amniotic-fluid cells and prenatal diagnosis of neural tube defects. Lancet. 2:99, 1979.

Harrod, M.J.E., Santos-Ramos, R., Cuarrino, G. and Maravilla, A.: Prenatal diagnosis of rhizomelic chondrodysplasia punctata. Proc. Greenwood Genet. Cent. 4:148, 1985.

Harsanyi, A., Toth, Z., Csecsei, K., Szeifert, G., Torok, O. and Papp, Z.: Prenatal diagnosis of midface defects associated with holoprosencephaly by ultrasound. Clin. Genet. 28:435, 1985.

Hart, P.S., Bodurtha, J., Redwine, F.O., Smeltzer, J.S., Kucera, L., McCall, J.B. and Brown, J.A.: Prenatal detection of non-cardiac rhabdomyosarcoma. Prenat. Diagn. 10:169, 1990.

Hartikainen-Sorri, A-L., Kirkinen, P. and Herva, R.: Prenatal detection of hydrolethalus syndrome. Prenat. Diagn. 3:219, 1983.

Hartsfield, J.K., Jr.: Intestinal hypoperistalsis, megacystic-microcolon type. In: Buyse, M.L. (Ed.), *Birth Defect Encyclopedia.* Dover, Mass.: Blackwell Scientific, 1990, p. 978.

Harzer, K.: Prenatal diagnosis of globoid cell leukodystrophy (Krabbe's disease): Third documented case. Hum. Genet. 35:193, 1977.

Harzer, K. and Schuster, I.: Prenatal enzymatic diagnosis of Krabbe disease (globoid-cell leukodystrophy) using chorionic villi. Pitfalls in the use of uncultured villi. Hum. Genet. 84:83, 1989.

Harzer, K., Hager, H.-D. and Tariverdian, G.: Prenatal enzymatic diagnosis and exclusion of Krabbe's disease (globoid-cell leukodystrophy) using chorionic villi in five risk pregnancies. Hum. Genet. 77:342, 1987.

Hashimoto, B.E., Mahony, B.S., Filly, R.A., Golbus, M.S., Anderson, R.L. and Callen, P.W.: Sonography, a complementary examination to alpha-fetoprotein testing for fetal neural tube defects. J. Ultrasound Med. 4:307, 1985.

Hashish, A.F., Monk, N.A., Lovell-Smith, M.P.F., Bardwell, L.M., Fiddes, T.M. and Gardner, R.J.M.: Trisomy 16 detected at chorion villus sampling. Prenat. Diagn. 9:427, 1989.

Haspeslagh, M., Fryns, J.P., van den Berghe, K., Goddeeris, P., Lauweryns, J. and Van den Berghe, H.: Hydrometrocolpos-polydactyly syndrome in a macerated female foetus. Eur. J. Pediatr. 136:307, 1981.

Hassani, S.N., Bard, R.L. and Barnes, D.A.: Fetal demise in third trimester: Ultrasonography and radiography. N.Y. State J. Med. 78:1260, 1978.

Hata, T., Makihara, K., Aoki, S., Kusakari, M., Hata, K., Kishida, K. and Kitao, M.: Prenatal diagnosis of valvar aortic stenosis by Doppler echocardiography and magnetic resonance imaging. Am. J. Obstet. Gynecol. 162:1068, 1990.

Hatjis, C.G., Horbar, J.D. and Anderson, G.G.: The in utero diagnosis of posterior fossa intracranial cyst (Dandy–Walker cyst). Am. J. Obstet. Gynecol. 140:473, 1981a.

Hatjis, C.G., Philip, A.G., Anderson, G.G. and Mann, L.I.: The in utero ultrasonographic appearance of Klippel–Trenaunay–Weber syndrome. Am. J. Obstet. Gynecol. 139:972, 1981b.

Hausser, I., Anton-Lamprecht, I. and Gustavii, B.: Prenatal diagnosis of junctional epidermolysis bullosa Herlitz type. Lancet. 2:1035, 1989.

Hausser, I. and Anton-Lamprecht, I.: Prenatal diagnosis of genodermatoses by ultrastructural diagnostic markers in extra-embryonic tissues: Defective hemidesmosomes in amnion epithelium of fetuses affected with epidermolysis bullosa Herlitz type (an alternative prenatal diagnosis in certain cases). Hum. Genet. 85:367, 1990.

Hayasaka, K., Tada, K., Fueki, N., Takahashi, I., Igarashi, A., Takabayashi, T. and Baumgartner, R.: Feasibility of prenatal diagnosis of nonketotic hyperglycinemia: Existence of the glycine cleavage system in placenta. J. Pediatr. 110:124, 1987.

Hayasaka, K., Tada, K., Fueki, N. and Aikaova, J.: Prenatal diagnosis of nonketotic hyperglycinemia: Enzymatic analysis of the glycine cleavage system in chorionic villi. J. Pediatr. 116:444, 1990.

Hayashi, Z., Orimo, H., Araki, T. and Shimada, T.: Prenatal diagnosis of steroid 21-hydroxylase deficiency by analysis of polymerase chain reaction single strand conformation polymorphism (PCR-SSCP) profiles. Prenat. Diagn. 17:435, 1997.

Haynor, D.R., Shuman, W.P., Brewer, D.K. and Mack, L.A.: Imaging of fetal ectopia cordis: Roles of sonography and computed tomography. J. Ultrasound Med. 3:25, 1984.

He, W., Voznyi, V., Huijmans, J.G.M., Geilen, G.C, Karpova, E.A., Dudukina, T.V., Zaremba, J., Van Diggelen, O.P. and Kleijer, W.J.: Prenatal diagnosis of Sanfilippo disease type C using a simple fluorometric enzyme assay. Prenat. Diagn. 14:17, 1994.

Hecht, F., Hecht, B.K. and O'Keeffe, D.: Sacrococcygeal teratoma: Prenatal diagnosis with elevated alphafetoprotein and acetylcholinesterase in amniotic fluid. Prenat. Diagn. 2:229, 1982.

Hecht, F., Grix, A., Jr., Hecht, B.K., Berger, C., Bixenman, H., Szucs, S., O'Keeffe, D. and Finberg, H.J.: Direct prenatal chromosome diagnosis of a malignancy. Cancer Genet. Cytogenet. 11:107, 1984.

Hedvall, G.: Congenital paroxysmal tachycardia—A report of three cases. Acta Paediatr. Scand. 62:550, 1973.

Hegmann, K.M., Spikes, A.S., Orr-Urtreger, A. and Shaffer, L.G.: Segregaton of a paternal insertional translocation results in partial 4q monosomy or 4q trisomy in two siblings. Am. J. Med. Genet. 61:10, 1996.

Heifetz, S.A.: Single umbilical arteries. A statistical analysis of 237 autopsy cases and review of the literature. Perspect. Pediatr. Pathol. 8:345, 1984.

Heikinheimo, M., Aula, P., Rapola, J., Wahlstrom, T., Jalanko, H. and Seppala, M.: Amniotic fluid pregnancy-specific beta$_1$-glycoprotein (SP$_1$) in Meckel's syndrome: A new test for prenatal diagnosis? Prenat. Diagn. 2:103, 1982.

Heikinheimo, M., Jalanko, H., Leisti, J., Kolho, K-L., Salonen, R., von Koskull, H. and Aula, P.: Amniotic fluid prenancy-specific beta$_1$-glycoprotein (SP$_1$) in fetal developmental disorders. Prenat. Diagn. 4:147, 1984.

Heilbronner, H., Wurster, K.G. and Harzer, K.: Pranatale diagnose der Gaucher-Krankheit. Dtsch. Med. Wschr. 106:652, 1981.

Hejtmancik, J.F., Harris, S.G., Tsao, C.C., Ward, P.A. and Caskey, C.T.: Carrier and prenatal diagnosis of Duchenne muscular dystrophy using DNA analysis. Am. J. Hum. Genet. 39(Suppl.):A94, 1986a.

Hejtmancik, J.F., Ward, P.A., Mansfield, T., Sifers, R.N., Harris, S. and Cox, D.W.: Prenatal diagnosis of alpha$_1$-antitrypsin deficiency by restriction fragment length polymorphisms, and comparison with oligonucleotide probe analysis. Lancet. 2:767, 1986b.

Helin, I., Axelsson, I. and Persson, P.-H.: Prenatal diagnosis of Potter's syndrome by ultrasound. Acta Paediatr. Scand. 72:939, 1983.

Heller, R.H., Adams, J.E., Hirschfeld, R.L. and Tapper, A.J.: Ultrasonic detection of an abnormal mass in a fetus later shown to have trisomy 18. Prenat. Diagn. 1:223, 1981.

Henderson, H.E. and Nelson, M.M.: Antenatal diagnosis of Hurler's syndrome. S. Afr. Med. J. 51:241, 1977.

Henderson, S.C., VanKolken, R.J. and Rahatzad, M.: Multicystic kidney with hydramnios. J. Clin. Ultrasound. 8:249, 1980.

Henrion, R. and Aubry, J.P.: Fetal cardiac abnormality and real-time ultrasound study: A case of Ivemark syndrome. Contrib. Gynecol. Obstet. 6:119, 1979.

Henrion, R., Oury, J.F., Aubry, J.P. and Aubry, M.C.: Prenatal diagnosis of ectrodactyly. Lancet. 2:319, 1980.

Henry, R.J.W. and Norton, S.: Prenatal ultrasound diagnosis of fetal scoliosis with termination of the pregnancy: Case report. Prenat. Diagn. 7:663, 1987.

Hensleigh, P.A., Moore, W.V., Wilson, K. and Tulchinsky, D.: Congenital X-linked adrenal hypoplasia. Obstet. Gynecol. 52:228, 1978.

Hentemann, M., Rauskolb, R., Ulbrich, R. and Bartels, I.: Abnormal pregnancy sonogram and chromosomal anomalies: Four years' experience with rapid karyotyping. Prenat. Diagn. 9:605, 1989.

Henthorn, P.S. and Whyte, M.P.: Infantile hypophosphatasia: Successful prenatal assessment by testing for tissue-non-specific alkaline phosphatase isoenzyme gene mutations. Prenat. Diagn. 15:1001, 1995.

Herin, P. and Thoren, C.: Congenital arrhythmias with supraventricular tachycardia in the perinatal period. Acta Obstet. Gynecol. Scand. 52:381, 1973.

Herreman, G., Betous, F., Batisse, P., Bessis, R., Lesavre, P. and Ferme, I.: Intrauterine detection of atrio-ventricular block in two children whose mother had Sjogren's syndrome. Nouv. Presse Med. 11:657, 1982.

Herrmann, J. and Opitz, J.M.: An unusual form of acrocephalosyndactyly. Birth Defects. 5(3):39, 1969.

Herrmann, U.J., Jr., and Sidiropoulos, D.: Single umbilical artery: Prenatal findings. Prenat. Diagn. 8:275, 1988.

Hersh, J.H. and Weisskopf, B.: Syndrome identification case report 94 fetal ascites and multiple congenital defects. J. Clin. Dysmorph. 1:26, 1983.

Hersh, J.H. and McChane, R.H.: Agnathia-midline malformation association. Proc. Greenwood Genet. Cent. 8:172, 1989.

Hersh, J.H., Dela Cruz, T.V., Pietrantoni, M., von Drasek-Ascher, G., Turnquest, M.A., Yacoub, O.A. and Joyce, M.R.: Mirror image duplication of the hands and feet: Report of a sporadic case with multiple congenital anomalies. Am. J. Med. Genet. 59:341, 1995.

Hersh, J.H., McChane, R.H., Rosenberg, E.M., Powers, W.H., Jr., Corrigan, C. and Pancratz, L.: Otocephaly-midline malformation association. Am. J. Med. Genet. 34:246, 1989.

Herva, R., Rapola, J., Rosti, J. and Karlson, H.: Cluster of severe amniotic adhesion malformations in Finland. Lancet. 1:818, 1980.

Herva, R., Leisti, J., Kirkinen, P. and Seppanen, U.: A lethal autosomal recessive syndrome of multiple congenital contractures. Am. J. Med. Genet. 20:431, 1985.

Herva, R., Conradi, N.G., Kalimo, H., Leisti, J. and Sourander, P.: A syndrome of multiple congenital contractures: Neuropathological analysis on five fetal cases. Am. J. Med. Genet. 29:67, 1988.

Herzberg, A.J., Effmann, E.L. and Bradford, W.D.: Variant of atelosteogenesis?: Report of a 20-week fetus. Am. J. Med. Genet. 29:883, 1988.

Higa, K., Dan, K. and Manabe, H.: Varicella-zoster virus infections during pregnancy: Hypothesis concerning the mechanisms of congenital malformations. Obstet. Gynecol. 69:214, 1987.

Hill, S.J. and Hirsch, J.H.: Sonographic detection of fetal hydrometrocolpos. J. Ultrasound Med. 4:323, 1985.

Hill, L.M., Breckle, R. and Gehrking, W.C.: The prenatal detection of congenital malformations by ultrasonography. Mayo Clin. Proc. 58:805, 1983a.

Hill, L.M., Breckle, R., Wolfgram, K.R. and O'Brien, P.C.: Oligohydramnios: Ultrasonically detected incidence and subsequent fetal outcome. Am. J. Obstet. Gynecol. 147:407, 1983b.

Hill, L., Pearce, M., Dilly, S. and Patton, M.: Prenatal diagnosis of mosaic trisomy 20 associated with an embryonic tumour. J. Med. Genet. 25:281, 1988a.

Hill, M.C., Lande, I.M. and Larsen, J.W., Jr.: Prenatal diagnosis of fetal anomalies using ultrasound and MRI. Radiol. Clin. North Am. 26:287, 1988b.

Hine, D.G., Hack, A.M., Goodman, S.I. and Tanaka, K.: Stable isotope dilution analysis of isovalerylglycine in amniotic fluid and urine and its application for the prenatal diagnosis of isovaleric acidemia. Pediatr. Res. 20:222, 1986.

Hirata, G.I., Matsunaga, M.L., Medearis, A.L., Dixon, P. and Platt, L.D.: Ultrasonographic diagnosis of a fetal abdominal mass: A case of a mesenchymal liver hamartoma and a review of the literature. Prenat. Diagn. 10:507, 1990.

Hirsch, M., Josefsberg, Z., Schoenfeld, A., Pertzelan, A., Merlob, P., Leiba, S., Kohn, G., Ovadia, J., Lubin, E. and Laron, Z.: Congenital hereditary hypothyroidism—Prenatal diagnosis and treatment. Prenat. Diagn. 10:491, 1990.

Hirschhorn, K. and LaBadie, G.U.: Prenatal diagnosis of Menkes disease. Am. J. Hum. Genet. 37(Suppl.):A220, 1985.

Hirschhorn, R., Beratis, N., Rosen, R.S., Parkman, R., Stern, R. and Polmar, S.: Adenosine-deaminase deficiency in a child diagnosed prenatally. Lancet. 1:73, 1975.

Hirst, M., Knight, S., Davies, K., Cross, G., Ocraft, K., Raeburn, S., Heeger, S., Eunpu, D., Jenkins, E.C. and Lindenbaum, R.: Prenatal diagnosis of fragile X syndrome. Lancet. 338:956, 1991.

Hoadley, S.D., Wallace, R.L., Miller, J.F. and Murgo, J.P.: Prenatal diagnosis of multiple cardiac tumors presenting as an arrhythmia. J. Clin. Ultrasound 14:639, 1986.

Hoag, R.W.: Fetomaternal hemorrhage associated with umbilical vein thrombosis. Am. J. Obstet. Gynecol. 154:1271, 1986.

Hoar, D.I., Haslam, D.B. and Starozik, D.M.: Improved direct molecular diagnosis and rapid fetal sexing. Prenat. Diagn. 4:241, 1984.

Hobbins, J.C. and Mahoney, M.J.: In utero diagnosis of hemoglobinopathies. N. Engl. J. Med. 290:1065, 1974.

Hobbins, J.C. and Mahoney, M.J.: Fetal blood drawing. Lancet. 2:107, 1975.

Hobbins, J.C. and Mahoney, M.J.: Skeletal dysplasia. In: Sanders, R.C. and James, A.E., Jr. (Eds.), *The Principles and Practice of Ultrasonography in Obstetrics and Gynecology.* 3rd ed. Norwalk, Conn.: Appleton-Century-Crofts, 1985, p. 267.

Hobbins, J.C., Grannum, P.A.T., Berkowitz, R.L., Silverman, R. and Mahoney, M.J.: Ultrasound in the diagnosis of congenital anomalies. Am. J. Obstet. Gynecol. 134:331, 1979.

Hobbins, J.C., Bracken, M.B. and Mahoney, M.J.: Diagnosis of fetal skeletal dysplasias with ultrasound. Am. J. Obstet. Gynecol. 142:306, 1982.

Hobbins, J.C., Romero, R., Grannum, P., Berkowitz, R.L., Cullen, M. and Mahoney, M.: Antenatal diagnosis of renal anomalies with ultrasound. I. Obstructive uropathy. Am. J. Obstet. Gynecol. 148:868, 1984.

Hobbins, J.C., Grannum, P.A., Romero, R., Reece, E.A. and Mahoney, M.J.: Percutaneous umbilical blood sampling. Am. J. Obstet. Gynecol. 152:1, 1985.

Hockey, A., Crowhurst, J. and Cullity, G.: Microcephaly, holoprosencephaly, hypokinesia—Second report of a new syndrome. Prenat. Diagn. 8:683, 1988.

Hockey, A., Knowles, S., Davies, D., Carey, W., Hurst, J. and Goldblatt, J.: Glutaric aciduria type II, an unusual cause of prenatal polycystic kidneys: Report of prenatal diagnosis and confirmation of autosomal recessive inheritance. Birth Defects. 29(1):373, 1993.

Hoefler, S., Hoefler, G., Moser, A.B., Watkins, P.A., Chen, W.W. and Moser, H.W.: Prenatal diagnosis of rhizomelic chondrodysplasia punctata. Prenat. Diagn. 8:571, 1988.

Hoff, N.R. and Mackay, I.M.: Prenatal ultrasound diagnosis of intracranial teratoma. J. Clin. Ultrasound 8:247, 1980.

Hofstaetter, C., Neumann, I., Lennert, T. Dudenhausen, J.W.: Prenatal diagnosis of diffuse mesangial glomerulosclerosis by ultrasonogrphy: A longitudinal study of a case in an affected family. Fetal Diagn. Ther. 11:126, 1996.

Hogdall, C., Siegel-Bartelt, J., Toi, A. and Ritchie, S.: Prenatal diagnosis of Opitz (BBB) syndrome in the second trimester by ultrasound detection of hypospadias and hypertelorism. Prenat. Diagn. 9:783, 1989.

Hogge, W.A., Schonberg, S.A., Glover, T.W., Hecht, F. and Golbus, M.S.: Prenatal diagnosis of fragile (X) syndrome. Obstet. Gynecol. 63:19S, 1984.

Hogge, W.A., Golabi, M., Filly, R.A., Douglas, R. and Golbus, M.S.: The lethal multiple pterygium syndromes: Is prenatal detection possible? Am. J. Med. Genet. 20:441, 1985.

Hogge, W.A., Vick, D.J., Schnatterly, P.A. and MacMillan, R.H.: Bilateral renal agenesis and mullerian anomalies in a 47,XXX fetus. Am. J. Med. Genet. 33:242, 1989a.

Hogge, W.A., Vick, D.J., Hogge, J.S. and Thiagarajah, S.: Prenatal detection of fetal cytomegalovirus (CMV) infection. Am. J. Hum. Genet. 45(Suppl.):A261, 1989b.

Hogge, W.A., Dungan, J.S., Brooks, M.P., Dilks, S.A., Abbitt, P.L., Thiagarajah, S. and Ferguson, J.E.: Diagnosis and management of prenatally detected myelomeningocele: A preliminary report. Am. J. Obstet. Gynecol. 163:1061, 1990.

Hogge, W.A., Buffone, G.J. and Hogge, J.S.: Prenatal diagnosis of cytomegalovirus (CMV) infection: A preliminary report. Prenat. Diagn. 13:131, 1993.

Hohlfeld, P, Vial, Y., Maillard-Brignon, C., Vaudaux, B. and Fawer, C-L.: Cytomegalovirus fetal infection: Prenatal diagnosis. Obstet. Gynecol. 78:615, 1991.

Hohlfeld, P., Daffos, F., Costa, J-M, Thulliez, P., Forestier, F. and Vidaud, M.: Prenatal diagnosis of congenital toxoplasmosis with a polymerase-chain reaction test on amniotic fluid. N. Engl. J. Med. 331:695, 1994.

Holbrook, K.A., Dale, B.A., Sybert, V.P. and Sagebiel, R.W.: Epidermolytic hyperkeratosis: Ultrastructure and biochemistry of skin and amniotic fluid cells from two affected fetuses and a newborn infant. J. Invest. Dermatol. 80:222, 1983.

Holbrook, K.A., Dale, B.A., Witt, D.R., Hayden, M.R. and Toriello, H.V.: Arrested epidermal morphogenesis in three newborn infants with a fatal genetic disorder (restrictive dermopathy). J. Invest. Dermatol. 88:330, 1987a.

Holbrook, H.R., Jr., Krovoza, A.M., Schelley, S. and Ferguson, J.E., II: Biamnial elevated alpha-fetoprotein and positive acetylcholinesterase in twins, one with anencephaly. Prenat. Diagn. 7:653, 1987b.

Holbrook, K.A., Wapner, R., Jackson, L. and Zaeri, N.: Diagnosis and prenatal diagnosis of epidermolysis bullosa herpetiformis (Dowling–Meara) in a mother, two affected children, and an affected fetus. Prenat. Diagn. 12:725, 1992.

Holliday, D.J., Juberg, R.C. and Hennessy, V.S.: Familial sex chromosomal mosaicism. Am. J. Hum. Genet. 43(Suppl.):A235, 1988.

Hollingsworth, D.R. and Alexander, N.M.: Amniotic fluid concentrations of iodothyronines and thyrotropin do not reliably predict fetal thyroid status in pregnancies complicated by maternal thyroid disorders or anencephaly. J. Clin. Endocrinol. Metab. 57:349, 1983.

Holm, J., Ponders, L. and Sweetman, L.: Prenatal diagnosis of propionic and methylmalonic acidaemia by stable isotope dilution analysis of amniotic fluid. J. Inher. Metab. Dis. 12(Suppl. 2):271, 1989.

Holmberg, L., Gustavii, B., Cordesius, E., Kristoffersson, A.-C., Ljung, R., Lofberg, L., Stromberg, P. and Nilsson, I.M.: Prenatal diagnosis of hemophilia B by an immunoradiometric assay of factor IX. Blood. 56:397, 1980.

Holmes, J.H.: Early diagnostic ultrasonography. J. Ultrasound Med. 2:33, 1983.

Holmes-Siedle, M., Ryynanen, M. and Lindenbaum, R.H.: Parental decisions regarding termination of pregnancy following prenatal detection of sex chromosome abnormality. Prenat. Diagn. 7:239, 1987.

Holmgren, G. and Sigurd, J.: Prenatal diagnosis of two cases of gastroschisis following alphafetoprotein (AFP) screening. Acta Obstet. Gynecol. Scand. 63:325, 1984a.

Holmgren, G., Forsell, A., Kaariainen H. and Maroteaux, P.: Semi-lethal bone dysplasia in three sibs: A new genetic disorder. Clin. Genet. 26:246, 1984b.

Holt, D.E., Howie, A.F., Beckett, G.J., Hurley, R. and Harvey, D.: Measurement of fetal plasma levels of glutathione S-transferase B_1 as an indicator of damage ot the liver caused by hypoxia in utero. Fetal Diagn. Ther. 10:11, 1995.

Holton, J.B., Allen, J.T. and Gillett, M.G.: Prenatal diagnosis of disorders of galactose metabolism. J. Inher. Metab. Dis. 12(Suppl. 1):202, 1989.

Holzgreve, W.: Prenatal diagnosis of persistent common cloaca with prune belly and anencephaly in the second trimester. Am. J. Med. Genet. 20:729, 1985.

Holzgreve W. and Golbus, M.S.: Amniotic fluid acetylcholinesterase as a prenatal diagnostic marker for upper gastrointestinal atresias. Am. J. Obstet. Gynecol. 147:837, 1983.

Holzgreve, W. and Golbus, M.S.: Prenatal diagnosis of ornithine transcarbamylase deficiency utilizing fetal liver biopsy. Am. J. Hum. Genet. 36:320, 1984.

Holzgreve, W., Beller, F.K. and Pawlowitzki, I.H.: Amniotic fluid acetylcholinesterase as a marker in prenatal diagnosis of esophageal atresia. Am. J. Obstet. Gynecol. 145:641, 1983.

Holzgreve, W., Anderson, R.L., Mahony, B.S., Filly, R.A., Harrison, M.R., Callen, P.W. and Golbus, M.S.: Fetal sacrococcygeal teratomas: Features and prognosis. Am. J. Hum. Genet. 36(Suppl.):190S, 1984.

Holzgreve, W., Winde, B., Willital, G.H. and Beller, F.K.: Prenatal diagnosis and perinatal management of a fetal ovarian cyst. Prenat. Diagn. 5:155, 1985a.

Holzgreve, W., Mahony, B.S., Glick, P.L., Filly, R.A., Harrison, M.R., Delorimier, A.A., Holzgreve, A.C., Muller, K.M., Callen, P.W., Anderson, R.L. and Golbus, M.S.: Sonographic demonstration of fetal sacrococcygeal teratoma. Prenat. Diagn. 5:245, 1985b.

Holzgreve, W., Holzgreve, B. and Curry, C.J.R.: Nonimmune hydrops fetalis: Diagnosis and management. Semin. Perinatol. 9:52, 1985c.

Honour J.W. and Rumsby, G.: Problems in diagnosis and management of congenital adrenal hyperplasia due to 21-hydroxylase deficiency. J. Steroid Biochem. Molec. Biol. 45:69, 1993.

Hood, V.D. and Robinson, H.P.: Diagnosis of closed neural tube defects by ultrasound in second trimester of pregnancy. Br. Med. J. 2:931, 1978.

Horn, N.: Copper incorporation studies on cultured cells for prenatal diagnosis of Menkes' disease. Lancet. 1:1156, 1976.

Horn, N.: Menkes X-linked disease: Prenatal diagnosis of hemizygous males and heterozygous females. Prenat. Diagn. 1:107, 1981.

Horn, N.: Menkes' X-linked disease: prenatal diagnosis and carrier detection. J. Inher. Metab. Dis. 6(Suppl. 1):59, 1983.

Horvath, K., Csecsei, K., Szeifert, G., Toth, Z., Torok, O. and Papp, Z.: Prenatal diagnosis of X-linked hydrocephalus without aqueductal stenosis. Clin. Genet. 28:437, 1985.

Horwell, D.H., Heaton, D.E. and Old, J.M.: Diagnosis of haemoglobinopathy using cultured chorionic villus cells. Lancet. 2:613, 1985.

Hoshide, R., Matsuura, T., Sagara, Y., Kubo, T. Shimadzu, M., Endo, F. and Matsuda, I.: Prenatal monitoring in a family at high risk for ornithine transcarbamylase (OTC) deficiency: A new mutation of an A- to -C transversion in position +4 of intron 1 of the OTC gene that is likely to abolish enzyme activity. Am. J. Med. Genet. 64:459, 1996.

Hosli, P., de Bruyn, C.H.M.M., Oerlemans, F.J.J.M., Verjaal, M. and Norbrega, R.E.: Rapid prenatal diagnosis of HG-PRT deficiency using ultra-microchemical methods. Hum. Genet. 37:195, 1977.

Hoshide, R., Matsuura, T., Sagara, Y., Kubo, T. Shimadzu, M., Endo, F. and Matsuda, I.: Prenatal monitoring in a family at high risk for ornithine transcarbamylase (OTC) deficiency: A new mutation of an A-to-C transversion in position +4 of intron 1 of the OTC gene that is likely to abolish enzyme activity. Am. J. Med. Genet. 64:459, 1996.

Hou, J-W. and Wang, T-R: Galloway–Mowat syndrome in Taiwan. Am. J. Med. Genet. 58:245, 1995.

Houlton, M.C.C., Sutton, M. and Aitken, J.: Antenatal diagnosis of duodenal atresia. J. Obstet. Gynaecol. Br. Commonw. 81:818, 1974.

Hovav, Y., Nadjari, M., Dagan, J., Kafka, E. and Yaffe, H.: Nonimmune hydrops fetalis in a 49,XXXXY fetus at 16 menstrual weeks. Am. J. Med. Genet. 47:529, 1993.

Hovnanian, A., Hilal, L., Blanchet-Bardon, C., Bodemer, C., de Prost, Y., Stark, C.A., Christiano, A.M., Dommergues, M., Terwilliger, J.D., Izquierdo, L., Conteville, P., Dumex, Y., Uitto, J. and Goossens, M.: DNA-based prenatal diagnosis of generalized recessive dystrophic epidermolysis bullosa in six pregnancies at risk for recurrence. J. Invest. Derm. 104:456, 1995.

Hoyer, L.W., Carta, C.A., Golbus, M.S., Hobbins, J.C. and Mahoney, M.J.: Prenatal diagnosis of classic hemophilia (hemophilia A) by immunoradiometric assays. Blood. 65:1312, 1985.

Hoyme, H.E., Musgrave, S.D., Jr., Browne, A.F. and Clemmons, J.J.: Congenital oral tumor associated with neurofibromatosis detected by prenatal ultrasound. Clin. Pediatr. 26:372, 1987.

Hsu, L.Y.F., Kaffe, S., Yahr, F., Serotkin, A., Giordano, F., Godmilow, L., Kim, H.J., David,

K., Kerenyi, T. and Hirschhorn, K.: Prenatal cytogenetic diagnosis: First 1000 successful cases. Am. J. Med. Genet. 2:365, 1978.

Hsu, L.Y.F., Kaffe, S. and Perlis, T.E.: Trisomy 20 mosaicism in prenatal diagnosis—A review and update. Prenat. Diagn. 7:581, 1987.

Hsu, L.Y.F., Kaffe, S. and Perlis, T.E.: A revisit of trisomy 20 mosaicism in prenatal diagnosis—An overview of 103 cases. Prenat. Diagn. 11:7, 1991.

Hsu, C-D., Feng, T.I., Crawford, T.O. and Johnson, T.R.B.: Unusual fetal movement in congenital myotonic dystrophy. Fetal Diagn. Ther. 8:200, 1993a.

Hsu, W.T., Garber, A., Carlson, D., Fischel-Ghodsian, N. Graham, J.M., Jr., Linn, S., Wheeler, M., Oztas, S. and Schreck, R.: Prenatal detected trisomy 16 in two phenotypically abnormal newborn. Am. J. Hum. Genet. 53(Suppl.):1419, 1993b.

Hu, L-J, Laporte, J., Kress, W. and Dahl, N.: Prenatal diagnosis of X-linked myotubular myopathy: Strategies using new and tightly linked DNA markers. Prenat. Diagn. 16:231, 1996.

Huang, S.-Z., Zhou, X.-D., Ren, Z.-R., Zeng, Y.-T. and Woo, S.L.C.: Prenatal detection of an ARG-TER mutation at codon 111 of the PAH gene using DNA amplification. Prenat. Diagn. 10:289, 1990.

Hubbard, A.E., Ayers, A.B., MacDonald, L.M. and James, C.E.: In utero torsion of the testis: Antenatal and postnatal ultrasonic appearances. Br. J. Radiol. 57:644, 1984.

Hubinont, C., Pratola, D., Rothschild, E., Rodesch, F. and Schwers, J.: Dicephalus: Unusual case of conjoined twins and its prepartum diagnosis. Am. J. Obstet. Gynecol. 149:693, 1984.

Hug, G., Schubert, W.K. and Soukup, S.: Prenatal diagnosis of type-II glycogenosis. Lancet. 1:1002, 1970.

Hug, G., Bove, K.E., Soukup, S., Ryan, M., Bendon, R., Babcock, D., Warren, N.S. and Dignan, P.St.J.: Increased serum hexosaminidase in a woman pregnant with a fetus affected by mucolipidosis II (I-cell disease). N. Engl. J. Med. 311:988, 1984a.

Hug, G., Soukup, S., Ryan, M. and Chuck, G.: Rapid prenatal diagnosis of glycogen-storage disease type II by electron microscopy of uncultured amniotic-fluid cells. N. Engl. J. Med. 310:1018, 1984b.

Hug, G., Chuck, G., Chen, Y-T., Kay, H.H. and Bossen, E.H.: Chorionic villus ultrastructure in type II glycogen storage disease (Pompe's disease). N. Eng. J. Med. 324:342, 1991.

Hughes, R.M. and Benzie, R.J.: Amniotic band syndrome causing fetal head deformity. Prenat. Diagn. 4:447, 1984.

Hughes, I.A. and Laurence, K.M.: Antenatal diagnosis of congenital adrenal hyperplasia. Lancet. 2:7, 1979.

Hughes, I.A. and Laurence, K.M.: Prenatal diagnosis of congenital adrenal hyperplasia due to 21-hydroxylase deficiency by amniotic fluid steroid analysis. Prenat. Diagn. 2:97, 1982.

Hughes, H.E. and Miskin, M.: Congenital microcephaly due to vascular disruption: In utero documentation. Pediatrics. 78:85, 1986.

Hughes, I.A., Dyas, J., Riad-Fahmy, D. and Laurence, K.M.: Prenatal diagnosis of congenital adrenal hyperplasia: Reliability of amniotic fluid steroid analysis. J. Med. Genet. 24:344, 1987.

Hughes-Benzie, R.M., Xuan, J.Y., Hurst, J.A., Pilia, G., Schlessinger, D. and MacKenzie, A.E.: Prenatal diagnosis of Simpson–Golabi–Behmel syndrome: Identification of an informative AT repeat sequence in the critical SGBS region. Am. J. Hum. Genet. 57(Suppl.):A281, 1995.

Huhta, J.C.., Carpenter, R.J., Jr., Moise, K.J., Jr., Deter, R.L., Ott, D.A. and McNamara, D.G.: Prenatal diagnosis and postnatal management of critical aortic stenosis. Circulation. 75:573, 1987a.

Huhta, J.C., Moise, K.J., Fisher, D.J., Sharif, D.S., Wasserstrum, N. and Martin, C.: Detection and quantitation of constriction of the fetal ductus arteriosus by Doppler echocardiography. Circulation. 75:406, 1987b.

Hullin, D.A., Elder, G.H., Laurence, K.M., Roberts, A. and Newcombe, R.G.: Amniotic fluid cholinesterase measurement as a rapid method for the exclusion of fetal neural-tube defects. Lancet. 2:325, 1981.

Hullin, D.A., Gregory, P.J., Dyer, C.L. and Dew, J.O.: Place of amniotic fluid AFP in prenatal diagnosis of trisomies. Lancet. 2:662, 1985.

Hume, R.F., Jr., Gingras, J.L., Martin, L.S., Hertzberg, B.S., O'Donnell, K. and Killam, A.P.: Ultrasound diagnosis of fetal anomalies associated with in utero cocaine exposure: Further support for cocaine-induced vascular disruption teratogenesis. Fetal Diagn. Ther. 9:239, 1994.

Hummel, M., Baker, J.C., Cunningham, M.E. and Willard, D.A.: Prenatal diagnosis of homozygous achondroplasia. Am. J. Med. Genet. 34:140, 1989.

Hunter O.B. Jr.,: Cortisone in the management of hemolytic disease in the newborn. N.Y. State J. Med. 55:1136, 1955.

Hunter, A., Hammerton, J.L., Baskett, T. and Lyons, E.: Raised amniotic fluid alpha-fetoprotein in Turner syndrome. Lancet. 1:598, 1976.

Hunter, A.G.W., DesLauriers, G.E., Gillieson, M.S. and Muggah, H.F.: Prenatal diagnosis of Turner's syndrome by ultrasonography. Can. Med. Assoc. J. 127:401, 1982.

Hunziker, U.A., Savoldelli, G., Boltshauser, E., Giedion, A. and Schinzel, A.: Prenatal diagnosis of Schwartz–Jampel syndrome with early manifestation. Prenat. Diagn. 9:127, 1989.

Hurst, J.A., Houlston, R.S., Roberts, A., Gould, S.J. and Tingey, W.G.: Transverse limb deficiency, facial clefting and hypoxic renal damage: An association with treatment of maternal hypertension? Clin. Dysmorph. 4:359, 1995.

Hutcheon, R.G., Nitowsky, H.M., Cho, S., Koenigsberg, M. and Goldman, D.: Prenatal diagnosis of the McKusick–Kaufman syndrome by ultrasound. Am. J. Hum. Genet. 36(Suppl.): 190S, 1984.

Hutton, E.M., Shuman, C., Boehm, C. and Kazazian, H.H., Jr.: False paternity as a problem in the use of restriction fragment length polymorphisms for prenatal diagnosis. Am. J. Hum. Genet. 37(Suppl.):A221, 1985.

Huu, T.P., Dumez, Y., Marquetty, C., Durandy, A., Boue, J. and Hakim, J.: Prenatal diagnosis of chronic granulomatous disease (GGD) in four high risk male fetuses. Prenat. Diagn. 7:253, 1987.

Hyett, J.A., Clayton, P.T., Moscoso, G. and Nicolaides, K.H.: Increased first trimester nuchal translucency as a prenatal manifestation of Smith–Lemli–Opitz syndrome. Am. J. Med. Genet. 58:374, 1995.

Iaccarino, M., Lonardo, F., Giugliano, M. and Bruna, M.D.: Prenatal diagnosis of Mohr syndrome by ultrasonography. Prenat. Diagn. 5:415, 1985.

Iafolla, A.K., McConkie-Rosell, A. and Chen, Y.T.: VACTERL with hydrocephalus reexamined: Report of survival with good neurologic outcome. Am. J. Hum. Genet. 45(Suppl.): A49, 1989.

Iafolla, A.K., McConkie-Rosell, A. and Chen, Y.T.: Vater and hydrocephalus: Distinct syndrome? Am. J. Med. Genet 38:46, 1991.

Ianniruberto, A. and Tajani, E.: Ultrasonographic study of fetal movements. Semin. Perinatol. 5:175, 1981.

Iavarone, A., Dolfin, G., Bracco, G., Zaffaroni, M., Gallina, M.R. and Bona, G.: First trimester prenatal diagnosis of Wolman disease. J. Inher. Metab. Dis. 12(Suppl. 2):299, 1989.

Ikeno, T., Minami, R., Wagatsuma, K., Fujibayashi, S., Nakao, T., Abo, K., Tsugawa, S., Taniguchi, S. and Takasago, Y.: Prenatal diagnosis of Hurlers syndrome—Biochemical studies on the affected fetus. Hum. Genet. 59:353, 1981.

Imamura, A., Suzuki, Y., Song, X-Q, Fukao, T. Shimozawa, N., Orii, T. and Kondo, N.: Prenatal diagnosis of adrenoleukodystrophy by means of mutation analysis. Prenat. Diagn. 16:259, 1996.

Impraim, C.C. and Teplitz, R.L.: Prenatal diagnosis by allele-specific oligonucleotide analysis of in vitro amplified genomic DNA. Am. J. Hum. Genet. 41(Suppl.):A277, 1987.

Insley, J., Bird, G.W.G., Harper, P.S. and Pearce, G.W.: Prenatal prediction of myotonic dystrophy. Lancet. 1:806, 1976.

Inui, K., Wenger, D.A., Furukawa, M. Suehara, N., Yutaka, Y., Okada, S., Tanizawa, O. and Yabuuchi, H.: Prenatal diagnosis of GM_2 gangliosidoses using a fluorogenic sulfated substrate. Clin. Chim. Acta. 154:145, 1986.

Ionasescu, V., Zelleger, H. and Cancilla, P.: Fetal serum-creatine-phosphokinase not a valid predictor of Duchenne muscular dystrophy. Lancet. 2:1251, 1978.

Isada, N.B., Paar, D.P., Johnson, M.P., Evans, M.I., Holzgreve, W., Qureshi, F. and Straus, S.E.: In utero diagnosis of congenital varicella zoster virus infection by chorionic villus sampling and polymerase chain reaction. Am. J. Obstet. Gynecol. 165:1727, 1991.

Isada, N.B., Hume, R.F., Jr., Reichler, A., Johnson, M.P., Klinger, K.W., Evans, M.I. and Ward, B.E.: Fluorescent in situ hybridization and second-trimester sonographic anomalies: Uses and limitations. Fetal Diagn. Ther. 9:397, 1994.

Ishikiriyama, S., Isobe, M., Kuroda, N., and Yamamoto, Y.: Japanese girl with Krause–Van Schooneveld–Kivlin syndrome: Peters anomaly with short-limb dwarfism: Peter-plus syndrome. Am. J. Med. Genet. 44:701, 1992.

Israel, J., Arjmand, A., Strassner, H., Kirz, D. and Birnholz, J.: Fetal triploidy associated with elevated maternal serum alpha feto protein. Am. J. Hum. Genet. 39(Suppl.):A256, 1986.

Itskovitz, J., Timor-Tritsch, I. and Brandes, J.M.: Intrauterine fetal arrhythmia: Atrial premature beats. Int. J. Gynaecol. Obstet. 16:419, 1979.

Ivarsson, S-A., Bjerre, I., Brun, A., Ljungberg, O., Maly, E. and Taylor, I.: Joubert syndrome associated with Leber amaurosis and multicystic kidneys. Am. J. Med. Genet. 45:542, 1993.

Ives, E.J. and Houston, C.S.: Autosomal recessive microcephaly and micromelia in Cree Indians. Am. J. Med. Genet. 7:351, 1980.

Ivinson, A.J., Elles, R.G., Read, A.P. and Harris, R.: Fetal sexing using the polymerase chain reaction technique. J. Med. Genet. 25:641, 1988.

Izquierdo, L.A., Kushnir, O., Aase, J., Lantz, P., Castellano, T. and Curet, L.B.: Antenatal ultrasonic diagnosis of dyssegmental dysplasia: A case report. Prenat. Diagn. 10:587, 1990.

Jacobson, C.B. and Barter, R.H.: Intrauterine diagnosis and management of genetic defects. Am. J. Obstet. Gynecol. 99:796, 1967.

Jaffa, A.J., Barak, S., Kaysar, N. and Peyser, M.R.: Antenatal diagnosis of bilateral congenital chylothorax with pericardial effusion. Acta Obstet. Gynecol. Scand. 64:455, 1985.

Jafri, S.Z.H., Bree, R.L., Silver, T.M. and Ouimette, M.: Fetal ovarian cysts: Sonographic detection and association with hypothyroidism. Radiology. 150: 809, 1984.

Jakobs, C.: Prenatal diagnosis of inherited metabolic disorders by stable isotope dilution GC-MS analysis of metabolites in amniotic fluid: Review of four years experience. J. Inher. Metab. Dis. 12(Suppl. 2):267, 1989.

Jakobs, C., Sweetman L., Nyhan, W.L. and Packman, S.: Stable isotope dilution analysis of 3-hydroxyisovaleric acid in amniotic fluid: Contribution to the prenatal diagnosis of inherited disorders of leucine catabolism. J. Inherit. Metab. Dis. 7:15, 1984a.

Jakobs, C., Sweetman, L., Wadman, S.K., Duran, M., Saudubray, J.-M. and Nyhan, W.L.: Prenatal diagnosis of glutaric aciduria type II by direct chemical analysis of dicarboxylic acids in amniotic fluid. Eur. J. Pediatr. 141:153, 1984b.

Jakobs, C., Warner, T.G., Sweetman, L. and Nyhan, W.L.: Stable isotope dilution analysis of galactitol in amniotic fluid: An accurate approach to the prenatal diagnosis of galacosemia. Pediatr. Res. 18:714, 1984c.

Jakobs, C., Kvittingen, E.A., Berger, R., Haagen, A., Kleijer, W. and Niermeijer, M.: Prenatal diagnosis of tyrosinaemia type I by use of stable isotope dilution mass spectrometry. Eur. J. Pediatr. 144:209, 1985.

Jakobs, C., Kleijer, W.J., Bakker, H.D., Van Gennip, A.H., Przyrembel, H. and Niermeijer, M.F.: Dietary restriction of maternal lactose intake does not prevent accumulation of galactitol in the amniotic fluid of fetuses affected with galactosaemia. Prenat. Diagn. 8:641, 1988.

Jakobs, C., Stellard, F., Kvittingen, I.A., Henderson, M. and Lilford, R.: First-trimester prenatal diagnosis of tyrosinemia type I by amniotic fluid succinylacetone determination. Prenat. Diagn. 10:133, 1990.

Jakobs, C., ten Brink, H.J., Divry, P. and Rolland, M.O.: Prenatal diagnosis of Canavan disease. Eur. J. Ped. 151:620, 1992.

Jakobs, C., Ogier, H., Rabier, D., and Gibson, K.M.: Prenatal detection of succinic semialdehyde dehydrogenase deficiency (4-hydroxybutyric aciduria). Prenat. Diagn. 13:150, 1993.

Jalal, S.M., Kukolich, M.K., Garcia, M., Benjamin, T.R. and Day, D.W.: Tetrasomy 9p: An emerging syndrome. Clin. Genet. 39:60, 1991.

Jalanko, H., Heikinheimo, M., Ryynanen, M., Ranta, T. and Aula, P.: Alkaline phosphatase activity in amniotic fluid in pregnancies with fetal disorders. Prenat. Diagn. 3:303, 1983.

Jandial, V., Thom, H. and Gibson, J.: Raised alpha-fetoprotein levels associated with minor congenital defect. Br. Med. J. 2:22, 1976.

Jarmas, A.L., Weaver, D.D., Padilla, L.M., Stecker, E. and Bender, H.A.: Hirschsprung disease: Etiologic implications of unsuccessful prenatal diagnosis. Am. J. Med. Genet. 16:163, 1983.

Jarvela, I., Rapola, J., Peltonen, L., Puhakka, L., Vesa, J., Ammala, P., Salonen, R., Ryynanen, M., Haring, P., Mustonen, A. and Santavuori, P.: DNA-based prenatal diagnosis of the infantile form of neuronal ceroid lipofuscinosis (INCL, CLN1). Prenat. Diagn. 11:323, 1991.

Jaspers, N.G.J., Van Der Kraan, M., Linssen, C.M.L., Macek, M., Seemanova, E. and Kleijer, W.J.: First-trimester prenatal diagnosis of the Nijemegen breakage syndrome and ataxia telangiectasia using an assay of radioresistant DNA synthesis. Prenat. Diagn. 10:667, 1990.

Jassani, M.N., Brennan, J.N. and Merkatz, I.R.: Prenatal diagnosis of single umbilical artery by ultrasound. J. Clin. Ultrasound 8:447, 1980.

Jassani, M.N., Gauderer, M.W.L., Fanaroff, A.A., Fletcher, B. and Merkatz, I.R.: A perinatal approach to the diagnosis and management of gastrointestinal malformations. Obstet. Gynecol. 59:33, 1982.

Jaswaney, Y., Clark, B.A., Ashmead, G.G., Ko, L., Powell, D., Cassidy, S.B. and Schwartz, S.: Prenatal diagnosis and birth outcome of a mosaic ring18/monosomy 18. Am. J. Hum. Genet. 57(Suppl.):A345, 1995.

Jauniaux, E., Donner, C., Thomas, C., Francotte, J., Rodesch, F. and Avni, F.E.: Umbilical cord pseudocyst in trisomy 18. Prenat. Diagn. 8:557, 1988.

Jauniaux, E., Vyas, S., Finlayson, C., Moscoso, G., Driver, M. and Campbell, S.: Early sono-graphic diagnosis of body stalk anomaly. Prenat. Diagn. 10:127, 1990.

Jeanty, P., Romero, R. and Hobbins, J.C.: Fetal limb volume: A new parameter to assess fetal growth and nutrition. J. Ultrasound Med. 4:273, 1985.

Jeffcoate, T.N.A., Fliegner, J.R.H., Russell, S.H., Davis, J.C. and Wade, A.P.: Diagnosis of the adrenogenital syndrome before birth. Lancet. 2:553, 1965.

Jeffrey, R.B., Jr., Laing, F.C., Wing, V.W. and Hoddick, W.: Sonography of the fetal duplex kidney. Radiology. 153:123, 1984.

Jenkins, E.C., Brown, W.T., Duncan, C.J., Brooks, J., Ben-Yishay, M., Giordano, F.M. and Nitowsky, H.M.: Feasibility of fragile X chromosome prenatal diagnosis demonstrated. Lancet. 2:1292, 1981.

Jenkins, E.C., Brown, W.T., Brooks, J., Duncan, C.J., Rudelli, R.D. and Wisniewski, H.M.: Experience with prenatal fragile X detection. Am. J. Med. Genet. 17:215, 1984.

Jenkins, E.C., Brown, W.T., Brooks, J., Duncan, C.J., Masia, A. and Krawczun, M.S.: The prenatal detection of the fragile X chromosome: 3 new cases, lack of detection in Chang medium, and summary of world experience. Am. J. Hum. Genet. 37(Suppl.):A99, 1985.

Jenkins, E.C., Brown, W.T., Wilson, M.G., Lin, M.S., Alfi, O.S., Wassman, E.R., Brooks, J., Duncan, C.J., Masia, A. and Krawczun, M.S.: The prenatal detection of the fragile X chromosome: Review of recent experience. Am. J. Med. Genet. 23:297, 1986.

Jenkins, E.C., Brown, W.T., Krawczun, M.S., Duncan, C.J., Lele, K.P., Cantu, E.S., Schonberg, S., Golbus, M.S., Sekhon, G.S., Stark, S., Kunaporn, S. and Silverman, W.P.: Recent experience in prenatal Fra(X) detection. Am. J. Med. Genet. 30:329, 1988.

Jenkins, E.C., Krawczun, M.S., Stark-Houck, S.L., Duncan, C.J., Kunaporn, S., Gu, H., Schwartz-Richstein, C., Howard-Peebles, P.N., Gross, A., Sherman, S.L. and Brown, W.T.: Improved prenatal detection of Fra(X)(q27.3): Methods for prevention of false negatives in chorionic villus and amniotic fluid cell cultures. Am. J. Med. Genet. 38:447, 1991.

Jenkinson, E.L., Pfisterer, W.H., Latteier, K.K. and Martin, M.: A prenatal diagnosis of osteopetrosis. Am. J. Roentgenol. Rad. Therapy 49:455, 1943.

Jensen, M., Zahnn, V., Rauch, A. and Loukopoulos, D.: Prenatal diagnosis of beta-thalassemia. Klin. Wochenschr. 57:37, 1979.

Jeppsson, J.-O., Cordesius, E., Gustavii, B., Lofberg, L., Franzen, B., Stromberg, P. and Sveger,

T.: Prenatal diagnosis of alpha$_1$-antitrypsin deficiency by analysis of fetal blood obtained by fetoscopy. Pediatr. Res. 15:254, 1981.

Jewel, A.F., Musgrave, D.L., Cuzzocrea, A.D., Dennis, L.G. and Keene, C.L.: Pseudoxanthoma elasticum in pregnancy associated with delayed fetal growth and placental changes. Am. J. Hum. Genet. 53(Suppl.):1421, 1993.

Johansen, K.S.: Nitroblue tetrazolium slide test. Acta Pathol. Microbiol. Immunol. Scand. [C] 91:349, 1983.

Johnson, S.R. and Elkins, T.E.: Ethical issues in prenatal diagnosis. Clin. Obstet. Gynecol. 31:408, 1988.

Johnson, A. and Godmilow, L.: Genetic amniocentesis at 14 weeks or less. Clin. Obstet. Gynecol. 31:345, 1988.

Johnson, V.P. and Holzwarth, D.R.: Prenatal diagnosis of Meckel syndrome: Case reports and literature review. Am. J. Med. Genet. 18:699, 1984.

Johnson, M.L., Dunne, M.G., Mack, L.A. and Rashbaum, C.L.: Evaluation of fetal intracranial anatomy by static and real-time ultrasound. J. Clin. Ultrasound 8:311, 1980a.

Johnson, W.G., Thomas, G.H., Miranda, A.F., Driscoll, J.M., Wigger, J.H., Yeh, M.N., Schwartz, R.C., Cohen, C.S., Berdon, W.E. and Koenigsberger, M.R.: Congenital sialidosis: Biochemical studies; clinical spectrum in four sibs; two successful prenatal diagnoses. Am. J. Hum. Genet. 32(Suppl.):43A, 1980b.

Johnson, T.R.B., Jr., Corson, V.L., Payne, P.A. and Stetten, G.: Late prenatal diagnosis of fetal trisomy 18 associated with severe intrauterine growth retardation. Johns Hopkins Med. J. 151:242, 1982a.

Johnson, V.P., Petersen, L.P., Holzwarth, D.R. and Messner, F.D.: Midtrimester prenatal diagnosis of short-limb dwarfism (Saldino–Noonan syndrome). Birth Defects. 18(3A): 133, 1982b.

Johnson, J.A., Rumack, C.M., Johnson, M.L., Shikes, R., Appareti, K. and Rees, G.: Cystic adenomatoid malformation: Antenatal demonstration. Am. J. Roentgenol. 142:483, 1984a.

Johnson, V.P., Yiu-Chiu, V.S., Wierda, D.R. and Holzwarth, D.R.: Midtrimester prenatal diagnosis of achondrogenesis. J. Ultrasound Med. 3:223, 1984b.

Johnson, A., Cowchock, S., Darby, M.J., Landis, K., Ingham, K. and Jackson, L.G.: First trimester maternal serum alpha-fetoprotein (AFP) and human chorionic gonadotropin (HCG) in autosomal aneuploidy. Am. J. Hum. Genet. 45(Suppl.):A261, 1989a.

Johnson, R.L., Finberg, H.J., Perelman, A.H. and Clewell, W.H.: Fetal goitrous hypothyroidism: A new diagnostic and therapeutic approach. Fetal Ther. 4:141, 1989b.

Johnston, K.M. and Weinstein, S.L.: Inborn errors of metabolism presenting with structural central nervous system anomalies in neonates. Proc. Greenwood Genet. Cent. 8:140, 1989.

Jones, K.L.: *Smith's Recognizable Patterns of Human Malformation,* 4th ed. Philadelphia: Saunders, 1988.

Jones, S.R. and Evans, S.E.: The use of gamma glutamyl transferase activity in amniotic fluid in the detection of fetal trisomy 21. Prenat. Diagn. 8:63, 1988.

Jones, J.R., McCormack, M., Dietzel, C., Tricomi, V. and Ramirez, F.: Antenatal diagnosis of sickle cell disease: Amniotic fluid cell DNA analysis. Obstet. Gynecol. 59:484, 1982.

Jorgensen, O.S.: Fetal neural tube defects detected by rocket-on-line immunoelectrophoresis of amniotic fluids. Clin. Chim. Acta. 124:179, 1982.

Jorgensen, C. and Andolf, E.: Four cases of absent ductus venosus: Three in combinaton with severe hydrops fetalis. Fetal Diagn. Ther. 9:395, 1994.

Jorgensen, O.S. and Norgaard-Pedersen, B.: The synaptic membrane D2-protein in amniotic fluid from pregnancies with fetal neural tube defects. Prenat. Diagn. 1:3, 1981.

Joseph, M., Pai, G.S., Holden, K.R. and Herman, G.: X-linked myotubular myopathy: Clinical observations in ten additional cases. Am. J. Med. Genet. 59:168, 1995.

Journel, H., Roussey, M., Plais, M.H., Milon, J., Almange, C. and Le Marec, B.: Prenatal diagnosis of familial tuberous sclerosis following detection of cardiac rhabdomyoma by ultrasound. Prenat. Diagn. 6:283, 1986.

Julien, C., Bazin, A., Guyot, B., Forestier, F. and Daffos, F.: Rapid prenatal diagnosis of

Down's syndrome with in-situ hybridisation of fluorescent DNA probes. Lancet. 2:863, 1986.

Jung, C., Wolff, G., Back, E. and Stahl, M.: Two unrelated children with developmental delay, short stature and anterior chamber cleavage disorder, cerebellar hypoplasia, endocrine disturbances and tracheostenosis: A new entity? Clin. Dysmorph. 4:44, 1995.

Junien, C., Leroux, A., Lostanlen, D., Reghis, A., Boue, J., Nicolas, H., Boue, A. and Kaplan, J.C.: Prenatal diagnosis of congenital enzymopenic methaemoglobinaemia with mental retardation due to generalized cytochrome b_5 reductase deficiency: First report of two cases. Prenat. Diagn. 1:17, 1981.

Kaback, M.M.: Antenatal diagnosis: Report of a consensus developmental conference. National Institutes of Health Publication No. 80-1973. 1973, p. 1.

Kaffe, S. and Hsu, L.Y.F.: Amniotic fluid AFP levels and chromosome abnormalities. Am. J. Hum. Genet. 37(Suppl.):A221, 1985.

Kaffe, S., Godmilow, L., Walker, B.A. and Hirschhorn, K.: Prenatal diagnosis of bilateral renal agenesis. Obstet. Gynecol. 49:478, 1977a.

Kaffe, S., Rose, J.S., Godmilow, L., Walker, B.A., Kerenyi, T., Beratis, N., Reyes, P. and Hirschhorn, K.: Prenatal diagnosis of renal anomalies. Am. J. Med. Genet. 1:241, 1977b.

Kaffe, S., Patel, B. and Hsu, L.Y.F.: Normal amniotic fluid acetylcholinesterase in anencephalic fetus. Am. J. Hum. Genet. 41(Suppl.):A278, 1987.

Kaffe, S., Perlis, T.E. and Hsu, L.Y.F.: Amniotic fluid alpha-fetoprotein levels and prenatal diagnosis of autosomal trisomies. Prenat. Diagn. 8:183, 1988.

Kaffe, S., Eliasen, C., Wan, L., Charles, N., Jansen, V., Greco, M.A. and Hsu, L.Y.F.: A rare case of 68,XX triploidy diagnosed by amniocentesis. Prenat. Diagn. 9:857, 1989.

Kaftory, A., Freundlich, E., Manaster, J., Shukri, A. and Hegesh, E.: Prenatal diagnosis of congenital methemoglobinemia with mental retardation. Isr. J. Med. Sci. 22:837, 1986.

Kagie, M.J., Kleijer, W.J., Huijmans, J.G.M., Maaswinkel-Mooy, P. and Kanhai, H.H.H.: β-Glucuronidase deficiency as a cause of fetal hydrops. Am. J. Med. Genet. 42:693, 1992.

Kaiser, I.H.: Brown amniotic fluid in congenital erythropoietic porphyria. Obstet. Gynecol. 56:383, 1980.

Kaitila, I., Ammala, P., Karjalainen, O., Liukkonen, S. and Rapola, J.: Early prenatal detection of diastrophic dysplasia. Prenat. Diagn. 3:237, 1983.

Kalimo, H., Lundberg, P.O. and Olsson, Y.: Familial subacute necrotizing encephalomyelopathy of the adult form (adult Leigh syndrome). Ann. Neurol. 6:200, 1979.

Kalousek, D.K.: Confined placental mosaicism and intrauterine development. Pediatr. Pathol. 10:69, 1990.

Kalousek, D.K. and Dill, F.J.: Chromosomal mosaicism confined to the placenta in human conceptions. Science. 221:665, 1983.

Kamoun, P.P. and Chadefaux, B.: Eleventh week amniocentesis for prenatal diagnosis of some metabolic diseases. Prenat. Diagn. 11:691, 1991.

Kamoun, P., Parvy, P.H., Pham Dinh, D., Boue, J. and Cathelineau, L.: Citrulline in amniotic fluid and the prenatal diagnosis of citrullinemia. Prenat. Diagn. 3:53, 1983.

Kamoun, P., Fensom, A.H., Shin, Y.S., Bakker, E., Colombo, J.P., Munnich, A. Bird, S., Canini, S., Huijmans, J.G.M., Chadefaux-Vekemans, B., Whitfeld, A.E. and Kleijer, W.J.: Prenatal diagnosis of the urea cycle diseases: A survey of the European cases. Am. J. Med. Genet. 55:247, 1995.

Kan, Y.W. and Dozy, A.M.: Antenatal diagnosis of sickle-cell anaemia by D.N.A. analysis of amniotic-fluid cells. Lancet. 2:910, 1978.

Kan, Y.W., Golbus, M.S. and Trecartin, R.: Prenatal diagnosis of homozygous beta-thalassaemia. Lancet. 2:790, 1975.

Kan, Y.W. Golbus, M.S. and Dozy, A.M.: Prenatal diagnosis of alpha-thalassemia: Clinical application of molecular hybridizations. N. Engl. J. Med. 295:1165, 1976.

Kan, Y.W., Golbus, M.S., Trecartin, R.F. and Filly, R.A.: Prenatal diagnosis of beta-thalassaemia and sickle cell anemia: Experience with 24 cases. Lancet. 1:269, 1977.

Kanaan, C., Habecker-Green, J. and Cohn, G.: Prenatal diagnosis of a unilateral pelvic multicystic dysplastic kidney in a fetus with a 47,XXY karyotype and congenital megacolon. Am. J. Hum. Genet. 57(Suppl.):A306, 1995.

Kang, K.W., Hissong, S.L. and Langer, A.: Prenatal ultrasonic diagnosis of epignathus. J. Clin. Ultrasound. 6:330, 1978.

Kanhai, H.H.H., Gravenhorst, J.B., van't Veer, M.B., Maas, C.J., Beverstock, G.C. and Bernini, L.F.: Chorionic biopsy in management of severe rhesus isoimmunisation. Lancet. 2:157, 1984.

Kanhai, H.H.H., van Rijssel, E.J.C., Meerman, R.J. and Bennebroek Gravenhorst, J.: Selective termination in quintuplet pregnancy during first trimester. Lancet. 1:1447, 1986.

Kaplan, C., Daffos, F., Forestier, F., Cox, W.L., Lyon-Caen, D., Dupuy-Montbrun, M.C., and Salmon, C.: Management of alloimmune thrombocytopenia: Antenatal diagnosis and in utero transfusion of maternal platelets. Blood. 72:340, 1988a.

Kaplan, J., Chauvet, M.-L., Briard, M.-L. and Gazengel, C.: Genetic counselling, carrier detection, and prenatal diagnosis in hemophilia: A service experience. Ann. Genet., 31:221, 1988b.

Kaplan, C., Daffos, F., Forestier, F., Tertian, G., Catherine, N., Pons, J.C. and Tchernia, G.: Fetal platelet counts in thrombocytopenic pregnancy. Lancet. 336:979, 1990.

Kapur, S. and Van Vloten, A.: Isolated congenital bowed long bones. Clin. Genet. 29:165, 1986.

Karaviti, L.P., Mercado, A.B., Mercado, M.B., Speiser, P.W., Buegeleisen, M., Crawford, C., Antonian, L., White, P.C. and New, M.I.: Prenatal diagnosis/treatment in families at risk for infants with steroid 21-hydroxylase deficiency (congenital adrenal hyperplasia). J. Steroid Biochem. Molec. 41:445, 1992.

Karjalainen, O., Aula, P., Seppala, M., Hartikainen-Sorri, A.-L. and Ryynanen, M.: Prenatal diagnosis of the Meckel syndrome. Obstet. Gynecol. 57:135, 1981.

Katayama, S., Montano, M., Slotnick, N., Lebo, R.V. and Golbus, M.S.: Prenatal diagnosis and carrier detection of Duchenne muscular dystrophy by restriction fragment length polymorphism analysis with pERT 87 deoxyribonucleic acid probes. Am. J. Obstet. Gynecol. 158:548, 1988.

Katayama, S., Takeshita, N., Yano, T., Katagiri, Y., Shirosita, Y., Kubo, H., Hirakawa, S. and Ubagai, T.: Prenatal diagnosis of Duchenne muscular dystrophy by polymerase chain reaction analysis. Fetal Diagn. Ther. 9:379, 1994.

Katz, Z., Lancet, M., Kassif, R. and Chemke, M.J.: Antenatal ultrasonic diagnosis of complete urethral obstruction in the fetus. Acta Obstet. Gynecol. Scand. 59:463, 1980.

Katz, M., Dreval, D., Meizner, I. and Maor, E.: Bizarre fetal heart rate associated with congenital heart malformation. Isr. J. Med. Sci. 22:473, 1986a.

Katz, V.L., Cefalo, R.C., McCune, B.K. and Moos, M.-K.: Elevated second trimester maternal serum alpha-fetoprotein and cytomegalovirus infection. Obstet. Gynecol. 68:580, 1986b.

Kaufman, G.E., D'Alton, M.E. and Crombleholme, T.M.: Decompression of fetal axillary lymphangioma to prevent dystocia. Fetal Diagn. Ther. 11:218, 1996.

Kawira, E.L. and Bender, H.A.: An unusual distal arthrogryposis. Am. J. Med. Genet. 20:425, 1985.

Kazazian, L.C., Baramki, T.A. and Thomas, R. L.: Triploid fetus: An important consideration in the evaluation of very high maternal serum alpha-fetoprotein. Prenat. Diagn. 9:27, 1989.

Kazy, Z., Stygar, A.M. and Bakharev, A.V.A.: Chorionic biopsy under immediate realtime (ultrasonic) control. Orvosi Hetilap. 121:2765, 1980.

Kazy, Z., Rozovsky, I.S. and Bakharev, V.A.: Chorion biopsy in early pregnancy: A method of early prenatal diagnosis for inherited disorders. Prenat. Diagn. 2:39, 1982.

Kazzi, G.M., Gross, T.L., Sokol, R.J. and Kazzi, N.J.: Detection of intrauterine growth retardation: A new use of sonographic placental grading. Am. J. Obstet. Gynecol. 145:733, 1983.

Keatinge, R.M. and Williams, E.S.: Prenatal screening for Down's syndrome. Br. Med. J. 303:55, 1991.

Keckstein, G., Tschurtz, S., Schneider, V., Hutter, W., Terinde, R. and Jonatha, W.-D.: Umbilical cord haematoma as a complication of intrauterine intravascular blood transfusion. Prenat. Diagn. 10:59, 1990.

Keirse, M.J.N.C. and Meerman, R.H.: Antenatal diagnosis of Potter syndrome. Obstet. Gynecol. 52:Suppl.:1:64, 1978.

Keller, E., Andreas, A., Scholz, S., Dorr, H.C. and Albert, E.D.: Prenatal diagnosis of 21-hydroxylase deficiency by RFLP analysis of the 21-hydroxylase, complement C4, and HLA class II genes. Prenat. Diagn. 11:827, 1991.

Kelley, R.I.: Prenatal detection of Canavan disease by measurement of N-acetyl-L-aspartate in amniotic fluid. J. Inher. Metab. Dis. 16:918, 1993.

Kelley, R.I., Moser, A. and Natowicz, M.: The clinical and biochemical spectrum of 7-dehydrocholesterolemia: Diagnosis and prenatal diagnosis of Smith–Lemli–Opitz syndrome. Int. Pediatr. 9(Suppl. 2):75, 1994.

Kenney, R.T., Malech, H.L., Epstein, N.D., Roberts, R.L. and Leto, T.L.: Characterization of the p67[phox] Gene: Genomic organization and restriction fragment length polymorphism analysis for prenatal diagnosis in chronic granulomatous disease. Blood. 82:3739, 1993.

Kerenyi, T.D. and Chitkara, U.: Selective birth in twin pregnancy with discordancy for Down's syndrome. N. Engl. J. Med. 304:1525, 1981

Kerenyi, T.D., Meller, J., Steinfeld, L., Gleicher, N., Brown, E., Chitkara, U. and Raucher, H.: Transplacental cardioversion of intrauterine supraventricular tachycardia with digitalis. Lancet. 2:393, 1980.

Kerr Wilson, R.H.J., Duncan, A., Hume, R. and Bain, A.D.: Prenatal pleural effusion associated with congenital pulmonary lymphangiectasia. Prenat. Diagn. 5:73, 1985.

Khajavi, A., Lachman, R., Rimoin, D., Schimke, R.N., Dorst, J., Handmaker, S., Ebbin, A. and Perreault, G.: Heterogeneity in the campomelic syndromes. Radiology. 120:641, 1976.

Khong, T.Y., Ford, W.D.A. and Haan, E.A.: Umbilical cord ulceration in association with intestinal atresia in a child with deletion 13q and Hirschsprung's disease. Arch. Dis. Child. 71:F212, 1994.

Khouzam, M.N. and Hooker, J.G.: The significance of prenatal diagnosis of choroid plexus cysts. Prenat. Diagn. 9:213, 1989.

Kidd, V.J., Golbus, M.S., Wallace, R.B., Itakura, K. and Woo, S.L.C.: Prenatal diagnosis of alpha$_1$-antitrypsin deficiency by direct analysis of the mutation site in the gene. N. Engl. J. Med. 310:639, 1984.

Kihara, H., Fluharty, A.L., Tsay, K.K., Bachman, R.P., Stephens, J.D. and Ng, W.G.: Prenatal diagnosis of pseudo arylsulphatase A deficiency. Prenat. Diagn. 3:29, 1983.

Killeen, A.A. and Bowers, L.D.: Fetal supraventricular tachycardia treated with high-dose quinidine: Toxicity associated with marked elevation of the metabolite, 3(S)-3-hydroxyquinidine. Obstet. Gynecol. 70:445, 1987.

Kim, M.-S. and Elyaderani, M.K.: Sonographic diagnosis of cerebroventricular hemorrhage in utero. Radiology. 142:479, 1982.

Kim, H.J., Costales, F., Bouzouki, M. and Wallach, R.C.: Prenatal diagnosis of dyssegmental dwarfism. Prenat. Diagn. 6:143, 1986a.

Kim, H., Uppal, V. and Wallach, R.: Apert syndrome and fetal hydrocephaly. Hum. Genet. 73:93, 1986b.

Kimball, M.E., Milunsky, A. and Alpert, E.: Prenatal diagnosis of neural tube defects. III. A reevaluation of the alpha-fetoprotein assay. Obstet. Gynecol. 49:532, 1977.

Kirkinen, P. and Jouppila, P.: Prenatal ultrasonic findings in congenital chloride diarrhoea. Prenat. Diagn. 4:457, 1984.

Kirkinen, P., Jouppila, P., Valkeakari, T. and Saukkonen, A-L.: Ultrasonic evaluation of the Dandy–Walker syndrome. Obstet. Gynecol. 59:18S, 1982.

Kirkinen, P., Herva, R. and Leisti, J.: Early prenatal diagnosis of a lethal syndrome of multiple congenital contractures. Prenat. Diagn. 7:189, 1987.

Kirkinen, P., Ryynanen, M., Haring, P., Torkkeli, H., Paakkonen, L. and Martikainen, A.: Prenatal activity of a fetus with early-onset, severe spinal muscular atrophy. Prenat. Diagn. 14:1076, 1994.

Kjoller, M., Holm-Nielsen, G., Meiland, H., Mauritzen, K., Berget, A. and Hancke, S.: Prenatal obstruction of the ileum diagnosed by ultrasound. Prenat. Diagn. 5:427, 1985.

Kleijer, W.J.: First-trimester diagnosis of genetic metabolic disorders. Contrib. Gynecol. Obstet. 15:80, 1986.

Kleijer, W.J., Wolfers, C.M., Hoogeveen, A. and Niermeijer, M.F.: Prenatal diagnosis of Maroteaux–Lamy syndrome. Lancet. 2:50, 1976.

Kleijer, W.J., Hoogeveen, A., Verheijen, F.W., Niermeijer, N.F., Galjaard, H., O'Brien, J.S. and Warner, T.G.: Prenatal diagnosis of sialidosis with combined neuraminidase and beta-galactosidase deficiency. Clin. Genet. 16:60, 1979.

Kleijer, W.J., Thompson, E.J. and Niermeijer, M.F.: Prenatal diagnosis of the Hurler syndrome: Report on 40 pregnancies at risk. Prenat. Diagn. 3:179, 1983.

Kleijer, W.J., Blom, W., Huijmans, J.G.M., Mooyman, M.C.T., Berger, R. and Niermeijer, M.F.: Prenatal diagnosis of citrullinemia: Elevated levels of citrulline in the amniotic fluid in the three affected pregnancies. Prenat. Diagn. 4:113, 1984a.

Kleijer, W.J., Thoomes, R., Galjaard, H., Wendel, U. and Fowler, B.: First-trimester (chorion biopsy) diagnosis of citrullinaemia and methylmalonicaciduria. Lancet. 2:1340, 1984b.

Kleijer, W.J., Van Diggelen, O.P., Janse, H.C., Galjaard, H., Dumez, Y. and Boue, J.: First trimester diagnosis of Hunter syndrome on chorionic villi. Lancet. 2:472, 1984c.

Kleijer, W.J., Mancini, G.M.S., Jahoda, M.G.J., Vosters, R.P.L., Sachs, E.S., Niermeijer, M.F. and Galjaard, H.: First-trimester diagnosis of Krabbe's disease by direct enzyme analysis of chorionic villi. N. Engl. J. Med. 311:1257, 1984d.

Kleijer, W.J., Huijmans, J.G.M., Blom, W., Gorska, D., Kubalska, J., Walasek, M. and Zaremba, J.: Prenatal diagnosis of Sanfilippo disease type B. Hum. Genet. 66:287, 1984e.

Kleijer, W.J., Horsman, D., Mancini, G.M.S., Fois, A. and Boue, J.: First-trimester diagnosis of maple syrup urine disease on intact chorionic villi. N. Engl. J. Med. 313:1608, 1985a.

Kleijer, W.J., Janse, H.C., Van Diggelen, O.P. and Niermeijer, M.F.: Amniotic fluid disaccharidases in the prenatal detection of cystic fibrosis. Prenat. Diagn. 5:135, 1985b.

Kleijer, W.J., Janse, H.C., Vosters, R.P.L., Niermeijer, M.F. and van de Kamp, J.J.P.: First-trimester diagnosis of mucopolysaccharidosis IIIA (Sanfilippo A disease). N. Engl. J. Med. 314:185, 1986a.

Kleijer, W.J., Janse, H.C., van Diggelen, O.P., Macek, M., Hajek, Z., Gillett, M.G. and Holton, J.B.: First-trimester diagnosis of galactosaemia. Lancet. 1:748, 1986b.

Kleijer, W.J., Hussaarts-Odijk, L.M., Sachs, E.S., Jahoda, M.G.J. and Niermeijer, M.F.: Prenatal diagnosis of Fabry's disease by direct analysis of chorionic villi. Prenat. Diagn. 7:283, 1987.

Kleijer, W.J., Hussaarts-Odijk, L.M., Los, F.J., Pijpers, L., DeBree, P.K. and Duran, M.: Prenatal diagnosis of purine nucleoside phosphorylase deficiency in the first and second trimesters of pregnancy. Prenat. Diagn. 9:401, 1989.

Kleijer, W.J., Van Der Kraan, M., Huijmans, J.G.M., Van Den Heuvel, C.M.M. and Jakobs, C.: Prenatal diagnosis of isovaleric acidaemia by enzyme and metabolite assay in the first and second trimesters. Prenat. Diagn. 15:527, 1995.

Kleijer, W.J., Karpova, E.A., Gielen, G.C., Keulemans, J.L.M., Huijmans J.G.M., Tsvetkova, I.V., Voznyi, Y.V. and Van Diggelen, O.P.: Prenatal diagnosis of Sanfilippo A syndrome: Experience in 35 pregnancies at risk and the use of a new fluorogenic substrate for the heparin sulphamidase assay. Prenat. Diagn. 16:829, 1996.

Klein, A.M., Holzman, I.R. and Austin, E.M.: Fetal tachycardia prior to the development of hydrops—Attempted pharmacologic cardioversion: Case report. Am. J. Obstet. Gynecol. 134:347, 1979.

Kleinman, C.S. and Santulli, T.V., Jr.: Ultrasonic evaluation of the fetal human heart. Semin. Perinatol. 7:90, 1983.

Kleinman, C.S., Hobbins, J.C., Jaffe, C.C., Lynch, D.C. and Talner, N.S.: Echocardiographic studies of the human fetus: Prenatal diagnosis of congenital heart disease and cardiac dysrhythmias. Pediatrics. 65:1059, 1980.

Kleinman, C.S., Donnerstein, R.L., DeVore, G.R., Jaffe, C.C., Lynch, D.C., Berkowitz, R.L., Talner, N.S. and Hobbins, J.C.: Fetal echocardiography for evaluation of in utero congestive heart failure. N. Engl. J. Med. 306:568, 1982.

Kleinman, C.S., Donnerstein, R.L., Jaffe, C.C., DeVore, G.R., Weinstein, E.M., Lynch, D.C.,

Talner, N.S., Berkowitz, R.L. and Hobbins, J.C.: Fetal echocardiography. A tool for evaluation of in utero cardiac arrhythmias and monitoring of in utero therapy: Analysis of 71 patients. Am. J. Cardiol. 51:237, 1983.

Klingensmith, W.C., III, and Cioffi-Ragan, D.T.: Schizencephaly: Diagnosis and progression in utero. Radiology. 159:617, 1986.

Knight, G.J., Kloza, E.M., Smith, D.E. and Haddow, J.E.: Efficiency of human placental lactogen and alpha-fetoprotein measurement in twin pregnancy detection. Am. J. Obstet. Gynecol. 141:585, 1981.

Knight, G.J., Palomaki, G.E., Haddow, J.E., Johnson, A.M., Osathanondh, R. and Canick, J.A.: Maternal serum levels of the placental products hCG, hPL, SPI, and progesterone are all elevated in cases of fetal Down syndrome. Am. J. Hum. Genet. 45(Suppl.):A263, 1989.

Knisely, A.S., Richardson, A., Abuelo, D., Casey, S. and Singer, D.B.: Lethal osteogenesis imperfecta associated with 46,XY,inv(7)(p13q22) karyotype. J. Med. Genet. 25:352, 1988.

Knops, J., Krassikoff, N., Cosper, P., Rainey, E., Jr., Davis, R.O. and Finley, S.C.: A phenotypically abnormal fetus with 46,XX/46,XY amniotic fluid karyotype with paternally derived 46,XX cell line: chimera or extra-embryonic tissue contamination? Am. J. Hum. Genet. 45(Suppl.):A263, 1989.

Knott, P.D. and Colley, N.V.: Can fetal gastroschisis always be diagnosed prenatally? Prenat. Diagn. 7:607, 1987.

Knowles, S., Winter, R. and Rimoin, D.: A new category of lethal short-limbed dwarfism. Am. J. Med. Genet. 24:41, 1986.

Ko, T-M., Shen, M-K, Hsieh, F-J and Lee, T-Y.: Prenatal diagnosis of hemophilia A by DNA analysis of chorionic villi. J. Formosan Med. Assoc. 89:194, 1990.

Ko, T-M., Hwa, H-L., Tseng, L-H., Hsieh, F.-J., Huang, S-F. and Lee, T-Y.: Prenatal diagnosis of X-linked hydrocephalus in a Chinese family with four successive affected pregnancies. Prenat. Diagn. 14:57, 1994.

Kobayashi, M., Kaplan, B.S., Bellah, R.D, Sartore, M., Rappaport, E., Steele, M.W., Mansfield, E., Gasparini, P., Surrey, S. and Fortina, P.: Infundibulopelvic stenosis, multicystic kidney, and calyectasis in a kindred: Clinical observations and genetic analysis. Am. J. Med. Genet. 59:218, 1995.

Koeberl, D.D., McGillivray, B. and Sybert, V. P.: Prenatal diagnosis of 45,X/46,XX mosaicism and 45,X: Implications for postnatal outcome. Am. J. Hum. Genet. 57:661, 1995.

Koenig, H.M., Vedvick, T.S., Dozy, A.M., Golbus, M.S. and Kan, Y.W.: Prenatal diagnosis of hemoglobin H disease. J. Pediatr. 92:278, 1978.

Koenigsberg, M., Factor, S., Cho, S., Herskowitz, A., Nitowsky, H. and Morecki, R.: Fetal Marfan syndrome: Prenatal ultrasound diagnosis with pathological confirmation of skeletal and aortic lesions. Prenat. Diagn. 1:241, 1981.

Kohn, G., Livni, N., Ornoy, A., Sekeles, E., Beyth, Y., Legum, C., Bach, G. and Cohen, M.M.: Prenatal diagnosis of mucolipidosis IV by electron microscopy. J. Pediatr. 90:62, 1977.

Kohn, G., Sekeles, E., Arnon, J. and Ornoy, A.: Mucolipidosis IV: Prenatal diagnosis by electron microscopy. Prenat. Diagn. 2:301, 1982.

Kolho, K.-L.: Kazal type trypsin inhibitor in amniotic fluid in fetal developmental disorders. Prenat. Diagn. 6:299, 1986.

Komaromy, B., Gaal, J. and Lampe, L.: Fetal arrhythmia during pregnancy and labour. Br. J. Obstet. Gynaecol. 84:492, 1977.

Komrower, G.M.: The philosophy and practice of screening for inherited diseases. Pediatrics. 53:182, 1974.

Kondo, E., Saito, K., Toda, T., Osawa, M., Yamamoto, T., Kobayashi, M. and Fukuyama, Y.: Prenatal disangosis of Fukuyama type congenital muscular dystrophy by polymorphism analysis. Am. J. Med. Genet. 66:169, 1996.

Koontz, W.L., Seeds, J.W., Adams, N.J., Johnson, A.M. and Cefalo, R.C.: Elevated maternal serum alpha-fetoprotein, second-trimester oligohydramnios, and pregnancy outcome. Obstet. Gynecol. 62:301, 1983.

Koontz, W.L., Layman, L., Adams, A. and Lavery, J.P.: Antenatal sonographic diagnosis of conjoined twins in a triplet pregnancy. Am. J. Obstet. Gynecol. 153:230, 1985.

Kourides, I.A., Berkowitz, R.L., Pang, S., Van Natta, C., Barone, C.M. and Ginsberg-Fellner, F.: Antepartum diagnosis of goitrous hypothyroidism by fetal ultrasonography and amniotic fluid thyrotropin concentration. J. Clin. Endocrinol. Metab. 59:1016, 1984.

Kousseff, B.G.: Unique brain anomalies in an offspring of a diabetic mother. Proc. Greenwood Genet. Cent. 9:116, 1990.

Kousseff, B.G., Matsuoka, L.Y., Stenn, K.S., Hobbins, J.C., Mahoney, M.J. and Hashimoto, K.: Prenatal diagnosis of Sjogren–Larsson syndrome. J. Pediatr. 101:998, 1982.

Kousseff, B.G., Gilbert-Barness, E. and Debich-Spicer, D.: Bronchopulmonary-foregut malformations, a continuum of paracrine anomalies. Am. J. Hum. Genet. 57(Suppl.):A282, 1995.

Kovats-Szabo, E., Horvath, I., Nagy, M. and Kadar, K.: Intrauterine treatment of fetal tachycardia causing circulatory failure. Orvosi Hetilap. 131:807, 1990.

Kovnar, E.H., Coxe, W.S. and Volpe, J.J.: Normal neurologic development and marked reconstitution of cerebral mantle after postnatal treatment of intrauterine hydrocephalus. Neurology. 34:840, 1984.

Kozlowski, K.J., Frazier, C.N. and Quirk, J.G., Jr.: Prenatal diagnosis of abdominal cystic hygroma. Prenat. Diagn. 8:405, 1988.

Kozma, C., Scribanu, N. and Gersh, E.: The microcephaly–lymphoedema syndrome: Report of an additional family. Clin. Dysmorph. 5:49, 1996.

Krantz, D.A., Spencer, K., Buchanan, P.D., Hallahan, T.W., Klein, V.R., Macri, J.N.: Identifying triplet pregnancies at increased risk with an atypicality index employing MSAFP and free beta (hCG). Am. J. Hum. Genet. 57(Suppl.):A345, 1995.

Krassikoff, N., Konick, L. and Gilbert, E.F.: The hydrolethalus syndrome. Birth Defects. 23(1):411, 1987.

Krauss, C.M., Richkind, K., Benacerraf, B. and Doubilet, P.: Prenatal diagnosis of lissencephaly in a fetus with an unresolved chromosome abnormality. Am. J. Hum. Genet. 43(Suppl.): A238, 1988.

Krause, S., Ebbesen, F. and Lange, A.P.: Polyhydramnios with maternal lithium treatment. Obstet. Gynecol. 75:504, 1990.

Kristiansen F.V. and Nielsen, V.T.: Intra-uterine fetal death and thrombosis of the umbilical vessels. Acta Obstet. Gynecol. Scand. 64:331, 1985.

Kuboto, T., Christina, S.L., Horsthemke, B. and Ledbetter, D.H.: Advances in both postnatal and prenatal diagnosis for Prader–Willi syndrome (PWS). Am. J. Med. Genet. 64:575, 1996.

Kudoh, T., Kikuchi, K., Nakamura, F., Yokoyama, S., Karube, K., Tsugawa, S., Minami, R. and Nakao, T.: Prenatal diagnosis of Gm_1-gangliosidosis: Biochemical manifestations in fetal tissues. Hum. Genet. 44:287, 1978.

Kulharya, A.S., Maberry, M., Kukolich, M.K., Day, D.W., Schneider, N.R., Wilson, G.N. and Tonk, V.: Interstitial deletions 4q21.1q25 and 4q25q27: Phenotypic variability and relation to Rieger anomaly. Am. J. Med. Genet. 55:165, 1995.

Kuller, J.A., McMahon, M.J., Chescheir, N.C., Wells, S.R., Wright, L.N. and Nakayama, D.K.: Preinatal management of a lingual teratoma. Am. J. Hum. Genet. 57(Suppl.):A282, 1995.

Kupferminc, J.M., Tamura, R.K., Sabbagha, R.E., Parilla, B.V., Cohen, L.S. and Pergament, E.: Isolated choroid plexus cyst(s): An indication for amniocentesis. Am. J. Obstet. Gynecol. 171:1068, 1994.

Kurjak, A. and Latin, V.: Ultrasound diagnosis of fetal abnormalities in multiple pregnancy. Acta Obstet. Gynecol. Scand. 58:153, 1979.

Kurtz, A.B. and Wapner, R.J.: Ultrasonographic diagnosis of second-trimester skeletal dysplasias: A prospective analysis in a high-risk population. J. Ultrasound Med. 2:99, 1983.

Kurtz, A.B., Wapner, R.J., Rubin, C.S., Cole-Beuglet, C., Ross, R.D. and Goldberg, B.B.: Ultrasound criteria for in utero diagnosis of microcephaly. J. Clin. Ultrasound 8:11, 1980.

Kurtz, A.B., Foy, P.M., Wapner, R.J., Rubin, C.S., Dubbins, P.A. and Cole-Beuglet, C.: Fetal ultrasound findings in alpha-thalassemia major. J. Clin. Ultrasound 9:257, 1981.

Kurtz, A.B., Filly, R.A., Wapner, R.J., Golbus, M.S., Rifkin, M.R., Callen, P.W. and Pasto, M.E.: In utero analysis of heterozygous achondroplasia: Variable time of onset as detected by femur length measurements. J. Ultrasound Med. 5:137, 1986.

Kustermann, A., Zoppini, C., Tassis, B., Della Morte, M., Colucci, G. and Nicolini, U.: Prenatal diagnosis of congenital varicella infection. Prenat. Diagn. 16:71, 1996.

Kustermann-Kuhn, B. and Harzer, K.: Prenatal diagnosis of Tay–Sachs disease: Reflectometry of hexosaminidase A, B, and C/S bands on zymograms. Hum. Genet. 65:172, 1983.

Kutzner, D.K., Wilson, W.G. and Hogge, W.A.: OEIS complex (cloacal exstrophy): Prenatal diagnosis in the second trimester. Prenat. Diagn. 8:247, 1988.

Kvittingen, E.A., Guibaud, P.P., Divry, P., Mandon, G., Rolland, M.O., Domenichini, Y., Jakobs, C. and Christensen, E.: Prenatal diagnosis of hereditary tyrosinaemia type I by determination of fumarylacetoacetase in chorionic villus material. Eur. J. Pediatr. 144: 597, 1986.

Kwi, N.K. and Hing, N.K.: A simple technique of intra-uterine transfusion of foetus in University Hospital, Kuala Lumpur. Med. J. Malay. 28:287, 1974.

Kwok, C., Weller, P.A., Guioli, S., Foster, J.W., Mansour, S., Zuffardi, O., Punnett, H.H., Dominguez-Steglich, M.A., Brook, J.D., Young, I.D., Goodfellow, P.N. and Schafer, A.J.: Mutations in SOX9, the gene responaible for campomelic dysplasia and autosomal sex reversal. Am. J. Hum. Genet. 57:1028, 1995.

Lachman, R. and Hall, J.: The radiographic prenatal diagnosis of the generalized bone dysplasias and other skeletal abnormalities. Birth Defects. 15(5A):3, 1979.

Ladonne, J-M., Gaillard, D., Carre-Pigeon, F. and Gabriel, R.: Fryns syndrome phenotype and trisomy 22. Am. J. Med. Genet. 61:68, 1996.

Lagercrantz, H., Sjoquist, B., Bremmer, K., Lunell, N. and Somell, C.: Catecholamine metabolites in amniotic fluid as indicators of intrauterine stress. Am. J. Obstet. Gynecol. 136:1067, 1980.

Lake, B.D., Young, E.P. and Nicolaides, K.: Prenatal diagnosis of infantile sialic acid storage disease in a twin pregnancy. J. Inher. Metab. Dis. 12:152, 1989.

Lamvu, G. and Kuller, J.A.: Prenatal diagnosis using fetal cells from the maternal circulation. Obstet. Gynecol. Surv. 52:433, 1997.

Lande, I.M. and Hamilton, E.F.: The antenatal sonographic visualization of cloacal dysgenesis. J. Ultrasound Med. 5:275, 1986.

Landy, H.J., Weiner, S., Corson, S.L., Batzer, F.R. and Bolognese, R.J.: The "vanishing twin": Ultrasonographic assessment of fetal disappearance in the first trimester. Am. J. Obstet. Gynecol. 155:14, 1986.

Lang, G.D. and Young, I.D.: Cranioectodermal dysplasia in sibs. J. Med. Genet. 28:424, 1991.

Lange, I.R. and Manning, F.A.: Antenatal diagnosis of congenital pleural effusions. Am. J. Obstet. Gynecol. 140:839, 1981.

Lange, A.P., Hebjorn, S., Moth, I., Fuglsang, E., Hasch, E., Bruun Peterson, G. and Norgaard-Pedersen, B.: Twin fetus papyraceous and alphafetoprotein: A clinical dilemma. Lancet. 2:636, 1979.

Langer, O., Kozlowski, S. and Brustman, L.: Abnormal growth patterns in diabetes in pregnancy: A longitudinal study. Isr. J. Med. Sci. 27:516, 1991.

Langer, B., Haddad, J., Gasser, B., Maubert, M. and Schlaeder, G.: Isolated fetal bilateral radial ray reduction associated with valproic acid usage. Fetal Diagn. Ther. 9:155, 1994.

Langlois, S., Yong, S.L., Wilson, R.D., Kwong, L.C. and Kalousek, D.K.: Prenatal and postnatal growth failure associated with maternal heterodisomy for chromosome 7. J. Med. Genet. 32:871, 1995.

Lau, Y.-F., Huang, J.C., Dozy, A.M. and Kan, Y.W.: A rapid screening test for antenatal sex determination. Lancet. 1:14, 1984.

Laudon, C.H. and Buchanan, P.D.: Prenatal diagnosis of mosaicism involving the pull deletion of the 8 short arm. Am. J. Hum. Genet. 53(Suppl.):1580, 1993.

Laughlin, C.L. and Lee, T.G.: The prominent falx cerebri: New ultrasonic observation in hypophosphatasia. J. Clin. Ultrasound. 10:37, 1982.

Laurence, K.M., Dew, J.O., Dyer, C. and Downey, K.H.: Amniocentesis carried out for neural tube indications in South Wales, 1973–1981: Outcome of pregnancies and findings in the malformed abortuses. Prenat. Diagn. 3:187, 1983.

Laurence, K.M., Elder, G., Evans, K.T., Hibbard, B.M., Hoole, M. and Roberts, C.J.: Should women at high risk of neural tube defect have an amniocentesis? J. Med. Genet. 22:457, 1985.

Lavedan, C., Hofmann, H., Shelbourne, P., Duros, C., Savoy, D., Johnson, K. and Junien, C.: Prenatal diagnosis of myotonic dystrophy using closely linked flanking markers. J. Med. Genet. 28:89, 1991.

Lawton, K.: Amniotic fluid acetylcholinesterase in amniotic fluid to test for neural tube defects. Lancet. 1:503, 1981.

Laxova, R., Ohara, P.T., Ridler, M.A.C. and Timothy, J.A.D.: Family with probable achondrogenesis and lipid inclusions in fibroblasts. Arch. Dis. Child. 48:212, 1973.

Lazaro, C., Gaona, A., Ravella, A., Volpini, V. and Estivill, X.: Prenatal diagnosis of neurofibromatosis type 1: From flanking RFLPS to intragenic microsatellite markers. Prenat. Diagn. 15:129, 1995.

Lazzarini, A., Cummings, E., Stahl, T., Kutosovik, A. and McCormack, M.K.: Occurrence of congenital diaphragmatic hernia (CDH) with an elevated amniotic fluid AFP. Am. J. Hum. Genet. 37(Suppl.):A133, 1985.

Lazzarini, A., Nagele, R., Ciesielski, J., Wesley, B., Nemiroff, R., Ashmead, J. and McCormack, M.K.: Fetal alcohol syndrome (FAS) in a 21 week fetus: Efficacy of combined service delivery systems in patient management. Am. J. Hum. Genet. 41(Suppl.):A198, 1987.

Leach, R.E., Ney, J.A. and Ory, S.J.: Selective embryo reduction of an interstitial heterotopic gestation. Fetal Diagn. Ther. 7:41, 1992.

Lebo, R.V., Koerper, M.A., Kim, J.H., Chueh, J. and Golbus, M.S.: Prenatal diagnosis of hemophilia involving grandpaternal mosaicism. Am. J. Med. Genet. 47:401, 1993a.

Lebo, R.V., Martelli, L., Su, Y., Li., L., Lynch, E., Mansfield, E., Pua, K-H., Watson, D.F., Chueh, J. and Hurko, O.: Prenatal diagnosis of Charcot–Marie–Tooth disease type 1A by multicolor in situ hybridization. Am. J. Med. Genet. 47:441, 1993b.

Le Bris-Quillevere, M.J., Riviere, D., Pluchon-Riviere, E., Chabaud, J.J., Parent, P., Volant, A. and Boog, G.: Prenatal diagnosis of del(15)(q11q13). Prenat. Diagn. 10:405, 1990.

LeChien, K.A. and Thomas, R.L.: Congenital cystic adenomatoid malformations of the lung and horseshoe kidney: A case report. Am. J. Hum. Genet. 57(Suppl.):A345, 1995.

Lecolier, B., Bercau, G., Gonzales, M., Afriat, R., Rambaud, D., Mulliez, N. and De Kermadec, S.: Radiographic, haematological, and biochemical findings in a fetus with Caffey disease. Prenat. Diagn. 12:637, 1992.

Lee, L.L. and McGahan, J.P.: Combined use of ultrasound and computed tomography in evaluation of intraabdominal pregnancy and fetal demise. J. Comput. Assist. Tomogr. 8:770, 1984.

Lee, T.G. and Newton, B.W.: Posterior fossa cyst: Prenatal diagnosis by ultrasound. J. Clin. Ultrasound. 4:29, 1976.

Lee, T.G. and Warren, B.H.: Antenatal ultrasonic demonstration of fetal bowel. Radiology. 124:471, 1977a.

Lee, T.G. and Warren, B.H.: Antenatal diagnosis of hydranencephaly by ultrasound: Correlation with ventriculography and computed tomography. J. Clin. Ultrasound. 5:271, 1977b.

Lee T.G., Knochel, J.O. and Kochenour, N.K.: Air as a contrast marker for ultrasound-guided fetal transfusions. Radiology. 138:490, 1981.

Leech, R.W., Bowlby, L.S., Brumback, R.A. and Schaefer, G.B., Jr.: Agnathia, holoprosencephaly, and situs inversus: Report of a case. Am. J. Med. Genet. 29:483, 1988.

Legge, M.: Amniotic fluid fibrinolytic system in fetal neural tube defects. Prenat. Diagn. 3:145, 1983.

Legge, M. and Rippon, P.: Prenatal diagnosis of intestinal obstruction in the third trimester using amniotic fluid bile acid analysis. Prenat. Diagn. 2:71, 1982.

Legius, E., Moerman, P., Fryns, J.P., Vandenberghe, K. and Eggermont, E.: Holzgreve–Wagner–Rehder syndrome: Potter sequence associated with persistent buccopharyngeal membrane. A second observation. Am. J. Med. Genet. 31:269, 1988.

Lehmann, A.R., Francis, A.J. and Giannelli, F.: Prenatal diagnosis of Cockayne's syndrome. Lancet. 1:486, 1985.

Leichtman, L.G.: Are cardio-facio-cutaneous syndrome and Noonan syndrome distinct? A case of CFC offspring of a mother with Noonan syndrome. Clin. Dysmorphol. 5:61, 1996.

Leidig, E., Dannecker, G., Pfeiffer, K.H., Salinas, R. and Peiffer, J.: Intrautaerine development of posthaemorrhagic hydrocephalus. Eur. J. Pediatr. 147:26, 1988.

Leighton, P.C., Kitau, M.J., Gordon, Y.B., Leck, A.E. and Chard, T.: Levels of alpha-fetoprotein in maternal blood as a screening test for fetal neural-tube defect. Lancet. 2:1012, 1975.

Leikin, E. and Randall, H.W., Jr.: Hydrocephalic fetus in an abdominal pregnancy. Obstet. Gynecol. 69:498, 1987.

Leithiser, R.E., Jr., Fyfe, D., Weatherby, E., III, Sade, R. and Garvin, A.J.: Prenatal sonographic diagnosis of atrial hemangioma. Am. J. Roentgenol. 147:1207, 1986.

Lemire, E.G., Evans, J.A., Giddins, N.G., Harman, C.R., Wiseman, N.E. and Chudley, A.E.: A familial disorder with duodenal atresia and tetralogy of Fallot. Am. J. Med. Genet. 66:39, 1996.

LeLann, D., Schiochet, F., Heintz, M., Winisdoerffer, G. and Dreyfus, J.: Diagnostic echographique antenatal du sexe masculin et feminin. Nouv. Presse Med. 8:2760, 1979.

Le Marec, B., Passarge, E., Dellenbach, P., Kerisit, J., Signargout, J., Ferrand, B., Senecal, J.: Lethal neonatal forms of chondroectodermal dysplasia. Apropos of 5 cases. Ann. Radiol. 16:19, 1973.

Lemos, M., Pinto, R., Ribeiro, G., Ribeiro, H., Lopes, L. and Sa Miranda, M.C.: Prenatal diagnosis of GM$_2$-gangliosidosis B1 variant. Prenat. Diagn. 15:585, 1995.

Lenz, S., Lund-Hansen, T., Band, J. and Christensen, E.: A possible prenatal evaluation of renal function by amino acid analysis on fetal urine. Prenat. Diagn. 5:259, 1985.

Leonard, C.O.: Prenatal diagnosis of the large for gestational age fetus. Proc. Greenwood Genet. Cent. 8:168, 1989.

Leonard, C.O. and Kazazian, H.H.: Prenatal diagnosis of hemoglobinopathies. Pediatr. Clin. North Am. 25:631, 1978.

Leonard, C.O., Sanders, R.C. and Lau, H.L.: Prenatal diagnosis of the Turner syndrome, a familial chromosomal rearrangement and achondroplasia by amniocentesis and ultrasonograph. Johns Hopkins Med. J. 145:25, 1979.

Leonard, C.O., Daikoku, N.H. and Winn, K.: Prenatal fetoscopic diagnosis of the Apert syndrome. Am. J. Med. Genet. 11:5, 1982.

Leonark, K., Byrne, J.L.B. and Elias, S.: Prenatal diagnosis of Wolf–Hirschorn syndrome associated with abnormal triple screen. Am. J. Hum. Genet. 57(Suppl.):A346, 1995.

Leschot, N.J., Heyting, C., Schaik, M.V. and Redeker, E.J.W.: Amniotic fluid gel acetylcholinesterase determination in prenatal diagnosis: Dark field illumination as a method for improving the detection of precipitation bands. Prenat. Diagn. 5:237, 1985.

Leschot, N.J., Wolf, H., Verjaal, M., van Prooijen-Knegt, A.C. and Boer, K.: Monosomy X found at first trimester CVS: A diagnostic and counselling dilemma. Clin. Genet. 37:236, 1990.

Lester, R.B., III, and Sty, J.R.: Prenatal diagnosis of cystic CNS lesions in neonatal isoimmune thrombocytopenia. J. Ultrasound Med. 6:479, 1987.

Levine, M.D., Kaback, M.M. and Griffin, C.: Prenatal genetic diagnosis (PGD) in North America—Results of a 1974 survey. Am. J. Hum. Genet. 27(Suppl.):58A, 1975.

Levinsky, R., Harvey, B., Nicolaides, K. and Rodeck, C.: Antenatal diagnosis of chronic granulomatous disease. Lancet. 1:504, 1986.

Levy, H.L., Lobbregt, D., Platt, L.D. and Benacerraf, B.R.: Fetal ultrasonography in maternal PKU. Prenat. Diagn. 16:599, 1996.

Lewinsky, R.M., Johnson, J.M., Lao, T.T., Winsor, E.J. and Cohen, H.: Fetal gastroschisis associated with monosomy 22 mosaicism and absent cerebral diastolic flow. Prenat. Diagn. 10:605, 1990.

Lewis, P.E., Cefalo, C.R. and Zaritsky, A.L.: Fetal heart block caused by cytomegalovirus. Am. J. Obstet. Gynecol. 36:967, 1980.

Lewis, K.E., Toriello, H.V. and Marsiglia, S.: Maternal serum hCG elevations and adverse pregnancy outcomes. Am. J. Hum. Genet. 57(Suppl.):A283, 1995.

Li, S-Y., Gibson, L.H., Gomez, K., Pober, B.R., Speer, J., Stiller, R. and Yang-Feng, T.L.: A familial dup (5)(q15q22) associated with normal and abnormal phenotypes. Am. J. Hum. Genet. 57(Suppl.):A283, 1995.

Liang, S.T., Woo, J.S.K. and Wong, V.C.W.: Chorioangioma of the placenta: An ultrasonic study. Case report. Br. J. Obstet. Gynaecol. 89:480, 1982.

Lidsky, A.S., Guttler, F. and Woo, S.L.C.: Prenatal diagnosis of classic phenylketonuria by DNA analysis. Lancet. 1:549, 1985.

Liebaers, I., DiNatale, P. and Neufeld, E.F.: Iduronate sulfatase in amniotic fluid: An aid in the prenatal diagnosis of the Hunter syndrome. J. Pediatr. 90:423, 1977.

Liechti-Gallati, S., Dionisi, C., Bachmann C., Wermuth, B. and Colombo, J.P.: Direct and indirect mutation analyses in patients with ornithine transcarbamylase deficiency. Enzyme. 45:81, 1991.

Lifson, A.R. and Rogers, M.F.: Vertical transmission of human immunodeficiency virus. Lancet. 2:337, 1986.

Liley, A.W.: Liquor amnii analysis in the management of the pregnancy complicated by rhesus sensitization. Am. J. Obstet. Gynecol. 82:1359, 1961.

Liley, A.W.: Intrauterine transfusion in haemolytic disease. Br. Med. J. 2:1107, 1963.

Lilford, R., Maxwell, D., Coleman, D., Czepulkowski, B. and Heaton, D.: Diagnosis, four hours after chorion biopsy, of female fetus in pregnancy at risk of Duchenne muscular dystrophy. Lancet. 2:1491, 1983.

Liming, W., Junwu, Z., Guanyun, W., Shenwu, W., Yu, F., Youwen, H., Letian, Z., Rongxin, W., Jidong, S., Nijia, Z., Guifang, L., Qi, L., Peng, Z., Rong, L. and Xu, L.: First-trimester prenatal diagnosis of severe alpha-thalassemia. Prenat. Diagn. 6:89, 1986.

Lin, C.-Y., Hwang, B., Hsiao, K.-J. and Jin Y.-R.: Pompe's disease in Chinese and prenatal diagnosis by determination of alpha-glucosidase activity. J. Inherit. Metab. Dis. 10:11, 1987.

Lin, A.E., Doshi, N., Flom, L., Teneholz, B. and Filkins, K.L.: Beemer–Langer syndrome with manifestations of an orofaciodigital syndrome. Am. J. Med. Genet. 39:247, 1991.

Lin, H.J., Cornford, M.E., Hu, B., Rutgers, J.K.L., Beall, M.H. and Lachman, R.S.: Occipital encephalocele and MURCS association: Case report and review of central nervous system anomalies in MURCS patients. Am. J. Med. Genet. 61:59, 1996.

Linch, D.C., Rodeck, C.H., Nicolaides, K., Jones, H.M. and Brent, L.: Attempted bone-marrow transplantation in a 17-week fetus. Lancet. 2:1453, 1986.

Lindenbaum, R.H., Ryynanen, M., Holmes-Siedle, M., Puhakainen, E., Jonasson, J. and Keenan, J.: Trisomy 18 and maternal serum and amniotic fluid alpha-fetoprotein. Prenat. Diagn. 7:511, 1987.

Lindhout, D., Hageman, G., Beemer, F.A., Ippel, P.F., Breslau-Siderius, L. and Willemse, J.: The Pena–Shokeir syndrome: Report of nine Dutch cases. Am. J. Med. Genet. 21:655, 1985.

Lipman, S.P., Pretorious, D.H., Rumack, C.M. and Manco-Johnson, M.L.: Fetal intracranial teratoma: US diagnosis of three cases and a review of the literature. Radiology. 157:491, 1985.

Lipson, M., Waskey, J., Rice, J., Adomian, G., Lachman, R., Filly, R. and Rimoin, D.: Prenatal diagnosis of asphyxiating thoracic dysplasia. Am. J. Med. Genet. 18:273, 1984.

Lissens, W., Van Lierde, M., Decaluwe, J., Foulon, W., Evrard, P., Van Hoof, F., Freund, M. and Liebaers, I.: Prenatal diagnosis of Hunter syndrome using fetal plasma. Prenat. Diagn. 8:59, 1988.

Lissens, W., Vercammen, M., Foulon, W., De Catte, L., Dab., I., Malfroot, A., Bonduelle, M. and Liebaers, I.: Prenatal diagnosis of cystic fibrosis using closely linked DNA probes. J. Inher. Metab. Dis. 12(Supp. 2):308, 1989.

Lissens, W. Dedobbeleer, G., Foulon, W., de Catte, L., Charels, K., Goossens, A. and Liebaers, I: Beta-glucuronidase deficiency as a cause of prenatally diagnosed non-immune hydrops fetalis. Prenat. Diagn. 11:405, 1991.

Lituania, M., Cordone, M., Zampatti, C., Passamonti, U. and Santi, F.: Prenatal diagnosis of a rare heteropagus. Prenat. Diagn. 8:547, 1988.

Lituania, M., Passamonti, U., Cordone, M.S., Magnano, G.M. and Toma, P.: Schizencephaly: Prenatal diagnosis by computed sonography and magnetic resonance imaging. Prenat. Diagn. 9:649, 1989.

Liu, J., Lissens, W., Silber, S.J., Devroey, P., Liebaers, I.. and Van Steirteghern, A.: Birth after preimplantation diagnosis of the cystic fibrosis delta F508 mutation of polymerase chain reaction in human embryos resulting from intracytoplasmic sperm injection with epididymal sperm. J. Am. Med. Assoc. 272:1858, 1994.

Livingston, B., Geller, E., Imagire, R. and Hershey, D.W.: Prenatal diagnosis of congenital nephrosis by repeat amniocentesis? Am. J. Hum. Genet. 57(Suppl.):A283, 1995.

Ljung, R., Holmberg, L., Gustavii, B., Philip, J. and Bang, J.: Haemophilia A and B—Two years experience of genetic counselling and prenatal diagnosis. Clin. Genet. 22:70, 1982.

Lobaccaro J-M., Belon, C., Lumbroso, S., Olewniczack, G., Carre-Pigeon, F., Job, J-C., Chaussain, J-L, Toublanc, J-E. and Sultan, C.: Molecular prenatal diagnosis of partial androgen insensitivity syndrome based on the Hind III polymorphism of the androgen receptor gene. Clin. Endocrinol. 40:297, 1994.

Lo Cicero, S., Capon, F., Melchionda, S., Gennarelli, M., Novelli, G., Dallapiccola, B.: First-trimester prenatal diagnosis of spinal muscular atrophy using microsatellite markers. Prenat. Diagn. 14:459, 1994.

Lockwood, C.J., Scioscia, A.L. and Hobbins, J.C.: Congenital absence of the umbilical cord resulting from maldevelopment of embryonic body folding. Am. J. Obstet. Gynecol. 155:1049, 1986.

Lockwood, C.J., Ghidini, A., Aggarwal, R., Hobbins, J.C.: Antenatal diagnosis of partial agenesis of the corpus callosum: A benign cause of ventriculomegaly. Am. J. Obstet. Gynecol. 159:184, 1988.

Loeuille, G.A., David, M. and Forest, M.G.: Prenatal treatment of congenital adrenal hyperplasia: Report of a new case. Eur. J. Pediatr. 149:237, 1990.

Lofberg, L. and Gustavii, B.: "Blind" versus direct vision technique for fetal skin sampling in cases for prenatal diagnosis. Clin. Genet. 25:37, 1984.

Loi, A., Pirastu, M., Cao, A., Ulbridh, R. and Hansmann, I.: Prenatal diagnosis of most common Mediterranean beta-thalassaemia mutants. Lancet. 1:274, 1986.

Longaker, M.T., Laberge, J-M., Dansereau, J., Langer, J.C., Crombleholme, T.M., Callen, P.W., Golbus, M.S. and Harrison, M.R.: Primary fetal hydrothorax: Natural history and management. J. Pediatr. Surg. 24:573, 1989.

Longo, N., Langley, S.D., Griffin, L.D. and Elsas, L.J.: Identification of two novel mutations in the insulin receptor gene of a patient with leprechaunism: Application to prenatal diagnosis. Am. J. Hum. Genet. 53(Suppl.):922, 1993.

Lopes, L.M., Cha, S.C., De Moraes, E.A. and Zugaib, M.: Echocardiographic diagnosis of fetal Marfan syndrome at 34 weeks' gestation. Prenat. Diagn. 15:183, 1995.

Loverro, G., Guanti, G., Caruso, G. and Selvaggi, L.: Robinow's syndrome: Prenatal diagnosis. Prenat. Diag. 10:121, 1990.

Lowden, J.A., Cutz, E., Conen, P.E., Rudd, N. and Doran, T.A.: Prenatal diagnosis of Gm_1-gangliosidosis. N. Engl. J. Med. 288:255, 1973.

Lowry, R.B., Machin, G.A., Morgan, K., Mayock, D. and Marx, L.: Congenital contractures, edema, hyperkeratosis, and intrauterine growth retardation: A fatal syndrome in Hutterite and Mennonite kindreds. Am. J. Med. Genet. 22:531, 1985.

Lurie, I.W., Gurevich, D.B., Binkert, F. and Schinzel, A.: Trisomy 17p11-pter: unbalanced pericentric inversion, inv(17)(p11q25) in two patients, unbalanced translocaitons t(4;17)(q27;p11) in a newborn and t(4;17)(p16;p11.2) in a fetus. Clin. Dysmorph. 4:25, 1995a.

Lurie, I.W., Magee, C.A., Sun, C.C.J. and Ferencz, C.: 'Microgastria-limb reduction' complex with congenital heart disease and twinning. Clin. Dysmorph. 4:150, 1995b.

Luthardt, F.W., Keitges, E.A., Shadoan, P.K., Flair, M., Beck, K. and Mains, A.: Prenatal diangosis of partial trisomy 13 resulting from a large monocentric r(13) and small mar(?13) identified by fluorescent in-situ hybridization (FISH). Am. J. Hum. Genet. 53(Suppl.): 1431, 1993.

Luthy, D.A., and Hirsch, J.H.: Infantile polycystic kidney disease: Observations from attempts at prenatal diagnosis. Am. J. Med. Genet. 20:505, 1985.

Luthy, D.A., Hall, J.G. and Graham, C.B.: Prenatal diagnosis of thrombocytopenia with absent radii. Clin. Genet. 15:495, 1979.

Lynch, L., Gilbert, F., Furst, E. and Berkowitz, R.L.: First trimester growth delay in trisomy 18. Am. J. Hum. Genet. 41(Suppl.):A280, 1987.

Lynch, L., Bussel, J., Goldberg, J.D., Chitkara, U., Wilkins, I., Macfarland, J. and Berkowitz, R.L.: The in utero diagnosis and management of alloimmune thrombocytopenia. Prenat. Diagn. 8:329, 1988.

Lynch, S.A., Gaunt, M.L. and Minford, A.M.B.: Campomelic dysplasia: Evidence of autosomal dominant inheritance. J. Med. Genet. 30:683, 1993.

Lynfield, R. and Eaton, R.B.: Teratogen update: Congenital toxoplasmosis. Teratology. 52:176, 1995.

Lyngbye, T., Haugaard, L. and Klebe, J.G.: Antenatal sonographic diagnoses of giant cystic hygroma of the neck. Acta Obstet. Gynecol. Scand. 65:873, 1986.

MacDonald, M.R., Schaefer, G.B., Olney, A.H., Tamayo, M. and Frias, J.L.: Brain magnetic resonance imaging findings in the Opitz G/BBB syndrome: Extension of the spectrum of midline brain anomalies. Am. J. Med. Genet. 46:706, 1993.

Macek, M., Anneren, G., Gustavson, K.H., Held, K., Tomasove, H., Hronkova, J., Burjankova, J. and Hrycejova, I.: Gamma-glutamyl transferase activity in the amniotic fluid of fetuses with chromosomal aberrations and inborn errors of metabolism. Clin. Genet. 32:403, 1987.

Mack, L., Gottesfeld, K. and Johnson, M.L.: Antenatal detection of ectopic fetal liver by ultrasound. J. Clin. Ultrasound 6:226, 1978.

MacKenzie, J., Chitayat, D., McLorie, G., Balfe, J.W., Pandit, P.B. and Blecher, S.R.: Penoscrotal transposition: A case report and review. Am. J. Med. Genet. 49:103, 1994.

MacLeod, P.M., Dolman, C.L., Nickel, R.E., Chang, E., Zonana, J. and Silvey, K.: Prenatal diagnosis of neuronal ceroid lipofuscinosis. N. Engl. J. Med. 310:595, 1984a.

MacLeod, P., Dolman, C., Nickel, R., Chang, E., Zonana, J., Nag, S. and Silvey, K.: The prenatal diagnosis with confirmation of the late-infantile form of neuronal ceroid lipofuscinoses—Jansky–Bielschowsky disease. Am. J. Hum. Genet. 36(Suppl.):193S, 1984b.

MacLeod, P.M., Dolman, C.L., Nickel, R.E., Chang, E., Nag, S., Zonana, J. and Silvey, K.: Prenatal diagnosis of neuronal ceroid-lipofuscinoses. Am. J. Med. Genet. 22:781, 1985.

MacLeod, P.M., Nag, S. and Berry, C.: Ultrastructural studies as a method of prenatal diagnosis of neuronal ceroid-lipofuscinosis. Am. J. Med. Genet. Suppl. 5:93, 1988.

Mac Mahon, R.A., Renou, P.M., Shekleton, P.A. and Paterson, P.J.: Severe urethral obstruction diagnosed at 14 weeks' gestation: variability of outcome with and without drainage. Fetal Diagn. Ther. 10:343, 1995.

MacMillan, R.H., Harbert, G.M., Davis, W.D. and Kelly, T.E.: Prenatal diagnosis of Pena–Shokeir syndrome, type 1. Am. J. Med. Genet. 21:279, 1985.

MacMillin, M.D., Larsen, J.W., Jr., Kent, S.G. and Rosenbaum, K.N.: Prenatal diagnosis of Beckwith–Wiedemann syndrome by ultrasound in three pregnancies. Am. J. Hum. Genet. 43(Suppl.):A239, 1988.

Macri, J.N., Weiss, R.R., Joshi, M.S. and Evans, M.I.: Antenatal diagnosis of neural-tube defects using cerebrospinal-fluid proteins. Lancet. 1:14, 1974.

Macri, J.N., Weiss, R.R., Libster, B. and Cagan, M.A.: Maternal serum-feto-protein and low birth-weight. Lancet. 1:660, 1978.

Macri, J.N., Baker, D.A. and Baim, R.S.: Diagnosis of neural tube defects by evaluation of amniotic fluid. Clin. Obstet. Gynecol. 24:1089, 1981.

Macri, J.N., Buchanan, P.D. and Gold, M.P.: Low alpha-fetoprotein and trisomy. Lancet. 2:405, 1986.

Macri, J.N., Kasturi, R.V., Cook, E.J. and Krantz, D.A.: Prenatal screening for Down's syndrome. Br. Med. J. 303:468, 1991.

Maddalena, A., Spence, W.C., Levinson, G. and Howard-Peebles, P.N.: Fragile X prenatal diagnosis in known carriers. Am. J. Hum. Genet. 53(Suppl.):88, 1993.

Madison, J.P., Sukhum, P., Williamson, D.P. and Campion, B.C.: Echocardiography and fetal heart sounds in the diagnosis of fetal heart block. Am. Heart J. 98:505, 1979.

Maggio, M., Callan, N.A., Hamod, K.A. and Sanders, R.C.: The first-trimester ultrasonographic diagnosis of conjoined twins. Am. J. Obstet. Gynecol. 152:833, 1985.

Mahoney, M.J. and Hobbins, J.C.: Prenatal diagnosis of chondroectodermal dysplasia (Ellis–van Creveld syndrome) with fetoscopy and ultrasound. N. Engl. J. Med. 297:258, 1977.

Mahoney, M.J., Rosenberg, L.E., Lindblad, B., Waldenstrom, J. and Zetterstrom, R.: Prenatal diagnosis of methylmalonic aciduria. Acta Paediatr. Scand. 64:44, 1975.

Mahoney, M.J., Haseltine, F.P., Hobbins, J.C., Banker, B.Q., Caskey, T. and Golbus, M.S.: Prenatal diagnosis of Duchenne's muscular dystrophy. N. Engl. J. Med. 297:968, 1977.

Mahony, B.S., Filly, R.A., Callen, P.W. and Golbus, M.S.: Thanatophoric dwarfism with the cloverleaf skull: A specific antenatal sonographic diagnosis. J. Ultrasound Med. 4:151, 1985a.

Mahony, B.S., Callen, P.W. and Filly, R.A.: Fetal urethral obstruction: US evaluation. Radiology. 157:221, 1985b.

Mahony, B.S., Petty, C.N., Nyberg, D.A., Luthy, D.A., Hickok, D.E. and Hirsch, J.H.: The "stuck twin" phenomenon: Ultrasonographic findings, pregnancy outcome, and management with serial amniocenteses. Am. J. Obstet. Gynecol. 163:1513, 1990.

Main, D., Mennuti, M.T., Cornfeld, D. and Coleman, B.: Prenatal diagnosis of adult polycystic kidney disease. Lancet. 2:337, 1983.

Main, D.M., Otto, C.E., Zneimer, S. and Shaffer, L.G.: Molecular genetic analysis: Confined placental trisomy 2 associated with severe intrauterine and postnatal growth deficiency. Am. J. Hum. Genet. 53(Suppl.):1434, 1993.

Maire, I., Mandon, G. and Mathieu, M.: First trimester prenatal diagnosis of glycogen storage disease type III. J. Inher. Metab. Dis. 12(Suppl. 2):292, 1989.

Maire, I., Epelbaum, S., Piraud, M., Mandon, G., Dumoulin, R. and Mathiew, M.: Second trimester prenatal diagnosis of Sanfilippo syndrome type C. J. Inher. Metab. Dis. 16:584, 1993.

Majoor-Krakauer, D.F., Wladimiroff, J.W., Stewart, P.A., van de Harten, J.J. and Niermeijer, M.F.: Microcephaly, micrognathia, and bird-headed dwarfism: Prenatal diagnosis of a Seckel-like syndrome. Am. J. Med. Genet. 27:183, 1987.

Makowski, E. L., Prem, K.A. and Kaiser, I.H.: Detection of sex of fetuses by the incidence of sex chromatin body in nuclei of cells in amniotic fluid. Science. 123:542, 1956.

Malcolm, S., Robertson, E., Harper, K., Fisher, J., Goldman, E., Rodeck, C.H., Mibashan, R.S. and Pembrey, M.E.: Prenatal assessment of haemophilia A using DNA probes. J. Med. Genet. 23:470, 1986.

Malinger, G., Rosen, N., Achiron, R. and Zakut, H.: Pierre Robin sequence associated with amniotic band syndrome ultrasonographic diagnosis and pathogenesis. Prenat. Diagn. 7:455, 1987.

Malpuech, G., Vanlieferinghen, P., Dechelotte, P., Gaulme, J., Labbe, A. and Guiot, F.: Isolated familial adrenocorticotropin deficiency: Prenatal diagnosis by maternal plasma estriol assay. Am. J. Med. Genet. 29:125, 1988.

Mancini, J., Philip, N., Chabrol, B., Divry, P., Rolland, M-O. and Pinsard, N.: Mevalonic aciduria in 3 siblings: A new recognizable metabolic encephalopathy. Pediatr. Neurol. 9:243, 1993.

Mandel, H., Berant, M., Gotfried, E. and Hochberg, Z.: Autosomal recessive hypothalmic corticotropin deficiency: A new entity and its metabolic consequences. Am. J. Hum. Genet 47(Suppl.):A66, 1990.

Mandell, J., Kinard, H.W., Mittelstaedt, C.A. and Seeds, J.W.: Prenatal diagnosis of unilateral hydronephrosis with early postnatal reconstruction. J. Urol. 132:303, 1984.

Mandell, R., Packman, S., Laframboise, R., Golbus, M.S., Schmidt, K., Workman, L., Saudubray, J.M. and Shih, V.E.: Use of amniotic fluid amino acids in prenatal testing for argininosuccinic aciduria and citrullinaemia. Prenat. Diagn. 16:419, 1996.

Mandelbaum, B., Pontarelli, D.A. and Brushenko, A.: Amnioscopy for prenatal transfusion. Am. J. Obstet. Gynecol. 98:1140, 1967.

Mann, L., Ferguson-Smith, M.A., Desai, M., Gibson, A.A.M. and Raine, P.A.M.: Prenatal assessment of anterior abdominal wall defects and their prognosis. Prenat. Diagn. 4:427, 1984.

Manning, N.J., Davies, N.P., Olpin, S.E., Carpenter, K.H., Smith, M.F., Pollitt, R.J., Duncan,

S.L.B., Larsson, A. and Carlsson, B.: Prenatal diagnosis of glutathione synthase deficiency. Prenat. Diagn. 14:475, 1994.

Manouvrier-Hanu, S., Devisme, L., Zelasko, M.C., Bourgeot, P., Vincent-Delorme, C., Valat-Rigot, A.A., Puech, F. and Farriaux, J.P.: Prenatal diagnosis of metatropic dwarfism. Prenat. Diagn. 15:753, 1995.

Mantagos, S., Weiss, R.R., Mahoney, M. and Hobbins, J.C.: Prenatal diagnosis of diastrophic dwarfism. Am. J. Obstet. Gynecol. 139:111, 1981.

Mantoni, M. and Pedersen, J.F.: Fetal growth delay in threatened abortion: An ultrasound study. Br. J. Obstet. Gynaecol. 89:525, 1982.

Mao, K. and Adams, J.: Antenatal diagnosis of intracranial arteriovenous fistula by ultrasonography: Case report. Br. J. Obstet. Gynaecol. 90:872, 1983.

Marchese, C., Savin, E., Dragone, E., Carozzi, F., De Marchi, M., Campogrande, M., Dolfin, G.C., Pagliano, G., Viora, E. and Carbonara, A.: Cystic hygroma: Prenatal diagnosis and genetic counselling. Prenat. Diagn. 5:221, 1985a.

Marchese, C.A., Carozzi, F., Mosso, R., Savin, E., Campogrande, M., Viora, E., LaProva, A., Dolfin, G.C. and Carbonara, A.O.: Fetal karyotype in malformations detected by ultrasound. Am. J. Hum. Genet. 37(Suppl.):A223, 1985b.

Marcus, E.S., Holcombe, J.H., Tulchinsky, D., Rich, R.R. and Riccardi, V.M.: Prenatal diagnosis of congenital adrenal hyperplasia. Am. J. Med. Genet. 4:201, 1979.

Marcus, S., Steen, A-M., Andersson, B., Lambert, B., Kristoffersson, U. and Francke, U.: Mutation analysis and prenatal diagnosis in a Lesch–Nyhan family showing non-random X-inactivation interfering with carrier detection tests. Hum. Genet. 89:395, 1992.

Mariona, F., McAlpin G., Zador, I., Philippart, A. and Jafri, S.Z.H.: Sonographic detection of fetal extrathoracic pulmonary sequestration. J. Ultrasound Med. 5:283, 1986.

Marles, S.L., Chodirker, B.N., Greenberg, C.R. and Chudley, A.E.: Evidence for Ritscher–Schinzel syndrome in Canadian native indians. Am. J. Med. Genet.56:343, 1995.

Maroteaux, P., Stanescu, V. and Stanescu, R.: Hypochondrogenesis. Eur. J. Pediatr. 141:14, 1983.

Marquet, J., Chadefaux, B., Bonnefont, J.P., Saudubray, J.M. and Zittoun, J.: Methylenetetrahydrofolate reductase deficiency: Prenatal diagnosis and family studies. Prenat. Diagn. 14:29, 1994.

Marquis, J.R. and Lee, J.K.: Extensive central nervous system calcification in a stillborn male infant due to cytomegalovirus infection. Am. J. Roentgenol. 127:665, 1976.

Marsac, C., Augereau, C., Boue, J. and Vidailhet, M.: Antenatal diagnosis of pyruvate-carboxylase deficiency. Lancet. 1:675, 1981.

Marsac, C., Augereau, Ch., Feldman, G., Wolf, B., Hansen, T.L. and Berger, R.: Prenatal diagnosis of pyruvate carboxylase deficiency. Clin. Chim. Acta 119:121, 1982.

Martens, P.R. and Rivas, M.L.: Analysis of amniotic fluid AFP levels in non-neural tube defect pregnancies. Am. J. Hum. Genet. 39(Suppl.):A260, 1986.

Martin, N.J., Hill, J.B., Cooper, D.H., O'Brien, G.D. and Masel, J.P.: Lethal multiple pterygium syndrome: Three consecutive cases in one family. Am. J. Med. Genet. 24:295, 1986.

Martincic, N.: Case reports: Osteopoikilie (spotted bones). Br. J. Radiol. 25:612, 1952.

Martinez-Roman, S., Torres, P.J. and Puerto, B.: Acardius acephalus after ovulation induction by clomiphene. Teratology. 51:231, 1995.

Matalon, R., Michals, K., Gashkoff, P. and Kaul, R.: Prenatal diagnosis of Canavan disease. J. Inher. Metab. Dis.: 15:392, 1992.

Matalon, R., Kaul, R., Gao, G.P., Michals, K., Gray, R.G.F., Bennett-Briton, S., Norman, A., Smith, M. and Jakobs, C.: Prenatal diagnosis for Canavan disease: The use of DNA markers. J. Inher. Metab. Dis. 18:215, 1995.

Matilla, T., Corral, J., Miranda, M., Troyano, J., Morrison, K., Volpini, V. and Estivill, X.: Prenatal diagnosis of Werdnig–Hoffmann disease: DNA analysis of a mummified umbilical cord using closely linked microsatellite markers. Prenat. Diagn. 14:219, 1994.

Matsumoto, N., Saito, N., Harada, N., Tanaka, K. and Niikawa, N.: DNA-based prenatal carrier detection for group A xeroderma pigmentosum in a chorionic villus sample. Prenat. Diagn. 15:675, 1995.

Mattison, D.R. and Angtuaco, T.: Magnetic resonance imaging in prenatal diagnosis. Clin. Obstet. Gynecol. 31:353, 1988.

Maxwell, K.D., Kearney, K.K., Johnson, J.W.C., Eagan, J.W., Jr., and Tyson, J.E.: Fetal tachycardia associated with intrauterine fetal thyrotoxicosis. Obstet. Gynecol. 55:18S, 1980.

Mayden, K.L., Tortora, M., Berkowitz, R.L., Bracken, M. and Hobbins, J.C.: Orbital diameters: A new parameter for prenatal diagnosis and dating. Am. J. Obstet. Gynecol. 144:289, 1982.

Mayden, K.L., Tortora, M., Chervenak, F.A. and Hobbins, J.C.: The antenatal sonographic detection of lung masses. Am. J. Obstet. Gynecol. 148:349, 1984.

Mbakop, A., Cox, J.N., Stormann, C. and Delozier-Blanchet, C.D.: Lethal multiple pterygium syndrome: Report of a new case with hydranencephaly. Am. J. Med. Genet. 25:575, 1986.

McAlister, W.H., Wright, J.R., Jr. and Crane, J.P.: Main-stem bronchial atresia: Intrauterine sonographic diagnosis. Am. J. Roentgenol. 148:364, 1987.

McCabe, R. and Remington, J.S.: Toxoplasmosis: The time has come. N. Engl. J. Med. 318:313, 1988.

McCormack, M.K.: Prenatal detection of the autosomal dominant type of congenital hydronephrosis by ultrasonography. Prenat. Diagn. 2:157, 1982.

McCormack, M.K., D'Aguillo, A. and Scully, J.: Autosomal dominant congenital hydronephrosis (CH): Prenatal diagnosis by ultrasound. Am. J. Hum. Genet. 33(Suppl.):85A, 1981.

McDonald, H. and Gordon, D.L.: Capnocytophaga species: A cause of amniotic fluid infection and preterm labour. Pathology. 20:74, 1988.

McDonnell, A., Hux, C., Wapner, R., Rupp, L. and Schneider, A.: Prenatal diagnosis of twins discordant for neural tube defect (NTD). Am. J. Hum. Genet. 45(Suppl.):A264, 1989.

McDowall, A.A., Blunt, S., Berry, A.C. and Fensom, A.H.: Prenatal diagnosis of a case of tetrasomy 9p. Prenat. Diagn. 9:809, 1989.

McFarland, B.L.: Congenital dislocation of the knee. J. Bone Joint Surg. 11:281, 1929.

McGahan, J.P. and Hanson, F.: Meconium peritonitis with accompanying pseudocyst: Prenatal sonographic diagnosis. Radiology. 148:125, 1983.

McGahan, J.P. and Schneider, J.M.: Fetal neck hemangioendothelioma with secondary hydrops fetalis: Sonographic diagnosis. J. Clin. Ultrasound 14:384, 1986.

McGaughran, J., Donnai, D., Clayton, P. and Mills, K.: Diagnosis of Smith–Lemli–Opitz syndrome. N. Engl. J. Med. 330:1685, 1994.

McGaughran, J.M., Clayton, P.T., Mills, K.A., Rimmer, S., Moore, L. and Donnai, D.: Prenatal diagnosis of Smith–Lemli–Opitz syndrome. Am. J. Med. Genet. 56:269, 1995.

McGillivray, B., Chitayat, D., Diamond, S., Wittmann, B.K. and Sandor, G.: Prenatal diagnosis of tuberous sclerosis. Am. J. Hum. Genet. 41(Suppl.):A280, 1987.

McGowan, K.D., Brewster, S.J., Correia, L., Fontana-Bitton, S., Pagnotto, M.A., Dailey, J.V. and Canick, J.A.: Association of very low maternal serum unconjugated estriol (uE3) levels with adverse pregnancy outcome and X-linked ichthyosis. Am. J. Hum. Genet. 57(Suppl.):A50, 1995.

McGuire, J., Manning, F., Lange, I., Lyons, E. and deSa, D.J.: Antenatel diagnosis of skeletal dysplasia using ultrasound. Birth Defects. 23(1):367, 1987.

McKeown, C.M.E. and Donnai, D.: Prune belly in trisomy 13. Prenat. Diagn. 6:379,1986.

McKinley, M.J., Kearney, L.U. and Nicolaides, K.: Prenatal diagnosis of fragile X syndrome by placental biopsy. J. Med. Genet., 25:131, 1988a.

McKinley, M.J., Kearney, L.U., Nicolaides, K.H., Gosden, C.M., Webb, T.P. and Fryns, J.P.: Prenatal diagnosis of fragile X syndrome by placental (chorionic villi) biopsy culture. Am. J. Med. Genet. 30:355, 1988b.

McKusick, V.A.: *Mendelian Inheritance in Man: Catalogs of Autosomal Dominant, Autosomal Recessive, and X-linked Phenotypes,* 7th ed. Baltimore: Johns Hopkins University Press, 1986.

McKusick, V.A.: *Mendelian Inheritance in Man: Catalogs of Autosomal Dominant, Autosomal Recessive, and X-linked Phenotypes,* 8th ed. Baltimore: Johns Hopkins University Press, 1988.

McKusick, V.A.: *Mendelian Inheritance in Man: Catalogs of Autosomal Dominant, Autosomal*

Recessive, and X-linked Phenotypes, 9th ed. Baltimore: Johns Hopkins University Press, 1990.

McKusick, V.A.: *Mendelian Inheritance in Man: Catalogs of Autosomal Dominant, Autosomal Recessive, and X-linked Phenotypes,* 10th ed. Baltimore: Johns Hopkins University Press, 1992.

McKusick, V.A.: Mendelian Inheritance in Man, 11th ed. Baltimore: The Johns Hopkins University Press, 1994.

McKusick, V.A.: Mendelian Inheritance in Man, 12th ed. The Johns Hopkins University, Cedars-Sinai Medical Center/University of California at Los Angeles, January, 1995.

McKusick, V.A.: Online Mendelian Inheritance in Man, OMIM. Center for Medical Gentics, Johns Hopkins Univeristy (Baltimore, MD) and National Center for Biotechnology Information, National Library of Medicine (Bethesda, MD). 1996. World Wide Web URL: http://www3.ncbi.nlm.nih.gov/omim/

McKusick, V.A.: Online Mendelian Inheritance in Man, OMIM. Center for Medical Gentics, Johns Hopkins Univeristy (Baltimore, MD) and National Center for Biotechnology Information, National Library of Medicine (Bethesda, MD). 1997. World Wide Web URL: http://www3.ncbi.nlm.nih.gov/omim/

McLaughlin, J.F., Marks, W.M. and Jones, G.: Prospective management of exstrophy of the cloaca and myelocystocele following prenatal ultrasound recognition of neural tube defects in identical twins. Am. J. Med. Genet. 19:721, 1984.

McLennan, A.C., Chitty, L.S., Rissik, J. and Maxwell, D.J.: Prenatal diagnosis of Blackfan– Diamond syndorme: Case report and reveiw of the literature. Prenat. Diagn. 16:349, 1996.

McMahon, M.J., Kuller, J.A. and Chescheir, N.C.: Gastrochisis: Intraabdominal bowel dilatation may predict short bowel syndrome. Am. J. Hum. Genet. 57(Suppl.):A284, 1995.

McMorrow, L.E., Lazzarini, A., Walgenbach, D., Kletz, T. and McCormack, M.K.: Three cases of Y/autosome translocation in amniotic fluid culture. Am. J. Hum. Genet. 41:A133, 1987.

McPherson, E.W., Clemens, M.M., Gibbons, R.J. and Higgs, D.R.: X-linked alpha-thalassemia/mental retadation (ATR-X) syndrome: A new kindred with severe genital anomalies and mild hematologic expression. Am. J. Med. Genet. 55:302, 1995.

Meaders, A.J., Clark, P. and Miller, W.A.: Prenatal diagnosis of femoral hypoplasia in a diabetic women. Am. J. Hum. Genet. 57(Suppl.):A346, 1995.

Medina-Gomez, P. and Bard, J.B.L.: Analysis of normal and abnormal amniotic fluid cells in vitro by cinemicrography. Prenat. Diagn. 3:311, 1983.

Medina-Gomez, P. and McBride, W.H.: Amniotic fluid macrophages from normal and malformed fetuses. Prenat. Diagn. 6:195, 1986.

Medlock, M.D., Rhead, W.J., Pollack, L., Meredith, J.T., Pearl, G. and Reece, C.: A case of glutaric acidemia type II (severe multiple acyl-CoA dehydrogenation disorder) with subsequent prenatal exclusion in a sibling. J. Perinatol. 11:227, 1991.

Meininger, M.G. and Christ, J.E.: Real-time ultrasonography for the prenatal diagnosis of facial clefts. Birth Defects. 18(1):161, 1982.

Meisner, L.F., Louie, R.R., Arya, S. and Gilbert, E.F.: Triploidy with an extra sex chromosome (70,XXYY) and elevated alpha-fetoprotein levels. Birth Defects. 23(1):333, 1987.

Meizner, I.: Pleuroamniotic shunting for decompression of fetal pleural effusions: Obstet. Gynecol. 73:298, 1989.

Meizner, I. and Bar-Ziv, J.: In utero prenatal ultrasonic diagnosis of a rare case of cloacal exstrophy. J. Clin. Ultrasound 13:500, 1985.

Meizner, I and Bar-Ziv, J.: *In Utero Diagnosis of Skeletal Disorders: An Atlas of Prental Sonographic and Postnatal Radiologic Correlation.* Boca Raton, Fla: CRC Press, 1993.

Meizner, I., Bar-Ziv, J., Holcberg, G. and Katz, M.: In utero prenatal diagnosis of fetal facial tumor-hemangioma. J. Clin. Ultrasound. 13:435, 1985.

Meizner, I., Carmi, R. and Bar-Ziv, J.: Congenital chylothorax—Prenatal ultrasonic diagnosis and successful post partum management. Prenat. Diagn. 6:217, 1986a.

Meizner, I., Bar-Ziv, J., Barki, Y. and Abeliovich, D.: Prenatal ultrasonic diagnosis of radial-ray aplasia and renal anomalies (Acro-renal syndrome). Prenat. Diagn. 6:223, 1986b.

Meizner, I., Bar-Ziv, J. and Insler, V.: Prenatal ultrasonic diagnosis of fetal thoracic and intrathoracic abnormalities. Isr. J. Med. Sci. 22:350, 1986c.

Meizner, I., Katz, M., Lunenfeld, E. and Insler, V.: Umbilical and uterine flow velocity wave forms in pregnancies complicated by major fetal anomalies. Prenat. Diagn. 7:491, 1987.

Meizner, I., Carmi, R., Katz, M. and Insler, V.: In utero prenatal diagnosis of Beckwith–Wiedemann syndrome: A case report. Eur. J. Obstet. Gynecol. Reprod. Biol. 32:259, 1989.

Melki, J., Abdelhak, S., Burlet, P., Raclin, V., Kaplan, J., Spiegel, R., Gilgenkrantz, S., Philip, N., Chauvet, M-L., Dumez, Y., Briard, M-L., Frezal, J. and Munnich, A.: Prenatal predication of Werdnig–Hoffmann disease using linked polymorphic DNA probes. J. Med. Genet. 29:171, 1992.

Melnick, M., Bixler, D., Silk, K., Yune, H. and Nance, W.E.: Autosomal dominant branchiootorenal dysplasia. Birth Defects. 11:(5)121, 1975.

Menashe, Y., Baruch, G.B., Rabinovitch, O., Shalev, Y., Katzenlson, M.B.M. and Shalev, E.: Exophthalmus—Prenatal ultrasonic features for diagnosis of Crouzon syndrome. Prenat. Diagn. 9:805, 1989.

Mendelsohn, D.B., Hertzanu, Y. and Butterworth, A.: In utero diagnosis of a vein of Galen aneurysm by ultrasound. Neuroradiology. 26:417, 1984.

Mercer, L.J., Petres, R.E. and Smeltzer, J.S.: Ultrasonic diagnosis of ectopia cordis. Obstet. Gynecol. 61:523, 1983.

Merkatz, I.R., Nitowsky, H.M., Macri, J.N. and Johnson, W.E.: An association between low maternal serum alpha-fetoprotein and fetal chromosomal abnormalities. Am. J. Obstet. Gynecol. 148:886, 1984.

Merlob, P., Schonfeld, A., Grunebaum, M., Mor, N. and Reisner, S.H.: Autosomal dominant cerebro-costo-mandibular syndrome: Ultrasonographic and clinical findings. Am. J. Med. Genet. 26:195, 1987.

Meschino, W.S., Siu, V.M., Miskin, M. and Smith, C.: Varicella embryopathy: a new cause for elevated MSAFP. Am. J. Hum. Genet. 53:1438, 1993.

Mibashan, R.S. and Millar, D.S.: Fetal haemophilia and allied bleeding disorders. Br. Med. Bull. 39:392, 1983.

Mibashan, R.S., Rodeck, C.H., Thumpston, J.K., Edwards, R.J., Singer, J.D., White, J.M. and Campbell, S.: Plasma assay of fetal factors VIIIC and IX for prenatal diagnosis of haemophilia. Lancet. 1:1309, 1979.

Mibashan, R.S., Peuke, I.R., Rodeck, C.H., Thumpston, J.K., Furlong, R.A., Gorer, R., Bains, L. and Bloom, A.L.: Dual diagnosis of prenatal haemophilia A by measurement of fetal factor VIIIC and VIIIC antigen (VIIIC Ag). Lancet. 2:994, 1980.

Mibashan, R.S., Millar, D.S., Rodeck, C.H., Nicolaides, K.H., Berger, A. and Seligsohn, U.: Prenatal diangosis of hereditary protein C deficiency. N. Eng. J. Med. 313:1607, 1985.

Micale, M.A., Wolff, D., Dickerman, L.H., Redline, R. and Schwartz, S.: Cytogenetic and molecular genetic characterization of trisomy 20 mosaicism in fetal blood and tissues. Am. J. Hum. Genet. 57(Suppl.):A284, 1995.

Michaud, J., Russo, P., Grignon, A., Dallaire, L., Bichet, D., Rosenblatt, D., Lamothe, E. and Lambert, M.: Expression of autosomal dominant polycystic kidney disease (ADPKD) during fetal life. Am. J. Hum. Genet. 53(Suppl.):1439, 1993.

Michaud, J., Filiatrault, D., Dalllaire, L., and Lambert, M.: New autosomal recessive form of amelia. Am. J. Med. Genet. 56:164, 1995.

Michell, R.C. and Bradley-Watson, P.J.: The detection of fetal meningocele by ultrasound B scan. J. Obstet. Gynaecol. Br. Commonw. 80:1100, 1973.

Mieler, W. and Weise, W.: Genetic counselling and prenatal diagnosis in split-hand/split-foot syndrome. Clin. Genet. 28:451, 1985.

Mievis, C., Claus, D., Clapuyt, P., Nyssen-Behets, C., Gosseye, S., Malvaux, P. and Verellen-Dumoulin, C.: A new familial short stature syndrome: Brussels type. Clin. Dysmorph. 5:9, 1996.

Migeon, C.J.: Comments about the need for prenatal treatment of congenital adrenal hyperplasia due to 21-hydroxylase deficiency. J. Clin. Endocrinol. Metab. 70:836, 1990.

Millard, D.D., Gidding, S.S., Socol, M.L., MacGregor, S.N., Dooley, S.L., Ney, J.A. and

Stockman, J.A.: Effects of intravascular, intrauterine transfusion on prenatal and postnatal hemolysis and erythropoiesis in severe fetal isoimmunization. J. Pediatr. 117:447, 1990.

Miller, C.H. and Hoyer, L.W.: Prenatal diagnosis of two "sporadic" cases of hemophilia. N. Engl. J. Med. 314:584, 1986.

Miller, C.H., Hilgartner, M.W. and Aledort, L.M.: Reproductive choices in hemophilic men and carriers. Am. J. Med. Genet. 26:591, 1987.

Miller, W., Peters, M., Cetrulo, C. and Lockwood, C.: Efficacy of fetal sonographic biometry in Down syndrome screening. Am. J. Hum. Genet. 45(Suppl.):A264, 1989.

Miller, I., Songster, G., Fontana, S. and Hsieh, C.-L.: Satellited 4q identified in amniotic fluid cells. Am. J. Med. Genet. 55:237, 1995.

Milunsky, A. (Ed.): *Genetic Disorders and the Fetus: Diagnosis, Prevention and Treatment,* 2nd ed. New York: Plenum Press, 1986.

Milunsky, A. and Nebiolo, L.: Maternal serum triple analyte screening and adverse pregnancy outcome. Am. J. Hum. Genet. 57(Suppl.):A284, 1995.

Milunsky, A. and Sapirstein, V.S.: Prenatal diagnosis of open neural tube defects using the amniotic fluid acetylcholinesterase assay. Obstet. Gynecol. 59:1, 1982.

Milunsky, J.M. and Skare, J.S.: Experience with molecular probes for diagnosis of myotonic muscular dystrophy (MD). Am. J. Hum. Genet. 45(Suppl.):A264, 1989.

Milunsky, A., Alpert, E., Frigoletto, F.D., Driscoll, S.G., McCluskey, R.T. and Colvin, R.B.: Prenatal diagnosis of the congenital nephrotic syndrome. Pediatrics. 59:770, 1977.

Milunsky, A., Blusztajn, J.K. and Zeisel, S.H.: Amniotic-fluid total cholinesterase and neural-tube defects. Lancet. 2:36, 1979.

Milunsky, A., Jick, H., MacLaughlin, D.S., Rothman, K.J., Willett, W., Borkowski, C. and Jick, S.: New epidemiologic predictive data for high and low maternal serum alpha-fetoprotein (MSAFP) screening. Am. J. Hum. Genet. 43(Suppl.):A241, 1988.

Milunsky, J.M., Wyandt, H.E., Huang, X-L., Kang, X-Z., Elias, E.R. and Milunsky, A.: Trisomy 15 mosaicism and uniparental disomy (UPD) in a liveborn infant. Am. J. Med. Genet. 61:269, 1996.

Minagawa, Y., Akaiwa, A., Hidaka, T., Tsuzaki, T., Tatsumura, M., Ito, T. and Maeda, K.: Severe fetal supraventricular bradyarrhythmia without fetal hypoxia. Obstet. Gynecol. 70:454, 1987.

Minelli, A., Danesino, C., Curto, F.L., Tenti, P., Zampatti, C., Simoni, G., Rossella, F. and Fois, A.: First trimester prenatal diagnosis of Sanfilippo disease (MPSIII) type B. Prenat. Diagn. 8:47, 1988.

Mingarelli, R., Iampieri, M.P., Gennarelli, M., Lo Cicero, S., Novelli, G. and Dallapiccola, B.: First trimester fetal diagnosis of X-linked retinitis. Prenat. Diagn. 12(Suppl.):S120, 1992.

Mintz, M.D., Arger, P.H. and Coleman, B.G.: In utero sonographic diagnosis of intracerebral hemorrhage. J. Ultrasound Med. 4:375, 1985.

Miny, P., Koppers, B., Dworniczak, B., Bogdanova, N., Holzgreve, W., Tercanli, S., Basaran, S., Rehder, H., Exeler, R. and Horst, J.: Parental origin of the extra haploid chromosome set in triploidies diagnosed prenatally. Am. J. Med. Genet. 57:102, 1995.

Miodovnik, M., Lavin, J.P., Gimmon, Z., Hill, J., Fischer, J.E. and Barden, T.P.: The use of amniotic fluid 3-methyl histidine to creatinine molar ratio for the diagnosis of intrauterine growth retardation. Obstet. Gynecol. 60:288, 1982.

Mirk, P., Calisti, A. and Fileni, A.: Prenatal sonographic diagnosis of bladder exstrophy. J. Ultrasound Med. 5:291, 1986.

Miskin, M.: Prenatal diagnosis of renal agenesis by ultrasonography and maternal pyelography. Am. J. Roentgenol. 132:1025, 1979.

Miskin, M., Rudd, N.L., Dische, M.R., Benzie, R. and Pirani, B.B.K.: Prenatal ultrasonic diagnosis of occipital encephalocele. Am. J. Obstet. Gynecol. 130:585, 1978.

Miskin, M., Rothberg, R., Rudd, N.L., Benzie, R.J. and Shime, J.: Arthrogryposis multiplex congenita—Prenatal assessment with diagnostic ultrasound and fetoscopy. J. Pediatr. 95:463, 1979.

Mitchell, G., Sandubray, J.M., Benoit, Y., Rocchiccioli, F., Charpentier, C., Ogier, H. and Boue, J.: Antenatal diagnosis of glutaricaciduria type II. Lancet. 1:1099, 1983.

Mitchell, G.A., Jakobs, C., Gibson, K.M.. Robert, M-F., Burlina, A., Dionisi-Vici, C. and Dallaire, L.: Molecular prenatal diagnosis of 3-hydroxy-3-methylglutaryl CoA lyase deficiency. Prenat. Diagn. 15:725, 1995.

Mizejewski, G.J., Polansky, S., Mondragon-Tiu, F.A. and Ellman, A.M.: Combined use of alpha-fetoprotein and ultrasound in the prenatal diagnosis of arteriovenous fistula in the brain. Obstet. Gynecol. 70:452, 1987.

Moerman, P., Fryns, J.P., Goddeeris, P., Lauweryns, J.M. and Van Assche, A.: Aberrant twinning (diprosopus) associated with anencephaly. Clin. Genet. 24:252, 1983.

Moerman, P., Fryns, J.-P., Vandenberghe, K., Devlieger, H. and Lauweryns, J.M.: The syndrome of diaphragmatic hernia, abnormal face and distal limb anomalies (Fryns syndrome): Report of two sibs with further delineation of this multiple congenital anomaly (MCA) syndrome. Am. J. Med. Genet. 31:805, 1988.

Moeschler, J.B., Amato, R.S., Corbin, S. and Willard, D.: Placental hemangioma elevates AFP. Am. J. Hum. Genet. 37(Suppl.):A223, 1985.

Momoi, T., Kikuchi, K., Shigematsu, Y., Sudo, M. and Tanioka, K.: Prenatal diagnosis of Tay–Sachs disease with heat-labile beta-hexosaminidase B. Clin. Chim. Acta. 133:331, 1983.

Monni, G., Rosatelli, C., Falchi, A.M., Scalas, M.T., Addis, M., Maccioni, L., Di Tucci, A., Tuveri, T. and Cao, A.: First trimester diagnosis of beta-thalassaemia in a twin pregnancy. Prenat. Diagn. 6:63, 1986.

Monni, G., Ibba, R.M., Olla, G., Rosatelli, C. and Cao, A.: Prenatal diagnosis of beta-thalassaemia by second-trimester chorionic villus sampling. Prenat. Diagn. 8:447, 1988.

Monros, E., Smeyers, P., Ramos, M.A., Prieto, F. and Palau, F.: Prenatal diagnosis of Friedreich ataxia: Improved accuracy by using new genetic flanking markers. Prenat. Diagn. 15:551, 1995.

Moola, S., Toi, A., Chitayat, D., Terespolsky, D, Johnson, J., Thomas, M., Cushing, D. and Sermer, M.: Prenatal diagnosis of the Holt–Oram syndrome. Am. J. Hum. Genet. 57(Suppl.):A346, 1995.

Moore, C.A., Harmon, J.P., Padilla, L.-M., Castro, V.B. and Weaver, D.D.: Neural tube defects and omphalocele in trisomy 18. Clin. Genet. 34:98, 1988.

Moore, C.A., Weaver, D.D. and Bull, M. J.: Fetal brain disruption sequence. J. Pediatr. 116:383, 1990.

Morgan, C.L., Haney, A., Christakos, A. and Phillips, J.: Antenatal detection of fetal structural defects with ultrasound. J. Clin. Ultrasound 3:287, 1975.

Morgan, C.L., Trought, W.S., Sheldon, G. and Barton, T.K.: B-scan and real-time ultrasound in the antepartum diagnosis of conjoined twins and pericardial effusion. Am. J. Roentgenol. 130:578, 1978.

Morgan-Capner, P., Rodeck, C.H., Nicolaides, K. and Cradock-Watson, J.E.: Prenatal diagnosis of rubella. Lancet. 2:343, 1984.

Morgan-Capner, P., Rodeck, C.H., Nicolaides, K.H. and Cradock-Watson, J.E.: Prenatal detection of rubella-specific IgM in fetal sera. Prenat. Diagn. 5:21, 1986.

Mori, M., Yamagata, T., Mori, Y., Nokubi, M., Saito, K., Fukushima, Y. and Momoi, Y.: Elastic fiber degeneration in Costello syndrome. Am. J. Med. Genet. 61:304, 1996.

Morin, P.R., Potier, M., Dallaire, L., Malancon, S.B. and Milunsky, A.: Prenatal detection of intestinal obstruction: Deficient amniotic fluid disaccharidases in affected fetuses. Clin. Genet. 18:217, 1980.

Morin, P.R., Potier, M., Dallaire, L., Melancon, S.B. and Boisvert, J.: Prenatal detection of the autosomal recessive type of polycystic kidney disease by trehalase assay in amniotic fluid. Prenat. Diagn. 1:75, 1981.

Morin, P.R., Potier, M., Lasalle, R., Melancon, S.B. and Dallaire, L.: Amniotic-fluid disaccharidases in the prenatal detection of cystic fibrosis. Lancet. 2:621, 1983.

Morin, P.R., Nguyen, H.V., Beauregard, G., Dallaire, L, Melancon, S.B. and Potier, M.: Present status of prenatal detection of cystic fibrosis with microvillar enzymes in amniotic fluid. Am. J. Hum. Genet. 36(Suppl.):16S, 1984a.

Morin, P.R., Potier, M., Dallaire, L. and Melancon, S.B.: Prenatal detection of the congenital nephrotic syndrome (Finnish type) by trehalase assay in amniotic fluid. Prenat. Diagn. 4:257, 1984b.

Morin, P.R., Melancon, S.B., Dallaire, L. and Potier, M.: Prenatal detection of intestinal obstructions, aneuploidy syndromes, and cystic fibrosis by microvillar enzyme assays (disaccharidases, alkaline phosphatase, and glutamyltransferase) in amniotic fluid. Am. J. Med. Genet. 26:405, 1987.

Morin, L.R.M., Herlicoviez, M., Loisel, J.C., Jacob, B., Feuilly, C. and Stanescu, V.: Prenatal diagnosis of lethal osteogenesis imperfecta in twin pregnancy. Clin. Genet. 39:467, 1991.

Mornet, E., Couillin, P., Boue, J., Cohen, D. and Boue, A.: First trimester prenatal diagnosis of 21-hydroxylase deficiency by linkage analysis of HLA class I and class II probes. Clin. Genet. 28:452, 1985.

Mornet, E., Boue, J., Raux-Demay, M., Couillin, P., Oury, J.F., Dumez, Y., Dausset, J., Cohen, D. and Boue, A.: First trimester prenatal diagnosis of 21-hydroxylase deficiency by linkage analysis to HLA-DNA probes and by 17-hydroxyprogesterone determination. Hum. Genet. 73:358, 1986.

Morocz, I., Szeifert, G.T., Molnar, P., Toth, Z., Csecsei, K. and Papp, Z.: Prenatal diagnosis and pathoanatomy of iniencephaly. Clin. Genet. 30:81, 1986.

Morris, C.A. and Hertel, G.A.: Metastatic hemangioendothelioma resulting in hydrops fetalis. Proc. Greenwood Genet. Cent. 8:219, 1989.

Morris, M., Nichols, W. and Benson, M.: Prenatal diagnosis of hereditary amyloidosis in a Portuguese family. Am. J. Med. Genet. 39:123, 1991.

Morrone, L.C., Shih, L.Y. and Silbey, E.: Elevated amniotic fluid alpha-fetoprotein associated with umbilical cord hemangioma. Am. J. Hum. Genet. 43(Suppl.):A241, 1988.

Morrow, G., III, Revsin, B., Lebowitz, J., Britt, W. and Giles, H.: Detection of errors in methylmalonyl-CoA metabolism by using amniotic fluid. Clin. Chem. 23:791, 1977.

Morse, R.P., Rawnsley, E., Sargent, S.K. and Graham, J.M., Jr.: Prenatal diagnosis of a new syndrome: Holoprosencephaly with hypokinesia. Prenat. Diagn. 7:631, 1987a.

Morse, R.P., Rawnsley, E., Crowe, H.C., Marin-Padilla, M. and Graham, J.M., Jr.: Bilateral renal agenesis in three consecutive siblings. Prenat. Diagn. 7:573, 1987b.

Moser, H.W., Moser, A.B., Powers, J.M., Nitowsky, H.M., Schaumburg, H.H., Norum, R.A. and Migeon, B.R.: The prenatal diagnosis of adrenoleukodystrophy: Demonstration of increased hexacosanoic acid levels in cultured amniocytes and fetal adrenal gland. Pediatr. Res. 16:172, 1982.

Moser, A.E., Singh, I., Brown, F.R., III, Solish, G.I., Kelley, R.I., Benke, P.J. and Moser, H.W.: The cerebrohepatorenal (Zellweger) syndrome: Increased levels and impaired degradation of very-long-chain fatty acids and their use in prenatal diagnosis. N. Engl. J. Med. 310:1141, 1984.

Moser, H.W. and Moser, A.B.: Adrenoleukodystrophy (X-linked). In: Scriver, C.R, Beaudet, A.L., Sly, W.S. and Valle, D. (Eds.), *The Metabolic Basis of Inherited Disease,* 6th ed. New York: McGraw-Hill, 1989, p. 1511.

Mossman, J. and Patrick, A.D.: Prenatal diagnosis of mucopolysaccharidosis by two-dimensional electrophoresis of amniotic fluid glycosaminoglycans. Prenat. Diagn. 2:169, 1982.

Mossman, J., Patrick, A.D., Fensom, A.H., Tansley, L.R., Benson, P.F., der Kaloustian, V.M. and Dudin, G.: Correct prenatal diagnosis of a Hurler fetus where amniotic fluid cell cultures were of maternal origin. Prenat. Diagn. 1:121, 1981.

Mossman, J., Young, E.P. and Patrick, A.D.: Prenatal tests for Sanfilippo disease type B in four pregnancies. Prenat. Diagn. 3:347, 1983.

Mostello, D., Hoechstetter, L, Bendon, R. Siddiqi, T. and Dignan, P.: Recurrence and prenatal diagnosis of lethal Larsen syndrome. Am. J. Hum. Genet. 45(Suppl.):A56, 1989.

Mostello, D., Hoechstetter, L., Bendon, R.W., Dignan, P.S.J., Oestreich, A.E. and Siddiqi, T.A.: Prenatal diagnosis of recurrent Larsen syndrome: Further definition of a lethal variant. Prenat. Diagn. 11:215, 1991.

Motulsky, A.G. and Murray, J.: Will prenatal diagnosis with selective abortion affect society's attitude toward the handicapped? Prog. Clin. Biol. Res. 128:277, 1983.

Mulcahy, M.T., Roberman, B. and Reid, S.E.: Chorion biopsy, cytogenetic diagnosis, and selective termination in a twin pregnancy at risk of haemophilia. Lancet. 2:866, 1984.

Mulder, A.F.P., van Eyck, J., Groenendaal, F. and Wladimiroff, J.W.: Trisomy 18 in monozygotic twins. Hum. Genet. 83:300, 1989.

Mulivor, R.A., Mennuti, M., Zackai, E.H. and Harris, H.: Prenatal diagnosis of hypophosphatasia: Genetic, biochemical, and clinical studies. Am. J. Hum. Genet. 30:271, 1978.

Mulivor, R.A., Mennuti, M.T., Punnett, H.H. and Harris, H.: Prenatal diagnosis of cystic fibrosis. Am. J. Hum. Genet. 37(Suppl.):A224, 1985.

Muller, F. and Boue, A.: A single chorionic gonadotropin assay for maternal serum screening for Down's syndrome. Prenat. Diagn. 10:389, 1990.

Muller, L.M. and de Jong, G.: Prenatal ultrasonographic features of the Pena–Shokeir I syndrome and the trisomy 18 syndrome. Am. J. Med. Genet. 25:119, 1986.

Muller, F., Frot, J.C., Aubry, M.C., Boue, J. and Boue, A.: Meconium ileus in cystic fibrosis fetuses. Lancet. 2:223, 1984a.

Muller, F., Berg, S., Frot, J.-F., Boue, J. and Boue, A.: Alkaline phosphatase isoenzyme assays for prenatal diagnosis of cystic fibrosis. Lancet. 1:572, 1984b.

Muller, F., Boue, J. and Boue, A.: Prenatal diagnosis of cystic fibrosis in 140 pregnancies with 1-in-4 risk. Clin. Genet. 28:452, 1985a.

Muller, F., Berg, S., Frot, J.C., Boue, J. and Boue, A.: Prenatal diagnosis of cystic fibrosis I: Prospective study of 51 pregnancies. Prenat. Diagn. 5:97, 1985b.

Muller, F., Aubry, M.C., Gasser, B., Duchatel, F., Boue, J. and Boue, A.: Prenatal diagnosis of cystic fibrosis II: Meconium ileus in affected fetuses. Prenat. Diagn. 5:109, 1985c.

Muller, L.M., de Jong, G. and Van Heerden, K.M.M.: The antenatal ultrasonographic detection of the Holt–Oram syndrome. S. Afr. Med. J. 68:313, 1985d.

Muller, L.M., de Jong, G., Mouton, S.C.E., Greeff, M.J., Kirby, P., Hewlett, R. and Jordaan, H.F.: A case of the Neu-Laxova syndrome: Prenatal ultrasonographic monitoring in the third trimester and the histopathological findings. Am. J. Med. Genet. 26:421, 1987.

Muller, F., Oury, J.F., Dumez, Y., Boue, J. and Boue, A.: Microvillar enzyme assays in amniotic fluid and fetal tissues at different stages of development. Prenat. Diagn. 8:189, 1988.

Muller, F. Oury, J.F., Bussiere, P., Lewin, F. and Boue, J.: First-trimester diagnosis of hypophosphatasia. Importance of gestational age and of purity of CV samples. Prenat. Diagn. 11:725, 1991.

Multon, O., Sibony, O., Carbillon, L., Guerin, J.M., Nessman, C. and Blot, P.: Sickle cell and thiamine deficiency: Case report of a fetal death. Fetal Diagn. Ther. 9:337, 1994.

Mundy, D.C., Schinazi, R.F., Gerber, A.R., Nahmias, A.J. and Randall, H.W., Jr.: Human immunodeficiency virus isolated from amniotic fluid. Lancet. 2:460, 1987.

Munoz, C., Filly, R.A. and Golbus, M.S.: Osteogenesis imperfecta type II: Prenatal sonographic diagnosis. Radiology. 174:181, 1990.

Murer-Orlando, M., Llerena, J.C., Jr., Birjandi, F. Gibson, R.A. and Mathew, C.G.: FACC gene mutations and early prenatal diagnosis of Fanconi's anaemia. Lancet. 342:686, 1993.

Murotsuki, J., Okamura, K., Iwamoto, M., Kosuge, S., Kimura, Y., Kobayashi, M., Takeyama, Y., Yano, M. and Yajima, A.: Hematological values in fetal blood by cordocentesis. Acta Obstet. Gynaecol. Jap. 44:638, 1992.

Murphy, P.D., Watson, M.S., Kidd, K.K. and Breg, W.R.: The fragile X syndrome: Molecular approaches to carrier detection and prenatal diagnosis. Am. J. Hum. Genet. 39(Suppl.): A127, 1986.

Murphy, J.L., Mendoza, S.A., Griswold, W.R. and Reznik, V.M.: Severe bilateral renal disease: Correlation of antenatal and autopsy findings. Prenat. Diagn. 9:119, 1989.

Murray, M., Habecker-Green, J., Kanaan, C., Pfleuger, S. and Cohn, G.: Prenatal diagnosis of an atypical case of OEIS complex. Am. J. Hum. Genet. 57(Suppl.):A346, 1995.

Myles, T.D., Burd, L., Font, G., McCorquodale, M. and McCorquodale, D.J.: Prenatal diagnosis of pentasomy X by fluorescent in situ hybridization in a fetus presenting with the Dandy–Walker malformation. Am. J. Hum. Genet. 57(Suppl.):A346, 1995.

Nada, M.A., Vianey-Saban, C., Roe, C.R., Ding. J-H., Mathieu, M., Wappner, R.S., Bialer,

M.G., McGlynn, J.A. and Mandon, G.: Prenatal diagnosis of mitochondrial fatty acid oxidation defects. Prenat. Diagn. 16:117, 1996.

Nadler, H.L.: Antenatal detection of hereditary disorders. Pediatrics. 42:912, 1968.

Nadler, H.L. and Egan, T.J.: Deficiency of lysosomal acid phosphatase: A new familial metabolic disorder. N. Engl. J. Med. 282:302, 1970.

Nadler, H.L. and Gerbie, A.B.: Role of amniocentesis in the intrauterine detection of genetic disorders. N. Engl. J. Med. 282:596, 1970.

Nadler, H.L. and Walsh, M.M.J.: Intrauterine detection of cystic fibrosis. Pediatrics. 66:690, 1980.

Nadler, H.L., Rembelski, P., Meserow, K. and Gerbie, A.B.: Prenatal detection of cystic fibrosis. Am. J. Obstet. Gynecol. 141:885, 1981a.

Nadler, H.L., Rembelski, P. and Mesirow, K.H.: Prenatal detection of cystic fibrosis. Lancet. 2:1226, 1981b.

Nagamani, M., McDonough, P.G., Ellegood, J.O. and Mahesh, V.B.: Maternal and amniotic fluid 17-alpha-hydroxyprogesterone levels during pregnancy: Diagnosis of congenital adrenal hyperplasia in utero. Am. J. Obstet. Gynecol. 130:791, 1978.

Nagashima, M., Asai, T., Suzuki, C., Matsushima, M. and Ogawa, A.: Intrauterine supraventricular tachyarrhythmias and transplacental digitalisation. Arch. Dis. Child. 61:996, 1986.

Naides, S.J. and Weiner, C.P.: Antenatal diagnosis and palliative treatment of non-immune hydrops fetalis secondary to fetal parvovirus B19 infection. Prenat. Diagn. 9:105, 1989.

Nakamoto, S.K., Dreilinger, A., Dattel, B., Mattrey, R.F. and Key, T.C.: The sonographic appearance of hepatic hemangioma in utero. J. Ultrasound Med. 2:239, 1983.

Nakamura, E., Rosenberg, L.E. and Tanaka, K.: Microdetermination of methylmalonic acid and other short chain dicarboxylic acids by gas chromatography: Use in prenatal diagnosis of methylmalonic acidemia and in studies of isovaleric acidemia. Clin. Chim. Acta. 68:127, 1976.

Nancarrow, P.A., Mattrey, R.F., Edwards, D.K. and Skram, C.: Fibroadhesive meconium peritonitis: In utero sonographic diagnosis. J. Ultrasound Med. 4:213, 1985.

Narayan, H., De Chazal, R., Barrow, M., McKeever, P. and Neale, E.: Familial congenital diaphragmatic hernia: Prenatal diagnosis, management, and outcome. Prenat. Diagn. 13:893, 1993.

Nathan, D.G., Alter, B.P. and Orkin, S.H.: Prenatal diagnosis of hemoglobinopathies. Clin. Perinatol. 6:275, 1979.

Nathan, L., Bohman, V.R., Sanchez, P.J., Leos, N.K., Twickler, D.M. and Wendel, G.D, Jr.: In utero infection with *Treponema pallidum* in early pregnancy. Prenat. Diagn. 17:119, 1997.

Natsuyama, E.: Sonographic determination of fetal sex from twelve weeks of gestation. Am. J. Obstet. Gynecol. 149:748, 1984.

Navon, R. and Padeh, B.: Prenatal diagnosis of Tay–Sachs genotypes. Br. Med. J. 4:17, 1971.

Navon, R., Sandbank, U., Frisch, A., Baram, D. and Adam, A.: Adult-onset GM_2 gangliosidosis diagnosed in a fetus. Prenat. Diagn. 6:169, 1986.

Navon, R., Timmerman, V., Lofgren, A., Liang, P., Nelis, E., Zeitune, M. and Van Broeckhoven, C.: Prenatal diangosis of Charcot–Marie–Tooth disease type 1A (CMT1A) using molecular genetic techniques. Prenat. Diagn. 15:633, 1995.

Naylor, G., Sweetman, L., Nyhan, W., Hornbeck, C., Griffiths, J. Morch, L. and Brandange, S.: Isotope dilution analysis of methylcitric acid in amniotic fluid for the prenatal diagnosis of propionic and methylmalonic acidemia. Clin. Chim. Acta. 107:175, 1980.

Nazzaro, V., Nicolini, U., De Luca, L., Berti, E. and Caputo, R.: Prenatal diagnosis of junctional epidermolysis bullosa associated with pyloric atresia. J. Med. Genet. 27:244, 1990.

Neidich, J.A., Hellman, F.N., Dillman, N.J., Ming, L.P., Cryer, D.R., Grumbach, K., McDonald, D., Schnur, R., Block, M.J., Huff, D., Rorke, L., Zackai, E.H. and Mennuti, M.T.: The spectrum of defects in Neu–Laxova syndrome including pathology and prenatal diagnosis. Am. J. Hum. Genet. 41(Suppl.):A76, 1987.

Nelson, L.H. and Reiff, R.H.: Megacystic-microcolon-hypoperistalsis syndrome and anechoic areas in the fetal abdomen. Am. J. Obstet. Gynecol. 144:464, 1982.

Nelson, M.M. and Petersen, E.M.: Prospective screening for Down syndrome using maternal serum AFP. Lancet. 1:1281, 1985.

Nelson, L.H., Clark, C.E., Fishburne, J.I., Urban, R.B. and Penry, M.F.: Value of serial sonography in the in utero detection of duodenal atresia. Obstet. Gynecol. 59:657, 1982a.

Nelson, P.A., Bowie, J.D., Filston, H.C. and Crane, L.M.: Sonographic diagnosis of omphalocele in utero. Am. J. Roentgenol. 138:1178, 1982b.

Nelson, L.M., Baker, J.S., Byme, J. and Ward, K.: Presymptomatic and prenatal DNA testing on 123 neurofibromatosis I families. Am. J. Hum. Genet. 53(Suppl.):1746, 1993.

Neu, R.L., Lockwood, D.H., Weinstein, M.E., Thomson, K.A., Gersen, S.L. and Jackson, J.A.: Chromosme abnormalities in 176 prenatal cases referred for cystic hygroma. Am. J. Hum. Genet. 53(Suppl.):1444, 1993.

Neufeld, E.F. and Muenzer, J.: The mucopolysaccaridoses. In: Scriver, C.R., Reaudet, A.L., Sly., W.S. and Valle, D. (Eds.), *The Metabolic Basis of Inherited Disease,* 6th ed. New York: McGraw-Hill, 1989. p. 1577.

Nevin, N.C. and Thomas, P.S.: Orofaciodigital syndrome type IV: Report of a patient. Am. J. Med. Genet. 32:151, 1989.

Nevin, N.C., Ritchie, A., McKeown, F. and Roberts, G.: Raised alpha-fetoprotein levels in amniotic fluid and maternal serum associated with distension of the fetal bladder caused by absence of urethra. J. Med. Genet. 15:61, 1978.

Nevin, N.C., Thompson, W., Davison, G. and Horner, W.T.: Prenatal diagnosis of the Meckel syndrome. Clin. Genet. 15:1, 1979.

Nevin, N.C., Nevin, J., Thompson, W. and O'Hara, M.D.: Cystic hygroma simulating an encephalocele. Prenat. Diagn. 3:249, 1983a.

Nevin, N.C., Nevin, J., Dunlop, J.M. and Gray, M.: Antenatal detection of grossly distended bladder owing to absence of the urethra in a fetus with trisomy 18. J. Med. Genet. 20:132, 1983b.

Nevin, N.C., Herron, B. and Armstrong, M.J.: An 18 week fetus with Elejalde syndrome (acrocephalopolydactylyous dysplasia). Clin. Dysmorph. 3:180, 1994.

New, M.I. Genetics disorders of adrenal hormone synthesis. Horm. Res. 37(Suppl. 3): 22, 1992.

Newburger, J.W. and Keane, J.F.: Intrauterine supraventricular tachycardia. J. Pediatr. 95:780, 1979.

Newburger, P.E., Cohen, H.J., Rothchild, S.B., Hobbins, J.C., Malawista, S.E. and Mahoney, M.J.: Prenatal diagnosis of chronic granulomatous disease. N. Engl. J. Med. 300:178, 1979.

Newman, G.C., Buschi, A.I., Sugg, N.K., Kelly, T.E. and Miller, J.Q.: Dandy–Walker syndrome diagnosed in utero by ultrasonography. Neurology. 32:180, 1982.

Newnham, J.P., Crues, J.V., III, Vinstein, A.L. and Medearis, A.L.: Sonographic diagnosis of thoracic gastroenteric cyst in utero. Prenat. Diagn. 4:467, 1984.

Ng, W.G., Donnell, G.N. and Alfi, O.: Prenatal diagnosis of galactosaemia. Lancet. 1:43, 1977a.

Ng, W.G., Donnell, G.N., Bergren, W.R., Alfi, O. and Golbus, M.S.: Prenatal diagnosis of galactosemia. Clin. Chim. Acta. 74:227, 1977b.

Nguyen The, H., Pescia, G., Deonna, T. and Bakaric, O.: Early prenatal diagnosis of genetic microcephaly. Prenat. Diagn. 5:345, 1985.

Nichols, J. and Gibson, G.G.: Antenatal diagnosis of the adrenogenital syndrome. Lancet. 2:1068, 1969.

Nicolaides, K.H. and Azar, G.B.: Thoraco-amniotic shunting. Fetal Diagn. Ther. 5:153, 1990.

Nicolaides, K.H., Johansson, D., Donnai, D. and Rodeck, C.H.: Prenatal diagnosis of mandibulofacial dysostosis. Prenat. Diagn. 4:201, 1984.

Nicolaides, K.H., Rodeck, C.H., Millar, D.S. and Mibashan, R.S.: Fetal haematology in rhesus isoimmunisation. Br. Med. J. 290:661, 1985.

Nicolaides, K.H., Rodeck, C.H. and Gosden, C.M.: Rapid karyotyping in non-lethal fetal malformations. Lancet. 1:283, 1986a.

Nicolaides, K.H., Soothill, P.W., Rodeck, C.H. and Warren, R.C.: Why confine chorionic villus (placental) biopsy to the first trimester? Lancet. 1:543, 1986b.

Nicolaides, K.H., Rodeck, C.H., Mibashan, R.S. and Kemp, J.R.: Have Liley charts outlived their usefulness? Am. J. Obstet. Gynecol. 155:90, 1986c.

Nicolaides, K.H., Soothill, P.W., Rodeck, C.H., Clewell, W.: Rh disease: Intravascular fetal blood transfusion by cordocentesis. Fetal Ther. 1:185, 1986d.

Nicolaides, K.H., Soothill, P.W., Rodeck, C.H. and Campbell, S.: Ultrasound-guided sampling of umbilical cord and placental blood to assess fetal wellbeing. Lancet. 2:1065, 1986e.

Nicolaides, K.H., Blott, M. and Greenough, A.: Chronic drainage of fetal pulmonary cyst. Lancet. 1:618, 1987.

Nicolini, U., Kochenour, N.K., Greco, P, Letsky, E. and Rodeck, C.H.: When to perform the next intra-uterine transfusion in patients with Rh allo-immunization: Combined intravascular and intraperitoneal transfusion allows longer intervals. Fetal Ther. 4:14, 1989a.

Nicolini, U., Santolaya, J., Hubinont, C., Fisk, N., Maxwell, D. and Rodeck, C.: Visualization of fetal intra-abdominal organs in second-trimester severe oligohydramnios by intraperitoneal infusion. Prenat. Diagn. 9:191, 1989b.

Nicolini, U., Tannirandorn, Y., Gonzalez, P., Fisk, N.M., Beacham, J., Letsky, E.A. and Rodeck, C. H.: Continuing controversy in alloimmune thrombocytopenia: Fetal hyperimmunoglobulinemia fails to prevent thrombocytopenia. Am. J. Obstet. Gynecol. 163: 1114, 1990.

Niederwieser, A., Shintaku, H., Hasler, T., Curtius, H.C., Lehmann, H., Guardamagna, O. and Schmidt, H.: Prenatal diagnosis of "dihydrobiopterin synthetase" deficiency, a variant form of phenylketonuria. Eur. J. Pediatr. 145:176, 1986.

Nielsen, J.S. and Moestrup, J.K.: Foetal electrocardiographic studies of cardiac arrhythmias and the heart rate. Acta Obstet. Gynecol. Scand. 47:247, 1968.

Nielsen, L.B., Nielsen, K.B. and Tommerup, N.: Fragile X demonstrated retrospectively in amniotic cells cultured in low folate medium. Prenat. Diagn. 3:367, 1983.

Nielsen, L.B., Bang, J. and Norgaard-Pedersen, B.: Prenatal diagnosis of omphalocele and gastroschisis by ultrasonography. Prenat. Diagn. 5:381, 1985.

Niermeijer, M.F., Koster, J.F., Jahodova, M., Fernandes, J., Heukels-Dully, M.J. and Galjaard, H.: Prenatal diagnosis of type II glycogenosis (Pompe's disease) using microchemical analyses. Pediatr. Res. 9:498, 1975.

Nimrod, C., Davies, D., Iwanicki, S., Harder, J., Persaud, D. and Nicholson, S.: Ultrasound prediction of pulmonary hypoplasia. Obstet. Gynecol. 68:495, 1986.

Nisani, R., Chemke, J., Cohen-Ankori, H. and Nissim, F.: Neural tube defects in trisomy 18. Prenat. Diagn. 1:227, 1981.

Nivelon-Chevallier, A., Mavel, A., Michiels, R. and Bethenod, M.: Syndrome de Wiedeman Beckwith-familial: Diagnostic antenatal echographique et confirmation histologique. J. Genet. Hum. 31:397, 1983.

Noia, G., De Santis, M., Tocci, A., Maussier, M.L., D'Errico, G., Bianchi, A., Romagnoli, C., Masini, L., Caruso, A. and Mancuso, S.: Early prenatal diangosis and therapy of fetal hypothyroid goiter. Fetal Diagn. Ther. 7:138, 1992.

Nolan, C.M. and Sly, W.s.: I-cell disease and pseudo-Hurler polydystrophy: Disorders of lysosomal enzyme phosphorylation and localization. In Scriver, C.J., Beudet, A.L., Sly, W.S. and Valle, D. (Eds.), *The Metabolic Basis of Inherited Disease,* 6th Ed. 1989. p. 1589.

Noonan, C.D.: Antenatal diagnosis of fetal abnormalities. Radiol. Clin. North Am. 12:13, 1974.

Nora, J.J., Zlotnik, L., Ozturk, G. and Walknowska, J.: An approach to prenatal diagnosis of paternity. Am. J. Med. Genet. 16:641. 1983.

Nores, J.A., Rotmensch, S., Romero, R., Avila, C., Inati, M. and Hobbins, J.C.: Atelosteogenesis type II: Sonographic and radiological correlation. Prenat. Diagn. 12:741, 1992.

Norman, A.M. and Donnai, D.: Response to Drs. Cohen and Gorlin. Am. J. Med. Genet. 39:336, 1991.

Norman, A.M., Floyd, J.L., Meredith, A.L. and Harper, P.S.: Presymptomatic detection and prenatal diagnosis for myotonic dystrophy by means of linked DNA markers. J. Med. Genet. 26:750, 1989.

Northrup, H., Beaudet, A.L. and O'Brien, W.E.: Prenatal diagnosis of citrullinemia using restriction fragment length polymorphisms from within the argininosuccinate synthetase (AS) gene. Am. J. Hum. Genet. 43(Suppl.):A242, 1988.

Northrup, H., Beaudet, A.L. and O'Brien, W.E.: Prenatal diagnosis of citrullinaemia: Review of a 10-year experience including recent use of DNA analysis. Prenat. Diagn. 10:771, 1990.

Novelli, G., Frontali, M., Baldini, D., Bosman, C., Dallapiccola, B., Pachi, A. and Torcia, F.: Prenatal diagnosis of adult polycystic kidney disease with DNA markers on chromosome 16 and the genetic heterogeneity problem. Prenat. Diagn. 9:759, 1989.

Novelli, G., Sangiuolo, G., Dallapiccola, B., Gasparini, P., Savoia, A., Pignatti, P.F., Fernandez, E., Benitez, J., Casals, T., Nunes, V., Manas, P. and Estivill, X.: Delta F508 gene deletion and prenatal diagnosis of cystic fibrosis in Italian and Spanish families. Prenat. Diagn. 10:413, 1990.

Nussbaum, R.L., Boggs, B.A., Beaudet, A.L., Doyle, S., Potter, J.L. and O'Brien, W.E.: New mutation and prenatal diagnosis in onithine transcarbamylase deficiency. Am. J. Hum. Genet. 38:149, 1986.

Nyberg, D.A., Mack, L.A., Hirsch, J., Pagon, R.O. and Shepard, T.H.: Fetal hydrocephalus: Sonographic detection and clinical significance of associated anomalies. Radiology. 163:187, 1987.

Nyberg, D.A., Fitzsimmons, J., Mack, L.A., Hughes, M., Pretorius, D.H., Hickok, D. and Shepard, T.H.: Chromosomal abnormalities in fetuses with omphalocele. J. Ultrasound Med. 8:299, 1989.

Nyberg, D.A., Kramer, D., Resta, R.G., Kapur, R., Mahony, B.S., Luthy, D.A. and Hickok, D.: Prenatal sonographic findings of trisomy 18: Review of 47 cases. J. Ultrasound Med. 2:103, 1993.

Nyland, M.H., Whiteman, D.A.H., Pettenati, M.J., Bennett, T.J., Nelson, L.H., Hopkins, M.B. and Burton, B.K.: High frequency mosaic tetraploidy in amniotic fluid cell culture: Culture artifact or placental contamination? Am. J. Hum. Genet. 41(Suppl.):A281, 1987.

O'Brien, J.S., Okada, S., Fillerup, D.L., Veath, M.L., Adornato, B., Brenner, P.H. and Leroy, J.G.: Tay–Sachs disease: Prenatal diagnosis. Science. 172:61, 1971.

O'Brien, G.D. and Queenan, J.T.: Ultrasound fetal femur length in relation to intrauterine growth retardation, Part II. Am. J. Obstet. Gynecol. 144:35, 1982.

O'Brien, G.D., Rodeck, C. and Queenan, J.T.: Early prenatal diagnosis of diastrophic dwarfism by ultrasound. Br. Med. J. 280:1300, 1980a.

O'Brien, W.F., Cefalo, R.C. and Bair, D.G.: Ultrasonographic diagnosis of fetal cystic hygroma. Am. J. Obstet. Gynecol. 138:464, 1980b.

Ogata, E.S., Sabbagha, R., Metzger, B.E., Phelps, R.L., Depp, R. and Freinkel, N.: Serial ultrasonography to assess evolving fetal macrosomia: Studies of 23 pregnant diabetic women. J. Am. Med. Assoc. 243:2405, 1980.

Ogier, H., Wadman, S.K., Johnson, J.L., Saudubray, J.M., Duran, M., Boue, J., Munnich, A. and Charpentier, C.: Antenatal diagnosis of combined xanthine and sulphite oxidase deficiencies. Lancet. 2:1363, 1983.

Ogur, G., Ogur, E., Celasun, B., Baser, I., Imirzalioglu, N., Ozturk, T. and Alemdaroglu, A.: Prenatal diagnosis of autosomal recessive osteopetrosis, infantile type, by X-ray evaluation. Prenat. Diagn. 15:477, 1995.

Ohba, S., Kidouchi, K., Toyama, J., Oda, T., Tsuboi, T., Ichiki, T., Sobajima, H., Sugiyama, N., Morishita, H., Kobayashi, M., Togari, H., Suzumori, K. and Wada, Y.: Quantitative analysis of amniotic fluid pyrimidines for the prenatal diagnosis of hereditary orotic aciduria. J. Inher. Metab. Dis. 16:872, 1993.

Ohdo, S., Madokoro, H., Sonoda, T., Takei, M., Yasuda, H. and Mori, N.: Association of tetra-amelia, ectodermal dysplasia, hypoplastic lacrimal ducts and sacs opening towards the exterior, peculiar face, and developmental retardation. J. Med. Genet. 24:609, 1987.

Ohlsson, A., Fong, K.W., Rose, T.H. and Moore, D.C.: Prenatal sonographic diagnosis of Pena–Shokeir syndrome type I, or fetal akinesia deformation sequence. Am. J. Med. Genet. 29:59, 1988.

Okamura, K., Murotsuki, J., Iwamoto, M., Endo, H., Watanabe, T., Ohashi, K. and Yajima, A.: A probable case of superfecundation. Fetal Diagn. Ther. 7:17, 1992.

Okamura, K., Murotsuki, J., Sakai, T., Matsumoto, K., Shirane, R. and Yajima, A.: Prenatal diagnosis of lissencephaly by magnetic resonance image. Fetal Diagn. Ther. 8:56, 1993.

Okazaki, J.R., Wilson, J.L., Holmes, S.M. and Vandermark, L.L.: Diprosopus: Diagnosis in utero. Am. J. Roentgenol. 149:147, 1987.

Okulski, T.A.: The prenatal diagnosis of lower urinary tract obstruction using beta scan ultrasound: A case report. J. Clin. Ultrasound. 5:268, 1977.

Old, J.M., Ward, R.H.T., Petrou, M., Karagozlu, F., Modell, B. and Weatherall, D.J.: First trimester fetal diagnosis for haemoglobinopathies: Three cases. Lancet. 2:1413, 1982.

Old, J.M., Heath, C., Fitches, A., Thein, S.L., Weatherall, D.J., Warren, R., McKenzie, C., Rodeck, C.H., Modell, B., Petrou, M. and Ward, R.H.T.: First-trimester fetal diagnosis for haemoglobinopathies: Report on 200 cases. Lancet. 2:763, 1986.

Olney, A., Andrews, R.V., Haggstrom, J.A. and Munroe, H.B.: Autosomal dominant distal arthrogryposis with short stature, normal palate, dislocated radial heads, and decreased facial expression. Proc. Greenwood Genet. Cent. 8:205, 1989a.

Olney, P.N., Izquierdo, L., Kushnir, O., Curet, B. and Olney, R.S.: Prenatal diagnosis of Noonan syndrome in a female with spontaneous resolution of cystic hygroma and hydrops. Am. J. Hum. Genet. 45(Suppl.):A265, 1989b.

Olney, P.N., Korotkin, J., Sanford Hanna, J.S., Lamb, A., Allitto, B.A., Hirsch, R. and Kupke, K.: Prenatal diagnosis of a 46,XX male with the SRY probe and FISH. Am. J. Hum. Genet. 57(Suppl.):A286, 1995.

Olson, R.W., Nishibatake, M., Arya, S. and Gilbert, E.F.: Nonimmunologic hydrops fetalis due to intrauterine closure of fetal foramen ovale. Birth Defects. 23(1):433, 1987.

Olund, A., Troell, S., Bistolette, P., Kraepelien, T. and Somell, C.: Diagnosis in utero of congenital hydrocephalus by sonography and computerized tomography. Acta Obstet. Gynaecol. Scand. 62:325, 1983.

Omenn, G.S., Hall, J.G., Graham, C.B. and Karp, L.E.: The use of radiographic visualization for prenatal diagnosis. Birth Defects. 13(3D):217, 1977.

Oorthuys, J.W.E. and Bleeker-Wagemakers, E.M.: A girl with the Pitt–Rogers–Danks syndrome. Am. J. Med. Genet. 32:140, 1989.

Opitz, J.M. and Lowry, R.B.: Lincoln vs. Douglas again: Comments on the papers by Curry et al., Greenberg et al., and Belmont et al.: Am. J. Med. Genet. 26:69, 1987.

Orimo, H., Nakajima, E., Hayashi, Z., Kijima, K., Watanabe, A., Tenjin, H., Araki, T. and Shimada, T.: First-trimester prenatal molecular diagnosis of infantile hypophosphatasia in a Japanese family. Prenat. Diagn. 16:559, 1996.

Orkin, S.H., Little, P.F.R., Kazazian, H.H., Jr., and Boehm, C.D.: Improved detection of the sickle mutation by DNA analysis. N. Engl. J. Med. 307:32, 1982.

Ornoy, A., Arnon, J., Grebner, E.E., Jackson, L.G. and Bach, G.: Early prenatal diagnosis of mucolipidosis IV. Am. J. Hum. Genet. 39(Suppl.):A261, 1986.

Ornoy, A., Arnon, J., Grebner, E.E., Jackson, L.G. and Bach, G.: Early prenatal diagnosis of mucolipidosis IV. Am. J. Med. Genet. 27:983, 1987.

Ostlere, S.J., Irving, H.C. and Lilford, R.J.: A prospective study of the incidence and significance of fetal choroid plexus cysts. Prenat. Diagn. 9:205, 1989.

Otano, L., Matayoshi, T., Lippold, S.E., Serafin, E., Scarpati, R. and Gadow, E.C.: Roberts syndrome: first trimester prenatal diagnosis by cytogenetic analysis and ultrasound in affected and non-affected fetuses. Am. J. Hum. Genet. 53:1445, 1993.

Oudejans, C.B.M., Konst, A., Mulders, M.A.M., van Vugt, J.M.G. and van Wijk, I.J.: PCR analysis of trophoblast cells enriched from the peripheral blood of pregnant women. Am. J. Hum. Genet. 57(Suppl.):A286, 1995.

Overhauser, J., Bengtsson, U., McMahon, J., Ulm, J., Butler, M.G., Santiago, L. and Wasmuth, J.J.: Prenatal diagnosis and carrier detection of a cryptic translocation by using DNA markers from the short arm of chromosome 5. Am. J. Hum. Genet. 45:296, 1989.

Ozand, P.T., Gascon, G.G., Aqeel, A.A., Nester, M.J., Feryal, R.R., Gleispach, H., Cook, J.D., Odaib, A.A. and Leis, H.J.: Prenatal detection of Canavan disease. Lancet. 337:735, 1991.

Pachi, A., Giancotti, A., Torcia, F., DeProsperi, V. and Maggi, E.: Meckel–Gruber syndrome ultrasonographic diagnosis at 13 weeks' gestational age in an at-risk case. Prenat. Diagn. 9:187, 1989.

Packman, S., Cowan, M.J., Golbus, M.S. and Caswell, N.M.: Prenatal treatment of biotin-responsive multiple carboxylase deficiency. Lancet. 1:1435, 1982.

Pagon, R.A., Stephens, T.D., McGillivray, B.C., Siebert, J.R., Wright, V.J., Hsu, L.L., Poland, B.J., Emanuel, I. and Hall, J.G.: Body wall defects with reduction limb anomalies: A report of 15 cases. Birth Defects. 15(5A):171, 1979.

Pallante, V.A., Walsh, M., Meyen, J.M., Redwine, F.O., Bodurtha, J.N., Jackson-Cook, C. and Vanner, L.: The clinical significance of fetal echogenic bowel. Am. J. Hum. Genet. 57(Suppl.):A286, 1995.

Palmer, A. and Gordon, R.R.: A critical review of intrauterine fetal transfusion. Br. J. Obstet. Gynaecol. 83:688, 1976.

Palmer, C.G., Miles, J.H., Howard-Peebles, P.N., Magenis, R.E., Patil, S. and Friedman, J.M.: Fetal karyotype following ascertainment of fetal anomalies by ultrasound. Prenat. Diagn. 7:551, 1987.

Palomaki, G.E., Haddow, J.E., Knight, G.J., Wald, N.J., Kennard, A., Canick, J.A., Saller, D.N., Jr., Blitzer, M.G., Dickerman, L.H., Fisher, R., Hansmann, D., Hansmann, M., Luthy, D.A., Summers, A.M. and Wyatt, P.: Risk-based prenatal screening for trisom 18 using alpha-fetoprotein, unconjugated oestriol and human chorionic gonadotropin. Prenat. Diagn. 15:713, 1995.

Palumbos, J.C. and Stierman, E.D.: Outcome of 86 cases of prenatally diagnosed hydrocephalus. Am. J. Hum. Genet. 45(Suppl.):A265, 1989.

Palumbos, J.C., Baty, B.J., Demsey, S.A., Cubberley, D.A. and Carey, J.C.: Fetal cystic hygroma: Implications for diagnosis and outcome. Am. J. Hum. Genet. 41(Suppl.): A282, 1987.

Pang, S. and Clark, A.: Newborn screening, prenatal diagnosis, and prenatal treatment of congenital adrenal hyperplasia due to 21-hydroxylase deficiency. Trends Endocrinol. Metab. 1:300, 1990.

Pang, S., Pollack, M.S., Loo, M., Green, O., Nussbaum, R., Clayton, G., Dupont, B. and New, M.I.: Pitfalls of prenatal diagnosis of 21-hydroxylase deficiency congenital adrenal hyperplasia. J. Clin. Endocrinol. Metab. 61:89, 1985.

Pang, S., Levine, L.S., Cederqvist, L.L., Fuentes, M., Riccardi, V.M., Holcombe, J.H., Nitowsky, H.M., Sachs, G., Anderson, C.E., Duchon, M.A., Owens, R., Merkatz, I. and New, M.E.: Amniotic fluid concentrations of delta^5 and delta^4 steroids in fetuses with congenital adrenal hyperplasia due to 21-hydroxylase deficiency and in anencephalic fetuses. J. Clin. Endocrinol. Metab. 51:223, 1986.

Pang, S., Pollack, M.S., Marshall, R.N. and Immken, L.: Prenatal treatment of congenital adrenal hyperplasia due to 21-hydroxylase deficiency. N. Engl. J. Med. 322:111, 1990.

Pang, S., Clark, A., Dolan, L. and Schulman, D.: Hormonal monitoring and side effects of prenatal dexamethasone treatment for 21-hydroxylase deficiency congenital adrenal hyperplasia. Clin. Courier. 11(11):5, 1993.

Pannone, N., Gatti, R., Lombardo, C. and Dinatale, P.: Prenatal diagnosis of Hunter syndrome using chorionic villi. Prenat. Diagn. 6:207, 1986.

Panny, S.R., Scott, A.F., Phillips, J.A., Smith, K.D., Kazazian, H.H., Charache, S. and Talbot, C.C.: Prenatal diagnosis of sickle cell disease by restriction endonuclease analysis: Limitation and advantages. Am. J. Hum. Genet. 31(Suppl.):58A, 1979.

Pao, C.C., Kao, S-M., Wang, H-C. and Lee, C.C.: Intraamniotic detection of *Chlamydia trachomatis* deoxyribonucleic acid sequences by polymerase chain reaction. Am. J. Obstet. Gynecol. 164:1295, 1991.

Paola Iampieri, M., Mingarelli, R., Le Guern, E., Novelli, G. and Dallapiccola, B.: Prenatal diagnosis of X-linked retinitis pigmentosa (RP) in five pregnancies at risk. Prenat. Diagn. 14:285, 1994.

Papenhausen, P.R., Mueller, O.T., Johnson, V.P., Sutcliffe, M., Diamond, T.M. and Kousseff, B.G.: Uniparental isodisomy of chromosome 14 in two cases: An abnormal child and a normal adult. Am. J. Med. Genet. 59:271, 1995.

Papp, Z. and Bell, J.E.: Uncultured cells in amniotic fluid from normal and abnormal foetuses. Clin. Genet. 16:282, 1979.

Papp, Z., Toth, Z., Szabo, M. and Szeifert, G.T.: Early prenatal diagnosis of cystic fibrosis by ultrasound. Clin. Genet. 28:356, 1985.

Papp, Z., Csecsei, K., Toth, Z, Polgar, K. and Szeifert, G.T.: Exencephaly in human fetuses. Clin. Genet. 30:440, 1986.

Pappas, J.G., Havens, G., Bogosian, V., Bhatt, J., Paka, D., Babu, A. and Penchaszadeh, V.B.: Trisomy 2 mosaicism. Am. J. Hum. Genet. 57(Suppl.):A286, 1995.

Park, H.K., Kay, H.H., McConkie-Rosell, A., Lanman, J. and Chen Y-T.: Prenatal diagnosis of Pompe's disease (type II glycogenosis) in chorionic villus biopsy using maltose as a substrate. Prenat. Diagn. 12:169, 1992.

Park, V.M., Bravo, R.R. and Shulman, L.P.: Double non-disjunction in maternal meiosis II giving rise to a fetus with 48,XXX, + 21. J. Med. Genet. 32:650, 1995.

Parvy, P., Rabier, D., Boue, J., Saudubray, J.M. and Kamoun, P.: Glycine/serine ratio and the prenatal diagnosis of nonketotic hyperglycinaemia. Prenat. Diagn. 10:303, 1990.

Patel, R.B., Gibson, J.Y., D'Cruz, C.A. and Burkhalter, J.L.: Sonographic diagnosis of cervical teratoma in utero. Am. J. Roentgenol. 139:1220, 1982.

Patel, Z.M., Shah, H.L., Madon, P.F. and Ambani, L.M.: Prenatal diagnosis of lethal osteogenesis imperfecta (OI) by ultrasonography. Prenat. Diagn. 3:261, 1983.

Patil, S.R., Weiner, C. and Williamson, R.: Rapid chromosome analysis and prenatal diagnosis using fluid from cystic hygromas. N. Engl. J. Med. 317:1159, 1987.

Patrick, J.E., Perry, T.B. and Kinch, R.A.H.: Fetoscopy and fetal blood sampling: A percutaneous approach. Am. J. Obstet. Gynecol. 119:539, 1974.

Patrick, A.D., Willcox, P., Stephens, R. and Kenyon, V.G.: Prenatal diagnosis of Wolman's disease. J. Med. Genet. 13:49, 1976.

Patrick, A.D., Young, E., Kleijer, W.J. and Niermeijer, M.F.: Prenatal diagnosis of Niemann–Pick disease type A using chromogenic substrate. Lancet. 2:144, 1977.

Patrick, A.D., Young, E.P. and Mossman, J.: First trimester diagnosis of cystinosis using intact chorionic villi. Prenat. Diagn. 7:71, 1987.

Patrick, A.D., Young, E., Ellis, C. and Rodeck, C.H.: Multiple sulphatase deficiency: Prenatal diagnosis using chorionic villi. Prenat. Diagn. 8:303, 1988.

Patten, R.M., Van Allen, M., Mack, L.A., Wilson, D., Nyberg, D., Hirsch, J. and Viamont, T.: Limb–body wall complex: In utero sonographic diagnosis of a complicated fetal malformation. Am. J. Roentgenogr. 146:1019, 1986.

Patterson, J.A., Gold, W.R., Jr., Sanz, L.E. and McCullough, D.C.: Antenatal evaluation of fetal hydrocephalus with computer tomography. Am. J. Obstet. Gynecol. 140:344, 1981.

Patton, M.A., Baraitser, M., Nickolaides, K., Rodeck, C.H. and Gamsu, H.: Prenatal treatment of fetal hydrops associated with the hypertelorism-dysphagia syndrome (Opitz-G syndrome). Prenat. Diagn. 6:109, 1986.

Payne, G. Jr., and Robie, G.: Selective hysterotomy birth of acardiac acephalic fetus. Am. J. Hum. Genet. 43(Suppl.):A243, 1988.

Payne, S.J., Maher, E.R., Barton, D.E., Bentley, E., McMahon, R., Quarrell, O.W.J. and Ferguson-Smith, M.A.: Prenatal diagnosis in von Hippel–Lindau disease. J. Med. Genet. 28:282, 1992.

Peake, I.R., Bowen, D., Bignell, P., Liddel, M.B., Sadler, J.E., Standen, G. and Bloom, A.L.: Family studies and prenatal diagnosis in severe von Willebrand disease by polymerase chain reaction amplification of a variable number tandem repeat region of the von Willebrand factor gene. Blood. 76:555, 1990.

Pearce, J.M., Griffin, D. and Campbell, S.: Cystic hygromata in trisomy 18 and 21. Prenat. Diagn. 4:371, 1984.

Pearl, W.: Cardiac malformations presenting as congenital atrial flutter. South. Med. J. 70:622, 1977.

Peeden, J.N., Jr., Rimoin, D.L., Lachman, R.S., Dyer, M.I., Gerard, D. and Gruber, H.E.: Spondylometaphyseal dysplasia, Sedaghatian type. Am. J. Med. Genet. 44:651, 1992.

Pekonen, F., Teramo, K., Makinen, T., Ikonen, E., Osterlund, K. and Lamberg, B.A.: Prenatal diagnosis and treatment of fetal thyrotoxicosis. Am. J. Obstet. Gynecol. 150:893, 1984.

Pekrun, A., Neubauer, B.A., Eber, S.W., Lakomek, M., Seidel, H. and Schroter, W.: Triosephosphate isomerase deficiency: Biochemical and molecular genetic analysis for prenatal diagnosis. Clin. Genet. 47:175, 1995.

Peled, Y., Hod, M., Friedman, S., Mashiach, R., Greenberg, N. and Ovadia, J.: Prenatal diagnosis of familial congenital pyloric atresia. Prenat. Diagn. 12:151, 1992.

Pembrey, M.E., Old, J.M., Leonard, J.V., Rodeck, C.H., Warren, R. and Davies, K.E.: Prenatal diagnosis of ornithine carbamoyl transferase deficiency using a gene specific probe. J. Med. Genet. 22:462, 1985.

Pena, S.D.J., Reis, D.D., Prado, V.F. and Farah, L.M.S.: Decreased levels of a 36,000 glycoprotein in the amniotic fluid from pregnancies of fetuses affected with Down syndrome. Am. J. Hum. Genet. 45(Suppl.):A265, 1989.

Penchaszadeh, V.B., Uppal, V.L., Costales, F., Zinberg, R. and Babu, A.: Prenatal diagnosis of campomelic dysplasia, short-limb type, and trisomy 21 in the same fetus. Am. J. Hum. Genet. 41(Suppl.):A283, 1987.

Penketh, R.J.A., Delhanty, J.D.A., Van Den Berghe, J.A., Finklestone, E.M., Handyside, A.H., Malcolm, S. and Winston, R.M.L.: Rapid sexing of human embryos by non-radioactive in-situ hybridization: Potential for preimplantation diagnosis of X-linked disorders. Prenat. Diagn. 9:489, 1989.

Penn, D. Schmidt-Sommerfeld, E., Jakobs, C. and Bieber, L.L.: Amniotic fluid propionylcarnitine in methylmalonic aciduria. J. Inher. Metab. Dis. 10:376, 1987.

Pennell, R.G. and Baltarowich, O.H.: Prenatal sonographic diagnosis of a fetal hemangioma. J. Ultrasound Med. 5:525, 1986.

Pepper, A.E., Middleton, L.A., I. Isakov and Puck, J.M.: Implementation of molecular prenatal and carrier diagnosis for X-linked severe combined immunodeficiency. Am. J. Hum. Genet. 57(Suppl.):A50, 1995.

Pereira, R.R. and Hasaart, T.: Hydramnios and observations in Bartter's syndrome. Acta Obstet. Gynecol. Scand. 61:477, 1982.

Perez-Cerda, C., Merinero, B., Sanz, P., Jimenez, A., Garcia, M.J., Urbon, A., Diaz Recasens, J., Ramos, C., Ayuso, C. and Ugarte, M.: Successful first trimester diagnosis in a pregnancy at risk for propionic acidaemia. J. Inher. Metab. Dis. 12(Suppl. 2):274, 1989.

Perez-Cerda, C., Merinero, B., Jimenez, A., Garcia, M.J., Sanz, P., Ulst, L., Wanders, R.J.A. and Ugarte, M.: First report of prenatal diagnosis of long-chain 3-hydroxyacyl-CoA dehydrogenase deficiency in a pregnancy at risk. Prenat. Diagn. 13:529, 1993.

Perlman, J.M., Burns, D.K., Twickler, D.M. and Weinberg, A.G.: Fetal hypokinesia syndrome in the monochorionic pair of a triplet pregnancy secondary to severe disruptive cerebral injury. Pediatrics. 96:521, 1995.

Perry, T.B., Holbrook, K.A., Hoff, M.S., Hamilton, E.F., Senikas, S. and Fisher, C.: Prenatal diagnosis of congenital non-bullous ichthyosiform erythroderma (lamellar ichthyosis). Prenat. Diagn. 7:145, 1987

Persutte, W.H., Kurczynski, T.W., Chaudhuri, K., Lenke, R.R., Woldenberg, L., and Brinker, R.A.: Prenatal diagnosis of autosomal dominant microcephaly and postnatal evaluation with magnetic resonance imaging. Prenat. Diagn. 10:631, 1990.

Pescia, G., Cruz, J.M. and Weihs, D.: Prenatal diagnosis of prune belly syndrome by means of raised maternal AFP levels. J. Genet. Hum. 30:271, 1982.

Pescia, G., Nguyen-The, H. and Deonna, T.: Prenatal diagnosis of genetic microcephaly. Prenat. Diagn. 3:363, 1983.

Pesonen, E., Haavisto, H., Ammala, P. and Teramo, K.: Intrauterine hydrops caused by premature closure of the foramen ovale. Arch. Dis. Child. 58:1015, 1983.

Peters, M.T. and Nicolaides, K.H.: Cordocentesis for the diagnosis and treatment of human fetal parvovirus infection. Obstet. Gynecol. 75:501, 1990.

Peters-Brown, T., Fry-Mehltretter, L., Decker-Phillips, M., Kahler, S.G. and Oumsiyeh, M.B.: Mild phenotype in a prenatally diagnosed case with de novo deletion for terminal 18q. Am. J. Hum. Genet. 57(Suppl.):A347, 1995.

Petrella, R., Rabinowitz, J.G., Steinmann, B. and Hirschhorn, K.: Long-term follow-up of two sibs with Larsen syndrome possible due to parental germ-line mosaicism. Am. J. Med. Genet. 47:187, 1993.

Petres, R.E. and Redwine, F.: Selective birth in twin pregnancy. N. Engl. J. Med. 305:1218, 1981.

Petres, R.E., Redwine, F.O. and Cruikshank, D.P.: Congenital bilateral chylothorax: Antepartum diagnosis and successful intrauterine surgical management. J. Am. Med. Assoc. 248:1360, 1982.

Petrikovsky, B.M., Nochimson, D.J., Campbell, W.A. and Vintzileos, A.M.: Fetal jejunoileal atresia with persistent omphalomesenteric duct. Am. J. Obstet. Gynecol. 158:173, 1988.

Pettit, B.R., King, G.S. and Blau, K.: Low glucose concentrations in amniotic fluids from anencephalic pregnancies. Lancet. 2:1288, 1977.

Pettit, B.R., Kvittingen, E.A. and Leonard, J.V.: Early prenatal diagnosis of hereditary tyrosinaemia. Lancet. 1:1038, 1985.

Petushkova, N.A.: First-trimester diagnosis of an unusual case of alpha-mannosidosis. Prenat. Diagn. 11:279, 1991.

Pfeiffer, R.A., Stoss, H., Voight, H.J. and Wundisch, G.F.: Absence of fibula and ulna with oligodactyly, contractures, right-angle bowing of femora, abnormal facial morphology, cleft lip/palate and brain malformation in two sibs: A possibly new lethal syndrome. Am. J. Med. Genet. 29:901, 1988.

Phadke, M.A., Kate, S.L., Mokashi, G.D., Khedkar, V.A. and Joshi, A.S.: Prenatal diagnosis of thalassaemia major. Lancet. 2:1143, 1979.

Phelan, M.C., Stevenson, R.E. and Schroer, R.J.: Double autosomal aneuploidy: 48,XY,+inv dup(15),+18. Proc. Greenwood Genet. Cent. 8:33, 1989.

Phelps-Sandall, B., Clark, R.D., Chun, N. and Berman, N.: Prenatal diagnosis of gastroschisis is associated with reduced morbidity. Am. J. Hum. Genet. 45(Suppl.):A266, 1989.

Philip, N., Guala, A., Moncla, A., Monlouis, M., Ayme, S. and Giraud, F.: Cerebrofaciothoracic dysplasia: A new family. J. Med. Genet. 29:497, 1992.

Philipson, E.H., Sokol, R.J. and Williams, T.: Oligohydramnios: Clinical associations and predictive value for intrauterine growth retardation. Am. J. Obstet. Gynecol. 146:271, 1983.

Phillips, D.G., Kazazian, H.H., Scott, A.F., Toole, J.J. and Antonarakis, S.E.: Hemophilia A: Experience with prenatal diagnosis using DNA analysis. Am. J. Hum. Genet. 37(Suppl.): A224, 1985.

Phillips, O.P., Tharapel, A.T., Park, V.M., Wachtel, S.S. and Shulman, L.P.: Risk of fetal mosaicism when placental mosaisism is diagnosed by chorionic villus sampling. Am. J. Hum. Genet. 57(Suppl.):A287, 1995.

Piceni Sereni, L.P., Bachmann, C., Pfister, U., Buscaglia, M. and Nicolini, U.: Prenatal diagnosis of carbamoyl-phosphate synthetase deficiency by fetal liver biopsy. Prenat. Diagn. 8:307, 1988.

Piepkorn, M., Karp, L.E., Hickok, D., Wiegenstein, L. and Hall, J.G.: A lethal neonatal dwarfing condition with short ribs, polysyndactyly, cranial synostosis, cleft palate, cardiovascular and urogenital anomalies and severe ossification defect. Teratology. 16:345, 1977.

Pierce, P., McGillivray, B. and Wittmann, B.K.: Ultrasound findings in triploid pregnancy. Am. J. Hum. Genet. 36(Suppl.):196S, 1984.

Pijpers, L., Jahods, M.G.J., Reuss, A., Sachs, E.S., Los, F.J. and Wladimiroff, J.W.: Selective birth in a dyzygotic twin pregnancy with discordancy for Down's syndrome. Fetal Ther. 4:58, 1989a.

Pijpers, L., Reuss, A., Stewart, P.A. and Wladimiroff, J.W.: Noninvasive management of isolated bilateral fetal hydrothorax. Am. J. Obstet. Gynecol. 161:330, 1989b.

Pijpers, L., Kleijer, W.J., Reuss, A., Jahoda, M.G.J., Los, F.J., Sachs, E.S. and Wladimiroff, J.W.: Transabdominal chorionic villus sampling in a multiple pregnancy at risk of argininosuccinic aciduria: A case report. Am. J. Med. Genet. 36:449, 1990.

Pilu, G., Reece, E.A., Romero, R., Bovicelli, L. Hobbins, J.C.: Prenatal diagnosis of craniofacial malformations with ultrasonography. Am. J. Obstet. Gynecol. 155:45, 1986.

Pilu, G., Romero, R., Rizzo, N., Jeanty, P., Bovicelli, L. and Hobbins, J.C.: Criteria for the prenatal diagnosis of holoprosencephaly. Am. J. Perinatol. 4:41, 1987.

Pina-Neto, J.M., Defino, H.L.A., Guedes, M.L. and Jorge, S.M.: Spondyloepimetaphyseal dysplasia with joint laxity (SEMDJL): A Brazilian case. Am. J. Med. Genet. 61:131, 1996.

Pirastu, M., Ristaldi, M.S. and Cao, A.: Prenatal diagnosis of beta-thalassaemia based on restriction endonuclease analysis of amplified fetal DNA. J. Med. Genet. 26:363, 1989.

Plant, R.K., and Steven R.A.: Complete A-V block in a fetus. Am. Heart. J. 30:615, 1945.

Platt, L.D., Keegan, K.A., Druzin, M.L., Gauthier, R.J., Evertson, L.R. and Manning F.A.: Intrauterine transfusion utilizing linear-array, real-time B scan: A preliminary report. Am. J. Obstet. Gynecol. 135:1115, 1979a.

Platt, L.D., Manning, F.A., Gray, C., Guttenburg, M. and Turkel, S.B.: Antenatal detection of fetal A-V dissociation utilizing real-time B-mode ultrasound. Obstet. Gynecol. 3:Suppl: 59S, 1979b.

Platt, L.D., Geierman, C.A., Turkel, S.B., Young, G. and Keegan, K.A.: Atrial hemangioma and hydrops fetalis. Am. J. Obstet. Gynecol. 141:107, 1981.

Platt, L.D., Golde, S.H., Artal, R., Frohlich, G., Alfi, O. and Ng, W.G.: False negative maternal serum alpha-fetoprotein determinations in myelodysplasia: The role of ultrasound. Am. J. Obstet. Gynecol. 144:352, 1982.

Platt, L.D., DeVore, G.R., Bieniarz, A., Benner, P. and Rao, R.: Antenatal diagnosis of acephalus acardia: A proposed management scheme. Am. J. Obstet. Gynecol. 146:857, 1983.

Platt, L.D., DeVore, G.R., Horenstein, J., Pavlova, Z., Kovacs, B. and Falk, R.E.: Prenatal diagnosis of tuberous sclerosis: The use of fetal echocardiography. Prenat. Diagn. 7:407, 1987.

Platt, L.D., Medearis, A.L., Horenstein, J., Devore, G.R., Carlson, D., Falk, R., Wassman, E.R. and Alfi, O.S.: Down syndrome screening with ultrasound appears premature. Am. J. Hum. Genet. 43(Suppl.):A244, 1988.

Plattner, G., Renner, W., Went, J., Beaudette, L. and Viau, G.: Fetal sex determination by ultrasound scan in the second and third trimesters. Obstet. Gynecol. 61:454, 1983.

Pletcher, B.A., Friedes, J.S., Breg, W.R. and Touloukian, R.J.: Familial occurrence of esophageal atresia with and without tracheoesophageal fistula: Report of two unusual kindreds. Am. J. Med. Genet. 39:380, 1991.

Poenaru, L., Dreyfus, J-C., Boue, J., Nicolesco, H.., Ravise, N. and Bamberger, J.: Prenatal diagnosis of fucosidosis. Clin. Genet. 10:260, 1976.

Poenaru, L., Girard, S., Thepot, F., Madelenat, P., Huraux-Rendu, C., Vinet, M.-C. and Dreyfus, J.-C.: Antenatal diagnosis of three pregnancies at risk for mannosidosis. Clin. Genet. 16:428, 1979.

Poenaru, L., Castelnau, L., Dumez, Y. and Thepot, F.: First trimester prenatal diagnosis of mucolipidosis II (I-cell disease) by chorionic biopsy. Am. J. Hum. Genet. 36:1379, 1984.

Poenaru, L., Castelnau, L, Besancon, A-M., Nicolesco, H., Akli, S. and Theophil, D.: First trimester prenatal diagnosis of metachromatic leukodystrophy on chorionic villi by 'immunoprecipitation-electrophoresis'. J. Inher. Metab. Dis. 11:123, 1988.

Poenaru, L., Mezard, C., Akli, S., Oury, J.-F., Dumez, Y. and Boue, J.: Prenatal diagnosis of mucolipidosis type II on first-trimester amniotic fluid. Prenat. Diagn. 10:231, 1990.

Polanska, N., Burgess, D.E., Hill, P., Bensted, J.P.M. and Landells, W.M.: Screening for neural tube defect: False positive findings on ultrasound and in amniotic fluid. Br. Med. J. 2:24, 1983.

Polgar, K., Sipka, S., Abel, G. and Papp, Z.: Neutral-red uptake by amniotic-fluid macrophages in neural-tube defects: A rapid test. N. Engl. J. Med. 310:1463, 1984.

Pollack, M.S., Maurer, D., Levine, L.S., New, M.I., Pang, S., Duchon, M., Owens, R.P., Merkatz, I.R., Nitowsky, H.M., Sachs, G. and Dupont, B.: Prenatal diagnosis of congenital adrenal hyperplasia (21-hydroxylase deficiency) by HLA typing. Lancet. 1:1107, 1979.

Pollack, M.S., Ochs, H.D. and Dupont, B.: HLA typing of cultured amniotic cells for the prenatal diagnosis of complement C4 deficiency. Clin. Genet. 18:197, 1980a.

Pollack, M.S., Schafer, I.A., Barford, D. and Dupont, B.: Prenatal identification of paternity: HLA typing helpful after rape. J. Am. Med. Assoc. 244:1954, 1980b.

Pollitt, R.J., Manning, N.J., Olpin, S.E. and Young, I.D.: Prenatal diagnosis of a defect in medium-chain fatty acid oxidation. J. Inher. Metab. Dis. 17:279, 1994.

Poll-The, B.T., Poulos, A., Sharp, P., Boue, J., Ogier, H., Odievre, M. and Saudubray, J.M.: Antenatal diagnosis of infantile Refsum's disease. Clin. Genet. 27:524, 1985.

Poll-The, B.T., Saudubray, J.M., Rocchiccioli, F., Scotto, J., Roels, F., Boue, J., Ogier, H., Dumez, Y., Wanders, R.J.A., Schutgens, R.B.H., Schram, A.W. and Tager, J.M.: Prenatal diagnosis and confirmation of infantile Refsum's disease. J. Inherit. Metab. Dis. 10(Suppl. 2):229, 1987.

Pons, J-C., Rozenberg, F., Imbert, M-C., Lebon, P., Olivennes, F., Lelaidier, C., Strub, N., Vial, M. and Frydman, R.: Prenatal diangosis of second-trimester congenital varicella syndrome. Prenat. Diagn. 12:975, 1992.

Poor, M.A., Alberti, O., Jr., Griscom, N.T., Driscoll, S.G. and Holmes, L.B.: Nonskeletal malformations in one of three siblings with Jarcho–Levin syndrome of vertebral anomalies. J. Pediatr. 103:270, 1983.

Porreco, R.P., Matson, M.R., Young, P.E., Bradshaw, C., Leopold, G. and Jones, O.W.: Diagnosis of a triploid fetus at genetic amniocentesis. Obstet. Gynecol. 56:115, 1980.

Potier, M., Dallaire, L. and Malancon, S.B.: Prenatal detection of intestinal obstruction by disaccharidase assay in amniotic fluid. Lancet. 2:982, 1977.

Potocki, L., Abuelo, D.N. and Oyer, C.E.: Cardiac malformation in two infants with hypochondrogenesis. Am. J. Med. Genet. 59:295, 1995.

Poulain, P., Odent, S., Maire, I., Milon, J., Proudhon, F.J., Jouan, H. and Le Marec, B.: Fetal ascites and oligohydramnios: Prenatal diagnosis of a sialic acid storage disease (index case). Prenat. Diagn. 15:864, 1995.

Poulos, A., van Crugten, C., Sharp, P., Carey, W.F., Robertson, E., Becroft, D.M.O., Saudubray, J.M., Poll-The, B.T., Christensen, E. and Brandt, N.: Prenatal diagnosis of Zellweger syndrome and related disorders: Impaired degradation of phytanic acid. Eur. J. Pediatr. 145:507, 1986.

Powell, I.C.: Intense plasmapheresis in the pregnant Rh-sensitized woman. Am. J. Obstet. Gynecol. 101:153, 1968.

Powledge, T.M. and Fletcher, J.: Guidelines for the ethical, social, and legal issues in prenatal diagnosis. N. Engl. J. Med. 300:168, 1979.

Preus, M., Kaplan, P. and Kirkham, T.H.: Renal anomalies and oligohydramnios in the cerebro-oculofacio-skeletal syndrome. Am. J. Dis. Child., 131:62, 1977.

Proesmans, W., Massa, G., Vandenberghe, K. and Van Assche, A.: Prenatal diagnosis of Bartter syndrome. Lancet. 1:394, 1987.

Purvis-Smith, S.G., Laing, S., Sutherland, G.R. and Baker, E.: Prenatal diagnosis of the fragile X—The Australasian experience. Am. J. Med. Genet. 30:337, 1988.

Quagliarello, J.R., Passalaqua, A.M., Greco, M.A., Zinberg, S. and Young, B.K.: Ballantyne's triple edema syndrome: Prenatal diagnosis with ultrasound and maternal renal biopsy findings. Am. J. Obstet. Gynecol. 132:580, 1978.

Quan, L. and Smith, D.W.: The VATER association, vertebral defects, anal atresia, T-E fistula with esophageal atresia, radial and renal dysplasia: A spectrum of associated defects. J. Pediatr. 82:104, l973.

Queenan, J.T.: Intrauterine transfusion: A cooperative study. Am. J. Obstet. Gynecol. 104: 397, 1969.

Queenan, J.T. and Adams, D.W.: Amniocentesis for prenatal diagnosis of erythroblastosis fetalis. Obstet. Gynecol. 25:302, 1965.

Queenan, J.T. and Douglas, R.G.: Intrauterine transfusion: A preliminary report. Obstet. Gynecol. 25:308, 1965.

Queenan, J.T. and Gadow, E.C.: Amniography for detection of congenital malformations. Obstet. Gynecol. 35:648, 1970.

Queenan, J.T. and Wyatt, R.H.: Intrauterine transfusion of fetus for severe erythroblastosis fetalis. Am. J. Obstet. Gynecol. 92:375, 1965.

Quigg, M.H., Evans, M.I., Zador, E.I., Budeu, I, Belsky, R., Niederlucke, D. and Nadler, H.L.: Ultrasonographic prenatal diagnosis of Langer-type mesomelic dwarfism. Am. J. Hum. Genet. 37(Suppl.):A225, 1985.

Quinlan, R.W., Cruz, A.C. and Martin, M.: Hydramnios: Ultrasound diagnosis and its impact on perinatal management and pregnancy outcome. Am. J. Obstet. Gynecol. 145:306, 1983.

Qumsiyeh, M.B., Tomasi, A. Taslimi, M.: Prenatal detection of short arm deletion and isochromosome 18 formation investigated by molecular techniques. J. Med. Genet. 32:991, 1995.

Qureshi, F. Jacques, S.M., Johnson, S.F., Johnson, M.P., Hume, R.F., Evans, M.I. and Yang, S.S.: Histopathology of fetal diastrophic dysplasia. Am. J. Med. Genet. 56:300, 1995.

Raas-Rothschild, A., Goodman, R.M., Meyer, S., Katznelson, M.B.-M., Winter, S.T., Gross, E., Tamarkin, M., Ben-Ami, T., Nebel, L. and Mashiach, S.: Pathological features and prenatal diagnosis in the newly recognised limb/pelvis-hypoplasia/aplasia syndrome. J. Med. Genet. 25:687, 1988.

Rabe, H., Brune, T., Rossi, R., Steinhorst, V., Jorch, G., Horst, J. and Wittwer, B.: Yunis–Varon syndrome: the first case of German origin. Clin. Dysmorph. 5:217, 1996.

Rajendra, B.R., Trabilcy, E.T., Manchigiah, K., Leinen, J. and Knight, G.: MS-AFP assay sensitivity and the detection of pregnancies at-risk for Down's syndrome. Am. J. Hum. Genet. 39(Suppl.):A263, 1986.

Raghunath, M., Steinmann, B., Delozier-Blanchet, C., Extermann, P. and Superti-Furga, A: Prenatal diagnosis of collagen disorders by direct biochemical analysis of chorionic villus biopsies. Pediatr. Res. 36:441, 1994.

Ram, S.P. and Noor, A.R.: Neonatal Proteus syndrome. Am. J. Med. Genet. 47:303, 1993.

Ramos, F.J., McDonald-McGinn, D.M., Emanuel, B.S. and Zackai, E.H.: Tricho-rhino-phalangeal syndrome type II (Langer–Giedion) with persistent cloaca and prune belly sequence in a girl with 8q interstitial deletion. Am. J. Med. Genet. 44:790, 1992.

Ramsden, G.H., Johnson, P.M., Hart, C.A. and Farquharson, R.G.: Listeriosis in immunocompromised pregnancy. Lancet. 1:794, 1989.

Ramzin, M.S. and Napflin, S.: Transient intrauterine supraventricular tachycardia associated with transient hydrops fetalis. Case report. Br. J. Obstet. Gynaecol. 89:965, 1982.

Randel, S.B., Filly, R.A., Callen, P.W., Anderson, R.L., and Golbus, M.S.: Amniotic sheets. Radiology. 166:633, 1988.

Rantamaki, T., Raghunath, M., Karttunen, L., Lonnqvist, L., Child, A. and Peltonen, L.: Prenatal diagnosis of Marfan syndrome: Identification of a fibrillin-1 mutation in chorionic villus sample. Prenat. Diagn. 15:1176, 1995.

Rao, K.W. and Atkin, J.F.: Low maternal serum alpha-fetoprotein and de novo structural rearrangements. Am. J. Hum. Genet. 43(Suppl.):A244, 1988.

Rapola, J., Salonen, R., Ammala, P. and Santavuori, P.: Prenatal diagnosis of infantile type of neuronal ceroid lipofuscinosis. Am. J. Hum. Genet. 43(Suppl.):A245, 1988.

Rapola, J., Salonen, R. Ammala, P. and Santavuori, P.: Prental diagnosis of the infantile type of neuronal ceroid lipofuscinosis by electron microscopic investigation of human chorionic villi. Prenat. Diagn. 10:553, 1990.

Rapola, J. Salonen, R., Ammala, P. and Santavuori, P.: Prenatal diagnosis of infantile neuronal ceroid-lipofuscinosis, INCL: Morphological aspects. J. Inher. Metab. Dis. 16:349, 1993.

Rasmussen, S.A., Bieber, F.R., Benacerraf, B.R., Lachman, R.S., Rimoin, D.L. and Holmes, L.B.: Epidemiology of osteochondrodysplasias: Changing trends due to advances in prenatal diagnosis. Am. J. Med. Genet. 61:49, 1996.

Rattazzi, M.C. and Davidson, R.G.: Prenatal diagnosis of metachromatic leukodystrophy by electrophoretic and immunologic techniques. Pediatr. Res. 11:1030, 1977.

Rattenbury, J.M., Blau, K., Sandler, M., Pryse-Davies, J., Clark, P.J. and Pooley, S.S.F.: Prenatal diagnosis of hypophosphatasia. Lancet. 1:306, 1976.

Raux-Demay, M., Mornet, E., Boue, J., Couillin, P., Oury, J.F., Ravise, N., Deluchat, C. and Boue, A.: Early prenatal diagnosis of 21-hydroxylase deficiency using amniotic fluid 17-hydroxyprogesterone determination and DNA probes. Prenat. Diagn. 9:457, 1989.

Ravia, Y., Nakash, Y., Shaki, R., Barkai, G. and Goldman, B.: Analysis of fetal cells in maternal blood by PCR. Am. J. Hum. Genet. 57(Suppl.):A287, 1995.

Rawnsley, E.R., Simmons, G.M., Graham, J.M., Jr., and Crow, H.C.: Prenatal diagnosis of X-linked hydrocephalus. Am. J. Hum. Genet. 37(Suppl.):A135, 1985.

Rawnsley, B.E., Charman, C.E., Crow, H. and Graham, J.M.: Prenatal diagnosis of Jeune syndrome. Am. J. Hum. Genet. 39:A263, 1986.

Rawnsley, E., Edwards, M.J. and Graham, J.M., Jr.: Cystic hygroma and lethal multiple pterygia. Am. J. Hum. Genet. 43(Suppl.):A245, 1988.

Ray, J.H., Sanz, M.M. Schlessel, J.S., Kunaporn, S., McKenna, C., Bialer, M.G., Alonso, M.L., Zaslav, A.L., Brown, W.T. and Pletcher, B.A.: Trisomy 16 mosaicism: Postnatal confirmation of two prenatally diagnosed cases in phenotypically abnormal liveborns. Am. J. Hum. Genet. 53(Suppl.):1452, 1993.

Rayburn, W.F.: Fetal drug therapy: An overview of selected conditions. Obstet. Gynecol. Surv. 47:1, 1991.

Raymond, J.J. and Simpson, N.E.: Acetylcholinesterase in amniotic fluid and open neural tube defects: Five years experience as a Canadian referral centre. Am. J. Hum. Genet. 43(Suppl.):A245, 1988.

Read, A.P., Fennell, S.J., Donnai, D. and Harris, R.: Amniotic fluid acetylcholinesterase: A retrospective and prospective study of the qualitative method. Br. J. Obstet. Gynaecol. 89:111, 1982a.

Read, A.P., Donnai, D. and Brandreth, C.: Abnormalities of the umbilical cord or membranes leading to raised amniotic AFP. J. Med. Genet. 19:64, 1982b.

Read, A.P., Donnai, D., Tracey, J. and Fennell, S.J.: Increased amniotic alpha-fetoprotein due to a holoacardium amorphous twin. Clin. Genet. 21:382, 1982c.

Reardon, W., Hockey, A., Silberstein, P., Kendall, B., Farag, T.I., Swash, M., Stevenson, R. and Baraitser, M.: Autosomal recessive congenital intrauterine infection-like syndrome of microcephaly, intracranial calcification, and CNS disease. Am. J. Med. Genet. 52:58, 1994.

Reddy, K.S., Stetten, G., Corson, V.L., Escallon, C.S., Cooper, L.F. and Blakemore, K.J.: Interpreting chromosomal mosaicism in chorionic villus samples (CVS). Am. J. Hum. Genet. 45(Suppl.):A267, 1989.

Redford, D.H.A., McNay, M.B., Ferguson-Smith, M.E. and Jamieson, M.E.: Aneuploidy and cystic hygroma detectable by ultrasound. Prenat. Diagn. 4:377, 1984.

Redwine, F.O. and Hays, P.M.: Selective birth. Semin. Perinatol. 10:73, 1986.

Redwine, F.O. and Petres, R.E.: Selective birth in a case of twins discordant for Tay Sachs disease. Acta Genet. Med. Gemellol. 33:35, 1984.

Redwine, P.O., Wright, L.E., Hays, P.M., Bodurtha, J.N. and Urick, C.: Low maternal serum alpha feto protein as in indication for genetic amniocentesis. Am. J. Hum. Genet. 43(Suppl.):A246, 1988.

Reece, E.A., Lockwook, C.J., Rizzo, N., Pilu, G., Bovicelli, L. and Hobbins, J.C.: Intrinsic intrathoracic malformations of the fetus: Sonographic detection and clinical presentation. Obstet. Gynecol. 70:627, 1987.

Reeders, S.T., Gal, A., Propping, P., Waldherr, R., Davies, K.E., Zerres, K., Hogenkamp, T., Schmidt, W., Dolata, M.M. and Weatherall, D.J.: Prenatal diagnosis of autosomal dominant polycystic kidney disease with a DNA probe. Lancet. 2:6, 1986.

Regec, S.P. and Bernstine, R.L.: Hydranencephaly in a twin gestation. Obstet. Gynecol. 54:369, 1979.

Rehder, H. and Labbe, F.: Prenatal morphology in Meckel's syndrome (with special reference to polycystic kidneys and double encephalocele). Prenat. Diagn. 1:161, 1981.

Reid, R.L., Pancham, S.R., Kean, W.F. and Ford, P.M.: Maternal and neonatal implications of congenital complete heart block in the fetus. Obstet. Gynecol. 54:470, 1979.

Rein, A.J.J.T., Lotan, C., Goiten, K.J. and Simcha, A.: Severe hydrops fetalis due to congenital supraventricular tachycardia. Eur. J. Pediatr. 144:511, 1986.

Reindollar, R.H., Lewis, J.B. White, P.C., Fernhoff, P.M., McDonough, P.G. and Whitney, J.B.: Prenatal diagnosis of 21-hydroxylase deficiency by the complementary deoxyribonucleic acid probe for cytochrome $P\text{-}450_{C\text{-}21OH}$. Am. J. Obstet. Gynecol. 158:545, 1988.

Reish, O., Berry, S.A. and Hirsch, B.: Partial monosomy of chromosome 1p36.3: Characterization of the critical region and delineation of a syndrome. Am. J. Med. Genet. 59:467, 1995.

Remes, A.M., Rantala, H., Hiltunen, J.K., Leisti, J. and Ruokonen, A.: Fumarase deficiency: Two siblings with enlarged cerebral ventricles and polyhydramnios in utero. Pediatrics. 89:730, 1992.

Renlund, M. and Aula, P.: Prenatal detection of Salla disease based upon increased free sialic acid in amniocytes. Am. J. Med. Genet. 28:377, 1987.

Reuss, A., Pijpers, L., Schampers, P.T.F.M., Wladimiroff, J.W. and Sachs, E.S.: The importance of chorionic villus sampling after first trimester diagnosis of cystic hygroma. Prenat. Diagn. 7:299, 1987a.

Reuss, A., Wladimiroff, J.W., Pijpers, L. and Provoost, A.P.: Fetal urinary electrolytes in bladder outlet obstruction. Fetal Ther. 2:148, 1987b.

Reuss, A., Wladimiroff, J.W., Scholtmeijer, R.J., Stewart, P.A., Sauer, P.J.J. and Niermeijer, M.F.: Prenatal evaluation and outcome of fetal obstructive uropathies. Prenat. Diagn. 8:93, 1988.

Reuss, A., den Hollander, J.C., Niermeijer, M.F., Wladimiroff, J.W., van Diggelen, O.P., Lindhout, D. and Los, F.J.: Prenatal diagnosis of cystic kidney disease with ventriculomegaly: A report of six cases in two related sibships. Am. J. Med. Genet. 33:385, 1989.

Reuter, K.L. and Lebowitz, R.L.: Massive vesicoureteral reflux mimicking posterior urethral valves in a fetus. J. Clin. Ultrasound 13:584, 1985.

Reuwer, P.J.H.M., Sijmons, E.A., Rietman, G.W., van Tiel, M.W.M. and Bruinse, H.W.: Intrauterine growth retardation: Prediction of perinatal distress by Doppler ultrasound. Lancet. 2:415, 1987.

Rey, E., Duperron, L., Gauthier, R., Lemay, M., Grignon, A. and LeLorier, J.: Transplacental treatment of tachycardia-induced fetal heart failure with verapamil and amiodarone: A case report. Am. J. Obstet. Gynecol. 153:311, 1985.

Reynolds, J.F. and Waldstein, G.: Aprosencephaly: Case report with neuropathology and review of the embryology. Proc. Greenwood Genet. Cent. 8:208, 1989.

Richardson, R.J. and Kirk, J.M.W.: Short stature, mental retardation, and hypoparathyroidism: a new syndrome. Arch. Dis. Child. 65:1113, 1990.

Richardson, M.M., Beaudet, A.L., Wagner, M.L., Malini, S., Rosenberg, H.S. and Lucci, J.A., Jr.: Prenatal diagnosis of recurrence of Saldino–Noonan dwarfism. J. Pediatr. 91:467, 1977.

Richkind, K.E., Mahoney, M.J., Evans, M.I., Willner, J. and Douglass, R.: Prenatal diagnosis and outcomes of five cases of mosaicism for an isochromosome of 20q. Prenat. Diagn. 11:371, 1991.

Rightmire, D.A., Nicolaides, K.H., Rodeck, C.H. and Campbell, S.: Fetal blood velocities in Rh isoimmunization: Relationship to gestational age and to fetal hematocrit. Obstet. Gynecol. 68:233, 1986.

Riis, P. and Fuchs, F.: Antenatal determination of foetal sex in prevention of hereditary diseases. Lancet. 2:180, 1960.

Rittler, M. and Orioli, I.M.: Achondrogenesis type II with polydactyly. Am. J. Med. Genet. 59:157, 1995.

Rittler, M., Menger, H., Spranger, J.: Chondrodysplasia punctata, tibia-metacarpal (MT) type. Am. J. Med. Genet. 37:200, 1990.

Rizzo, G., Arduini, D., Pennestri, F., Romanini, C. and Mancuso, S.: Fetal behaviour in growth retardation: Its relationship to fetal blood flow. Prenat. Diagn. 7:229, 1987a.

Rizzo, N., Gabrielli, S., Gianluigi, P., Perolo, A., Cacciari, A., Domini, R. and Bovicelli, L.: Prenatal diagnosis and obstetrical management of multicystic dysplastic kidney disease. Prenat. Diagn. 7:109, 1987b.

Rizzo, N., Gabrielli, S., Perolo, A., Pilu, G., Cacciari, A., Domini, R. and Bovicelli, L.: Prenatal diagnosis and management of fetal ovarian cysts. Prenat. Diagn. 9:97, 1989.

Rizzo, G., Nicolaides, K.H., Arduini, D. and Campbell, S.: Effects of intravascular fetal blood transfusion on fetal intracardiac doppler velocity waveforms. Am. J. Obstet. Gynecol. 163:1231, 1990.

Rizzo, W.B., Craft, D.A., Kelson, T.L., Bonnefont,, J.P., Saudubray, J.M., Schulman, J.D., Black, S.H., Tabsh, K. and Di Rocco, M.: Prenatal diagnosis Sjogren–Larsson syndrome in the first and second trimester using enzymatic methods. Am. J. Hum. Genet. 53(Suppl.):89, 1993.

Robbins-Furman, P., Hecht, J.T., Hocklin, M., Maklad, N. and Wilkins, I.: Report of prenatal diagnosis of Freeman–Sheldon syndrome (whistling face syndrome). Am. J. Hum. Genet. 53(Suppl.):1453, 1993.

Robbins-Furman, P., Drinkwater, B., Crino, J.P. and Elder, F.F.B.: Tetrasomy 1q, mosaic tetrasomy 1q, and mosaic partial tetrasomy 1q diagnosed prenatally. Am. J. Hum Genet. 57(Suppl.):A287, 1995.

Roberts, C.: Intrauterine diagnosis of omphalocele. Radiology. 127:762, 1978.

Roberts, R.M.: Management of human parvovirus infection in pregnancy. Am. J. Hum. Genet. 43(Suppl.):A246, 1988.

Roberts, A.B. and Campbell, S.: Small biparietal diameter of fetuses with spina bifida: Implications for antenatal screening. Br. J. Obstet. Gynaecol. 87:927, 1980.

Roberts, D.F. and Coleman, D.V.: A case of prenatal paternity discrimination. Prenat. Diagn. 2:319, 1982.

Roberts, S.H., Duckett, D.P., Little, E. and Laurence, K.M.: Prenatal detection of a male pseudohermaphrodite resulting from an X;Y translocation. J. Med. Genet. 24:248, 1987.

Robertson, E.G., Brown, A., Ellis, M.I. and Walker, W.: Intrauterine transfusion in the management of severe Rhesus isoimmunization. Br. J. Obstet. Gynaecol. 83:694, 1976.

Robie, G.F., Payne, G.G., Jr., and Morgan, M.A.: Selective delivery of an acardiac, acephalic twin. N. Engl. J. Med. 320:512, 1989.

Robinow, M., Sonek, J., Buttino, L. and Veghte, A.: Femoral-facial syndrome-prenatal diagnosis—Autosomal dominant inheritance. Am. J. Med. Genet. 57:397, 1995.

Robinson, B.H., Toone, J.R., Benedict, R.P., Dimmick, J.E., Oei, J. and Applegarth, D.A.: Prenatal diagnosis of pyruvate carboxylase deficiency. Prenat. Diagn. 5:67, 1985.

Robinson, L.P., Worthen, N.J., Lachman, R.S., Adomian, G.E. and Rimoin, D.L.: Prenatal diagnosis of osteogenesis imperfecta type III. Prenat. Diagn. 7:7, 1987.

Robinson, L, Grau, P. and Crandall, B.F.: Pregnancy outcomes after different MS-AFP elavations. Am. J. Hum. Genet. 43(Suppl.):A247, 1988.

Robinson, L.P., Lieber, C., Shih, L.Y., Rappaport, R., Rakow, J., Peters, S. and Desposito, F.: Familial postaxial polydactyly, craniofacial anomalies and hypopituitarism: Case report and prenatal diagnosis. Am. J. Hum. Genet. 45(Suppl.):A60, 1989.

Rocchi, M., Pecile, V., Archidiacono, N., Monni, G., Dumez, Y. and Filippi, G.: Prenatal diagnosis of the fragile-X in male monozygotic twins: Discordant expression of the fragile site in amniocytes. Prenat. Diagn. 5:229, 1985.

Rocchiccioli, F., Aubourg, P. and Choiset, A.: Immediate prenatal diagnosis of Zellweger syndrome by direct measurement of very long chain fatty acids in chorionic villus cells. Prenat. Diagn. 7:349, 1987.

Rodan, B.A. and Bean, W.J.: Chorioangioma of the placenta causing intrauterine fetal demise. J. Ultrasound Med. 2:95, 1983.

Rodeck, C.H. and Campbell, S.: Early prenatal diagnosis of neural-tube defects by ultrasound-guided fetoscopy. Lancet. 1:1128, 1978.

Rodeck, C.H. and Campbell, S.: Umbilical-cord insertion as source of pure fetal blood for prenatal diagnosis. Lancet. 1:1244, 1979.

Rodeck, C.H. and Roberts, L.J.: Successful treatment of fetal cardiac arrest by left ventricular exchange transfusion. Fetal Diagn. Ther. 9:213, 1994.

Rodeck, C.H., Eady, R.A.J. and Gosden, C.M.: Prenatal diagnosis of epidermolysis bullosa letalis. Lancet. 1:949, 1980.

Rodeck, C.H., Kemp, J.R., Holman, C.A., Whitmore, D.N., Karnicki, J. and Austin, M.A.: Direct intravascular fetal blood transfusion by fetoscopy in severe Rhesus isoimmunisation. Lancet. 1:625, 1981.

Rodeck, C.H., Patrick, A.D., Pembrey, M.E., Tzannatos, C. and Whitfield, A.E.: Fetal liver biopsy for prenatal diagnosis of ornithine carbamyl transferase deficiency. Lancet. 2:297, 1982a.

Rodeck, C.H., Mibashan, R.S., Abramowicz, J. and Campbell, S.: Selective feticide of the affected twin by fetoscopic air embolism. Prenat. Diagn. 2:189, 1982b.

Rodeck, C.H., Nicolaides, K.H., Warsof, S.L., Fysh, W.J., Gamsu, H.R. and Kemp, J.R.: The management of severe rhesus isoimmunization by fetoscopic intravascular transfusions. Am. J. Obstet. Gynecol. 150:769, 1984.

Rodeck, C.H., Gill, D., Rosenberg, D.A. and Collins, W.P.: Testosterone levels in midtrimester maternal and fetal plasma and amniotic fluid. Prenat. Diagn. 5:175, 1985.

Rodeck, C.H., Fisk, N.M., Fraser, D.I. and Nicolini, R.: Long-term in utero drainage of fetal hydrothorax. N. Engl. J. Med. 319:1135, 1988.

Rodis, J.F., Vintzileos, A.M., Campbell, W.A., Deaton, J.L., Fumia, F. and Nochimson, D.J.: Antenatal diagnosis and management of monoamniotic twins. Am. J. Obstet. Gynecol. 157:1255, 1987.

Rodriguez, P.L., Heredero, B., Oliva, R.J. and Zaldivar, G.O.: Maternal serum AFP screening in Havana, Cuba. Am. J. Hum. Genet. 41(Suppl.):A284, 1987a.

Rodriguez, P.L., Heredero, B., Oliva, R.J. and Zaldivar, G.O.: Prenatal diagnosis of neural tube defects by measurement of serum alpha-fetoprotein in Havana City. Prenat. Diagn. 7:657, 1987b.

Rodriguez, J.I., Palacios, J., Omenaca, F. and Lorente, M.: Polyasplenia, caudal deficiency, and agenesis of the corpus callosum. Am. J. Med. Genet. 38:99, 1991.

Rogers, J.G. and Danks, D.M.: Prenatal diagnosis of sex-linked hydrocephalus. Prenat. Diagn. 3:269, 1983.

Rogers, R.C. and Phelan M.C.: Neural tube defects associated with chromosome aberrations. Proc. Greenwood Genet. Cent. 8:50, 1989.

Rolland, M., Sarramon, M.F. and Bloom, M.C.: Astomia-agnathia-holoprosencephaly association. Prenatal diagnosis of a new case. Prenat. Diagn. 11:199, 1991.

Rolland, M.O., Divry, P., Mandon, G., Thoulon, J.M., Fiumara, A. and Mathieu, M.: First-trimester prenatal diagnosis of Canavan disease. J. Inher. Metab. Dis. 16:581, 1993a.

Rolland, M.O., Mandon, G. and Mathieu, M.: First-trimester prenatal diagnosis of non-ketotic hyperglycinemia by a micro assay of glycine cleavage enzyme. Prenat. Diagn. 13:771, 1993b.

Romano, V., Dianzani, I., Ponzone, A.A., Zammarchi, E., Eisensmith, R., Ceratto, N., Bosco, P. and Indelicato, A.: Prenatal diagnosis by minisatellite analysis of three Italian PKU families. Int. Pediatr. 9(Suppl. 2):84, 1994.

Romero, R., Chervenak, F.A., DeVore, G., Tortora, M. and Hobbins, J.C.: Fetal head deformation and congenital torticollis associated with a uterine tumor. Am. J. Obstet. Gynecol. 141:839, 1981.

Romero, R., Chervenak, F.A., Coustan, D., Berkowitz, R.L. and Hobbins, J.C.: Antenatal sonographic diagnosis of umbilical cord laceration. Am. J. Obstet. Gynecol. 143:719, 1982a.

Romero, R., Chervenak, F.A., Berkowitz, R.L. and Hobbins, J.C.: Intrauterine fetal tachypnea. Am. J. Obstet. Gynecol. 144:356, 1982b.

Romero, R., Pilu, G., Philippe, J., Ghidini, A. and Hobbins, J.D. (Eds.). *Prenatal Diagnosis of Congenital Anomalies.* Norwalk, Conn, Appleton and Lagce, 1988.

Romke, C., Froster-Iskenius, U., Heyne, K., Hohn, W., Hof, M., Grzejszczyk, G., Rauskolb, R., Rehder, H. and Schwinger, E.: Roberts syndrome and SC phocomelia: A single genetic entity. Clin. Genet. 31:170, 1987.

Rosatelli, C., Falchi, A.M., Tuveri, T., Scalas, M.T., DiTucci, A., Monni, G. and Cao, A.: Prenatal diagnosis of beta-thalassaemia with the synthetic-oligomer technique. Lancet. 1:241, 1985.

Rosatelli, M.C., Tuveri, T., Scalas, M.T., Di Tucci, A., Leoni, G.B., Furbetta, M., Monni, G. and Cao, A.: Prenatal diagnosis of beta-thalassaemia by oligonucleotide analysis in Mediterranean populations. J. Med. Genet. 25:762, 1988.

Rose V., Wilson, G. and Steiner, G.: Familial hypercholesterolemia: Report of coronary death at age 3 in a homozygous child and prenatal diagnosis in a heterozygous sibling. J. Pediatr. 100:757, 1982.

Rosen, R.S. and Bocian, M.: Hydrops fetalis in the McKusick–Kaufman syndrome. Proc. Greenwood Genet. Cent. 8:180, 1989a.

Rosen, R.S. and Bocian, M.E.: Non-immune hydrops fetalis in the McKusick–Kaufman syndrome. Am. J. Hum. Genet. 45(Suppl.):A61, 1989b.

Rosenak, D., Ariel, I., Arnon, J., Diamant, Y.Z., Ben Chetrit, A., Nadjari, M., Zilberman,

R., Yaffe, H., Cohen, T. and Ornoy, A.: Recurrent tetraamelia and pulmonary hypoplasia with multiple malformations in sibs. Am. J. Med. Genet. 38:25, 1991.

Rosenberg, J.C., Chervenak, F.A., Walker, B.A., Chitkara, U. and Berkowitz, R.L.: Antenatal sonographic appearance of omphalomesenteric duct cyst. J. Ultrasound Med. 5:719, 1986.

Rosenblatt, D.S., Cooper, B.A., Schmutz, S.M., Zaleski, W.A. and Casey, R.E.: Prenatal vitamin B_{12} therapy of a fetus with methylcobalamin deficiency (cobalamin E disease). Lancet. 1:1127, 1985.

Rosenblum-Vos, L.S., Roberson, A.E., Meyers, C.M., and Cohen, M.M.: Trisomy 16 mosaicism identified in mid-trimester amniocentesis and confirmed in fetal tissues. Am. J. Hum. Genet. 53(Suppl.):1808, 1993.

Rosengren, S.S., Quinn, D.L. and Rodis, J.F.: Risk of adverse outcome in pregnancies infected with human parvovirus B19. Am. J. Hum. Genet. 43(Suppl.):A247, 1988.

Rosler, A., Leiberman, E., Rosenmann, A., Ben-Uzilio, R. and Weidenfeld, J.: Prenatal diagnosis of 11 beta-hydroxylase deficiency congenital adrenal hyperplasia. J. Clin. Endocrinol. Metab. 49:546, 1979.

Rossbach, H-C., Sutcliffe, M.J., Haag, M.M., Grana, N.H., Rossi, A.R. and Barbosa, J.L.: Fanconi anemia in brothers initially diagnosed with VACTERL association with hydrocephalus, and subsequently with Baller–Gerold syndrome. Am. J. Med. Genet. 61:65, 1996.

Rosser, E.M., Wilkinson, A.R., Hurst, J.A., McGaughran, J.M. and Donnai, D.: Geleophysic dysplasia: A report of three affected boys—Prenatal ultrasound does not detect recurrence. Am. J. Med. Genet. 58:217, 1995.

Rosser, L.M., Hall, C.M., Harper, J. Lacour, M. and Baraitser, M.: Nance–Sweeney chondrodysplasia—A further case? Clin. Dysmorph. 5:207, 1996.

Rossi, R., Hozgreve, W. and Rehder, H.: Extreme hypotrophy of the lower body pole, extensive hypoplasia of the spinal column and multiple anomalies of abdominal organs: A maximal variant of the caudal regression sequence? Clin. Dysmorph. 4:87, 1995.

Rossiter, J.P., Hofman, K.J. and Kelley, R.I.: Detection of 7-dehydrocholesterol in amniotic fluid: A potential method for prenatal diagnosis of Smith–Lemli–Opitz syndrome. Am. J. Med. Genet. 52:377, 1994.

Rossiter, J.P., Hofman, K.J. and Kelley, R.I.: Smith–Lemli–Opitz syndrome: Prenatal diagnosis by quantification of cholesterol precursors in amniotic fluid. Am. J. Med. Genet. 56:272, 1995.

Roth, K.S., Yang, W., Allan, L., Saunders, M., Gravel, R.A. and Dakshinamurti, K.: Prenatal administration of biotin in biotin responsive multiple carboxylase deficiency. Pediatr. Res. 16:126, 1982.

Rotmensch, S., Liberati, M., Luo, J-S., Tallini, G., Mahoney, M.J. and Hobbins, J.C.: Prenatal diagnosis of a fetus with terminal deletion of chromosome 1 (q41). Prenat. Diagn. 11:867, 1991.

Rouyer-Fessard, P.H., Beuzard, Y., Vidaud, M., John, P. and Mibashan, R.S.: Prenatal diagnosis of beta thalassaemia by reverse phase HPLC. Prenat. Diagn. 7:171, 1987.

Rouyer-Fessard, P., Plassa, F., Blouquit, Y., Vidaud, M., Varnavides, L., Mibashan, R.S., Bellingham, A. and Beuzard, Y.: Prenatal diagnosis of haemoglobinopathies by ion exchange HPLC of haemoglobins. Prenat. Diagn. 9:19, 1989.

Rowley, K.A.: Coronal cleft vertebra. J. Fac. Radiol. 6:267, 1955.

Rubin, E.M. and Kan, Y.W.: A simple sensitive prenatal test of hydrops fetalis caused by alpha-thalassaemia. Lancet. 1:75, 1985.

Rudd, N.L., Miskin, M., Hoar, D.I., Benzie, R. and Doran, T.A.: Prenatal diagnosis of hypophosphatasia. N. Engl. J. Med. 295:146, 1976.

Ruddick, W. and Wilcox, W.: Operating on the fetus. Hastings Cent. Rep. 12(5):10, 1982.

Ruitenbeek, W., Sengers, R., Albani, M., Trijbels, F., Janssen, A., van Diggelen, O. and Bakkeren, J.: Prenatal diagnosis of cytochrome c oxidase deficiency by biopsy of chorionic villi. N. Engl. J. Med. 319:1095, 1988.

Ruitenbeek, W., Wendel, U., Hamel, B.C.J. and Trubels, J.M.F.: Genetic counselling and prenatal diagnosis in disorders of the mitochondrial energy metabolism. J. Inher. Metab. Dis. 19:581, 1996.

Rupp, L., McDonnell, A., Hux, C. and Schneider, A.: Prenatal diagnosis of triploidy presenting as oligohydramnios and intra-uterine growth retardation. Am. J. Hum. Genet. 45(Suppl.): A268, 1989.

Russ, P.D., Zavitz, W.R., Pretorius, D.H., Manco-Johnson, M.L., Rumack, C.M., Pfister, R.R. and Greenholz, S.K.: Hydrometrocolpos, uterus didelphys, and septate vagina: An antenatal sonographic diagnosis. J. Ultrasound Med. 5:211, 1986.

Russell, J.G.B.: Radiology in the diagnosis of fetal abnormalities. J. Obstet. Gynaecol. Br. Commonw. 76:345, 1969.

Russell, J.G.B.: *Radiology in Obstetrics and Antenatal Paediatrics.* London: Butterworths, 1973, p. 79.

Russell, J.G.B. and Hill, L.F.: True fetal rickets. Br. J. Radiol. 47:732, 1974.

Russell, L.J., Weaver, D.D., Bull, M.J. and Weinbaum, M.: In utero brain destruction resulting in collapse of the fetal skull, microcephaly, scalp rugae, and neurologic impairment: The fetal brain disruption sequence. Am. J. Med. Genet. 17:509, 1984.

Russo, R., D'Armiento, M., Martinelli, P. and Ventruto, V.: Neu–Laxova syndrome: Pathological, radiological, and prenatal findings in a stillborn female. Am. J. Med. Genet. 32:136, 1989.

Rutledge, J.C., Friedman, J.M., Harrod, M.J.E., Currarino, H.G., Wright, C.G., Pinckney, L. and Chen, H.: A "new" lethal multiple congenital anomaly syndorme: Joint contractures, cerebellar hypoplasia, renal hypoplasia, urogenital anomalies, tongue cysts, shortness of limbs, eye abnormalities, defects of the heart, gallbladder agenesis, and ear malformations. Am. J. Med. Genet. 19:255, 1984.

Rutledge, J.C., Weinberg, A.G., Friedman, J.M., Harrod, M.J. and Santos-Ramos, R.: Anatomic correlates of ultrasonographic prenatal diagnosis. Prenat. Diagn. 6:51, 1986.

Ruvinsky, E.D., Wiley, T.L., Morrison, J.C. and Blake, P.G.: In utero diagnosis of umbilical cord hematoma by ultrasonography. Am. J. Obstet. Gynecol. 140:833, 1981.

Ryynanen, M., Castren, O., Rapola, J., Aula, P. and Seppala, M.: Prenatal screening for congenital nephrosis. Lancet. 2:991, 1978.

Ryynanen, M., Seppala, M., Kuusela, P., Rapola, J., Aula, P., Seppa, A., Jokela, V. and Castren, O.: Antenatal screening for congenital nephrosis in Finland by maternal serum alpha-fetoprotein. Br. J. Obstet. Gynaecol. 90:437, 1983.

Saal, H.M., Deutsch, L., Herson, V., Cassidy, S.B., Greenstein, R.M. and Poole, A.E.: The RAG syndrome: A new autosomal recessive syndrome with Robin sequence, aniridia, and profound growth and development delays. Am. J. Hum. Genet. 34(Suppl.):A78, 1986.

Saal, H.M., Bulas, D.I., Allen, J.F., Vezina, L.G., Walton, D. and Rosenbaum, K.N.: Patient with craniosynotosis and marfanoid phenotype (Shprintzen–Goldberg syndrome) and cloverleaf skull. Am. J. Med. Genet. 57;573, 1995.

Sabbagha, R.E., Tamura, R.K., Dal Compo, S., Elias, S., Salvino, C., Shkolnik, A. and Gerbie, A.B.: Fetal cranial and craniocervical masses: Ultrasound characteristics and differential diagnosis. Am. J. Obstet. Gynecol. 138:511, 1980.

Sabbagha, R.E., Tamura, R.K. and Dal Compo, S.: Antenatal ultrasonic diagnosis of genetic defects: Present status. Clin. Obstet. Gynecol. 24:1103, 1981.

Sachs, L., Fourcroy, J.L., Wenzel, D.J., Austin, M. and Nash, J.D.: Prenatal detection of umbilical cord allantoic cyst. Radiology. 145:445, 1982.

Sagot, P., Nomballais, M.F., David, A., Yvinec, M., Beaujard, M.P., Barriere, P. and Boog, G.: Prenatal diagnosis of tetrapliody. Fetal Diagn. Ther. 8:182, 1993.

Sahakian, V., Weiner, C.P., Naides, S.J., Williamson, R.A. and Scharosch, L.L.: Intrauterine transfusion treatment of nonimmune hydrops fetalis secondary to human parvovirus B19 infection. Am. J. Obstet. Gynecol. 164:1090, 1991.

Saifer, A., Schneck, L., Perle, G., Valenti, C. and Volk, B.W.: Caveats of antenatal diagnosis of Tay–Sachs disease. Am. J. Obstet. Gynecol. 115:553, 1973.

Sakuma, T., Sugiyama, N. Ichiki, T. Kobayashi, M., Wada, Y. and Nohara, D.: Analysis of acylcarnitines in maternal urine for prenatal diagnosis of glutaric aciduria type 2. Prenat. Diagn. 11:77, 1991.

Saller, D.N., Jr., Mullins Keene, C.L., Raffel, L.J., Kostrubiak, I.S. and Sun, C.C.: Prenatal diagnosis of severe hydrocephalus in a case of hemifacial microsomia. Am. J. Hum. Genet. 43(Suppl.):A248, 1988.

Salonen, R., Herva, R. and Norio, R.: The hydrolethalus syndrome: Delineation of a "new," lethal malformation syndrome based on 28 patients. Clin. Genet. 19:321, 1981.

Saltzman, D.H., Benacerraf, B.R. and Frigoletto, F.D.: Diagnosis and management of fetal facial clefts. Am. J. Obstet. Gynecol. 155:377, 1986.

Salvo, A.F.: In utero diagnosis of Kleeblattschadel (cloverleaf skull). Prenat. Diagn. 1:141, 1981.

Sameshima, H., Nishibatake, M., Ninomiya, Y. and Tokudome, T.: Antenatal diagnosis of tetralogy of Fallot with absent pulmonary valve accompanid by hydrops fetalis and polyhydramnios. Fetal Diag. Ther. 8:305, 1993.

Samn, M., Lewis, K. and Blumberg, B.: Monozygotic twins discordant for Russell–Silver syndrome. Proc. Greenwood Genet. Cent. 8:221, 1989.

Samn, M., Lewis, K. and Blumberg, B.: Monozygotic twins discordant for the Russell–Silver syndrome. Am. J. Med. Genet. 37:543, 1990.

Samuel N., Dicker, D., Landman, J., Feldberg, D. and Goldman, J.A.: Early diagnosis and intrauterine therapy of meconium plug syndrome in the fetus: Risks and benefits. J. Ultrasound Med. 5:425, 1986.

Samueloff, A., Navot, D., Birkenfeld, A. and Schenker, J.G.: Fryns syndrome: A predictable, lethal pattern of multiple congenital anomalies. Am. J. Obstet. Gynecol. 156:86, 1987.

Sanders, S.P., Chin, A.J., Parness, I.A., Benacerraf, B., Greene, M.F., Epstein, M.F., Colan, S.D. and Frigoletto, F.D.: Prenatal diagnosis of congenital heart defects in thoracoabdominally conjoined twins. N. Engl. J. Med. 313:370, 1985.

Sandlin, C., Howard, R., Grube, G. and Lu, A.: Second trimester ultrasonic diagnosis of two cases of X-linked recessive hydrocephalus. Birth Defects. 17(1):159, 1981.

Sanguinetti, N., Marsh, J., Jackson, M., Fensom, A.H., Warren, R.C. and Rodeck, C.H.: The arylsulphatases of chorionic villi: Potential problems in the first-trimester diagnosis of metachromatic leucodystrophy and Maroteaux–Lamy disease. Clin. Genet. 30:302, 1986.

Sankaran, K., Sheridan, M., Singh, M., Cheema, G.S. and Laxdal, V.A.: Abnormal amniotic fluid spectrophotometry in a pregnancy associated with fetal duodenal atresia. Am. J. Obstet. Gynecol. 148:1140, 1984.

Santos, H.G. and Saraiva, J.M.: Opsismodysplasia: Another case and literature review. Clin. Dysmorph. 4:222, 1995.

Santos-Ramos, R. and Duenhoelter, J.H.: Diagnosis of congenital fetal abnormalities by sonography. Obstet. Gynecol. 45:279, 1975.

Sarti, D.A., Crandall, B.F., Winter, J., Robertson, R.D., Kaback, M.M. and Karp, L.E.: Correlation of fetal body diameter to BPD from 12 to 26 weeks gestation. Meeting of the American Institute Ultrasound Medicine, New Orleans, 1980, paper no. 513.

Sasagasako, N., Miyahara, S., Saito, N., Shinnoh, N., Kobayashi, T. and Goto, I.: Prenatal diagnosis of congenital sialidosis. Clin. Genet. 44:8, 1993.

Sassa, S., Solish, G., Levere, R.D. and Kappas, A.: Studies in porphyria: IV. Expression of the gene defect of acute intermittent porphyria in cultured skin fibroblasts and amniotic cells: Prenatal diagnosis of the porphyric trait. J. Exp. Med. 142:722, 1975.

Saul, R.A.: Prenatal documentation of craniofacial teratomas. Proc. Greenwood Genet. Cent. 1:34, 1982.

Savary, J.B., Vassseur, F., Vinatier, D. Manouvrier, S., Thomas, P. and Deminatti, M.M.: Prenatal diagnosis of PHIBIDS. Prenat. Diagn. 11:859, 1991.

Savoldelli, G. and Schinzel, A.: Prenatal ultrasound detection of humero-radial synostosis in a case of Antley–Bixler syndrome. Prenat. Diagn. 2:219, 1982.

Savoldelli, G., Schmid, W. and Schinzel, A.: Prenatal diagnosis of cleft lip and palate by ultrasound. Prenat. Diagn. 2:313, 1982.

Scarbrough, P.R., Files, B., Carroll, A.J., Quinlan, R.W., Finley, S.C. and Finley, W. H.: Interstitial deletion of chromosome [del(1)(q25q32)] in an infant with prune belly sequence. Prenat. Diagn. 8:169, 1988.

Schaffer, R.M., Cabbad, M., Minkoff, H., Schiller, M., Haller, J.O. and Shapiro, A.J.: Sonographic diagnosis of fetal cardiac rhabdomyoma. J. Ultrasound Med. 5:531, 1986.

Schatz, F.: Eine besondere Art von einseitiger Polyhydramnie mit anderseitiger Oligohydromie bei eineiigen Zwillingen. Arch Gynak. 19:329, 1882.

Scherer, A., Rodriguez, G., Dorjo, I. and Desposito, F.: Integration of genetic services into a Hispanic community health center. Am. J. Hum. Genet. 45(Suppl.):A126, 1989.

Scheuerle, A., Zenger-Hain, J.L., Van Dyke, D.L., Ledbetter, D.H., Greenberg, F. and Shaffer, L.G.: Replication banding and molecular studies of a mosaic, unbalanced dic(X;15) (Xpter->Xq26.1 :: 15p11->15qter). Am. J. Med. Genet. 56:403, 1995.

Schiff, I., Driscoll, S.G. and Naftolin, F.: Calcification of the umbilical cord. Am. J. Obstet. Gynecol. 126:1046, 1976.

Schimke, R.N., Claflin, K.S., Seguin, J.H., Bennett, T.L., Finley, B.E., Levitch, L.M. and Newcomb, W.M.: Hypomandibular faciocranial dysostosis: Report of an affected sib and follow-up. Am. J. Med. Genet. 41:102, 1991.

Schimmenti, L.A., Higgins, R.R., Mendelsohn, N.J., Casey, T.M., Steinberger, J., Mammel, M.C. and Wiesner, G.L.: Monosomy 9p24 → pter and trisomy 5q31 → qter: Case report and review of two cases. Am. J. Med. Genet. 57:52, 1995.

Schinzel, A. and Litschgi, M.: Autosomal recessive severe congenital microcephaly: Antenatal ultrasonographic diagnosis and head growth from 15 to 24 weeks of gestation. J. Med. Genet. 21:355, 1984.

Schinzel, A. and Savoldelli, G.: Prenatal ultrasonographic diagnosis of asphyxiating thoracic dysplasia (Jeune syndrome). Proc. Greenwood Genet. Cent. 4:136, 1985.

Schinzel, A., Savoldelli, G., Briner, J. and Schubiger, G.: Prenatal sonographic diagnosis of Jeune syndrome. Radiology. 154:777, 1985.

Schleifer, R.A., Bradley, D.A., Dowman, A.C., and Horwitz, J.A.: Early prenatal identification of placental steroid sulfatase deficiency by maternal serum triple marker screening. Am. J. Hum. Genet. 53(Suppl.):1455, 1993.

Schmid, W.: Cytogenetical problems in prenatal diagnosis. Hereditas. 86:37, 1977.

Schmidt, A.: Prenatal diagnosis of fragile X-syndrome. Clin. Genet. 27:334, 1985.

Schmidt, W. and Kubli, F.: Early diagnosis of severe congenital malformations by ultrasonography. J. Perinatol. Med. 10:233, 1982.

Schmidt, A., Passarge, E., Seemanova, E. and Macek, M.: Prenatal detection of a fetus hemizygous for the fragile X-chromosome. Hum. Genet. 62:285, 1982a.

Schmidt, W., Schroeder, T.M., Buchinger, G. and Kubli, F.: Genetics, pathoanatomy, and prenatal diagnosis of Potter I syndrome and other urogenital tract diseases. Clin. Genet. 22:105, 1982b.

Schmidt, W., Harms, E. and Wolf, D.: Successful prenatal treatment of non-immune hydrops fetalis due to congenital chylothorax: Case report. Br. J. Obstet. Gynaecol. 92:685, 1985.

Schnatterly, P.T. and Hogge, W.A.: Alpha fetoprotein (AFP) and acetylcholinesterase (AChE) levels in twins discordant for neural tube defects: Dependence on type of fetal membranes. Am. J. Hum. Genet. 43(Suppl.):A249, 1988.

Schneider, E.L., Ellis, W.G., Brady, R.O., McCulloch, J.R. and Epstein, C.J.: Infantile (type II) Gaucher's disease: In utero diagnosis and fetal pathology. J. Pediatr. 81:1134, 1972.

Schneider, J.A., Verroust, F.M., Kroll, W.A., Garvin, A.J., Horger, E.O., III, Wong, V.G., Spear, G.S., Jacobson, C., Pellett, O.L. and Becker, F.L.A.: Prenatal diagnosis of cystinosis. N. Engl. J. Med. 290:878, 1974.

Schneider, K., Scioscia, A., DiMaio, M., Baumgarten, A. and Mahoney, M.: Should ultrasound redating be employed in low MSAFP assessment? Am. J. Hum. Genet. 43(Suppl.): A249, 1988.

Schneiderman, H., Wu, A.Y.-Y., Campbell, W.A., Forouhar, F., Yamase, H., Greenstein, R. and Grant-Kels, J.M.: Congenital melanoma with multiple prenatal metastases. Cancer. 60:1371, 1987.

Schnittger, A. and Kjessler, B.: The outcome of a uniform program for alpha-fetoprotein screening in early pregnancy in seven regions in Sweden. Acta Obstet. Gynecol. Scand. Suppl. 119:9, 1984.

Schnittger, A., Liedgren, S., Radberg, C., Johansson, S.G.O. and Kjessler, B.: Raised maternal serum and amniotic fluid alpha-fetoprotein levels associated with a placental haemangioma. Br. J. Obstet. Gynaecol. 87:824, 1980.

Schoene, W.C. and Holmes, L.B.: The face predicts the brain: Sometimes. Teratology. 39:479, 1989.

Schoenfeld, A., Edelstein, T. and Joel-Cohen, S.J.: Prenatal ultrasonic diagnosis of fetal teratoma of the neck. Br. J. Radiol. 51:742, 1978.

Schoenfeld, A., Ovadia, J., Neri, A., Abramovici, A. and Klibanski, C.: Chemical and biochemical studies in fetuses affected with Nieman–Pick disease type A. Prenat. Diagn. 2:177, 1982.

Schoenfeld, M., Mahoney, M.J., Greenstein, R.M., Saal, H.M. and Baumgarten, A.: Maternal serum alpha-fetoprotein (MSAFP) concentration and risk for Down syndrome (DS). Am. J. Hum. Genet. 37(Suppl.):A226, 1985.

Scholl, H.W.: In utero diagnosis of agnathia, microstomia and synotia. Obstet. Gynecol. 49(Suppl.):81S, 1977.

Schorderet, D.F., Huber, M., Laurini, R.N., Von Moos, G., Gianadda, B., Deleze, G. and Hohl, D.: Prenatal diangosis of lamellar ichthyosis by direct mutational analysis of the keratinocyte transglutaminase gene. Prenat. Diagn. 17:483, 1997.

Schotten, A.G. and Giese, C.: The "female echo": Prenatal determination of the female fetus by ultrasound. Am. J. Obstet. Gynecol. 138:463, 1980.

Schuster, V., Seidenspinner, S. and Kreth, H.W.: Prenatal diagnosis of X linked lymphoproliferative disease using multiplex polymerase chain reaction. J. Med. Genet. 32:756, 1995.

Schutgens, R.B.H., Schrakamp, G., Wanders, R.J.A., Heymans, H.S.A., Moser, H.W., Moser, A.E., Tager, J.M., Bosch, H.V.D. and Aubourg, P.: The cerebro-hepato-renal (Zellweger) syndrome. Prenat. Diagn. 5:337, 1985.

Schutgens, R.B.H., Schrakamp, G., Wanders, R.J.A., Heymans, H.S.A., Tager, J.M. and van den Bosch, H.: Prenatal and perinatal diagnosis of peroxisomal disorders. J. Inher. Metab. Dis. 12(Suppl. 1):118, 1989.

Schwanitz, G., Zerres, K., Niesen, M., Haverkamp, F. and Schmid, G.: Hydrops fetalis as an indication for prenatal chromosome analysis with the example of the diagnosis of a duplication 15q11 and 17q25 due to a familial translocation 15/17. Ann. Genet. 31:186, 1988.

Schwartz, M. and Brandt, N.J.: False-negative results with methylumbelliferylguanidinobenzoate reactive proteases in cystic fibrosis pregnancies. Lancet. 2:1226, 1981.

Schwartz, M. and Brandt, N.J.: Disaccharidase deficiency in amniotic fluid from cases of cystic fibrosis. Prenat. Diagn. 5:145, 1985.

Schwartz, M., Scheibel, E. and Din, N.: Clinical use of DNA markers (RFLP) in genetic counseling and prenatal diagnosis of haemophilia A and B. Clin. Genet. 29:472, 1986.

Schwartz, M., Super, M., Schmidtke, J., Buys, C., Farrall, M., Halley, D., Krawczak, M., Poncin, J.E., Loukopoulos, D. and Devoto, M.: Prenatal diagnosis of cystic fibrosis using linked DNA probes. Prenat. Diagn. 8:619, 1988.

Schwartz, S., Raffel, L.J., Sun C.-C.J. and Chisum, R.: An unusual mosaic karyotype detected through prenatal diagnosis with duplication of 1q and 19q and associated teratoma development. Am. J. Hum. Genet. 45(Suppl.):A91, 1989a.

Schwartz, S., Ashai, S., Meijboom, E.J., Schwartz, M.F., Sun, C.C.-J. and Cohen, M.M.: Prenatal detection of trisomy 9 mosaicism. Prenat. Diagn. 9:549, 1989b.

Schwarz, T.F., Roggendorf, M. and Simader, R.: Assoziation eines nicht immunologisch bedingten Hydrops Fetalis mit einer Parvovirus-B19-Infektion. Geburtsh. u. Frauenheilk. 47: 572, 1987.

Schwarz, T.F., Roggendorf, M., Hottentrager, B., Deinhardt, F., Enders, G., Gloning, K.P., Schramm, T. and Hansmann, M.: Human parvovirus B19 infection in pregnancy. Lancet. 2:566, 1988.

Scioscia, A., Green, J., Robinson, J., Blakemore, K., Mahoney, M. and Baumgarten, A.: Maternal serum alpha-fetoprotein in normal first trimester pregnancies with fetal anomalies. Am. J. Hum. Genet. 41(Suppl.):A285, 1987.

Scott, C.I., Louro, J.M., Laurence, K.M., Tolarova, M., Hall, J.G., Reed, S. and Curry, C.J.R.: Comments on the Neu–Laxova syndrome and CAD complex. Am. J. Med. Genet. 9:165, 1981.

Scrimgeour, J.: Other techniques for antenatal diagnosis. In: Emery, A.E.H., (Ed.). *Antenatal Diagnosis of Genetic Disease.* Baltimore: Williams & Wilkins, 1973.

Seale, T.W. and Rennert, O.M.: Current status of prenatal diagnosis and heterozygote detection of cystic fibrosis. Ann. Clin. Lab. Sci. 12:415, 1982.

Seashore, J.H., Collins, F.S., Markowitz, R.I. and Seashore, M.R.: Familial apple peel jejunal atresia: Surgical, genetic, and radiographic aspects. Pediatrics. 80:540, 1987.

Seeds, J.W. and Bowes, W.A., Jr.: Results of treatment of severe fetal hydrothorax with bilateral pleuroamniotic catheters. Obstet. Gynecol. 68:577, 1986.

Seeds, J.W. and Cefalo, R.C.: Technique of early sonographic diagnosis of bilateral cleft lip and palate. Obstet. Gynecol. 62(Suppl. 3):2S, 1983.

Seeds, J.W. and Jones, F.D.: Lipomyelomeningocele: Prenatal diagnosis and management. Obstet. Gynecol. 67:34S, 1986.

Seeds, J.W., Cefalo, R.C., Lies, S.C. and Koontz, W.L.: Early prenatal sonographic appearance of rare thoraco-abdominal eventration. Prenat. Diagn. 4:437, 1984.

Seelen, J., Van Kessel, H., Eskes, T., Van Leusden, H., Been, J., Evers, J., Van Gent, I., Peeters, L., Van Der Velden, W. and Zonderland, F.: A new method of exchange transfusion in utero: Cannulation of vessels on the fetal side of the human placenta. Am. J. Obstet. Gynecol. 95:872, 1966.

Seligsohn, U., Mibashan, R.S., Rodeck, C.H., Nicolaides, K.H., Millar, D.S. and Coller, B.S.: Prenatal diagnosis of Glanzmann's thrombasthenia. Lancet. 2:1419, 1985.

Seller, M.J.: Amniotic fluid alpha-fetoprotein and Turner's syndrome. Lancet. 1:955, 1977.

Seller, M.J.: Meckel syndrome and the prenatal diagnosis of neural tube defects. J. Med. Genet. 15:462, 1978.

Seller, M.J.: Prenatal screening for Down syndrome. Lancet. 1:1359, 1984.

Seller, M.J. and Cole, K.J.: Polyacrylamide gel electrophoresis of amniotic fluid cholinesterase: A good prenatal test for neural tube defects. Br. J. Obstet. Gynaecol. 87:1103, 1980.

Seller, M.J., Russell, J. and Tint, G.S.: Unusual case of Smith–Lemli–Opitz syndrome "type II." Am. J. Med. Genet. 56:265, 1995.

Seller, M.J., Berry, A.C., Maxwell, D., McLennan, A. and Hall, C.M.: A new lethal chondrodysplasia with platyspondyly, long bone angulation and mixed bone density. Clin. Dysmorph. 5:213, 1996.

Seoud, M., Santos-Ramos, R. and Friedman, J.M.: Early prenatal ultrasonic findings in Klippel–Trenaunay–Weber syndrome. Prenat. Diagn. 4:227, 1984.

Seppala, M.: Increased alpha-fetoprotein amniotic fluid associated with a congenital esophageal atresia of the fetus. Obstet. Gynecol. 42:613, 1973.

Seppala, M.: Fetal pathophysiology of human alpha-fetoprotein. Ann. N.Y. Acad. Sci. 259: 59, 1975.

Seppala, M.: The use of alpha-fetoprotein in prenatal diagnosis. Int. J. Gynaecol. Obstet. 14:308, 1976.

Seppala, M. and Ruoslahti, E.: Alphafetoprotein in maternal serum: A new marker for detection of fetal distress and intrauterine death. Am. J. Obstet. Gynecol. 115:48, 1973.

Seppala, M. and Unnerus, H.A.: Elevated amniotic fluid alpha fetoprotein in fetal hydrocephaly. Am. J. Obstet. Gynecol. 119:270, 1974.

Seppala, M., Rapola, J., Huttunen, N.-P., Aula, P., Karjalainen, O. and Ruoslahti, E.: Congenital nephrotic syndrome: Prenatal diagnosis and genetic counseling by estimation of amniotic-fluid and maternal serum alpha-fetoprotein. Lancet. 2:123, 1976.

Serr, D.M., and Margolis, E.: Diagnosis of fetal sex in a sex-linked hereditary disorder. Am. J. Obstet. Gynecol. 88:230, 1964.

Serr, D.M., Sachs, L. and Danon, M.: Diagnosis of sex before birth using cells from amniotic fluid. Bull. Res. Counc. Israel. 5B:137, 1955.

Sewell, A.C. and Pontz, B.F.: Prenatal diagnosis of galactosialidosis. Prenat. Diagn. 8:151, 1988.

Seydel, F.D. and Eglinton, G.S.: Unusual low triple screen profile associated with major placental infarction and prematurity. Am. J. Hum. Genet. 57(Suppl.):A347, 1995.

Shaff, M.I., Fleicher, A.C., Battino, R., Herbert, C. and Boehm, F.H.: Antenatal sonographic diagnosis of thanatophoric dysplasia. J. Clin. Ultrasound. 8:363, 1980.

Shagina, I., Dadali, H.L., Sitnikov, V.P., Pugachev, V.V., Malygina, N.A. and Evgrafov, O.V.: Prenatal diagnosis of spinal muscular atrophy in Russia. Prenat. Diagn. 15:27, 1995.

Shah, H.O., Brown, W.T., Silverberg, G., Shaham, M. and Davis, J.G.: Correlation between low maternal serum alpha-fetoprotein (MSAFP) and cytogenetically abnormal fetuses. Am. J. Hum. Genet. 45(Suppl.):A126, 1989.

Shaham, M., Voss, R., Becker, Y., Yarkoni, S., Ornoy, A. and Kohn, G.: Prenatal diagnosis of ataxia telangiectasia. J. Pediatr. 100:134, 1982.

Shalev, J., Frankel, Y., Avigad, I. and Mashiach, S.: Spontaneous intestinal perforation in utero: Ultrasonic diagnostic criteria. Am. J. Obstet. Gynecol. 144:855, 1982.

Shalev, E., Weiner, E. and Zuckerman, H.: Prenatal ultrasound diagnosis of intestinal calcifications with imperforate anus. Acta Obstet. Gynecol. Scand. 62:95, 1983a.

Shalev, J., Navon, R., Urbach, D., Mashiach, S. and Goldman, B.: Intestinal obstruction and cystic fibrosis: Antenatal ultrasound appearance. J. Med. Genet. 20:229, 1983b.

Shalev, J., Ben-Rafael, Z., Goldman, B., Engelberg, I. and Mashiach, S.: Mid-trimester diagnosis of bladder neck obstruction by ultrasound and paracentesis. J. Med. Genet. 20:223, 1983c.

Shalev, E., Weiner, E., Feldman, E., Sudarsky, M., Shmilowitz, L. and Zuckerman, H.: External bladder–amniotic fluid shunt for fetal urinary tract obstruction. Obstet. Gynecol. 63:31S, 1984.

Shapiro, L.R. and Wilmot, P.L.: Prenatal diagnosis of the fra(X) syndrome. Am. J. Med. Genet. 23:325, 1986.

Shapiro, J.E., Phillips, J.A., III, Byers, P.H., Sanders, R., Holbrook, K.A., Levin, S.L., Dorst, J., Barsh, G.S., Peterson, K.E. and Goldstein, P.: Prenatal diagnosis of lethal perinatal osteogenesis imperfecta (OI Type II). J. Pediatr. 100:127, 1982a.

Shapiro, L.R., Wilmot, P.L., Brenholz, P., Leff, A., Martino, M., Harris, G., Mahoney, M.J. and Hobbins, J.C.: Prenatal diagnosis of fragile X chromosome. Lancet. 1:99, 1982b.

Shapiro, L.R., Wilmot, P.L. and Brenholz, P.: The fragile X syndrome: Experience with prenatal diagnosis. Am. J. Hum. Genet. 36(Suppl.):196S, 1984.

Shapiro, L.R., Wilmot, P.L., Murphy, P.D. and Breg, W.R.: Multiple approaches to the prenatal diagnosis of the fragile X syndrome: Amniotic fluid, chorionic villi, fetal blood, and molecular methods. Am. J. Hum. Genet. 41(Suppl.):A285, 1987.

Shapiro, L.R., Wilmot, P.L., Murphy, P.D. and Breg, W.R.: Experience with multiple approaches to the prenatal diagnosis of the fragile X syndrome: Amniotic fluid, chorionic villi, fetal blood and molecular methods. Am. J. Med. Genet. 30:347, 1988.

Shapiro, L.R., Wilmot, P.L. and Murphy, P.D.: Prenatal diagnosis of the fragile X syndrome: End of the experimental status. Am. J. Hum. Genet. 45(Suppl.):A269, 1989.

Shapiro, L.R., Wilmot, P.L. and Marinello, M.J.: Non-induced fragile X chromosomes detected in routine amniotic fluid cell culture: Determinatin of significance. Am. J. Hum. Genet. 57(Suppl.):A288, 1995.

Sharf, M., Abinader, E.G., Shapiro, I., Rosenfeld, T. and Eibschitz, I.: Prenatal echocardiographic diagnosis of Ebstein's anomaly with pulmonary atresia. Am. J. Obstet. Gynecol. 147:300, 1983.

Sharland, M., Hill, L., Patel, R. and Patton, M.: Pallister–Killian syndrome diagnosed by chorionic villus sampling. Prenat. Diagn. 11:477, 1991.

Sharony, R., Browne, C., Lachman, R.S. and Rimoin, D.L.: Prenatal diagnosis of the skeletal dysplasias. Am. J. Obstet. Gynecol. 169:668, 1993.

Shaub, M. and Wilson, R.: Erythroblastosis fetalis: Ultrasonic diagnosis. J. Clin. Ultrasound 4:19, 1976.

Sheldon, T.A. and Simpson, J.: Appraisal of a new scheme for prenatal screening for Down's syndrome. Br. Med. J. 302:1133, 1991a.

Sheldon, T.A. and Simpson, J.: Prenatal screening for Down's syndrome. Br. Med. J. 303:55, 1991b.

Shenker, L.: Fetal cardiac arrhythmias. Obstet. Gynecol. Surv. 34:561, 1979.

Shenker, L., Anderson, W. and Anderson, C.: Ultrasound demonstration of masses in a 15 week fetus: Hydrops in a fetus with umbilical cord occlusion. Prenat. Diagn. 1:217, 1981.

Shenker, L., Reed, K., Anderson, C., Hauck, L. and Spark, R.: Syndrome of camptodactyly, ankyloses, facial anomalies, and pulmonary hypoplasia (Pena–Shokeir syndrome): Obstetric and ultrasound aspects. Am. J. Obstet. Gynecol. 152:303, 1985.

Shen-Schwarz, S. and Dave, H.: Meckel syndrome with polysplenia: Case report and review of the literature. Am. J. Med. Genet. 31:349, 1988.

Shen-Schwarz, S., Hill, L.M., Surti, U. and Marchese, S.: Deletion of terminal portion of 6q: Report of a case with unusual malformations. Am. J. Med. Genet. 32:81, 1989.

Shepard, M.K., Linman, S.K. and Cavazos, A.: Familial thymic aplasia with intrauterine growth retardation and fetal death: A new syndrome or a variant of DiGeorge syndrome. Birth Defects. 12(6):123, 1976.

Shephard, B.A., Berlin, B.M., McCauley, R.G. and Irons, M.: Bowed long bones, unusual hands, narrow chest, dysmorphic facies, and cystic hygroma: A new, autosomal recessive skeletal dysplasia. Am. J. Hum. Genet. 57(Suppl.):A103, 1995.

Sherer, D.M., Wang, N., Thompson, H.O., Peterson, J.C., Miller, M.E., Metlay, L.A. and Abramowicz, J.S.: An infant with trisomy 9 mosaicism presenting as a complete trisomy 9 by amniocentesis. Prenat. Diagn. 12:31, 1992.

Sherowsky, R.C., Williams, C.H., Nichols, V.B. and Singh, K.B.: Prenatal ultrasonographic diagnosis of a sacrococcygeal teratoma in twin pregnancy. J. Ultrasound Med. 4:159, 1985.

Shettles, L.B.: Nuclear morphology of cells in human amniotic fluid in relation to sex of infant. Am. J. Obstet. Gynecol. 71:834, 1956.

Shih, L.Y., Filkins, K., Suslak, L., Lieber, C., Roth, J.A. and Desposito, F.: Dwarfism associated with prenatal ventriculomegaly. Prenat. Diagn. 3:69, 1983.

Shih, L.Y., Chen, T.H., Lieber, C., Desposito, F. and Ainbender, E.: Abnormal second trimester amniotic fluid alpha-fetoprotein and acetylcholinesterase associated with fetal intestinal atresia. Am. J. Hum. Genet. 36(Suppl.):196S, 1984.

Shih, V.E., Laframboise, R., Mandell, R. and Pichette, J.: Neonatal form of the hyperornithinaemia, hyperammonaemia, and homocitrullinuria (HHH) syndrome and prenatal diagnosis. Prenat. Diagn. 12:717, 1992.

Shimozawa, N., Suzuki, Y., Orii, T. and Hashimoto, T.: Immunoblot detection of enzyme proteins of peroxisomal beta-oxidation in fibroblasts, amniocytes, and chorionic villous cells. Possible marker for prenatal diagnosis of Zellweger's syndrome. Prenat. Diagn. 8:287, 1988.

Shimozawa, N., Suzuki, Y., Orii, T., Tsukamoto, T. and Fujiki, Y.: Prenatal diagnosis of Zellweger syndrome using DNA analysis. Prenat. Diagn. 13:149, 1993.

Shin, Y.S., Endres, W., Rieth, M. and Schaub, J.: Prenatal diagnosis of galactosemia and properties of galactose-1-phosphate uridyltransferase in erythrocytes of galactosemic variants as well as in human fetal and adult organs. Clin. Chim. Acta. 128:271, 1983.

Shin, Y.S., Rieth, M., Tausenfreund, J. and Endres, W.: First trimester diagnosis of glycogen storage disease type II and type III. J. Inher. Metab. Dis. 12(Suppl.2):289, 1989.

Shintaku, H., Hsiao, K.J., Liu, T.T., Imamura, T., Hase, Y., Chen, R.G., Isshiki, G. and Oura, T.: Prenatal diagnosis of 6-pyruvoyl tetrahydropterin synthase deficiency in seven subjects. J. Inher. Metab. Dis. 17:163, 1994.

Shipley, J., Rodeck, C.H., Garrett, C., Galbraith, J. and Giannelli, F.: Mitomycin C induced chromosome damage in fetal blood cultures and prenatal diagnosis of Fanconi's anaemia. Prenat. Diagn. 4:217, 1984.

Shivashankar, L., Whitney, E., Colmorgen, G., Young, T., Munshi, G., Wilmoth, D., Byrne, K., Reeves, G., Borgaonkar, D.S., Picciano, S.R. and Martin-Deleon, P.A.: Prenatal diagnosis of tetrasomy 47,XY,+i(12p) confirmed by in situ hybridization. Prenat. Diagn. 8:85, 1988.

Shohat, M., Rimoin, D.L., Gruber, H.E. and Lachman, R.S.: Perinatal lethal hypophosphatasia: Clinical, radiologic and morphologic findings. Pediatr. Radiol. 21:421, 1991.

Shohat, M., Lachman, R., Gruber, H.E., Hsia, Y.E., Golbus, M.S., Witt, D.R., Bodell, A., Bryke, C.R., Hogge, W.A. and Rimoin, D.L.: Desbuquois syndorme: Clinical, radiographic, and morphologic characterization. Am. J. Med. Genet. 52:9, 1994.

Shulman, L.P., Mace, P.C., Raafat, N.A., Emerson, D.S., Gross, S.J., Simpson, J.L., and Elias, S., Isolated first-trimester cystic hygroma: Clinical course, newborn outcome and infant development. Am. J. Hum. Genet. 53(Suppl.):1456, 1993.

Sibony, O., Fondacci, C., Oury, J-F., Benard, C., Vuillard, E. and Blot, P.: In utero fetal cerebral intraparenchymal hemorrhage associated with an abnormal cerebral doppler. Fetal Diagn. Ther. 8:126, 1993.

Siebert, J.R., Warkany, J. and Lemire, R.J.: Atelencephalic microcephaly in a 21-week human fetus. Teratology. 34:9, 1986.

Sieck, U.V. and Ohlsson, A.: Fetal polyuria and hydramnios associated with Bartter's syndrome. Obstet. Gynecol. 63:22S, 1984.

Silber, D.L. and Durnin, R.E.: Intrauterine atrial tachycardia. Am. J. Dis. Child. 117:722, 1969.

Silver, M., Nowaczyk, M. Chitayat, D., Jay, V., Toi, A., Lehotey, D., Solomon, L. and Thomas, M.: Congenital nephrotic syndrome and brain dysgenesis: A new syndrome? Am. J. Hum. Genet. 57(Suppl.):A103, 1995.

Silverman, N.H., Enderlein, M.A. and Golbus, M.S.: Ultrasonic recognition of aortic valve atresia in utero. Am. J. Cardiol. 53:391, 1984.

Simmonds, H.A., Fairbanks, L.D., Webster, D.R., Rodeck, C.H., Linch, D.C. and Levinsky, R.J.: Rapid prenatal diagnosis of adenosine deaminase deficiency and other purine disorders using foetal blood. Biosci. Rep. 3:31, 1983.

Simoni, G., Brambati, B., Danesino, C., Rossella, F., Terzoli, G.L., Ferrari, M. and Fraccaro, M.: Efficient direct chromosome analyses and enzyme determinations from chorionic villi samples in the first trimester of pregnancy. Hum. Genet. 63:349, 1983.

Simoni, G., Brambati, B., Danesino, C., Terzoli, G.L., Romitti, L., Rossella, F. and Fraccaro, M.: Diagnostic application of first trimester trophoblast sampling in 100 pregnancies. Hum. Genet. 66:252, 1984.

Simoni, G., Gimelli, G., Cuoco, C., Romitti, L., Terzoli, G., Guerneri, S., Rossella, F., Pescetto, L., Pezzolo, A., Porta, S., Brambati, B., Porro, E. and Fraccaro, M.: First trimester fetal karyotyping: One thousand diagnoses. Hum. Genet. 72:203, 1986.

Simpson, J.L. and Martin. A.O.: Prenatal diagnosis of cytogenetic disorders. Clin. Obstet. Gynecol. 19:841, 1976.

Simpson, J.L. and Elias, S.: Isolating fetal cells in maternal circulation. Hum. Reprod. Update. 1:409, 1995.

Simpson, N.E., Bone, M. and Girard, K.: Measurement of cholinesterase in amniotic fluid using naphthyl acetate as substrate: A possible initial test for prenatal diagnosis of open neural tube defects. Prenat. Diagn. 2:273, 1982.

Simpson, G.F., Edwards, M.S.B., Callen, P., Filly, R.F., Anderson, R.L. and Golbus, M.S.: Pressure, biochemical, and culture characteristics of CSF associated with the in utero drainage of various fetal CNS defects. Am. J. Med. Genet. 29:343, 1988.

Sindic, C.J.M., Freund, M., Van Regemorter, N., Verellen-Dumoulin, C. and Masson, P.L.: S-100 protein in amniotic fluid of anencephalic fetuses. Prenat. Diagn. 4:297, 1984.

Singer, N., Gersen, S. and Warburton, D.: The value of chromosome analysis in cases of neural tube defects: A case of anencephaly associated with fetal dup(2)(p24pter). Prenat. Diagn. 7:567, 1987.

Singsen, B.H., Akhter, J.E., Weinstein, M.M. and Sharp, G.C.: Congenital complete heart block and SSA antibodies: Obstetric implications. Am. J. Obstet. Gynecol. 152:655, 1985.

Slotnick, R.N., McGahan, J., Milio, L., Schwartz, M. and Ablin, D.: Antenatal diagnosis and treatment of fetal bronchopulmonary sequestration. Fetal Diagn. Ther. 5:33, 1990.

Smart, P.J., Schwarz, C. and Kelsey, A.: Ultrasonographic and biochemical abnormalities associated with the prenatal diagnosis of epignathus. Prenat. Diagn. 10:327, 1990.

Smidt-Jensen, S. and Hahnemann, N.: Transabdominal fine needle biopsy from chorionic villi in the first trimester. Prenat. Diagn. 4:163, 1984.

Smith, D.W.: *Recognizable Patterns of Human Malformation: Genetic, Embryologic, and Clinical Aspects,* 3rd ed. Philadelphia: Saunders, 1982.

Smith, J.J., Schwartz, E.D.and Blatman, S.: Fetal bradycardia—Fetal distress or cardiac abnormality? Obstet. Gynecol. 15:761, 1960.

Smith, A.D., Wald, N.J., Cuckle, H.S., Stirrat, G.M., Bobrow, M. and Lagercrantz, H.: Amniotic-fluid acetylcholinesterase as a possible diagnostic test for neural-tube defects in early pregnancy. Lancet. 1:685, 1979.

Smith, H.J., Hanken, H. and Brundelet, P.J.: Ultrasound diagnosis of interstitial pregnancy. Acta Obstet. Gynecol. Scand. 60:413, 1981a.

Smith, W.L., Breitweiser, T.D. and Dinno, N.: In utero diagnosis of achondrogenesis, Type I. Clin. Genet. 19:51, 1981b.

Smith, M.L., Pellett, O.L., Cass, M.M.J., Kennaway, N.G., Buist, N.R.M., Buckmaster, J., Golbus, M., Spear, G.S. and Schneider, J.A.: Prenatal diagnosis of cystinosis utilizing chorionic villus sampling. Prenat. Diagn. 7:23, 1987.

Smith, E.E., Surti, U., Leger, W.J. and Hogge, W.A.: Can triploidy and its parental origin be predicted based on maternal serum screening and ultrasound? Am. J. Hum. Genet. 57(Suppl.):A289, 1995.

Smooker, P.M., Cotton, R.G.H. and Lipson, A.: Prenatal diagnosis of DHPR deficiency by direct detection of mutation. Prenat. Diagn. 13:881, 1993.

Smurl, J.F. and Weaver, D.D.: Presymptomatic testing for Huntington chorea: Guidelines for moral and social accountability. Am. J. Med. Genet. 26:247, 1987.

Smythe, A.R.: Ultrasonic detection of fetal ascites and bladder dilation with resulting prune belly. J. Pediatr. 98:978, 1981.

Snijders, R.J.M., Shawa, L. and Nicolaides, K.H.: Fetal choroid plexus cysts and trisomy 18: Assessment of risk based on ultrasound findings and maternal age. Prenat. Diagn. 14:1119, 1994.

Socol, M.L., Sabbagha, R.E., Elias, S., Tamura, R.K., Simpson, J.L., Dooley, S.L. and Depp, R.: Prenatal diagnosis of congenital muscular dystrophy producing arthrogryposis. N. Engl. J. Med. 313:1230, 1985.

Soda, H., Ohura, T., Yoshida, I., Aramaki, S., Aoki, K., Inokuchi, T., Mikami, H. and Narisawa, K.: Prenatal diagnosis and therapy for a patient with vitamin B_{12}-responsive methylmalonic acidaemia. J. Inher. Metab. Dis. 18:295, 1995.

Sokol, R.J., Hutchison, P., Krouskop, R.W., Brown, E.G., Reed, G. and Vasquez, H.: Congenital complete heart block diagnosed during intrauterine fetal monitoring. Am. J. Obstet. Gynecol. 120:1115, 1974.

Sokol, R.J., Kazzi, G.M., Kalhan, S.C. and Pillay, S.K.: Identifying the pregnancy at risk for intrauterine growth retardation: Possible usefulness of the intravenous glucose tolerance test. Am. J. Obstet. Gynecol. 143:220, 1982.

Solish, G.I., Moser, H.W., Ringer, L.D., Moser, A.E., Tiffany, C. and Schutta, E.: The prenatal diagnosis of the cerebro-hepato-renal syndrome of Zellweger. Prenat. Diagn. 5:27, 1985.

Solomons, C.C. and Gottesfeld, K.: Prenatal biochemistry of osteogenesis imperfecta. Birth Defects. 15(5A):69, 1979.

Soong, B.-W., Tsai, T-F., Su, C-H., Kao, K-P, Hsiao, K-J and Su, T-S.: DNA polymorphisms and deletion analysis of the Duchenne–Becker muscular dystrophy gene in the Chinese. Am. J. Med. Genet. 38:593, 1991.

Soothill, P.: Intrauterine blood transfusion for non-immune hydrops fetalis due to parvovirus B19 infection. Lancet. 336:121, 1990.

Soothill, P.W., Nicolaides, K.H. and Campbell, S.: Prenatal asphyxia, hyperlacticaemia, hypoglycaemia, and erythroblastosis in growth retarded fetuses. Br. Med. J. 294:1051, 1987.

Spahr, R.C., Botti, J.J., MacDonald, H.M. and Holzman, I.R.: Nonimmunologic hydrops fetalis: A review of 19 cases. Int. J. Gynaecol. Obstet. 18:303, 1980.

Spanta, R., Roffman, L.E., Grissom, T.J., Newland, J.R. and McManus, B.M.: Abdominal pregnancy: Magnetic resonance identification with ultrasonographic follow-up of placental involution. Am. J. Obstet. Gynecol. 157:887, 1987.

Spear, G.S. and Porto, M.: 47,XXX chromosome constitution, ovarian dysgenesis, and genitourinary malformation. Am. J. Med. Genet. 29:511, 1988.

Spearritt, D.J., Tannenberg, A.E.G. and Payton, D.J.: Lethal multiple pterygium syndrome: Report of a case with neurological anomalies. Am. J. Med. Genet. 47:45, 1993.

Speer, A., Bollman, R., Michel, A. Neumann, R., Bommer, C., Hanke, R., Riess, O., Cobet, G. and Coutelle, C.: Prenatal diagnosis of classical phenylketonuria by linked restriction fragment length polymorphism analysis. Prenat. Diagn. 6:447, 1986.

Speiser, P.W., Laforgia, N., Kato, K., Pareira, J., Khan, R., Yang, S.Y., Whorwood, C., White,

P.C., Elias, S., Schriock, E., Schriock, E., Simpson, J.L., Taslimi, M., Najjar, J., May, S., Mills, G., Crawford, C. and New, M.I.: First trimester prenatal treatment and molecular genetic diagnosis of congenital adrenal hyperplasia (21-hydroxylase deficiency). J. Clin. Endocrinol. Metab. 70:838, 1990.

Spence, J.E., Buffone, G.J., Rosenbloom, C.L., Fernbach, S.D., Curry, M.R., Carpenter, R.J., O'Brien, W.E. and Beaudet, A.L.: Prenatal diagnosis of cystic fibrosis using linked DNA markers and amniotic fluid intestinal enzyme analysis. Am. J. Hum. Genet. 39(Suppl.): A266, 1986.

Spence, J.E., Maddalena, A., O'Brien, W.E., Fernbach, S.D. Batshaw, M.L., Leonard, C.O. and Beaudet, A.L.: Prenatal diagnosis and heterozygote detection by DNA analysis in ornithine transcarbamylase deficiency. J. Pediatr. 114:582, 1989.

Spencer, K., Aitken, D. and Macri, J.N.: Urine free beta hCG and beta core in pregnancies affected by trisomy 21. Am. J. Hum. Genet. 57(Suppl.):289A, 1995.

Sperber, G.H. and Machin, G.A.: Microscopic study of midline determinants in Janiceps twins. Birth Defects. 23(1):243, 1987.

Spikes, A.S., Hegmann, K., Smith, J.L. and Shaffer, L.G.: Use of fluorescence in situ hybridization to clarify a complex chromosomal rearrangement in a child with multiple congenital anomalies. Am. J. Med. Genet. 57:31, 1995.

Spinner, N.B., Eunpu, D.L., Austria, J.R. and Mamunes, P.: Holoprosencephaly in a newborn girl with 46,XX,i(18q). Am. J. Med. Genet. 39:11, 1991.

Spinner, N.B., Gibas, Z., Kline, R., Berger, B. and Jackson, L.: Placental mosaicism in a case of 46,XY,-22,+t(22;22)(p11;q11) or i(22q) diagnosed at amniocentesis. Prenat. Diagn. 12:47, 1992.

Spirt, B.A., Gordon, L., Cohen, W.N. and Yambao, T.: Antenatal diagnosis of chorioangioma of the placenta. Am. J. Roentgenol. 135:1273, 1980.

Spirt, B.A., Kagan, E.H., Gordon, L.P. and Massad, L.S.: Antepartum diagnosis of a succenturiate lobe: Sonographic and pathologic correlation. J. Clin. Ultrasound 9:139, 1981.

Spirt, B.A., Gordon, L.P. and Oliphant, M.: In: *Prenatal Ultrasound: A Color Atlas With Anatomic and Pathologic Correlation.* New York: Churchill Livingstone, 1987.

Spranger, J.: "Spur-limbed" dwarfism identified as hypophosphatasia. Dysmorph. Clin. Genet. 2:123, 1988.

Sprecher, S., Soumenkoff, G., Puissant, F. and Degueldre, M.: Vertical transmission of HIV in 15-week fetus. Lancet. 2:288, 1986.

Stangenberg, M., Lingman, G., Roberts, G. and Ozand, P.: Mucopolysaccharidosis VII as a cause of fetal hydrops in early pregnancy. Am. J. Med. Genet. 44:42, 1992.

Stanley, W.S., Pai, G.S., Horger E.O., III., Yongshan, Y. and McNeal, K.S.: Incidental detection of premature centromere separation in amniocytes associated with a mild form of Roberts syndrome. Prenat. Diagn. 8:565, 1988.

States, B., Blazer, B., Harris, D. and Segal, S.: Prenatal diagnosis of cystinosis. J. Pediatr. 87:558, 1975.

Steele, M.W. and Breg, W.R.: Chromosome analysis of human amniotic-fluid cells. Lancet. 1:383, 1966.

Steele, P.S., Bodurtha, J., Redwine, F.E., Smeltzer, J.S., Kucera, L., McCall, J.B. and Brown, J.A.: Prenatal detection of non-cardiac rhabdomyosarcoma. Am. J. Hum. Genet. 43(Suppl.):A250, 1988.

Steele, D., Hill, L., Gorin, M., Nussbaum, R. and Hogge, W.A.: Prenatal diagnosis of presumed Lowe syndrome in the absence of a living affected proband. Am. J. Hum. Genet. 53(Suppl.):1461, 1993.

Steele, C.D., Wapner, R.J., Smith, J.B., Haynes, M.K. and Jackson, L.G.: Prenatal diagnosis using fetal cells isolated from maternal peripheral blood: A review. Clin. Obstet. Gynecol. 39:801, 1996.

Steinfeld, L., Rappaport, H.L., Rossbach, H.C. and Martinez, E.: Diagnosis of fetal arrhythmias using echocardiographic and Doppler techniques. J. Am. Coll. Cardiol. 9:1425, 1986.

Steinmann, B., Gitzelmann, R., Kvittingen, E.A. and Stokke, O.: Prenatal diagnosis of hereditary tyrosinemia. N. Engl. J. Med. 310:855, 1984.

Stempel, L.E. and Lott, J.A.: Diagnosis of fetal death in utero with amniotic fluid creatine kinase. Am. J. Obstet. Gynecol. 138:1173, 1980.

Stephens, J.D.: Prenatal diagnosis of testicular feminisation. Lancet. 2:1038, 1984.

Stephens, J.D. and Sherman, S.: Determination of fetal sex by ultrasound. N. Engl. J. Med. 309:984, 1983.

Stephens, J.D., Filly, R.A., Callen, P.W. and Golbus, M.S.: Prenatal diagnosis of osteogenesis imperfecta type II by real-time ultrasound. Hum. Genet. 64: 191, 1983.

Stephenson, S.R. and Weaver, D.D.: Prenatal diagnosis—A compilation of diagnosis conditions. Am. J. Obstet. Gynecol. 141:319, 1981.

Stevens, C.A. and Qumsiyeh, M.B.: Syndromal frontonasal dysostosis in a child with a complex translocation involving chromosomes 3, 7, and 11. Am. J. Med. Genet. 55:494, 1995.

Stevenson, R.E., Jones, K.L., Phelan, M.C., Jones, M.C., Barr, M., Jr., Clericuzio, C., Harley, R.A. and Benirschke, K.: Vascular steal: The pathogenetic mechanism producing sirenomelia and associated defects of the viscera and soft tissues. Pediatrics. 78:451, 1986.

Stevenson, R.E., Phelan, M.C., Stanislovitis, P., Klinger, K. and Schwartz, C.E.: Interstitial deletion of 7q22 in a fetus with anencephaly. Proc. Greenwood Genet. Cent. 8:56, 1989.

Stewart, P.A., Tonge, H.M. and Wladimiroff, J.W.: Arrhythmia and structural abnormalities of the fetal heart. Br. Heart J. 50:550, 1983a.

Stewart, P.A., Wladimiroff, J.W. and Essed, C.E.: Prenatal ultrasound diagnosis of congenital heart disease associated with intrauterine growth retardation: A report of 2 cases. Prenat. Diagn. 3:279, 1983b.

Stewart, P.A., Buis-Liem, T., Verwey, R.A. and Wladimiroff, J.W.: Prenatal ultrasonic diagnosis of familial asymmetric septal hypertrophy. Prenat. Diagn. 6:249, 1986.

Stibler, H. and Skovby, F.: Failure to diagnose carbohydrate-deficient glycoprotein syndrome prenatally. Pediatr. Neurol. 11:71, 1994.

Stierman, E.D., Kochenour, N.K., Lee, T.G., Carey, J.C. and Leonard, C.O.: The prenatal diagnosis of amniotic bands. Am. J. Hum. Genet. 37(Suppl.):A227, 1985.

Still, K., Kolatat, T., Corbett, T. and Byrne, P.: Early third trimester selective feticide of a compromising twin. Fetal Ther. 4:83, 1989.

Stioui, S., DeSilvestris, M., Molinari, A., Stripparo, L., Ghisoni, L. and Simoni, G.: Trisomic 22 placenta in a case of severe intrauterine growth retardation. Prenat. Diagn. 9:673, 1989.

Stioui S., Privitera, O., Brambati, B., Zuliani, G., Lalatta, F. and Simoni, G.: First-trimester prenatal diagnosis of Roberts syndrome. Prenat. Diagn. 12:145, 1992.

Stirling, J.L., Robinson, D., Fensom, A.H., Benson, P.F., Baker, J.E. and Button, L.R.: Prenatal diagnosis of two Hurler fetuses using an improved assay for methylumbelliferyl-alpha-L-iduronidase. Lancet. 2:37, 1979.

Stoll, C., Willard, D., Czernichow, P. and Boue, J.: Prenatal diagnosis of primary pituitary dysgenesis. Lancet. 1:932, 1978.

Stoll, C., Manini, P., Bloch, J. and Roth, M.-P.: Prenatal diagnosis of hypochondroplasia. Prenat. Diagn. 5:423, 1985.

Storlazzi, E., Vintzileos, A.M., Campbell, W.A., Nochimson, D.J. and Weinbaum, P.J.: Ultrasonic diagnosis of discordant fetal growth in twin gestations. Obstet. Gynecol. 69:363, 1987.

Stout, J.T., Jackson, L.G. and Caskey, C.T.: First trimester diagnosis of Lesch–Nyhan syndrome: Application to other disorders of purine metabolism. Prenat. Diagn. 5:183, 1985.

Strachan, T.: Molecular pathology of 21-hydroxylase deficiency. Clin. Courier. 11(11):4, 1993.

Strasberg, P., Chitayat, D., Moola, S., Toi, A., Sermer, M., Gardner, A., Farrell, S., Summers, A., Thomas, M., Ray, R. and Van Allen, M.: Fetal echogenic bowel: Etiology, significance and outcome. Am. J. Hum. Genet. 57(Suppl.):A289, 1995.

Stratakis, C.A. and Garnica, A.: Premature infant with Wiedemann–Beckwith syndrome: Postnatal changes in facial appearance and somatic phenotype. Am. J. Med. Genet. 57:635, 1995.

Stratton, R.F. and Patterson, R.M.: DNA confirmation of congenital myotonic dystrophy in non-immune hydrops fetalis. Prenat. Diagn. 13:1027, 1993.

Stratton, R.F., Dobyns, W.B., Airhart, S.D. and Ledbetter, D.H.: New chromsomal syndrome: Miller–Dieker syndrome and monosomy 17p13. Hum. Genet. 67:193, 1984.

Straussberg, R., Amir, J., Harel, L. and Djaldetti, M.: Ultrastrucural alterations of the amnio-cytes in 2 patients with rubella during the first trimester of pregnancy. Fetal Diagn. Ther. 10:60, 1995.

Streade Nielsen, J. and Moestrup, J.K.: Foetal electrocardiographic studies of cardiac arrhyth-mias and the heart rate. Acta. Obstet. Gynecol. Scand. 47:247, 1968.

Strecker, J.R. and Jonatha, W.: Prenatal diagnosis of obstructions of the upper intestinal tract—A new endocrinological method. J. Perinatol. Med. 10:85, 1982.

Streit, J.A., Penick, G.D., Williamson, R.A., Weiner, C.P. and Benda, J.: Prolonged elevation of alphafetoprotein and detectable acetylcholinesterase after death of an anomalous twin fetus. Prenat. Diagn. 9:1, 1989.

Strom, C.M., Verlinsky, Y., Milayeva, S., Evsikov, S., Cieslak, J., Lifchez, A., Valle, J., Moise, J., Ginsberg, N. and Applebaum, M.: Preconception genetic diagnosis of cystic fibrosis. Lancet. 336:306, 1990.

Strom, C.M., Rechitsky, S., Ginsberg, N., Verlinsky, O. and Verlinsky, Y.: Prenatal paternity testing in the 1st trimester using AMPFLP technology. Am. J. Hum. Genet. 57(Suppl.): A289, 1995.

Stuart, B., Drumm, J., Fitzgerald, D.E. and Duignan, N.M.: Fetal blood velocity waveforms in normal pregnancy. Br. J. Obstet. Gynaecol. 87:780, 1980.

Subramaniam, R., Sadasivan, T., Rao, M.R. and Reddy, S.B.: An association between maternal serum alpha-fetoprotein and fetal autosomal trisomies. Am. J. Hum. Genet. 43(Suppl.): A250, 1988.

Suchy, S.F. and Yeager, M.T.: Maternal serum human chorionic gonadotropin screening for Down syndrome in women under 35. Am. J. Hum. Genet. 45(Suppl.):A271, 1989.

Suchlandt, G., Schlote, W. and Harzer, K.: Ultrastrukturelle Befunde bei 9 Feten nach prana-taler Diagnose von Neurolipidosen. Arch. Psychiatr. Nervenkr. 232:407, 1982.

Sugarman, R.G., Rawlinson, K.F. and Schifrin, B.S.: Fetal arrhythmia. Obstet. Gynecol. 52:301, 1978.

Sugino, S., Fujishita, S., Kamimura, N., Matsumoto, T., Wapenaar, M.C., Deng, H-X. Shibuya, N., Miike, T. and Niikawa, N.: Molecular-genetic study of Duchenne and Becker muscular dystrophies: Deletion analyses of 45 Japanese patients and segregation analyses in their families with RFLP's based on the data from normal Japanese females. Am. J. Med. Genet. 34:555, 1989.

Sugita, T., Ikenaga, M., Suehara, N., Kozuka, T., Furuyama, J. and Yabuuchi, H.: Prenatal diagnosis of Cockayne syndrome using assay of colony-forming ability in ultraviolet light irradiated cells. Clin. Genet. 22:137, 1982.

Sugiyama, N., Kidouchi, K. Kobayashi, M. and Wada, Y.: Carnitine deficiency in inherited organic acid disorders and Reye syndrome. Acta Paediatr. Jap. 32:410, 1990.

Sulak, L.E. and Dodson, M.G.: The vanishing twin: Pathologic confirmation of an ultrasono-graphic phenomenon. Obstet. Gynecol. 68:811, 1986.

Sulisalo, T., Sillence, D., Wilson, M., Ryynanen, M. and Kaitila, I.: Early prenatal diagnosis of cartilage-hair hypoplasia (CHH) with polymorphic DNA markers. Prenat. Diagn. 15:135, 1995.

Summers, M.C. and Donnenfeld, A.E.: Dandy–Walker malformation in the Meckel syndrome. Am. J. Med. Genet. 55:57, 1995.

Sunden, B.: On the dianostic value of ultrasound in obstetrics and gynaecology. Acta Obstet. Gynecol. Scand. 43:1, 1964.

Super, M., Ivinson, A., Schwarz, M., Giles, L., Elles, R.G., Read, A.P. and Harris, R.: Clinic experience of prenatal diagnosis of cystic fibrosis by use of linked DNA probes. Lancet. 2:782, 1987.

Sutcliffe, M.J., Mueller, O.T., Gallardo, L.A., Papenhausen, P.R. and Tedesco, T.A.: Maternal isodisomy 16 in a normal 46,XX following trisomic conception. Am. J. Hum. Genet. 53(Suppl.):1464, 1993.

Sutherland, G.R., Baker, E., Purvis-Smith, S., Hockey, A., Krumins, E. and Eichenbaum, S.Z.: Prenatal diagnosis of the fragile X using thymidine induction. Prenat. Diagn. 7:197, 1987.

Sutherland, G.R., Gedeon, A., Kornman, L., Donnelly, A., Byard, R.W., Mulley, J.C., Kremer,

E., Lynch, M., Pritchard, M., Yu, S. and Richards, R.I.: Prenatal diagnosis of fragile X syndrome by direct detection of the unstable DNA sequence. N. Engl. J. Med. 325:1720, 1991.

Sutro, W.H., Tuck, S.M., Loesevitz, A., Novotny, P.L., Archbald, F. and Irwin, G.A.: Prenatal observation of umbilical cord hematoma. Am. J. Roentg. 142:801, 1984.

Suzuki, K., Schneider, E.L. and Epstein, C.J.: *In utero* diagnosis of globoid cell leukodystrophy (Krabbe's disease). Biochem. Biophys. Res. Commun. 45:1363, 1971.

Suzuki, K., Minei, L.J. and Schnitzer, L.E.: Ultrasonographic measurement of fetal heart volume for estimation of birthweight. Obstet. Gynecol. 43:867, 1974.

Suzuki, Y., Shimozawa, N., Kawabata, I., Yajima, S., Inoue, K., Uchida, Y., Izai, K., Tomatsu, S., Kondo, N. and Orii, T.: Prenatal diagnosis of peroxisomal disorders: Biochemical and immunocytochemical studies on peroxisomes in human amniocytes. Brain Developm. 16:27, 1994.

Suzumori, K. and Yagami, Y.: Diagnosis of human fetal abnormalities by fetography. Teratology. 12:303, 1975.

Svennerholm, L., Hakanssen, G., Lindsten, J., Wahlstrom, J. and Dreborg, S.: Prenatal diagnosis of Gaucher disease: Assay of the beta-glucosidase activity in amniotic fluid cells cultivated in two laboratories with different cultivation conditions. Clin. Genet. 19:16, 1981.

Sweet, L., Reid, W.D. and Roberton, N.R.C.: Hydrops fetalis in association with chorioangioma of the placenta. J. Pediatr. 82:91, 1973.

Sweetman, L.: Prenatal diagnosis of the organic acidurias. J. Inherit. Metab. Dis. 7(Suppl. 1):18, 1984.

Sweetman, L.: Prenatal diagnosis of the organic acidurias by stable isotope dilution GC/MS analysis of amniotic fluid, prenatal therapy, and identification of a new disorder, mevalonic aciduria. Jpn. Med. Mass Spectrom. 10:17, 1985.

Sweetman, L.: Branched-chained organic aciduria. In: Scriver, C.R., Beaudet, A.L., Sly, W.S. and Valle, D., (Eds.). *The Metabolic Basis of Inherited Disease,* 6th ed. New York: McGraw-Hill, 1989, p. 791.

Sweetman, L.: Carboxylase deficiency, holocarboxylase deficiency type. In: Buyse, M.L. (Ed.). *Birth Defects Encyclopedia.* Cambridge, Mass.: Blackwell Scientific, 1990, p. 280.

Sweetman, L., Weyler, W., Shafai, T., Young, P.E. and Nyhan, W.L.: Prenatal diagnosis of propionic acidemia. J. Am. Med. Assoc. 242:1048, 1979.

Sweetman, L., Naylor, G., Ladner, T., Holm, J., Nyhan, W.L., Hornbeck, C., Griffiths, Morch, J. L., Brandange, S., Gruenke, L. and Craig, J.C.: Prenatal diagnosis of propionic and methylmalonic acidemia by stable isotope dilution analysis of methylcitric and methylmalonic acids in amniotic fluids. In: Schmidt, H.L., Forstel, H., and Heinzinge, K. (Eds.). *Stable Isotopes.* Amsterdam: Elsevier, 1982, p. 287.

Swinford, A.E., Higgins, J.V., Foster, K.W., Jr., Freimanis, A.K. and Strate, S.M.: Pregnancy monitoring of extended family members in familial bilateral renal agenesis. Am. J. Hum. Genet. 37:A137, 1985.

Swinford, A.E., Bernstein, J., Toriello, H.V. and Higgins, J.V.: Renal tubular dysgenesis: Delayed onset of oligohydramnios. Am. J. Med. Genet. 32:127, 1989.

Szabo, M., Teichmann, F. and Papp, Z.: Low trehalase activity in amniotic fluid: A marker for cystic fibrosis. Clin. Genet. 25:475, 1984.

Szabo, M., Varga, P., Zalatnai, A., Hidvegi J., Toth, Z. and Papp, Z.: Sacrococcygeal teratoma and normal alphafetoprotein concentration in amniotic fluid. J. Med. Genet. 22:405, 1985a.

Szabo, M., Teichmann, F., Szeifert, G.T., Toth, M., Toth, Z., Torok, O. and Papp, Z.: Prenatal diagnosis of cystic fibrosis by trehalase enzyme assay in amniotic fluid. Clin. Genet. 28:16, 1985b.

Szymonowicz, W., Preston, H. and Yu, V.Y.H.: The surviving monozygotic twin. Arch. Dis. Child. 61:454, 1986.

Tabor, A., Bang, J. and Philip, J.: 45,X karyotype: May the diagnosis be suspected on ultrasonic examination in the second trimester of pregnancy? Prenat. Diagn. 1:281, 1981.

Tabor, A., Norgaard-Pedersen, B. and Jacobsen, J.C.: Low maternal serum AFP and Down syndrome. Lancet. 2:161, 1984.

Tachdjian, G., Fondaccl, C., Tapia, S., Huten, Y., Blot, P. and Nessmann, C.: The Wolf–Hirschhorn syndrome in fetuses. Clin. Genet. 42:281, 1992.

Tachdjian, G., Cacheux, V., Kiefer, H., Druart, L., Lapierre, J-M., Oury, J-F., Blot, P. and Metezeau, P.: Prenatal diagnosis of a (X;X) translocation by fluorescence in situ hybridization and laser scanning image cytometry. Fetal Diagn. Ther. 10:387, 1995.

Tada, K., Kure, S., Takayanagi, M., Kume, A. and Narisawa, K.: Non-ketotic hyperglycinemia: A life-threatening disorder in the neonate. Early Hum. Develop. 29:75, 1992.

Tadmor, O.P., Hammerman, C., Rabinowitz, R., Fisher, D., Itzchaki, M., Aboulafia, Y. and Diamant, Y.Z.: Femoral hypoplasia-unusual facies syndrome: Prenatal ultrasonographic observations. Fetal Dign. Ther. 8:279, 1993.

Takashima, T., Maeda, H., Koyanagi, T., Nishimura, J. and Nakano, H.: Prenatal diagnosis and obstetrical management of May–Hegglin anomaly: A case report. Fetal Diagn. Ther. 7:186, 1992.

Tamas, D.E., Mahony, B.S., Bowie, J.D., Woodruff, W.W. and Kay, H.H.: Prenatal sonographic diagnosis of hemifacial microsomia (Goldenhar–Gorlin syndrome). J. Ultrasound Med. 5:461, 1986.

Tamura, R.K., Sabbagha, R.E. and Depp, R.: Diagnosis of intrauterine growth retardation. Clin. Obstet. Gynecol. 20:309, 1977.

Taubert, H.-D., Bastert, G. and Dericks-Tan, J.S.E.: Maternal serum alpha-fetoprotein levels in a triplet pregnancy with 2 papyraceous fetuses. Arch. Gynecol. 237:127, 1986.

Tchobroutsky, C., Breat, G.L., Rambaud, D.C. and Henrion, R.: Correlation between fetal defects and early growth delay observed by ultrasound. Lancet. 1:706, 1985.

Terespolsky, D. and Weksberg, R.: Hepatoblastoma and cardiomyopathy: Fatal outcome in a 4.5 month old girl. Am. J. Hum. Genet. 57(Suppl.):A104, 1995.

Terespolsky, D., Farrell, S.A., Siegel-Bartelt, J. and Weksberg, R.: Infantile lethal variant of Simpson–Golabi–Behmel syndorme associated with hydrops fetalis. Am. J. Med. Genet. 59:329, 1995.

Teteris, N.J., Chisholm, J.W. and Ullery, J.C.: Antenatal diagnosis of congenital heart block: Report of a case. Obstet. Gynecol. 32:851, 1968.

Theil, A.C., Schutgens, R.B.H., Wanders, R.J.A. and Heymans, H.S.A.: Clinical recognition of patients affected by a peroxisomal disorder: A retrospective study in 40 patients. Eur. J. Pediatr. 151:117, 1992.

Theodoropoulos, D.S., Cowan, J.M., Elias, E.R. and Cole, C.: Physical findings in 21q22 deletion suggest critical region for 21q- phenotype in q22. Am. J. Med. Genet. 59:161, 1995.

Therkelsen, A.J., Jensen, P.K.A., Hertz, J.M., Smidt-Jensen, S. and Hahnemann, N.: Prenatal cytogenetic diagnosis after transabdominal chorionic villus sampling in the first trimester. Prenat. Diagn. 8:19, 1988.

Thiede, H.A., Creasman, W.T. and Metcalfe, S.: Antenatal analysis of the human chromosomes. Am. J. Obstet. Gynecol. 94:589, 1966.

Thies, U., Zuhlke, C., Bockel, B. and Schroder, K.: Prenatal diagnosis of Huntington's disease (HD): Experiences with six cases and PCR. Prenat. Diagn. 12:1055, 1992.

Thom, H., Buckland, C.M. and Campbell, A.G.M.: Maternal serum alpha fetoproteinin monozygotic and dizygotic twin pregnancies. Prenat. Diagn. 4:341, 1984.

Thomas, C.R., Lang, E.K. and Lloyd, F.P.: Fetal pyelography—A method for detecting fetal life. Obstet. Gynecol. 22:335, 1963.

Thomas, R.L., Hess, W.L. and Johnson, T.R.B.: Prepartum diagnosis of limb-shortening defects with associated hydramnios. Am. J. Perinatol. 4:293, 1987.

Thomas, M., Chitayat, D., Toi, A., Barrett, J., Waye, J., Chui, D., Pauzner, D., Morrow, R. and Ryan, G.: Sonographic findings in homozygous alpha thalassemia prior to the onset of hydrops. Am. J. Hum. Genet. 53(Suppl.):1813, 1993.

Thompson, P.J., Greenough, A. and Nicolaides, K.H.: Respiratory function in infancy following pleuro-amniotic shunting. Fetal Diagn. Ther. 8:79, 1993.

Thomson, G.S.M., Reynolds, C.P. and Cruickshank, J.: Antenatal detection of recurrence of Majewski dwarf (short rib-polydactyly syndrome type II Majewski). Clin. Radiol. 33:509, 1982.

Tick, D.B., Greenberg, F., Reiter, A., Redman, J., Foster, S., Hawkins, E. and Armstrong, D.: Prenatal detection of telencephalic hypoplasia. Proc. Greenwood Genet. Cent. 9:127, 1990.

Tiller, G.E., Weis, MA., Polumbo, P.A., Gruber, H.E., Rimoin, D.L., Cohn, D.H. and Eyre, D.R.: An RNA-splicing mutation ($G^{+5IVS20}$) in the type II collagen gene (CPL2A1) in a family with spondyloepiphyseal dysplasia congenita. Am. J. Hum. Genet. 56:388, 1995.

Tilley, L.D., Wade, R.V. and Grass, F.S.: Prenatal diagnosis of transient myeloproliferative disorder in a stillborn fetus with Down syndrome. Am. J. Hum. Genet. 53(Suppl.):1814, 1993.

Timor-Tritsch, I.E., Monteagudo, A., Haratz-Rubinstein, N. and Levine, R.U.: Transvaginal sonographic detection of adducted thumbs, hydrocephalus, and agenesis of the corpus callosum at 22 postmenstrual weeks: The MASA spectrum or L1 spectrum. A case report and review of the literature. Prenat. Diagn. 16:543, 1996.

Tint, G.S., Irons, M., Elias, E.R., Batta, A.K., Frieden, R., Chen, T.S. and Salen, G.: Defective cholesterol biosynthesis associated with the Smith–Lemli–Opitz syndrome. N. Engl. J. Med. 330:107, 1994a.

Tint, G.S., Salen, G. and Irons, M.: Diagnosis of Smith–Lemli–Opitz syndome. N. Engl. J. Med. 330:1687, 1994b.

Tischfield, J. Schafer, I.A., Dickerman, L.H., Trill, J., Mulivor, R.A., Greene, A.E. and Coriell, L.L.: Lesch–Nyhan syndrome. Repository identification Nos. GM-2290, 2291, 2292, 2338, 3115, 3116 and 3117. Cytogenet. Cell Genet. 24:199, 1979.

Toftager-Larsen, K. and Benzie, R.J.: Fetoscopy in prenatal diagnosis of the Majewski and the Saldino–Noonan types of the short rib-polydactyly syndromes. Clin. Genet. 26:56, 1984.

Toftager-Larsen, K., Kjaersgaard, E., Jacobsen, J.C. and Norgaard-Pedersen, B.: Reactivity of amniotic fluid alpha-fetoprotein with concanavalin A in relation to gestational age: Clinical implications. Clin. Chem. 26:1656, 1980.

Toftager-Larsen, K., Benzie, R.J., Doran, T.A., Miskin, M., Allen, L.C. and Becker, L.: Alpha-fetoprotein and ultrasound scanning in the prenatal diagnosis of Turner's syndrome. Prenat. Diagn. 3:35, 1983.

Toftager-Larsen, K., Wandrup, J. and Norgaard-Pedersen, B.: Amniotic fluid analysis in prenatal diagnosis of neural tube defects: A comparison between six biochemical tests supplementary to the measurement of amniotic fluid alpha-fetoprotein. Clin. Genet. 26:406, 1984.

Toi, A., Chitayat, D., Blazer, S. Moore, L., Leet, C. and Becker, L.: Prenatal diagnosis of the Dandy–Walker variant. An abnormality or a transient finding? Am. J. Hum. Genet. 53(Suppl.):1465, 1993.

Toi, A., Chitayat, D., Blaser, S., Semer, M., Moola, S., Johnson, J., Solomon, L. and Teshima, I.: Omphalocele: A prenatally detectable abnormality in Miller–Dieker syndrome. Am. J. Hum. Genet. 57(Suppl.):A289, 1995.

Tolarova, M. and Zwinger A.: The use of fetoscopy by inborn morphological anomalies. Acta Chirurgiae Plasticae. 23:3, 1981.

Tolkendorf, E., Mehner, G. and Prager, B.: Partial trisomy 22q12 → qter in prenatal diagnosis. Prenat. Diagn. 11:339, 1991.

Tolmie, J.L., Mortimer, G., Doyle, D., McKenzie, R., McLaurin, J. and Neilson, J.P.: The Neu–Laxova syndrome in female sibs: Clinical and pathological features with prenatal diagnosis in the second sib. Am. J. Med. Genet. 27:175, 1987a.

Tolmie, J.L., Whittle, M.J., McNay, M.B., Gibson, A.A.M. and Connor, J.M.: Second trimester prenatal diagnosis of the Jarcho–Levin syndrome. Prenat. Diagn. 7:129, 1987b.

Tolmie, J.L., Ferguson-Smith, M.E., Gilmore, D. and Ferguson-Smith, M.A.: Normal development in two six-year old boys born after prenatal diagnosis of trisomy 20 mosaicism. Prenat. Diagn. 7:597, 1987c.

Tolmie, J.L., Patrick, A. and Yates, J.R.W.: A lethal multiple pterygium syndrome with apparent X-linked recessive inheritance. Am. J. Med. Genet. 27:913, 1987d.

Tolmie, J.L., McNay, M., Stephenson, J.B.P., Doyle, D. and Connor, J.M.: Microcephaly: Genetic counselling and antenatal diagnosis after the birth of an affected child. Am. J. Med. Genet. 27:583, 1987e.

Tomlinson, M.W., Johnson, M.P., Gonclaves, L., King, M., Freedman, A., Smith, C., Hume, R.F., Jr. and Evans, M.I.: Correction of hemodynamic abnormalities by vesicoamniotic shunting in familial congenital megacystis. Fetal Diagn. Ther. 11:46, 1996.

Tommerup, N.: The fragile X chromosome: Prenatal diagnosis. Clin. Genet. 29:475, 1986.

Tommerup, N., Sondergaard, F., Tonnesen, T., Kristensen, M., Arveiler, B. and Schinzel, A.: First trimester prenatal diagnosis of a male fetus with fragile X. Lancet. 1:870, 1985.

Tommerup, N., Aula, P., Gustavii, B., Heibert, A., Holmgren, G., von Koskull, H., Leisti, J., Mikkelsen, M., Mitelman, F., Nielsen, K.B., Steinbach, P., Stengel-Rutkowski, S., Wahlstrom, J., Zang, K. and Zankl, M.: Second trimester prenatal diagnosis of the fragile X. Am. J. Med. Genet. 23:313, 1986.

Tonnesen T. and Horn, N.: Prenatal and postnatal diagnosis of Menkes disease, an inherited disorder of copper metabolism. J. Inher. Metab. Dis. 12:(Suppl. 1):207, 1989.

Tonnesen, T., Horn, N., Sondergaard, F., Mikkelsen, M., Boue, J., Damsgaard, E. and Heydorn, K.: Measurement of copper in chorionic villi for first-trimester diagnosis of Menkes' disease. Lancet. 1:1038, 1985.

Tonnesen, T., Horn, N., Sondergaard, F., Jensen, O.A., Gerdes, A.-M., Girard, S. and Damsgaard, E.: Experience with first trimester prenatal diagnosis of Menkes disease. Prenat. Diagn. 7:497, 1987a.

Tonnesen, T., Horn, N., Sondergaard, F. and Jensen, O.A.: Experience with first trimester prenatal diagnosis of Menkes disease. Curr. Probl. Dermatol. 16:175, 1987b.

Tonnesen, T., Gerdes, A.-M., Damsgaard, E., Miny, P., Holzgreve, W., Sondergaard, F. and Horn, N.: First-trimester dianosis of Menkes disease: Intermediate copper values in chorionic villi from three affected male fetuses. Prenat. Diagn. 9:159, 1989.

Toone, J.R. and Applegarth, D.A.: Use of placental enzyme analysis in assessment of the newborn at risk for nonketotic hyperglycinaemia (NKH). J. Inherit. Metab. Dis. 12:281, 1989.

Toone, J.R., Applegarth, D.A. and Levy, H.L.: Prenatal diagnosis of non-ketotic hyperglycinaemia. J. Inher. Metab. Dis. 15:713, 1992.

Toone, J.R., Applegarth, D.A. and Levy, H.L.: Prenatal diagnosis of non-ketotic hyperglycinaemia: Experience in 50 at-risk pregnancies. J. Inher. Metab. Dis. 17:342, 1994.

Toriello, H.V. and Higgins, J.V.: Craniodigital syndromes: Report of a child with Filippi syndrome and discussion of differential diagnosis. Am. J. Med. Genet. 55:200, 1995.

Toriello, H.V., Bauserman, S.C. and Higgins, J.V.: Sibs with the fetal akinesia sequence, fetal edema, and malformations: A new syndrome? Am. J. Med. Genet. 21:271, 1985.

Torok, O., Norregaard-Hansen, K., Szokol, M., Csecsei, K., Harsanyi, A. and Papp, Z.: Prenatal diagnosis of Duchenne muscular dystrophy by radioimmunoassay of myoglobin in amniotic fluid. Clin. Genet. 21:354, 1982.

Tortora, M., Chervenak, F.A., Mayden, K. and Hobbins, J.C.: Antenatal sonographic diagnosis of single umbilical artery. Obstet. Gynecol. 63:693, 1984.

Toth-Fejel, S., Magenis, R.E., Leff, S., Brown, M.G., Comegys, B., Lawce, H., Berry, T., Kesner, D., Webb, M.J. and Olson, S.: Prenatal diagnosis of chromosome 15 abormalities in the Prader–Willi/Angelman syndrome region by traditional and molecular cytogenetics. Am. J. Med. Genet. 55:444, 1995.

Trefz, F.K., Schmidt, H., Tauscher, B., Depene, E., Baumgartner, R., Hammersen, G. and Kochen, W.: Improved prenatal diagnosis of methylmalonic acidemia: Mass fragmentography of methylmalonic acid in amniotic fluid and maternal urine. Eur. J. Pediatr. 137:261, 1981.

Trigg, M.E., Hitchems, J., Geier, M.R. and Hutchinson, G.: Low maternal serum AFP and Down syndrome. Lancet. 2:161, 1984.

Triggs-Raine, B.L., Archibald, A., Gravel, R.A. and Clarke, J.T.R.: Prenatal exclusion of Tay–Sachs disease by DNA analysis. Lancet. 1:1164, 1990.

Tromans, P.M., Coulson, R., Lobb, M.O. and Abdulla, U.: Abdominal pregnancy associated with extremely elevated serum alpha-fetoprotein. Case report. Br. J. Obstet. Gynaecol. 91:296, 1984.

Trunca, C., Watson, M., Auerbach, A., Kaplan, C., Mahoney, M. and Baker, D.: Prenatal diagnosis of Fanconi anemia in a fetus not known to be at risk. Am. J. Hum. Genet. 36(Suppl.):198S, 1984.

Tsukahara, M., Sase, M., Tateishi, H., Saito, T., Kato, H. and Furukawa, S.: Skeletal manifestations in Fryns syndrome. Am. J. Med. Genet. 55:217, 1995.

Tsutsumi, O., Satoh, K., Sakamoto, S., Suzuki, Y. and Kato, T.: Application of a galactosylceramidase microassay method to early prenatal diagnosis of Krabbe's disease. Clin. Chim. Acta. 125:265, 1982.

Tuck, S.M., Slack, J. and Buckland, G.: Prenatal diagnosis of Conradi's syndrome: Case report. Prenat. Diagn. 10:195, 1990.

Tuerilings, J.H.A.M. and Nijhuis, J.G.: False negative and false positive result after amniocentesis. Am. J. Hum. Genet. 57(Suppl.):A290, 1995.

Tumer, Z, Tonnesen, T., Bohmann, J., Marg, W. and Horn, N.: First trimester prenatal diagnosis of Menkes disease by DNA analysis. J. Med. Genet. 31:615, 1994.

Turco, A.E., Padovani, E.M., Chiaffoni, G. P., Peissel, B., Rossetti, S., Marcolongo, A., Gammaro, L., Maschio, G. and Pignatti, P.F.: Molecular genetic diagnosis of autosomal dominant polycystic kidney disease in a newborn with bilateral cystic kidneys detected prenatally and multiple skeletal malformations. J. Med. Genet. 30:419, 1993.

Turner, R.J., Hankins, G.D.V., Weinreb, J.C., Ziaya, P.R., Davis, T.N., Lowe, T.W. and Gilstrap, L.C., III: Magnetic resonance imaging and ultrasonography in the antenatal evaluation of conjoined twins. Am. J. Obstet. Gynecol. 155:645, 1986.

Turnpenny, P.D., Davidson, R., Stockdale, E.J.N., Tolmie, J.L. and Sutton, A.M.: Severe prenatal infantile cortical hyperostosis (Caffey's disease). Clin. Dysmorph. 2:81, 1993.

U.K. Collaborative Study on Alpha-Fetoprotein in Relation to Neural-Tube Defects: Amniotic-fluid alpha-fetoprotein measurement in antenatal diagnosis of anencephaly and open spina bifida in early pregnancy. Lancet. 2:651, 1979.

Upadhyaya, M., Fryer, A., MacMillan, J., Broadhead, W., Huson, S.M. and Harper, P.S.: Prenatal diagnosis and presymptomatic detection of neurofibromatosis type 1. J. Med. Genet. 29:180, 1992.

Urig, M.A., Clewell, W.H. and Elliott, J.P.: Twin–twin transfusion syndrome. Am. J. Obstet. Gynecol. 163:1522, 1990.

Urioste, M., Arroyo, I., Villa, A., Lorda-Sanchez, I., Barrio, R., Lopez-Cuesta, M-J. and Rueda, J.: Distal deletion of chromosome 13 in a child with the "Opitz" GBBB syndrome. Am. J. Med. Genet. 59:114, 1995.

Ursell, W.: Hydramnios associated with congenital microstomia, agnathia, and synotia. J. Obstet. Gynaecol. Br. Commonw. 79:185, 1972.

Utter, G.O., Socol, M.L., Dooley, S.L., MacGregor, S.N. and Millard, D.D.: Is intrauterine transfusion associated with diminished fetal growth? Am. J. Obstet. Gynecol. 163:1781, 1990.

Valenti, C.: Endoamnioscopy and fetal biopsy: A new technique. Am. J. Obstet. Gynecol. 114:561, 1972.

Valenti, C.: Antenatal detection of hemoglobinopathies: A preliminary report. Am. J. Obstet. Gynecol. 115:851, 1973.

Valenti, C., Schutta, E.J. and Kehaty, T.: Prenatal diagnosis of Down's syndrome. Lancet. 2:220, 1968.

Valenti, C., Kassner, E.G., Yermakov, V. and Cromb, E.: Antenatal diagnosis of a fetal ovarian cyst. Am. J. Obstet. Gynecol. 123:216, 1975.

Valentin, L., Marsal, K. and Wahlgren, L.: Subjective recording of fetal movements. III. Screening of a pregnant population: The clinical significance of decreased fetal movement counts. Acta Obstet. Gynecol. Scand. 65:753, 1986.

Vamos, E., Pratola, D., Van Regemorter, N., Freunds, M., Flament-Durand, J. and Rodesch, F.: Prenatal diagnosis and fetal pathology of partial trisomy 20p-monosomy 4p resulting from paternal translocation. Prenat. Diagn. 5:209, 1985.

Vamos, E., Libert, J., Elkhazen, N., Jauniaux, E., Hustin, J. and Wilkin, P.: Prenatal diagnosis and confirmation of infantile sialic acid storage disease. Prenat. Diagn. 6:437, 1986.

Van Allen, M.I., Toi, A., Johnson, J., Shuman, C., Greer, W. and Ray, P.N.: A new approach to ultrasound scan diagnosis of cystic fibrosis. Am. J. Hum. Genet. 45(Suppl.):A272, 1989.

Van Allen, M.I., Toi, A., Johnson, J.M., Ray, P., Ritchie, S.: Congenital abnormalities in 18 fetuses with highly echogenic meconium on ultrasound. Clin. Res. 40:56A, 1992.

Van den Hof, M.C., Nicolaides, K.H., Campbell, J. and Campbell, S.: Evaluation of the lemon and banana signs in one hundred thirty fetuses with open spina bifida. Am. J. Obstet. Gynecol. 162:322, 1990.

van der Hagen, C.B., Borresen, A-L, Molne, K., Oftedal, G., Bjoro, K. and Berg, K.: Metachromatic leukodystrophy 1. Prenatal detection of arylsulphatase A deficiency. Clin. Genet. 4:256, 1973.

Van Diggelen, O.P., Janse, H.C. and Kleijer, W.J.: Disaccharidases in amniotic fluid as possible prenatal marker for cystic fibrosis. Lancet. 1:817, 1983.

van Diggelen, O.P., Von Koskull, H., Ammala, P., Vredeveldt, G.T.M., Janse, H.C. and Kleijer, W.J.: First trimester diagnosis of Wolman's disease. Prenat. Diagn. 8:661, 1988.

Van Dyke, D.L., Fluharty, A.L., Schafer, I.A., Shapiro, L.J., Kihara, H. and Weiss, L.: Prenatal diagnosis of Maroteaux–Lamy syndrome. Am. J. Med. Genet. 8:235, 1981.

Van Dyke, D.L., Marcy, A., Craig, B.M., Babu, V.R. and Roberson, J.R.: Chromosome 1 deletion associated with increased nuchal fold thickness in the second trimester. Prenat. Diagn. 9:140, 1989.

Van Egmond-Linden, A., Wladimiroff, J.W., Jahoda, M.G.J., Niermeijer, M.F., Sachs, E.S. and Stefanko, S.: Prenatal diagnosis of X-linked hydrocephaly. Prenat. Diagn. 3:245, 1983.

Vanesian, R., Grossman, M., Metherell, A., Flynn, J.J. and Louscher, S.: Antepartum ultrasonic diagnosis of congenital hydrocele. Radiology. 126:765, 1978.

Van Hemel, J.O., Schaap, C., Van Opstal, D., Mulder, M.P., Niermeijer, M.F. and Meijers, J.H.C.: Recurrence of DiGeorge syndrome: Prenatal detection by FISH of a molecular 22q11 deletion. J. Med. Genet. 32:657, 1995.

Van Herle, A.J., Young, R.T., Fisher, D.A., Uller, R.P. and Brinkmann, III, C.R.: Intrauterine treatment of a hypothyroid fetus. J. Clin. Endocrinol Metab. 40:474, 1975.

Van Hoesen, K.B., Camporesi, E.M., Moon, R.E., Hage, M.L. and Piantadosi, C.A.: Should hyperbaric oxygen be used to treat the pregnant patient for acute carbon monoxide poisoning? A case report and literature review. J. Am. Med. Assoc. 261:1039, 1989.

Van Hove, J.L.K., Chace, D.H., Kahler, S.G. and Millington, D.S.: Acylcarnitines in amniotic fluid: Application to the prenatal diagnosis of propionic acidaemia. J. Inher. Metab. Dis. 16:361, 1993.

Vanier, M.T., Boue, J. and Dumez, Y.: Niemann–Pick disease type B: First-trimester prenatal diagnosis on chorionic villi and biochemical study of a foetus at 12 weeks of development. Clin. Genet. 28:348, 1985.

Vanier, M.T., Rousson, R.M., Mandon, G., Choiset, A., Lake, B.D. and Pentchev, P.G.: Diagnosis of Niemann–Pick disease type C on chorionic villus cells. Lancet. 1:1014, 1989.

Vanier, M.T., Rodriguez-Lafrasse, C., Rousson, R., Mandon, G., Boue, J., Choiset, A., Peyrat, M-F, Dumontel, C., Juge, M-C., Pentchev, P.G., Revol, A. and Louisot, P.: Prenatal diagnosis of Niemann–Pick type C disease: Current strategy form an experience of 37 pregnancies at risk. Am. J. Hum. Genet. 51:111, 1992.

Van Maldergem, L., Jauniaux, E. and Gillerot, Y.: Morphological features of a case of retinoic acid embryopathy. Prenat. Diagn. 12:699, 1992.

Vanneuville, F. J., Leroy, J.G. and Van Elsen, A.F.: Alkaline phosphatase in cultured amniotic-fluid cells: Implications for prenatal diagnosis of hypophosphatasia. J. Inher. Metab. Dis. 5(Suppl. 1):39, 1982.

Van Regemorter, N., Wilkin, P., Englert, Y., El Khazen, N., Alexander, S., Rodesch, F. and Milaire, J.: Lethal multiple pterygium syndrome. Am. J. Med. Genet. 17:827, 1984.

van Rijn, M., Christiaens, G.C.M.L. and Hagenaars, A.M.: Low maternal serum alfa-fetoprotein levels in pregnancies with anus imperforatus as an outcome. Am. J. Hum. Genet. 57(Suppl.):A290, 1995.

Varadi, V., Csecsei, K., Szeifert, G.T., Toth, Z. and Papp, Z.: Prenatal diagnosis of X linked hydrocephalus without aqueductal stenosis. J. Med. Genet. 24:207, 1987.

Vats, S., Filkins, K., Russo, J. and Garver, K.: First trimester incidence of cystic hygromas. Am. J. Hum. Genet. 45(Suppl.):A272, 1989.

Vejerslev, L.O., Dueholm, M. and Nielsen, F.H.: Hydatidiform mole: Cytogenetic marker analysis in twin gestation. Am. J. Obstet. Gynecol. 155:614, 1986.

Venter, P.A., Coetzee, D.J., Badenhorst, A., Marx, M.P., Hof, J.O., Behari, D., Wilmot, J. and Battson, S.A.: A confirmed prenatal diagnosis of a female fetus with the fragile X chromosome. Prenat. Diagn. 4:473, 1984.

Verhoeven, N.M., Kulik, W., van den Heuvel, C.M.M. and Jakobs, C.: Pre- and postnatal diagnosis of peroxisomal disorders using stable-isotope dilution gas chromatography-mass spectrometry. J. Inher. Metab. Dis. 18(Suppl. 1):45, 1995.

Verjaal, M., Meyer, A.H., Becker-Bloemkolk, M.J., Leschot, N.J., der Weduwen, J.J. and Gras., J.G.F.M.: Oligohydramnios hampering prenatal diagnosis of Meckel syndrome. Am. J. Med. Genet. 7:85, 1980.

Verloes, A., Narcy, F. and Fallet-Bianco, C.: Syndromal hypothalamic hamartoblastoma with holoprosencephaly sequence, microphthalmia, pulmonary malformations, radial hypoplasia and Mullerian regression: Further delineation of a new syndrome. Clin. Dysmorph. 4:33, 1995.

Verma, I.C., Bhargava, S. and Agarwal, S.: An autosomal recessive form of lethal chondrodystrophy with severe thoracic narrowing, rhizoacromelic type of micromelia, polydactyly, and genital anomalies. Birth Defects. 11(6):167, 1975.

Verma, U., Weiss, R.R., Almonte, R., Macri, J.N., Tejani, N., Balsam, D. and Tuck, S.: Early prenatal diagnosis of soft-tissue malformations. Obstet. Gynecol. 53:660, 1979.

Vermesh, M., Mayden, K.L., Confino, E., Giglia, R.V. and Gleicher, N.: Prenatal sonographic diagnosis of Hirschsprung's disease. J. Ultrasound Med. 5:37, 1986.

Verp, M.S., Milunsky, A., Simpson, J.L., Graham, A. and Sabbagha, R.: Elevated alphafetoprotein and acetylcholinesterase associated with hydrocele. Am. J. Med. Genet. 19:651, 1984.

Verp, M.S., Rosinsky, B., Sheikh, Z. and Amarose, A.P.: Non-mosaic trisomy 16 confined to villi. Lancet. 2:915, 1989a.

Verp, M.S., Sheikh, Z., Amarose, A.P. and Cibils, L.A.: Cystic hygroma and 45,X/46,XY mosaicism. Am. J. Med. Genet. 33:402, 1989b.

Verp, M.S., Lindgren, V., Knutel, T., Christian, S. and Ledbetter, D.H.: Prospective prenatal detection of uniparental disomy 15. Am. J. Med. Genet. 57(Suppl.):A290, 1995.

Vesa, J., Hellsten, E., Makela, T.P., Jarvela, I., Airaksinen, T., Santavuori, P. and Peltonen, L.: A single PCR marker in strong allelic association with the infantile form of neuronal ceroid lipofuscinosis facilitates reliable prenatal diagnostics and disease carrier identification. Eur. J. Hum. Genet. 1:125, 1993.

Vezina, W.C., Morin, F.R. and Winsberg, F.: Megacystic-microcolon-intestinal hypoperistalsis syndrome: Antenatal ultrasound appearance. Am. J. Roentgenol. 133:749, 1979.

Vidaud, M., Chabret, C., Dumez, Y., Daffos, F. and Goossens, M.: First-trimester fetal diagnosis of hemoglobinopathies and hemophilias by DNA analysis: A three years experience. Contrib. Gynecol. Obstet. 15:104, 1986.

Vieira-Rush, P.W., Dickerman, L.H., Jassani, M.N. and Silverman, R.A.: Elevations of maternal serum alpha-fetoprotein (MSAFP), amniotic fluid alpha-fetoprotein (AFAFP), and acetylcholinesterase (AChE) associated with congenital cutis aplasia. Am. J. Hum. Genet. 43(Suppl.):A252, 1988.

Vielhaber, E., Sommer, S.S. and Freedenberg, D.: Mutation detection, prenatal testing, and delineation of the germline origin in a family with sporadic hemophilia B and no living hemophiliacs. Am. J. Med. Genet. 49:257, 1994.

Vinson, P.C., Goldenberg, R.L., Davis, R.O., Finley, S.C., Milunsky, A., Chase, T.M. and Nagendran, S.S.: Fetal bladder-neck obstruction and elevated amniotic-fluid alpha fetoprotein. N. Engl. J. Med. 297:1351, 1977.

Vinters, H.V., Murphy, J., Wittmann, B. and Norman, M.G.: Intracranial teratoma: Antenatal diagnosis at 31 weeks' gestation by ultrasound. Acta Neuropathol. 58:233, 1982.

Vintzileos, A.M., Nochimson, D.J., Walzak, M.P., Conrad, F.U. and Lillo, N.L.: Unilateral fetal hydronephrosis: Successful in utero surgical management. Am. J. Obstet. Gynecol. 145:885, 1983.

Vintzileos, A.M and Egan, J.F.X.: Adjusting the risk for trisomy 21 on the basis of second-trimester ultrasonograpy. Am. J. Obstet. Gynecol. 172:837, 1995.

Viscarello, R.R., Thio, C., Sokol, R., Gallagher, R. and Hobbins, J.C.: Can fetal alcohol syndrome be detected in utero by ultrasound? Preliminary findings. Am. J. Obstet. Gynecol. 164:340, 1991.

Visser, G.H.A., Desmedt, M.C.H. and Meijboom, E.J.: Altered fetal cardiac flow patterns in pure red cell anaemia (The Blackfan–Diamond syndrome). Prenat. Diagn. 8:525, 1988.

Voigtlander, T. and Vogel, F.: Low alpha-fetoprotein and serum albumin levels in Morbus Down may point to a common regulatory mechanism. Hum. Genet. 71:276, 1985.

Voigtlander, T., Friedl, W., Cremer, M., Schmidt, W. and Schroeder, T.M.: Quantitative and qualitative assay of amniotic-fluid acetylcholinesterase in the prenatal diagnosis of neural tube defects. Hum. Genet. 59:227, 1981.

von Dobeln, U. Venizelos, N., Westgren, M. and Hagenfeldt, L.: Long-chain 3-hydroxyacyl-CoA dehydrogenase in chorionic villi, fetal liver and fibroblasts and prenatal diagnosis of 3-hydroxyacyl-CoA dehydrogenase deficiency. J. Inher. Metab. Dis. 17:185, 1994.

von Figura, K., van de Kamp, J.J. and Niermeijer, M.F.: Prenatal diagnosis of Morquio's disease type A (N-acetylgalactosamine 6-sulphate sulphatase deficiency). Prenat. Diagn. 2:67, 1982.

von Koskull, H.: Rapid identification of glial cells in human amniotic fluid with indirect immunofluorescence. Acta Cytol. 28:393, 1984.

von Koskull, H., Virtanen, I., Lehto, V., Vartio, T., Dahl, D. and Aula, P.: Glial and neuronal cells in amniotic fluid of anencephalic pregnancies. Prenat. Diagn. 1:259, 1981.

von Koskull, H., Aula, P., Ammala, P., Nordstrom, A.-M. and Rapola, J.: Improved technique for the expression of fragile-X in cultured amniotic fluid cells. Hum. Genet. 69:218, 1985.

von Koskull, H. Gahmberg, N., Salonen, R., Salo, A. and Peippo, M.: FRAXA locus in fragile X diagnosis: Family studies, prenatal diagnosis, and diagnosis of sporadic cases of mental retardation. Am. J. Med. Genet. 51:486, 1994.

von Lennep, E., El Khazen, N., De Pierreux, G., Amy, J.J., Rodesch, F. and Van Regemorter, N.: A case of partial sirenomelia and possible vitamin A teratogenesis. Prenat. Diagn. 5:35, 1985.

Vulsma, T., Gons, M.H. and de Vijlder, J.J.M.: Maternal–fetal transfer of thyroxine in congenital hypothyroisism due to a total organification defect or thyroid agenesis. N. Engl. J. Med. 321:13, 1989.

Wachtel, S., Sammons, D., Manley, M., Wachtel, G., Utermohlen, J., Phillips, O., Shulman, L.P.. Addis, K., Porreco, R., Murata-Collins, J., Parker, N. and McGavran, L.: Culturing of fetal cells recovered from maternal blood by charge flow separation. Am. J. Hum. Genet. 57(Suppl.):A33, 1995.

Waites, K.B., Tully, J.G., Rose, D.L., Marriott, P.A., Davis, R.O., and Cassell, G.H.: Isolation of Acholeplasma oculi from human amniotic fluid in early pregnancy. Curr. Microbiol. 15:325, 1987.

Wajner, M., Gaidzinski, D., Wannmacher, C.M.D., Fontana, M.H., Jones, M., Mistry, J. and Chalmers, R.A.: Methylmalonic aciduria unresponsive to vitamin B_{12}: Description of two cases and prenatal diagnosis in a Brazilian family. Rev. Brasil. Genet. 9:693, 1986.

Wald, N.J. and Cuckle, H.S.: Maternal serum-alpha-fetoprotein measurement in antenatal screening for anencephaly and spina bifida in early pregnancy: Report of the U.K. Collaborative Study of Alpha-Fetoprotein in Relation to Neural-Tube Defects. Lancet. 1:1323, 1977.

Wald, N.J. and Cuckle, H.S.: Amniotic fluid acetylcholinesterase electrophoresis as a secondary test in the diagnosis of anencephaly and open spina bifida in early pregnancy: Report of the Collaborative Acetylcholinesterase Study. Lancet. 2:321, 1981.

Wald, N., Cuckle, H., Stirrat, G.M., Bennett, M.J. and Turnbull, A.C.: Maternal serum-alpha-fetoprotein and low birth-weight. Lancet. 2:268, 1977.

Wald, N., Cuckle, H., Boreham, J. and Stirrat, G.: Small biparietal diameter of fetuses with spina bifida: Implications for antenatal screening. Br. J. Obstet. Gynaecol. 87:219, 1980.

Waldherr, R., Zerres, K., Gall, A. and Enders, H.: Polycystic kidney disease in the fetus. Lancet. 2:274, 1989.

Walkinshaw, S., Pilling, D and Spriggs, A.: Isolated choroid plexus cysts—The need for routine offer of karyotyping. Prenat. Diagn. 14:663, 1994a.

Walkinshaw, S.A., Welch, C.R., McCormack, J. and Walsh, K.: In utero pacing for fetal congenital heart block. Fetal Diagn. Ther. 9:183, 1994b.

Waller, K.D., Lustig, L.S., Hook, E.B., Golbus, M.S. and Arnopp, J.J.: Maternal serum alpha-fetoprotein in 639 pregnancies ending in fetal death. Am. J. Hum. Genet. 45(Suppl.): A282, 1989.

Wallerstein, R., Wade, R.V., Young, S.R. and Pai, S.: Maternal serum alpha-fetoprotein (MS-AFP) and congenital amputations. Am. J. Med. Genet. 41:A286, 1987.

Wallis, J., Shaw, J., Wilkes, D., Farrall, M., Williamson, R., Chamberlain, S., Skare, J.C. and Milunsky, A.: Prenatal diagnosis of Friedreich ataxia. Am. J. Med. Genet. 34:458, 1989.

Walters, W.A.W., Renou, P.M., Campbell, A.J., Buttery, B.W., Matthews, R.N. and Sharma, R.S.: Antenatal intrauterine diagnosis of fetal thalassaemia. Med. J. Aust. 140:260, 1984.

Wanders, R.J.A., Schrakamp, G., van den Bosch, H., Tager, J.M. and Schutgens, R.B.H.: A prenatal test for the cerebro-hepato-renal (Zellweger) syndrome by demonstration of the absence of catalase-containing particles (peroxisomes) in cultured amniotic fluid cells. Eur. J. Pediatr. 145:136, 1986a.

Wanders, R.J.A., Schrakamp, G., van den Bosch, H., Tager, J.M., Moser, H.W., Moser, A.E., Aubourg, P., Kleijer, W.J. and Schutgens, R.B.H.: Pre- and postnatal diagnosis of the cerebro-hepato-renal (Zellweger) syndrome via a simple method directly demonstrating the presence or absence of peroxisomes in cultured skin fibroblasts, amniocytes or chorionic villi fibroblasts. J. Inher. Metab Dis. 9(Suppl. 2):317, 1986b.

Wanders, R.J.A., Shutgens, R.B.H. and Zoeters, B.H.M.: Prenatal diagnosis of 3-hydroxy-3-methylglutaric aciduria via enzyme activity measurements in chorionic villi, chorionic villous fibroblasts or amniocytes using a simple spectrophotometric method. J. Inher. Metab. Dis. 11:430, 1988.

Wanders, R.J.A., Wiemer, E.A.C., Brul, S., Schutgens, R.B.H., van den Bosch, H. and Tager, J.M.: Prenatal diagnosis of Zellweger syndrome by direct visualization of peroxisomes in chorionic villus fibroblasts by immunofluorescence microscopy. J. Inher. Metab. Dis. 12(Suppl. 2):301, 1989.

Wanders, R.J.A., van Roermund, C.W.T., Schutgens, R.B.H., Barth, P.G., Heymans, H.S.A., van den Bosch, H. and Tager, J.M.: The inborn errors of peroxisomal beta oxidation: A review. J. Inherited Metab. Dis. 13:4, 1990.

Wanders, R.J.A., Schutgens, R.B.H., van den Bosch, H., Tager, J.M. and Kleijer, W.J.: Prenatal diagnosis of inborn errors in peroxisomal beta-oxidation. Prenat. Diagn. 11:253, 1991.

Wanders, R.J.A., Ofman, R., Romeijn, G.J., Schutgens, R.B.H., Mooijer, P.A.W., Dekker, C. and van den Bosch, H.: Measurement of dihydroxyacetone-phosphate acyltransferase (DHAPAT) in chorionic villous samples, blood cells and cultured cells. J. Inher. Metab. Dis. 18(Suppl. 1):90, 1995.

Wanders, R.J.A., Barth, P.G., Schutgens, R.B.H. and Heymans, H.S.A.: Peroxisomal disorders: Post- and prenatal diagnosis based on a new classification with flowcharts. Int. Pediatr. 11:203, 1996.

Wang, H., Hunter, A.G.W., Clifford, B., McLaughlin, M. and Thompson, D.: VACTERL with hydrocephalus: Spontaneous chromosome breakage and rearrangement in a family showing apparent sex-linked recessive inheritance. Am. J. Med. Genet. 47:114, 1993a.

Wang, H-S., Surh, L.C., Aubrey, H.L., Janes, L., Thompson, D. and Hunter, A.G.W.: Two prenatal diagnoses of different chr 15 cytogenetic abnormalities from the same individual. Am. J. Hum. Genet. 53(Suppl.):1472, 1993b.

Wang, M., Mata, J., Price, C.E., Iversen, P.L. and Godfrey, M.: Prenatal and presymptomatic diagnosis of the Marfan syndrome using fluorescence PCR and an automated sequencer. Prenat. Diagn. 15:499, 1995.

Wapner, R.J., Kurtz, A.B., Ross, R.D. and Jackson, L.G.: Ultrasonographic parameters in the prenatal diagnosis of Meckel syndrome. Obstet. Gynecol. 57:388, 1981.

Ward, A.M.: Maternal serum alpha-fetoprotein screening for the early antenatal detection of neural tube defects. Ric. Clin. Lab. 12:189, 1982.

Ward, P.A., Hejtmancik, J.F., Baumbach, L.L., Gunnell, S.L., Witkowski, J.A. and Caskey, C.T.: Prenatal diagnosis of Duchenne muscular dystrophy by DNA analysis: Predictions and outcomes. Am. J. Hum. Genet. 41(Suppl.):A109, 1987.

Ward, P.A., Hejtmancik, J.F., Witkowski, J.A., Baumbach, L.L., Gunnell, S., Speer, J., Hawley, P., Tantravahi, U. and Caskey, C.T.: Prenatal diagnosis of Duchenne muscular dystrophy: Prospective linkage analysis and retrospective dystrophin cDNA analysis. Am. J. Hum. Genet. 44:270, 1989.

Ward, B.E., Wright, M., Silver, M.P. and Theve, R.: Identification of Robertsonian translocation trisomies for chromosomes 21 and 13 during rapid prenatal aneuploidy detection by fluorescence in situ hybridization (FISH). Am. J. Hum. Genet. 57(Suppl.):A290, 1995.

Warkany, J., Beaudry, P.H. and Hornstein, S.: Attempted abortion with aminopterin (4-amino-pteroylglutamic acid). Am. J. Dis. Child. 97:274, 1959.

Warner, R.W., Sharma, S. and Fox, H.E.: Ultrasound diagnosis of quintuplets following clomiphene-induced ovulation. J. Clin. Ultrasound 7:379, 1979.

Warner, T.G., Robertson, A.D., Mock, A.K., Johnson, W.G. and O'Brien, J.S.: Prenatal diagnosis of Gm_1 gangliosidosis by detection of galactosyl-oligosaccharides in amniotic fluid with high-performance liquid chromatography. Am. J. Hum. Genet. 35:1034, 1983.

Warner, T.G., Turner, M.W., Toone, J.R. and Applegarth, D.: Prenatal diagnosis of infantile GM_2 gangliosidosis type II (Sandhoff disease) by detection of N-acetylglucosaminyl-oligosaccharides in amniotic fluid with high-performance liquid chromatography. Prenat. Diagn. 6:393, 1986.

Warner, A.A., Pettenati, M.J. and Burton, B.K.: Is chromosome analysis indicated when amniocentesis is performed because of elevated maternal serum alpha-fetoprotein (MSAFP)? Am. J. Hum. Genet. 43(Suppl.):A252, 1988.

Warren, R.C., McKenzie C.F., Rodeck, C.H., Moscoso, G., Brock, D.J.H. and Barron, L.: First trimester diagnosis of hypophosphatasia with a monoclonal antibody to the liver/bone/kidney isoenzyme of alkaline phosphatase. Lancet. 2:856, 1985.

Warsof, S.L., Cooper, D.J., Little, D. and Campbell, S.: Routine ultrasound screening for antenatal detection of intrauterine growth retardation. Obstet. Gynecol. 67:33, 1986.

Warsos, S.L., Larsen, J.W., Kent, S.G., Rosenbaum, K.N., August, G.P., Migeon, C.J. and Schulman, J.D.: Prenatal diagnosis of congenital adrenal hyperplasia. Obstet. Gynecol. 55:751, 1980.

Wasmuth, J.J., McMahan, J., Santiago, L., Bengsston, U., Overhauser, J., Ulm, J. and Butler, M.: DNA probes in the prenatal detection of 5p monosomy and trisomy in a family with a subtle translocation unresolved by cytogenetic analysis. Am. J. Hum. Genet. 43(Suppl.): A99, 1988.

Waters, B.L. and West, B.R.: Lethal congenital non-spherocytic, non-immune hemolytic anemia with genital and other anomalies in two brothers. Am. J. Med. Genet. 55:319, 1995.

Watson, J.D., Ward, B.E., Peakman, D. and Henry, G.: Trisomy 16 and 12 confined chorionic mosaicism in liveborn infants with multiple anomalies. Am. J. Hum. Genet. 43(Suppl.): A252, 1988.

Watson, W.J., Thorp, J.M., Jr. and Seeds, J.W.: Familial cystic hygroma with normal karyotype. Prenat. Diagn. 10:37, 1990a.

Watson, W.J., Thorp, J.M., Jr., Miller, R.C., Chescheir, N.C., Katz, V.L. and Seeds, J.W.: Prenatal diagnosis of laryngeal atresia. Am. J. Obstet. Gynecol. 163:1456, 1990b.

Wax, J.R., Blakemore, K.J., Blohm, P. and Callan, N.A.: Stuck twin with cotwin nonimmune hydrops: Successful treatment by amniocentesis. Fetal Diagn. Ther. 6:126, 1991.

Weatherall, D.J., Old, J.M., Thein, S.L., Wainscoat, J.S. and Clegg J.B.: Prenatal diagnosis of the common haemoglobin disorders. J. Med. Genet. 22:422, 1985.

Weaver, D.D.: *Catalog of Prenatally Diagnosed Conditions,* 2nd ed. Baltimore: Johns Hopkins University Press, 1992.

Weaver, D.D., Mapstone, C.L. and Yu, P.-L.: The VATER association: Analysis of 46 patients. Am. J. Dis. Child. 140:225, 1986.

Webb, B., Richardson, S.J., Garry, R. and Atkins, J.: Particulate acetylcholinesterase in amniotic fluid and its implications for neural tube defect screening. Ann. Clin. Biochem. 18:299, 1981a.

Webb, T., Butler, D., Insley, J., Weaver, J.B., Green, S. and Rodeck, C.: Prenatal diagnosis of Martin–Bell syndrome associated with fragile site at Xq27-28. Lancet. 2:1423, 1981b.

Webb, T., Gosden, C.M., Rodeck, C.H., Hamill, M.A. and Eason, P.E.: Prenatal diagnosis of X-linked mental retardation with fragile (X) using fetoscopy and fetal blood sampling. Prenat. Diagn. 3:131, 1983.

Webb, T.P., Bundey, S., Thake, A. and Todd, J.: The frequency of the fragile X chromosome among school children in Coventry. J. Med. Genet. 23:396, 1986.

Webb, T.P., Rodeck, C.H., Nicolaides, K.H. and Gosden, C.M.: Prenatal diagnosis of the fragile X syndrome using fetal blood and amniotic fluid. Prenat. Diagn. 7:203, 1987.

Webb, A.L., Sturgiss, S., Robson, S.C., Goodship, J.A. and Wolstenholme, J.: Severe growth retardation in association with trisomy 2 in the placenta. Am. J. Hum. Genet. 57(Suppl.): A290, 1995.

Webster, R.D., Cudmore, D.W. and Gray, J.: Fetal bradycardia without fetal distress. Obstet. Gynecol. 50:50s, 1977.

Wehnert, M., Shukova, E.L., Surin, V.I., Schroder, W., Solovjev, G.Y. and Herrmann, F.H.: Prenatal diagnosis of hemophilia A by the polymerase chain reaction using the intragenic Hind III polymorphism. Prenat. Diagn. 10:529, 1990.

Weier, H.U.G., Grifo, J., Cohen, J. and Munne, S.: Differentiation between aneuploidy and polyploidy in single human interphase blastomeres by multiple probe FISH. Am. J. Hum. Genet. 53(Suppl.);1474, 1993.

Weinberg, A.G., Milunsky, A. and Harrod, M.J.: Elevated amniotic-fluid alpha-fetoprotein and duodenal atresia. Lancet. 2:496, 1975.

Weiner, C.P.: Cordocentesis for diagnostic indications: Two years' experience. Obstet. Gynecol. 70:664, 1987.

Weiner, C.P.: The role of cordocentesis in fetal diagnosis. Clin. Obstet. Gynecol. 31:285, 1988.

Weiner, D.L., Lovinger, R.D., Ghatak, N.R. and Redwine, F.D.: Ultrasound detection of abnormalities in a fetus with congenital hypothyroidism. Am. J. Hum. Genet. 32(Suppl.): 136A, 1980a.

Weiner, S., Scharf, J.I., Bolognese, R.J. and Librizzi, R.J.: Antenatal diagnosis and treatment of a fetal goiter. J. Reprod. Med. 24:39, 1980b.

Weiner, C., Varner, M., Pringle, K., Hein, H., Williamson, R. and Smith, W.L.: Antenatal diagnosis and palliative treatment of nonimmune hydrops fetalis is secondary to pulmonary extralobar sequestration. Obstet. Gynecol. 68:275, 1986.

Weinraub, Z., Langer, R., Bukovsky, I., Schneider, D. and Caspi, E.: Ultrasonographic diagnosis of fetal ascites in a twin pregnancy. Acta Obstet. Gynecol. Scand. 58:217, 1979.

Weinraub, Z., Gembruch, U., Fodisch, H.J. and Hansmann, M.: Intrauterine mediastinal teratoma associated with non-immune hydrops fetalis. Prenat. Diagn. 9:369, 1989.

Weinreb, J.C., Lowe, T., Cohen, J.M. and Kutler, M.: Human fetal anatomy: MR imaging. Radiology. 157:715, 1985.

Weinstein, L. and Anderson, C.: In utero diagnosis of Beckwith–Wiedemann syndrome by ultrasound. Radiology. 134:474, 1980.

Weisman, Y., Jaccard, N., Legum, C., Spirer, Z., Yedwab, G., Even, L., Edelstein, S., Kaye, A.M. and Hochberg, Z.: Prenatal diagnosis of vitamin D-dependent rickets, type II: Response to 1,25 dihydroxyvitamin D in amniotic fluid cells and fetal tissues. J. Clin. Endocrinol. Metab. 71:937, 1990.

Weiss, R.R., Macri, J.N. and Merskey, C.: F.D.P. in amniotic fluid as marker for neural-tube defects. Lancet. 1:304, 1976.

Weiss, R.R., Macri, J.N. and Balsam, D.: Amniography in the prenatal diagnosis of neural tube defects. Obstet. Gynecol. 51:299, 1978.

Weiss, P.A.M., Purstner, P., Winter, R. and Lichtenegger, W.: Insulin levels in amniotic fluid of normal and abnormal pregnancies. Obstet. Gynecol. 63:371, 1984.

Weiss, P.A.M., Hofmann, H., Winter, R., Purstner, P. and Lichtenegger, W.: Amniotic fluid glucose values in normal and abnormal pregnancies. Obstet. Gynecol. 65:333, 1985.

Weldner, B.M., Persson, P.H. and Ivarsson, S.A.: Prenatal diagnosis of dwarfism by ultrasound screening. Arch. Dis. Child. 60:1070, 1985.

Wendel, U. and Claussen, U.: Antenatal diagnosis of maple-syrup-urine disease. Lancet. 1:161, 1979.

Wendel, U., Claussen, U. and Diekmann, E.: Prenatal diagnosis for methylenetetrahydrofolate reductase deficiency. J. Pediatr. 102:939, 1983.

Wendt, L.V., Simila, S., Roukonen, A. and Hartikainen-Sorri, A.-L.: Problems of prenatal diagnosis of non-ketotic hyperglycinaemia. J. Inherit. Metab. Dis. 6:112, 1983.

Wenger, D.A., Wharton, C., Sattler, M. and Clark, C.: Niemann–Pick disease: Prenatal diagnoses and studies of sphingomyelinase activities. Am. J. Med. Genet. 2:345, 1978.

Wenger, D.A., Kudoh, T., Sattler, M., Palmieri, M. and Yudkoff, M.: Niemann–Pick disease Type B: Prenatal diagnosis and enzymatic and chemical studies on fetal brain and liver. Am. J. Hum. Genet. 33:337, 1981.

Wenstrom, K.D., Williamson, R.A., Hoover, W.W. and Grant, S.S.: Achondrogenesis type II (Langer–Saldino) in association with jugular lymphatic obstruction sequence. Prenat. Diagn. 9:527, 1989.

Wenstrom, K.D., Weiner, C.P., Williamson, R.A. and Grant, S.S.: Prenatal diagnosis of fetal hyperthyroidism using funipuncture. Obstet. Gynecol. 76:513, 1990.

Werner, H., Jr., Mirlesse, V., Jacquemard, F., Sonigo, P., Delezoide, A.L., Gonzales, M., Brunelle, F., Fermont, L. and Daffos, F.: Prenatal diagnosis of tuberous sclerosis. Use of magnetic resonance imaging and its implications for prognosis. Prenat. Diagn. 14:1151, 1994.

Wertz, D.C. and Fletcher, J.C.: Ethical problems in prenatal diagnosis: A cross-cultural survey of medical geneticists in 18 nations. Prenat. Diagn. 9:145, 1989.

Wester, H.-A., Grimm, G. and Lehmann, F.: Echokardiographischer Nachweis einer fetalen Herzinsuffizienz infolge supraventrikularer Tachykardie. Z. Kardiol. 73:405, 1984.

Westergaard, J.G., Chemnitz, J., Teisner, B., Poulsen, H.K., Ipsen, L., Beck, B. and Grudzinskas, J.G.: Pregnancy-associated plasma protein A: A possible marker in the classification and prenatal diagnosis of Cornelia de Lange syndrome. Prenat. Diagn. 3:225, 1983.

Westgren, M., Eastham, W.N., Ghandourah, S. and Woodhouse, N.: Intrauterine hypercalcaemia and non-immune hydrops fetalis—relationship to the Williams syndrome. Prenat. Diagn. 8:333, 1988.

Westin, B.: Hysteroscopy in early pregnancy. Lancet. 2:872, 1954.

Weston, P.J., Ives, E.J., Honore, R.L.H., Lees, G.M., Sinclair, D.B. and Schiff, D.: Monochorionic diamniotic minimally conjoined twins: A case report. Am. J. Med. Genet. 37:558, 1990.

Wheeler, M., Peakman, D. and Henry, G.: Elevated maternal serum alpha fetoprotein associated with sex chromosome abnormalities. Am. J. Hum. Genet. 41(Suppl.):A287, 1987.

Wheeler, M., Peakman, D., Robinson, A. and Henry, G.: 45,X/46,XY mosaicism: Contrast of prenatal and postnatal diagnosis. Am. J. Med. Genet. 29:565, 1988.

White, P.R. and Stewart, J.H.: Radiological diagnosis of foetal foregut abnormalities. Br. J. Radiol. 46:706, 1973.

Whitelaw, A.G.L., Rogers, P.A., Hopkinson, D.A., Gordon, H., Emerson, P.M., Darley, J.M., Reid, C. and Crawfurd, M. d'A.: Congenital haemolytic anaemia resulting from glucose phosphate isomerase deficiency: Genetics, clinical picture, and prenatal diagnosis. J. Med. Genet. 16:189, 1979.

Whitelaw, A., Haines, M.E., Bolsover, W. and Harris, E.: Factor V deficiency and antenatal intraventricular haemorrhage. Arch. Dis. Child. 59:997, 1984.

Whitfield, C.R.: A three-year assessment of an action line method of timing intervention in rhesus isoimmunization. Am. J. Obstet. Gynecol. 108:1239, 1970.

Whitley, C.B., Burke, B.A., Granroth, G. and Gorlin, R.J.: de la Chapelle dysplasia. Am. J. Med. Genet. 25:29, 1986.

Whittle, M.J., Gilmore, D.H., McNay, M.B., Turner, T.L. and Raine, P.A.M.: Diaphragmatic hernia presenting in utero as a unilateral hydrothorax. Prenat. Diagn. 9:115, 1989.

Wiesmann, U.N., Meier, C., Spycher, M.A., Schmid, W., Bischoff, A., Gautier, E. and Herschkowitz, N.: Prenatal metachromatic leukodystrophy. Helv. Paediatr. Acta. 30:31, 1975.

Wiggins, J.W., Bowes, W., Clewell, W., Manco-Johnson, M., Manchester, D., Johnson, R., Appareti, K. and Wolfe, R.: Echocardiographic diagnosis and intravenous digoxin management of fetal tachyarrhythmias and congestive heart failure. Am. J. Dis. Child. 140:202, 1986.

Wildemeersch, D. and Raven, E.: Fetal atrial arrhythmia. Case report. Z. Geburtsh. Perinat. 179:57, 1975.

Williams, R.A. and Barth, R.A.: In utero sonographic recognition of diastematomyelia. Am. J. Roentgenol. 144:87, 1985.

Williams, H., Brown, C.S., Thomas, N.S.T., Harper, P.S., Roberts, A., Ppadhyaya, M. and Gosden, J.R.: First trimester fetal sexing in pregnancy at risk for Duchenne muscular dystrophy. Lancet. 2:568, 1983.

Williams, J., Wang, B., Rubin, C., Clark, R. and Mohandas, T.: Apparent non-mosaic trisomy 16 in chorionic villi: Diagnostic dilemma or clinically significant finding? Am. J. Hum. Genet. 45(Suppl.):A273, 1989.

Williamson, R.A., Weiner, C.P., Grant, S.S. and Patil, S.R.: Evaluation of the severely growth retarded fetus by cordocentesis: Implications for pregnancy management. Am. J. Hum. Genet. 43(Suppl.):A253, 1988.

Willner, J.P., Radu, M., Hobbins, J.C., Kereny, T., Strauss, L. and Desnick, R.J.: Robert syndrome: Prenatal diagnosis by cytogenetic and ultrasonic studies. Pediatr. Res. 13: 428, 1979.

Wilson, M.G. and Marchese, C.A.: Prenatal diagnosis of fragile X in a heterozygous female fetus and postnatal follow-up. Prenat. Diagn. 4:61, 1984.

Wilson, G.N., Stout, J.P., Schneider, N.R., Zneimer, S.M., Gilstrap, L.C. and Richards, C.S.: Balanced chromosome 12/13 translocation in mother and fetus with situs abnormalities in the fetus: Transection of a maternal effect gene regulating early pattern? Am. J. Hum. Genet. 45(Suppl.):A95, 1989.

Wilson, G.N., Stout, J.P., Schneider, N.R., Zneimer, S.M. and Gilstrap, L.C.: Balanced chromosome 12/13 translocation in mother and fetus with situs abnormalities in the fetus: Transection of a maternal effect gene regulating early pattern formation? Proc. Greenwood Genet. Cent. 9:61, 1990.

Wilson, R.D., Johnson, J.A. and Dansereau, J.: Pregnancy outcome following amniocentesis at 11–14 versus 16–19 weeks' gestation. Obstet. Gynecol. 88:638, 1996.

Winchester, B.: Prenatal diagnosis of enzyme defects. Arch. Dis. Child. 65:59, 1990.

Windeband, K.P., Bridges, N.A., Ostman-Smith, I. and Stevens, J.E.: Hydrops fetalis due to abnormal lymphatics. Arch. Dis. Child. 62:198, 1987.

Winsberg, F.: Echocardiography of the fetal and newborn heart. Invest. Radiol. 7:152, 1972.

Winship, I., Cremin, B. and Beighton, P.: Boomerang dysplasia. Am. J. Med. Genet. 36:440, 1990.

Winsor, E.J.T., St. John Brown, B., Luther, E.R., Heifetz, S.A. and Welch, J.P.: Deceased co-twin as a cause of false positive amniotic fluid AFP and AChE. Prenat. Diagn. 7:485, 1987.

Winter, R.M. and Baraitser, M.: *The London Dysmorpholoy Database.* Oxford, Oxford University Press, 1990.

Winter, R., Rosenkranz, W., Hofmann, H., Zierler, H., Becker, H. and Borkenstein, M.: Prenatal diagnosis of campomelic dysplasia by ultrasonography. Prenat. Diagn. 5:1, 1985.

Winter, S.C., Curry, C.J.R., Smith, J.C., Kassel, S., Miller, L. and Andrea, J.: Prenatal diagnosis of the Beckwith–Wiedmann syndrome. Am. J. Med. Genet. 24:137, 1986.

Winter, R.M., Campbell, S., Wigglesworth, J.S. and Nevrkla, E.J.: A previously undescribed syndrome of thoracic dysplasia and communicating hydrocephalus in two sibs, one diagnosed prenatally by ultrasound. J. Med. Genet. 24:204, 1987.

Wirth, B., Rudnik-Schoneborn, S., Hahnen, E., Rohrig, D. and Zerres, K.: Prenatal prediction in families with autosomal recessive proximal spinal muscular atrophy (5q11.2-q13.3): Molecular genetics and clinical experience in 109 cases. Prenat. Diagn. 15:407, 1995.

Wishart, J.G.: Prenatal screening for Down's syndrome. Br. Med. J. 303:54, 1991a.

Wishart, J.G.: Prenatal screening for Down's syndrome. Br. Med. J. 303:468, 1991b.

Wisser, J., Schreiner, M., Diem, H. and Roithmeier, A.: Neonatal hemochromatosis: A rare cause of nonimmune hydrops fetalis and fetal anemia. Fetal Diagn. Ther. 8:273, 1993.

Wiswell, T.E., Rawlings, J.S., Wilson, J.L. and Pettett, G.: Megacystis-microcolon-intestinal hypoperistalsis syndrome. Pediatrics. 63:805, 1979.

Witt, D., Hall, J., Lau, A., McGillivray, B. and Manchester, D.: Prenatal diagnosis and fetal edema in Noonan syndrome. Am. J. Hum. Genet. 36(Suppl.)82S, 1984.

Witt, D.R., Hoyme, H.E., Zonana, J., Manchester, D.K., Fryns, J.P., Stevenson, J.G., Curry, C.J.R. and Hall, J.G.: Lymphedema in Noonan syndrome: Clues to pathogenesis and prenatal diagnosis and review of the literature. Am. J. Med. Genet. 27:841, 1987.

Witt, D.R., Yen-Batey, A., Uitto, J., McGuire, J. and Christiano, A.: Prenatal diagnosis and mutation detection in recessive dystrophic epidermolysis bullosa. Am. J. Hum. Gen. 57(Suppl.):A291, 1995.

Witter, F.R. and Molteni, R.A.: Intrauterine intestinal volvulus with hemoperitoneum presenting as fetal distress at 34 weeks' gestation. Am. J. Obstet. Gynecol. 155:1080, 1986.

Wittmann, B.K., Baldwin, V.J. and Nichol, B.: Antenatal diagnosis of twin transfusion syndrome by ultrasound. Obstet. Gynecol. 58:123, 1981a.

Wittmann, B.K., Fulton, L., Cooperberg, P.L., Lyons, E.A., Miller, C. and Shaw, D.: Molar pregnancy: Early diagnosis by ultrasound. J. Clin. Ultrasound 9:153, 1981b.

Wittmann, B.K., Farquharson, D.F., Thomas, W.D.S., Baldwin, V.J. and Wadsworth, L.D.: The role of feticide in the management of severe twin transfusion syndrome. Am. J. Obstet. Gynecol. 155:1023, 1986.

Wladimiroff, J.W., Niermeijer, M.F., Laar, J., Jahoda, M. and Stewart, P.A.: Prenatal diagnosis of skeletal dysplasia by real-time ultrasound. Obstet. Gynecol. 63:360, 1984.

Wladimiroff, J.W., Beemer, F.A., Scholtmeyer, R.J., Stewart, P.A., Spritzer, R. and Wolff, E.D.: Failure to detect fetal obstructive uropathy by second-trimester ultrasound. Prenat. Diagn. 5:41, 1985a.

Wladimiroff, J.W., Niermeijer, M.F., Van Der Harten, J.J., Stewart, P.A., Versteegh, F.G.A., Blom, W. and Huijmans, J.G.M.: Early prenatal diagnosis of congenital hypophosphatasia: Case report. Prenat. Diagn. 5:47, 1985b.

Wladimiroff, J.W., Sachs, E.S., Reuss, A., Stewart, P.A., Pijpers, L. and Niermeijer, M.F.: Prenatal diagnosis of chromosome abnormalities in the presence of fetal structural defects. Am. J. Med. Genet. 29:289, 1988a.

Wladimiroff, J.W., Stewart, P.A. and Tonge, H.M.: Fetal bradyarrhythmia: Diagnosis and outcome. Prenat. Diagn. 8:53, 1988b.

Wladimiroff, J.W., Stewart, P.A., Reuss, A. and Sachs, E.S.: Cardiac and extra-cardiac anomalies as indicators for trisomies 13 and 18: A prenatal ultrasound study. Prenat. Diagn. 9:515, 1989.

Wolf, L.M., Kelly, T.G., Austin, J.S., Senagore, P.K. and Netzloff, M.L.: Antley–Bixler syndrome: A case report and prenatal diagnosis in a subsequent pregnancy. Am. J. Hum. Genet. 57(Suppl.):A347, 1995.

Wolff, D.W., Ferre, M., Raffel, L.J., Blitzer, M.G. and Schwartz, S.: An inherited 18p duplication ascertained prenatally associated with a normal phenotype. Am. J. Hum. Genet. 45(Suppl.):A96, 1989.

Wolfson, R.N., Zador, I.E., Pillay, S.K., Timor-Tritsch, I.E. and Hertz, R.H.: Antenatal investigation of human fetal systolic time intervals. Am. J. Obstet. Gynecol. 129:203, 1977.

Wolstenholme, J., Hoogwerf, A.M., Sheridan, H., Maher, E.J. and Little, D.J.: Practical experience using transabdominal chorionic villus biopsies taken after 16 weeks' gestation for rapid prenatal diagnosis of chromosomal abnormalities. Prenat. Diagn. 9:357, 1989.

Wong, L-J. C.: Prenatal diagnosis of glycogen storage disease type 1a by direct mutation detection. Prenat. Diagn. 16:105, 1996.

Wong, W.S. and Filly, R.A.: Polyhydramnios associated with fetal limb abnormalities. Am. J. Roentgenol. 140:1001, 1983.

Wong, P.W.K. and Lessick, M.L.: Midtrimester prenatal diagnosis of adrenogenital syndrome due to 11 beta hydroxylase deficiency. Am. J. Hum. Genet. 43(Suppl.):A253, 1988.

Wong, V., Ma, H.K., Todd, D., Golbus, M.S., Dozy, A.M. and Kan, Y.W.: Diagnosis of homozygous alpha-thalassemia in cultured amniotic-fluid fibroblasts. N. Engl. J. Med. 298:669, 1978.

Wong, P.Y., Doran, T.A., Falk, M., Taylor, G.W. and Mee, A.V.: Prenatal diagnosis of fetal sex by amniotic fluid testosterone and FSH, and their potential use in detecting sex linked disorders. Clin. Biochem. 13:135, 1980.

Woo, J.S.K., Wan, C.W., Fang, A., Au, K.L., Tang, L.C.H. and Ghosh, A.: Is fetal femur length a better indicator of gestational age in the growth-retarded fetus as compared with biparietal diameter? J. Ultrasound Med. 4:139, 1985.

Wood, S., Shukin, R.J., Yong, S.L., Wilson, D., Kalousek, D. and Chudley, A.: Prenatal diagnosis in Becker muscular dystrophy. Clin. Genet. 31:45, 1987.

Worthen, N.J., Lawrence, D. and Bustillo, M.: Amniotic band syndrome: Antepartum ultrasonic diagnosis of discordant anencephaly. J. Clin. Ultrasound 8:453, 1980.

Wright, E.V., McIntosh, A.S. and Foulds, J.W.: Importance of routine fetoprotein estimations. Lancet. 2:769, 1975.

Wu, M-H., Kuo, P-L. and Lin, S-J.: Prenatal diagnosis of recurrence of short rib-polydactyly syndrome. Am. J. Med. Genet. 55:279, 1995.

Wulff, K., Wehnert, M., Schutz, M., Seidlitz, G. and Herrmann, F.H.: Prenatal diagnosis of phenylketonuria by haplotype analysis. Prenat. Diagn. 9:421, 1989.

Wyatt, P.R. and Cox, D.M.: Utilization of electron microscopy in the prenatal diagnosis of genetic disease. Hum. Hered. 27:22, 1977.

Wyvill, P.C., Hullin, D.A., Elder, G.H. and Laurence, K.M.: A prospective study of amniotic fluid cholinesterases: Comparison of quantitative and qualitative methods for the detection of open neural tube defects. Prenat. Diagn. 4:319, 1984.

Yacoub, T., Campbell, C.A., Gordon, Y.B., Kirby, J.D. and Kitau, M.J.: Maternal serum and amniotic fluid concentrations of alphafetoprotein in epidermolysis bullosa simplex. Br. Med. J. 1:307, 1979.

Yamaguchi, S., Shimizu, N., Orii, T., Fukao, T., Suzuki, Y., Maeda, K., Hashimoto, T., Previs, S.F. and Rinaldo, P.: Prenatal diagnosis and neonatal monitoring of a fetus with glutaric aciduria type II due to electron transfer flavoprotein (β-subunit) deficiency. Pediatr. Res. 30:439, 1991.

Yang, B.-Z., Ding, J.-H., Brown, B.I. and Chen, Y.-T.: Definitive prenatal diagnosis for type III glycogen storage disease. Am. J. Hum. Genet. 47:735, 1990.

Yang, S.S., Roth, J.A. and Langer, L.O., Jr.: Short rib syndrome Beemer–Langer type with polydactyly: A multiple congenital anomalies syndrome. Am. J. Med. Genet. 39:243, 1991.

Yapar, E.G., Ekici, E. and Gokmen, O.: Sonographic diagnosis of epignathus (oral teratoma), prosencephaly, meromelia and oligohydramnios in a fetus with trisomy 13. Clin. Dysmorph. 4:266, 1995.

Yapijakis, C., Kapaki, E., Boussiou, M., Vassilopoulos, D. and Papageorgiou, C.: Prenatal diagnosis of X-linked spinal and bulbar muscular atrophy in a Greek family. Prenat. Diagn. 16:262, 1996.

Yarberry-Allen, P., Abdel-Latif, N. and Cederqvist, L.L.: Prenatal diagnosis of congenital listeriosis. Am. J. Reprod. Immunol. Microbiol. 3:111, 1983.

Yong, S.L., Applegarth, D.A., Toone, J.R., Wilson, R.D. and Baldwin, V.J.: Morquio disease presenting as hydrops fetalis and enzyme analysis of chorionic villus tissue in a subsequent pregnancy. Am. J. Hum. Genet. 41(Suppl.):A288, 1987.

Young, L.W., Haimovici, H., LaVigne, R.J. and Howard, T.T.: Radiological case of the month: Hygroma (cystic lymphangioma)—Diagnosis by ultrasound. Am. J. Dis. Child. 134:311, 1980.

Young, R.S.K., Towfighi, J. and Marks, K.H.: Focal necrosis of the spinal cord in utero. Arch. Neurol. 40:654, 1983.

Young, I.D., McKeever, P.A., Brown, L.A. and Lang, G.D.: Prenatal diagnosis of the megacystis-microcolon-intestinal hypoperistalsis syndrome. J. Med. Genet. 26:403, 1989.

Young, K., Barth, C.K., Moore, C. and Weaver, D.D.: Otopalatodigital syndrome type II associated with omphalocele: Report of three cases. Am. J. Med. Genet. 45:481, 1993.

Yu, C.W., and Stephens, J.D.: Continuation or termination of pregnancy: Decision making in prenatal diagnosis. Am. J. Hum. Genet. 41(Suppl.):A288, 1987.

Zamah, N.M., Gillieson, M.S., Walters, J.H. and Hall, P.F.: Sonographic detection of polyhydramnios: A five-year experience. Am. J. Obstet. Gynecol. 143:523, 1982.

Zaragoza, M.V., Keep, D., Redline, R.W. and Hassold, T.: Molecular studies of the origin of very early complete hydatidiform moles. Am. J. Hum. Genet. 57(Suppl.):A292, 1995.

Zaremba, J., Kleijer, W.J., Huijmans, J.G.M., Poorthuis, B., Fidzianska, E. and Glogowska, I.: Chromsomes 14 and 21 as possible candidates for mapping the gene for Sanfilippo disease type IIIC. J. Med. Genet. 29:514, 1992.

Zass, R., Leupold, D., Fernandez, M.A. and Wendel, U.: Evaluation of prenatal treatment in newborns with cobalamin-responsive methylmalonic acidaemia. J. Inher. Metab. Dis. 18:100, 1995.

Zeigler, M., Bargal, R., Suri, V., Meidan B. and Bach, G.: Mucolipidosis type IV: Accumulation of phospholipids and gangliosides in cultured amniotic cells. A tool for prenatal diagnosis. Prenat. Diagn. 12:1037, 1992.

Zeitune, M., Fejgin, M.D., Abramowicz, J., Aderet, N.B. and Goodman, R.M.: Prenatal diagnosis of the pterygium syndrome. Prenat. Diagn. 8:145, 1988.

Zelante, L. and Dallapiccola, B.: Umbilical cord pseudocyst in trisomy 13. Prenat. Diagn. 9:448, 1989.

Zeng, Y.-T. and Huang, S.Z.: Alpha-globin gene organization and prenatal diagnosis of alpha-thalassaemia in Chinese. Lancet. 1:304, 1985.

Zeng, Y.-T., Zhang, M.-L., Ren, Z.-R., Chen, S.-R., Wang, H.-L., Wang, Z.-Y. and Tong, J.-H.: Prenatal diagnosis of haemophilia B in the first trimester. J. Med. Genet. 24:632, 1987.

Zerres, K., Weiss, H., Bulla, M. and Roth, B.: Prenatal diagnosis of an early manifestation of autosomal dominant adult-type polycystic kidney disease. Lancet. 2:988, 1982.

Zerres, K., Volpel, M.-C. and Weiss, H.: Cystic kidneys: Genetics, pathologic anatomy, clinical picture, and prenatal diagnosis. Hum. Genet. 68:104, 1984.

Zerres, K., Hansmann, M., Knopfle, G. and Stephan, M.: Prenatal diagnosis of genetically determined early manifestation of autosomal dominant polycystic kidney disease? Hum. Genet. 71:368, 1985.

Zerres, K., Hansmann, M., Mallmann, R. and Gembruch, U.: Autosomal recessive polycystic kidney disease. Problems of prenatal diagnosis. Prenat. Diagn. 8:215, 1988.

Zerres, K., Schuler, H., Gembruch, U., Bald, R., Hansmann, M. and Schwanitz, G.: Chromosomal findings in fetuses with prenatally diagnosed cysts of the choroid plexus. Hum. Genet. 89:301, 1992.

Zhao, H., Van Diggelen, O.P., Thoomes, R., Huijmans, J., Young, E., Mazurczak, T. and Kleijer, W.J.: Prenatal diagnosis of Morquio disease type A using a simple fluorometric enzyme assay. Prenat. Diagn. 10:85, 1990.

Zhao, J., Gordon, P.L., Wilroy, R.S. Jr., Martens, P.R., Tarleton, J., Shulman, L.P., Simpson, J.L., Elias, S. and Tharapel, A.T.: Characterization of an unbalanced de novo rearrangement by microsatellite polymorphism typing and by fluorescent in situ hybridization. Am. J. Med. Genet. 56:398, 1995.

Ziegler, J.B., van de Weyden, M.B., Lee, C.H. and Daniel, A.: Prenatal diagnosis for adenosine deaminase deficiency. J. Med. Genet. 18:154, 1981.

Zimmer, E.Z. and Divon, M.Y.: Sonographic diagnosis of IUGR-macrosomia. Clin. Obstet. Gynecol. 35:172, 1992.

Zimmer, E.Z., Jakobi, P., Goldstein, I. and Gutterman, E.: Cardiotocographic and sonographic findings in two cases of antenatally diagnosed intrauterine fetal brain death. Prenat. Diagn. 12:271, 1992.

Zimmerman, H.B.: Prenatal demonstration of gastric and duodenal obstruction by ultrasound. J. Can. Assoc. Radiol. 29:138, 1978.

Zimran, A., Elstein, D., Abrahamov, A., Kuhl, W., Brown, .K.H. and Beutler, E.: Prenatal molecular diagnosis of Gaucher disease. Prenat. Diagn. 15:1185, 1995.

Zinn, A.B., Hine, D.G., Mahoney, M.J. and Tanaka, K.: The stable isotope dilution method for measurement of methylmalonic acid: A highly accurate approach to the prenatal diagnosis of methylmalonic acidemia. Pediatr. Res. 16:740, 1982.

Zlotogora, J. and Bach, G.: Hunter syndrome: Prenatal diagnosis in maternal serum. Am. J. Hum. Genet. 38:253, 1986.

Zonana, J., Schinzel, A., Upadhyaya, M., Thomas, N.S.T., Anton-Lamprect, I. and Harper, P.S.: Prenatal diagnosis of X-linked hypohidrotic ectodermal dysplasia by linkage analysis. Am. J. Med. Genet. 35:132, 1990.

Index

NUMERICAL LISTING